Electrocardiogram in Clinical Medicine

Electrocardiogram in Clinical Medicine

Edited by

William J. Brady, MD
Professor of Emergency Medicine and Medicine
University of Virginia
Charlottesville, VA, USA

Michael J. Lipinski, MD, PhD
Cardiovascular Associates of Charlottesville
Charlottesville, VA, USA

Andrew E. Darby, MD, FHRS
Associate Professor of Cardiovascular Medicine
University of Virginia Health System
Charlottesville, VA, USA

Michael C. Bond, MD, FACEP, FAAEM
Associate Professor of Emergency Medicine
University of Maryland School of Medicine
Baltimore, MD, USA

Nathan P. Charlton, MD
Associate Professor of Emergency Medicine
Division of Medical Toxicology
University of Virginia
Charlottesville, VA, USA

Korin Hudson, MD
Associate Professor of Emergency Medicine
MedStar Georgetown University Hospital
Georgetown University School of Medicine
Washington, DC, USA

Kelly Williamson, MD
Assistant Residency Program Director
Advocate Christ Medical Center Emergency Medicine Residency;
Clinical Associate Professor of Emergency Medicine
University of Illinois at Chicago
Chicago, IL, USA

WILEY Blackwell

Registered Office(s)
John Wiley & Sons, Inc., 111 River Street, Hoboken, NJ 07030, USA
John Wiley & Sons Ltd, The Atrium, Southern Gate, Chichester, West Sussex, PO19 8SQ, UK

Editorial Office
9600 Garsington Road, Oxford, OX4 2DQ, UK

For details of our global editorial offices, customer services, and more information about Wiley products, visit us at www.wiley.com.

Wiley also publishes its books in a variety of electronic formats and by print-on-demand. Some content that appears in standard print versions of this book may not be available in other formats.

Limit of Liability/Disclaimer of Warranty
The contents of this work are intended to further general scientific research, understanding, and discussion only and are not intended and should not be relied upon as recommending or promoting scientific method, diagnosis, or treatment by physicians for any particular patient. In view of ongoing research, equipment modifications, changes in governmental regulations, and the constant flow of information relating to the use of medicines, equipment, and devices, the reader is urged to review and evaluate the information provided in the package insert or instructions for each medicine, equipment, or device for, among other things, any changes in the instructions or indication of usage and for added warnings and precautions. While the publisher and authors have used their best efforts in preparing this work, they make no representations or warranties with respect to the accuracy or completeness of the contents of this work and specifically disclaim all warranties, including without limitation any implied warranties of merchantability or fitness for a particular purpose. No warranty may be created or extended by sales representatives, written sales materials or promotional statements for this work. The fact that an organization, website, or product is referred to in this work as a citation and/or potential source of further information does not mean that the publisher and authors endorse the information or services the organization, website, or product may provide or recommendations it may make. This work is sold with the understanding that the publisher is not engaged in rendering professional services. The advice and strategies contained herein may not be suitable for your situation. You should consult with a specialist where appropriate. Further, readers should be aware that websites listed in this work may have changed or disappeared between when this work was written and when it is read. Neither the publisher nor authors shall be liable for any loss of profit or any other commercial damages, including but not limited to special, incidental, consequential, or other damages.

Library of Congress Cataloging-in-Publication Data

Names: Brady, William, 1960– editor.
Title: Electrocardiogram in clinical medicine / edited by William J. Brady,
    Michael J. Lipinski, Andrew E. Darby, Michael C. Bond, Nathan P. Charlton,
    Korin Hudson, Kelly Williamson.
Description: Hoboken, NJ : Wiley-Blackwell, 2021. | Includes
    bibliographical references and index.
Identifiers: LCCN 2020001252 (print) | LCCN 2020001253 (ebook) | ISBN
    9781118754559 (paperback) | ISBN 9781118754535 (adobe pdf) | ISBN
    9781118754542 (epub)
Subjects: MESH: Electrocardiography–methods | Heart Diseases–diagnosis
Classification: LCC RC683.5.E5 (print) | LCC RC683.5.E5 (ebook) | NLM WG
    140 | DDC 616.1/207547–dc23
LC record available at https://lccn.loc.gov/2020001252
LC ebook record available at https://lccn.loc.gov/2020001253

Cover Design: Wiley
Cover Image: © pedrosala/Shutterstock

Set in 9.5/12.5pt STIX Two Text by SPi Global, Pondicherry, India

Printed and bound by CPI Group (UK) Ltd, Croydon, CR0 4YY

10 9 8 7 6 5 4 3 2 1

Contents

List of Contributors

Seth O. Althoff, MD
Attending Emergency Physician
Grandview Hospital
Sellersville, PA, USA

Yasir Akhtar, MD
Division of Cardiovascular Medicine
University of Virginia Health System
Charlottesville, VA, USA

Paul Basel, MD
Emergency Medicine Physician
United States Air Force

Rahul Bhat
Associate Professor
Department of Emergency Medicine
Georgetown University & MedStar Health
Washington, DC, USA

Heather A. Borek, MD
Associate Professor
Division of Medical Toxicology
Department of Emergency Medicine
University of Virginia
Charlottesville, VA, USA

Michael C. Bond, MD, FACEP, FAAEM
Associate Professor
Department of Emergency Medicine
University of Maryland School of Medicine
Baltimore, MD, USA

Matthew Borloz
Associate Professor
Department of Emergency Medicine
Carilion Clinic

Virginia Tech Carilion School of Medicine
Roanoke, VA, USA

Jeffrey Brown, MD
Unity Point Health
Rock Island, IL, USA

Kirsti A. Campbell, MD
Harvard Medical School
Boston, MA, USA

David J. Carlberg, MD
Assistant Professor
Department of Emergency Medicine
Georgetown University & MedStar Health
Washington, DC, USA

Andrea Carlson, MD
Associate Residency Program Director
Advocate Christ Medical Center Emergency
Medicine Residency;
Clinical Assistant Professor
University of Illinois
Chicago, IL, USA

Nathan P. Charlton, MD
Associate Professor
Division of Medical Toxicology
Department of Emergency Medicine
University of Virginia
Charlottesville, VA, USA

Sarah Chuzi, MD
Division of Cardiology
Department of Medicine
Northwestern University Feinberg School of Medicine
Chicago, IL, USA

Michael Cirone, MD
Assistant Residency Program Director
Advocate Christ Medical Center Emergency Medicine Residency;
Clinical Assistant Professor of Emergency Medicine
University of Illinois at Chicago
Chicago, IL, USA

Andrew E. Darby, MD, FHRS
Associate Professor
Division of Cardiovascular Medicine
University of Virginia Health System
Charlottesville, VA, USA

B. Elizabeth Delasobera
Assistant Professor
Medical Director, MedStar Health Urgent Care
Department of Emergency Medicine
Georgetown University & MedStar Health
Washington, DC, USA

Will Dresen, MD
Cardiovascular Medicine
University of Virginia Health System
Charlottesville, VA, USA

Ali Farzad, MD
Department of Emergency Medicine
Baylor University Medical Center
Dallas, TX, USA

Victor F. Froelicher, MD
Division of Cardiovascular Medicine
Stanford University/Palo Alto Veterans Affairs Health Care System
Palo Alto, CA, USA

Robert Gibson, MD
Division of Cardiovascular Medicine
University of Virginia Health System
Charlottesville, VA, USA

George F. Glass, MD
Assistant Professor
Department of Emergency Medicine
University of Virginia
Charlottesville, VA, USA

Tress Goodwin
Assistant Professor
Department of Emergency Medicine & Pediatrics
Children's National Hospital
George Washington School of Medicine
Washington, DC, USA

Kari Gorder
Clinical Instructor
Department of Anesthesia
University of Cincinnati Hospital
University of Cincinnati School of Medicine
Cincinnati, OH, USA

Munish Goyal
Assistant Professor
Department of Emergency Medicine
Georgetown University & MedStar Health
Washington, DC, USA

Lewis S. Hardison, DO
Clinical Assistant Professor
College of Pharmacy
University of South Carolina;
Faculty, Emergency Medicine
Prisma Health Richland Hospital
Columbia, SC, USA

Nicholas D. Hartman, MD
Associate Professor
Department of Emergency Medicine
Wake Forest School of Medicine
Winston-Salem, NC, USA

Christopher P. Holstege, MD, FAACT, FACMT
Professor
Departments of Emergency Medicine and Pediatrics
University of Virginia
Charlottesville, VA, USA

Korin Hudson, MD
Associate Professor
Department of Emergency Medicine
MedStar Georgetown University Hospital
Georgetown University School of Medicine
Washington, DC, USA

Meagan R. Hunt, MD
Medical Director and Assistant Professor
Department of Emergency Medicine
Wake Forest School of Medicine
Winston-Salem, NC, USA

Robert Katzer
Associate Clinical Professor
Department of Emergency Medicine
University of California
Irvine, CA, USA

Erich Kiehl, MD
Cardiovascular Medicine
Cleveland Clinic Foundation
Cleveland, OH, USA

Brian Kessen, MD
Emergency Physician
Emergency Care Consultants
Minneapolis, MN, USA

Feras Khan, MD
Department of Emergency Medicine
University of Maryland School of Medicine
Baltimore, MD, USA

Joshua D. King, MD
Assistant Professor
Medicine and Pharmacy
University of Maryland;
Medical Director
Maryland Poison Center
Baltimore, MD, USA

Benjamin J. Lawner, DO, MS, EMT-P
Department of Emergency Medicine
University of Maryland School of Medicine
Baltimore, MD, USA

Thibault Lhermusier, MD, PhD
Division of Cardiology
Centre Hospitalo Universitaire de Toulouse Rangueil
Toulouse, France

Michael J. Lipinski, MD, PhD
Cardiovascular Associates of Charlottesville
Charlottesville, VA, USA

Adrián I. Löffler, MD
Cardiovascular Medicine
University of Virginia Health System
Charlottesville, VA, USA

Mitchell Lorenz, MD
Emergency Physician
Advocate Good Samitarian Hospital
Downer's Grove, IL, USA

Heather T. Lounsbury, MD
Assistant Professor
Department of Emergency Medicine
University of Virginia
Charlottesville, VA, USA

Rachel Villacorta Lyew, MD
Assistant Professor
Department of Emergency Medicine
Tripler Army Medical Center
Honolulu, HI, USA

Mark Marinescu, MD
Cardiovascular Medicine
Ohio State University
Columbus, OH, USA

Norine McGrath
Assistant Professor
Department of Emergency Medicine
Georgetown University & MedStar Health
Washington, DC, USA

Augustus E. Mealor, MD
Assistant Professor
University of Tennessee College of Medicine
Erlanger Heart and Lung Institute
Chattanooga, TN, USA

Anders Messersmith, DO
Emergency Physician
Envision Physician Services

Michele Murphy, MD
Cardiovascular Medicine
University of Virginia Health System
Charlottesville, VA, USA

Emma Nash, MD
Department of Anesthesiology
University of Nebraska
Omaha, Nebraska

Tu Carol Nguyen, DO
Department of Emergency Medicine
University of Maryland School of Medicine
Baltimore, MD, USA

Adriana Segura Olson, MD
Emergency Physician
University of Chicago
Chicago, IL, USA

Nathan Olson, MD, MAEd
Assistant Professor
Section of Emergency Medicine
University of Chicago
Chicago, IL, USA

Amit Anil Kumar Pandit, MD
Assistant Professor
Department of Emergency Medicine
University of Mississippi Medical Center
Jackson, MS, USA

Ashley Pastore, MD
Emergency Physician
Ochsner Medical Center
New Orleans, LA, USA

Trale Permar, MD
Medical Director
Yavapai Regional Medical Center
Prescott, AZ, USA

Amy West Pollak, MD
Division of Cardiovascular Medicine
Mayo Clinic Florida
Jacksonville, FL, USA

Peter M. Pollak, MD
Division of Cardiovascular Medicine
Mayo Clinic Florida
Jacksonville, FL, USA

Michael Ragosta, MD
Division of Cardiovascular Medicine
University of Virginia Health System
Charlottesville, VA, USA

Justin Rizer, MD
Clinical Instructor
Division of Medical Toxicology
Department of Emergency Medicine
University of Virginia
Charlottesville, VA, USA

Matthew Robinson, MD
Emergency Physician
Woodhull Hospital
Brooklyn, NY, USA

William F. Rushton, MD
Associate Professor
Department of Emergency Medicine
University of Alabama;
Medical Director
Regional Poison Control Center of Children's of
Alabama
Birmingham, AL, USA

Benjamin Shepple, MD
Division of Cardiology
University of Tennessee Medical Center
Knoxville, TN, USA

Sanjay Shewakramani
Associate Professor
Department of Emergency Medicine
University of Cincinnati West Chester Hospital
University of Cincinnati School of Medicine
Cincinnati, OH, USA

Janet Smereck
Associate Professor
Department of Emergency Medicine
Georgetown University & MedStar Health
Washington, DC, USA

Amita Sudhir, MD
Associate Professor
Department of Emergency Medicine
University of Virginia
Charlottesville, VA, USA

Karis Tekwani, MD
Emergency Physician
Advocate Christ Medical Center;
Clinical Assistant Professor of Emergency Medicine
University of Illinois at Chicago
Chicago, IL, USA

Semhar Tewelde, MD
Department of Emergency Medicine
University of Maryland School of Medicine
Baltimore, MD, USA

Lane Thaut, DO
Emergency Medicine Physician
United States Air Force

Lisa B. Van Wagner, MD, MSc, FAST, FAHA
Assistant Professor of Medicine
Division of Gastroenterology & Hepatology and
Preventive Medicine
Northwestern University Feinberg School of Medicine
Chicago, IL, USA

Jane Wilcox, MD
Assistant Professor of Medicine-Cardiology
Northwestern University Feinberg School of Medicine
Chicago, IL, USA

Kelly Williamson, MD
Assistant Residency Program Director
Advocate Christ Medical Center Emergency Medicine Residency;
Clinical Associate Professor of Emergency Medicine
University of Illinois at Chicago
Chicago, IL, USA

Matthew Wilson
Assistant Professor
Department of Emergency Medicine
Georgetown University & MedStar Health
Washington, DC, USA

Natasha Wheaton, MD
Assistant Residency Program Director
Associate Professor
University of California-Los Angeles
Los Angeles, CA, USA

Michael Ybarra
Assistant Professor
Department of Emergency Medicine
Georgetown University & MedStar Health
Washington, DC, USA

Scott Young, DO
Assistant Professor
Department of Emergency Medicine
Madigan Army Medical Center
Tacoma, WA, USA

Section I

The ECG in Clinical Practice

1

The ECG in Clinical Medicine

Brian Kessen[1] and Kelly Williamson[2,3]

[1] *Emergency Physician, Emergency Care Consultants, Minneapolis, MN, USA*
[2] *Advocate Christ Medical Center Emergency Medicine Residency, Chicago, IL, USA*
[3] *Department of Emergency Medicine, University of Illinois at Chicago, Chicago, IL, USA*

Introduction

Electrocardiography, the interpretation of the electrical activity of the heart using rhythm monitoring techniques involving single or multiple lead analysis as well as the 12-lead electrocardiogram (ECG), has emerged as one of the most widely utilized diagnostic tools in today's medical practice. The ECG, once solely valued for the detection of cardiac arrhythmias, was deemed most appropriate for use by cardiologists at its advent. However, with technological advancements as well as with increased education surrounding use of testing, this tool has expanded into a variety of clinical settings. In the emergency department (ED), physicians encounter patient presentations of varying acuity, and the tools that allow providers to determine those patients who require immediate care are invaluable. Utilization of the ECG for patients with certain presenting complaints can aid in this process and dramatically improve patient safety as well as operational efficiency. The ECG further affects a patient's medical care by enhancing the ability of emergency physicians to make diagnoses, monitor management strategies, and allow for the timely disposition of patients. The impact of this diagnostic tool has led to the majority of healthcare providers being trained on its applications and interpretation.

The ECG as a Clinical Tool

The ECG is a point-of-care diagnostic study that is readily available to emergency physicians. This testing initially evolved when it was discovered that one could record a tracing of the action potential generated within the myocardium and is now utilized in the detection, diagnosis, and management of medical conditions from a patient's pre-hospital presentation to disposition post-ED visit. Improvements in the simplicity of design of ECG machines have allowed physicians to screen patients in multiple settings, thereby reducing the time it takes to diagnose and treat life-threatening conditions.

The technology has now become so advanced that the machines are compact enough to be placed in primary care clinics, urgent care centers, and on Advanced Life Support ambulances. Utilization of the ECG by emergency medical services (EMS) providers is a particular area of practice in which use of the ECG has dramatically increased within the past several decades. In part because of the diagnostic equipment available to these providers, pre-hospital management of critically ill patients has dramatically improved over the past 50 years. The 12-lead ECG, now more compact and portable, has proven to be of significant value in pre-hospital patient management (Figure 1.1.1). Standing protocols to obtain pre-hospital ECGs in the appropriate patient population can significantly affect patient outcomes. As EMS systems now allow for the acquisition and transmission of a pre-hospital ECG, activation of the cardiac catheterization team can occur prior to a patient's arrival in the ED. This process has been very effective in decreasing door-to-balloon time [1]. Time to treatment is also critically important when an arrhythmia is detected, as certain medications can be administered by EMS providers that may lead to termination of a life-threatening rhythm even prior to ED arrival.

The ideal diagnostic test would have the following characteristics: 100% sensitivity and specificity, provide delivery of immediate results, and be inexpensive and easy to obtain. Unfortunately, this ideal remains elusive. Like many other diagnostic studies, the ECG is excellent at detecting certain

Electrocardiogram in Clinical Medicine, First Edition. Edited by William J. Brady, Michael J. Lipinski, Andrew E. Darby, Michael C. Bond, Nathan P. Charlton, Korin Hudson, and Kelly Williamson.

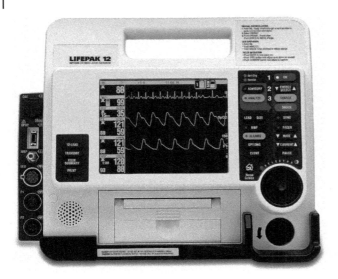

Figure 1.1.1 The Lifepak 12 is a portable device with functionality that includes defibrillation, pacing, and 12 lead electrocardiography. Figure obtained with permission from Physio-control.

conditions and disease processes yet is relatively poor at providing a specific diagnosis in other situations.

Multiple studies have investigated the utility of the ECG in specific situations. In a study examining the utilization of the ECG within emergency medicine, only 8% of applications provided a specific diagnosis, yet the testing was noted to be very helpful in ruling out various syndromes when interpreted within a clinical context [2]. It is therefore the responsibility of clinicians to determine the most appropriate utilization and interpretation of the ECG. For instance, chest pain and shortness of breath are the most frequent reasons for obtaining an ECG in the ED, as certain characteristic patterns emerge in the setting of cardiac injury. The presence of these patterns is inconsistent, however, and the ECG must be interpreted within the context of the clinical presentation. A 12-lead ECG demonstrating normal sinus rhythm with normal ST segments will likely be interpreted differently based on the presenting patient: this normal ECG will be very reassuring in a stable 29-year-old male with reproducible sharp anterior chest pain, yet may represent the early stages of a significant coronary event in a 68-year-old female with diaphoresis, substernal chest pressure, and dyspnea. As an ECG must always be interpreted within the context of a particular clinical presentation, we must use this test to the best of our abilities but also recognize its limitations.

Since emergency physicians evaluate a diverse range of patient complaints, the ECG is particularly useful in aiding in the detection of those patients requiring emergency management. For instance, when physicians assess a critically ill patient, namely one complaining of chest pain, dyspnea, or lightheadedness, the ECG can aid in the diagnosis of immediate life-threatening events. As there are many pathologic conditions that can disturb the electrical conduction of the heart, the ECG can be used to detect abnormalities prior to the results of any laboratory testing. Treatment can be initiated immediately, in attempts to prevent progression toward a fatal arrhythmia. Since the ECG is a dynamic rather than a static test, repeated tracings may also demonstrate an improvement in real time as management is initiated and serve as a guide as treatment continues.

The ECG is also invaluable in establishing appropriate timely disposition for ED patients; when applied in the appropriate clinical setting, the ECG can aid physicians in making disposition decisions earlier in a patient's ED course. This testing is especially helpful when a practitioner encounters delays in obtaining laboratory studies and diagnostic imaging. Regardless of the results of adjunctive testing, when faced with a concerning ECG, a physician can immediately recognize the necessity of admission and begin this process.

Clinical Presentations and the ECG

Emergency physicians evaluate patients with a diverse range of chief complaints that may represent a variety of underlying pathology. The ECG can be applied to many clinical scenarios, including patients presenting with chest pain, dyspnea, syncope, and toxic ingestions, as well as those with electrolyte abnormalities and pacemakers, in order to help the ED physician provide the most appropriate clinical care.

There are three broad classification systems under which a patient may receive ECG testing. The first is a symptom-based approach, in which patients presenting with certain chief complaints, most often chest pain, dyspnea, and syncope, undergo electrocardiography in order to evaluate for immediate life-threatening pathology and then to direct further workup. These symptom-based considerations are the most frequently encountered reason for obtaining an ECG in the ED. The other two classifications are systems-related indications, such as triage ECG protocols and preoperative clearance, as well as a diagnostic-based approach.

Chest Pain

When the ECG was first introduced as a diagnostic tool in the ED, a primary utilization was in the evaluation of patients who were experiencing chest pain, and it remains an essential component of this process. While an initial priority in the management of patients who present with this complaint is to detect those patients experiencing an acute myocardial infarction (AMI), the ECG provides

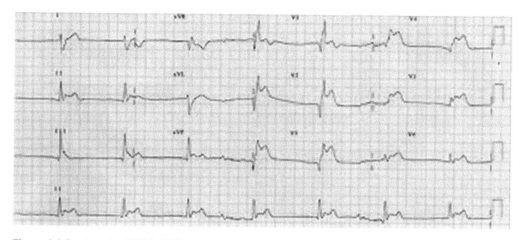

Figure 1.1.2 Anterior STEMI. ECG demonstrating acute ST-segment elevation in leads V2, V3, and V4. *Source:* Image obtained with permission from http://Lifeinthefastlane.com.

information that ultimately impacts a patient's clinical care in approximately one-third of patients presenting to the ED with chest pain [2]. Arguably the most time-sensitive application of this testing is the detection of an ST-segment elevation myocardial infarction, a disease process detected with relatively high sensitivity and specificity [3]. Acute anatomically oriented ST-segment elevation in a patient with chest pain is the major indication for acute reperfusion therapy (Figure 1.1.2) [4].

As the ECG is a dynamic test, ED physicians are able to follow changes to detect evolution in pathology. For instance, a patient presenting to the ED with chest pain may have a normal initial ECG and then subsequent ECGs that demonstrate an ischemia or infarction pattern. Serial ECGs obtained during the initial two to three hours of a patient's ED course will significantly increase the sensitivity for diagnosing an acute MI [3]. Without the ability to obtain repeat ECGs, a patient could experience a longer duration of infarcting myocardium prior to detection and intervention.

Even in the absence of ST-segment elevation infarctions, physicians can use the ECG to guide management decisions for chest pain patients. While patients experiencing non-ST-segment elevation (NSTEMI) myocardial infarction may not require emergent reperfusion, their diagnosis remains critically important. While the ECG changes in this disease process may be less specific than those previously discussed, the testing can still provide valuable information. For instance, a patient with chest pain who has anatomically oriented ST or T-wave changes, such as hyperacute T waves, T-wave inversions, or ST-segment depressions, may be a candidate for antiplatelet, anticoagulant, and anti-anginal therapies in order to optimize medical care and outcomes.

The ECG can also be used to risk-stratify patients presenting to the ED with chest pain, as it has great implications in terms of identifying those low-risk patients who may be safely discharged and those at higher risk who require a more extensive evaluation. The area of continued debate surrounds the management of patients who are at intermediate risk for acute coronary syndromes. The Standardized Reporting Criteria Working Group of the Emergency Medicine Cardiovascular Research and Education Group studied the association between the initial ECG and the outcomes of death, AMI, or the need for revascularization within 30 days of initial presentation in chest pain patients. The authors concluded that the relationship between the initial ECG, when classified into one of six categories, was highly associated with 30-day outcome [5]. While ED physicians must consider NSTEMI in the appropriate patient population even in the absence of ECG changes, in those patients in which an alternate diagnosis seems much more likely, a normal ECG can be quite reassuring.

Dyspnea

The chief complaint of dyspnea represents the second most frequently encountered indication to obtain an ECG in the ED. As discussed in the preceding section, an ECG can quickly aid in the diagnosis of myocardial ischemia as the etiology of dyspnea, or it may lead the treating physician to explore an alternate pathology, such as pulmonary embolism.

The diagnosis of pulmonary embolism (PE) relies on a combination of appropriate clinical suspicion paired with the interpretation of available diagnostic studies. While there is not one specific ECG change that can automatically confirm this diagnosis, there are some commonly associated electrical abnormalities. The most prevalent

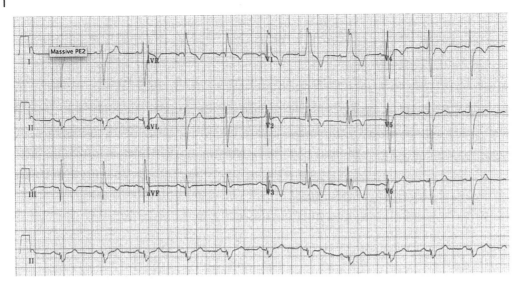

Figure 1.1.3 S1Q3T3 pattern associated with pulmonary embolism. *Source:* Image obtained with permission from http://Lifeinthefastlane.com.

ECG finding in patients with pulmonary embolism (PE) is sinus tachycardia, though up to 15–30% of patients with PE have normal ECGs [6]. Other characteristically associated patterns are those revealing evidence of right heart strain, including right axis deviation, a right bundle branch block (RBBB), and the often-referenced "S1Q3T3" (presence of a prominent S wave in lead I, and a Q wave and inverted T wave in lead III) (Figure 1.1.3). This S1Q3T3 finding, suggestive of acute cor pulmonale, was first reported by McGinn and White in 1935 [7]. The ECG may begin to show this finding when the PE causes the right ventricular pressures to exceed 40 mmHg, yet can be deceiving in those patients with preexisting pulmonary hypertension [3]. Unfortunately, the relatively low sensitivities and specificities of the various electrocardiographic findings limit the use of this study as a definitive diagnostic tool. However, in high-risk patients, such as those with risk factors for a hypercoagulable state, dyspnea, and hypoxemia, the presence of these findings may prompt a physician to initiate anticoagulation prior to obtaining further confirmatory testing.

Syncope

During their lifetime, up to a third of all individuals experience a syncopal event, defined as the sudden loss of postural tone and consciousness, and an additional third of these patients suffer an injury from this event. This presentation is another common indication for electrocardiography. It is the responsibility of the emergency healthcare provider to screen for serious abnormalities that would

require further management. Since syncope can result from any number of causes, ranging from benign vasovagal events to life-threatening arrhythmias, these presentations represent a diagnostic challenge to the ED physician. If a syncopal event is the result of alterations in the electrical conduction system of the heart, then timely diagnosis of the abnormality is critically important in order to restore a perfusing rhythm. For instance, an ECG that is diagnostic for third-degree heart block in an unstable patient mandates pacemaker placement, while one demonstrating supraventricular tachycardia would prompt the clinician to administer adenosine [3]. Other morphologic findings suggestive of certain disease processes that predispose to syncope include the ST-segment and T-wave abnormalities noted in ACS, ventricular hypertrophy suggestive of hypertrophic cardiomyopathy, ventricular pre-excitation seen in the Wolff-Parkinson-White syndrome, a prolonged QT interval, and the characteristic ST segments of Brugada syndrome.

While ECG findings such as bradycardia, AV block, and tachydysrhythmias may provide an etiology for the syncopal event [3], a patient often presents to the ED having returned to a normal state of health. As a result, a normal ECG in the ED does not exclude a cardiac event, given the often transient nature of arrhythmias. Therefore, investigators have studied the utility of the ECG in patients presenting with syncope in order to perform risk stratification for a future adverse event. In a review of 612 patients, Martin et al. endeavored to develop and validate such a risk classification system for those patients presenting to the ED with syncope. An abnormal ECG upon presentation was associated with arrhythmia or death with an odds ratio of

3 : 2; other factors suggestive of a poor outcome included a history of congestive heart failure (CHF) and ventricular arrhythmia [8]. Further work by Sarasin et al. examined outcomes in patients with syncope that remained unexplained after ED evaluation. In the 344 patients studied, an abnormal ECG was associated with future arrhythmia with an odds ratio of 8 : 1; other factors significantly associated with adverse outcome included older age and a history of CHF [9]. Finally, the San Francisco syncope rule, a commonly utilized clinical decision rule, incorporates the ECG into the risk stratification of patients presenting with syncope. The study investigators determined that an abnormal ECG, especially when taken in combination with factors such as dyspnea, low hematocrit, and hypotension, is a predictor of poor outcome [10].

Therefore, the most appropriate use of the ECG in relation to patients presenting with syncope is in the initial detection of a malignant dysrhythmia, followed by the utilization of the ECG for further risk stratification. As a normal ECG does not exclude a possible transient conduction disturbance, adjunctive devices such as Holter monitors can aid in the detection of cardiac events over the course of days to weeks, allowing a patient to resume their daily activities while still being screened for dangerous conduction abnormalities.

Toxicology

The diagnostic approach to the poisoned patient is multifaceted, including elucidation of the history surrounding the ingestion, performance of a thorough physical examination, with an emphasis on assessment for characteristic toxidromes, and evaluation of selected diagnostic studies, including the ECG. The ingestion of toxic substances can cause shifts in electrolytes leading to significant metabolic disturbances that may affect the electrical activity of the heart. Any patient who has sustained a toxic exposure or ingestion must undergo ECG screening to assess for cellular ischemia, conduction blockade, or prolongation of the intervals that can lead to fatal arrhythmias.

Characteristic ECG patterns may emerge with certain toxic exposures, and these changes can serve as a helpful guide toward the correct diagnosis if a patient is not forthcoming with historical details. A study by Homer et al. examined the range of ECG abnormalities encountered in poisoned patients, reviewing the ECGs of 277 patients evaluated for ingestion by the toxicology service at a tertiary care referral center who underwent electrocardiographic evaluation within six hours of ingestion. Of the patients studied, only 32% had a normal ECG. Of the 68% of patients with an abnormal ECG, 62% had rhythm disturbances (sinus tachycardia, sinus bradycardia, atrial-ventricular block, non-sinus atrial tachycardia, and nodal bradycardia) while 38% had morphologic abnormalities (abnormal QRS configuration, QRS complex widening, QT interval prolongation, PR interval prolongation, ST segment abnormality, and T wave inversion). Not surprisingly, the degree of abnormality was noted to be related to the number of toxins ingested. A more unexpected conclusion is that cardioactive medications such as beta-adrenergic blockers and calcium channel antagonists were no more likely to produce electrocardiographic abnormalities than the noncardiovascular substances such as sedative-hypnotic agents or stimulants [11].

The electrocardiographic changes associated with tricyclic antidepressant (TCA) overdose have been thoroughly delineated, including dysrhythmia, QRS complex widening, QT interval prolongation, and, perhaps most specifically, the QRS complex configuration with a prominent terminal R wave in lead aVR (Figure 1.1.4). This RSR prime pattern in lead aVR is particularly indicative of severe toxicity placing the patient at risk for seizures and ventricular arrhythmia; progressively larger R prime (R′) waves are associated with increasing degrees of toxicity [12]. Therefore, when a clinician notices the RSR prime morphology in lead aVR combined with a clinical suspicion for TCA overdose, it is an important signal to begin treatment with intravenous bicarbonate for this overdose and titrate to effect based on repeat ECGs (Figure 1.1.5).

Another commonly prescribed medication that demonstrates characteristic ECG changes in overdose is digoxin, associated with bradycardia, complete heart block, and atrial fibrillation with slow ventricular response as well as a characteristic downsloping of the ST segments [3] (Figures 1.1.6 and 1.1.7). The presence of these significant ECG changes can prompt the emergency physician of the possible need to administer Fab fragments prior to the availability of a digoxin level.

Finally, antipsychotic medications can also adversely affect the electrical conduction system of the heart. QT prolongation is particularly common, especially noted with thioridazine, pimozide, and intravenous haloperidol, and can lead to the life-threatening arrhythmia torsades de pointes [3]. Therefore, a baseline ECG obtained in patients presenting to the ED with acute psychosis can screen for preexisting QT prolongation and direct the physician toward safe medication choices.

Electrolyte Abnormalities

Critically ill patients, and especially those with underlying renal disease, frequently suffer from electrolyte abnormalities. Electrolytes such as sodium, potassium, and calcium

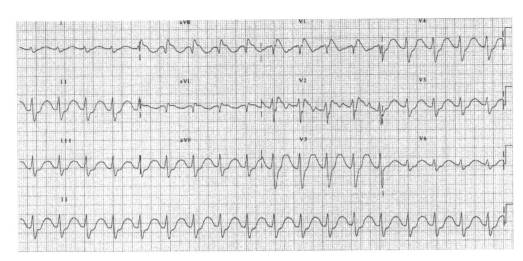

Figure 1.1.4 TCA toxicity noted by positive R wave in lead aVR, Sinus tachycardia, and widened QRS. *Source:* Image obtained with permission from http://Lifeinthefastlane.com.

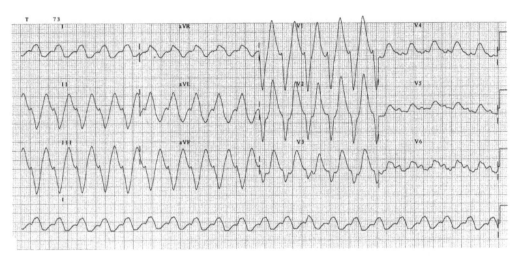

Figure 1.1.5 Progression of ECG changes in TCA toxicity in same patient. Marked QRS broadening. *Source:* Image obtained with permission from http://Lifeinthefastlane.com.

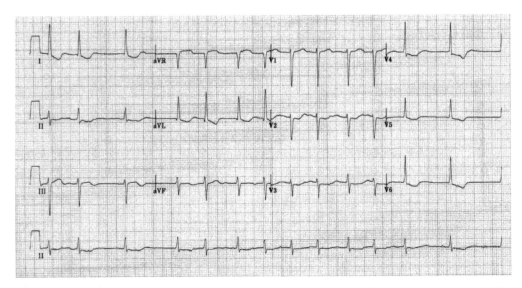

Figure 1.1.6 Digoxin effect. Evidence of digoxin noted by the swooping ST segments in the leads V4–V6 and I and aVL. Also noted to be similar to Salvador Dali's moustache. *Source:* Image obtained with permission from http://Lifeinthefastlane.com.

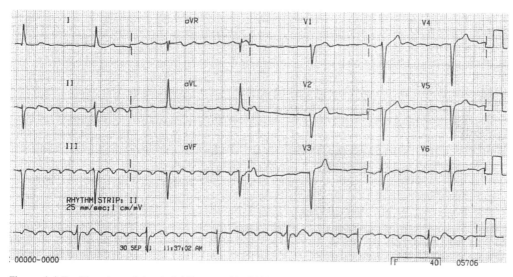

Figure 1.1.7 Digoxin toxicity. Atrial flutter with AV block with slow ventricular response. Classic findings for digoxin toxicity on an ECG: atrial supraventricular tachycardia with a slow ventricular response. *Source:* Image obtained with permission from http://Lifeinthefastlane.com.

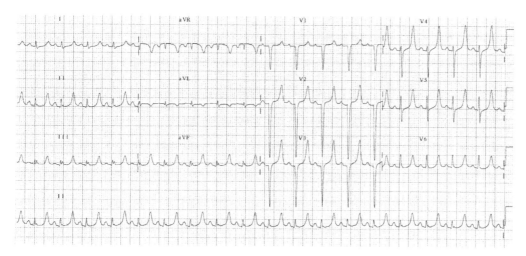

Figure 1.1.8 Hyperkalemia. Tall elevated and symmetrical peaked T waves. Pt had K level of 7.0. *Source:* Image obtained with permission from http://Lifeinthefastlane.com.

need to be in balance for optimal cellular functioning. There is a spectrum of physiologic changes that occur with toxic levels of the different electrolytes that may directly affect the cardiac conduction system.

Both hypo- and hyperkalemia are commonly encountered electrolyte abnormalities that have significant effects on the cardiac conduction system; appropriate levels of potassium, the most abundant cation in the intracellular fluid, are essential for both muscle and nerve activity. Severe derangements may result in ventricular fibrillation, complete heart block, and asystole [3]. Hyperkalemia is most often encountered in patients with end-stage renal disease, though it may also be caused by certain medications as well

as with rhabdomyolysis. It can lead to a characteristic ECG pattern with the presence of peaked T waves that progress to a sine wave pattern if left untreated (Figure 1.1.8) [4]. This finding, combined with appropriate clinical suspicion, can allow for the prompt arrangement of emergent treatment.

Within the cardiac myocytes, a deficiency in potassium levels leads to hyperpolarization of the resting membrane potential and requirement of a greater than normal stimulus to initiate the next action potential. Hypokalemia, which in severe states can lead to respiratory depression, arrhythmias, and cardiac arrest, also reveals notable changes on an ECG. While flat or inverted T waves, ST

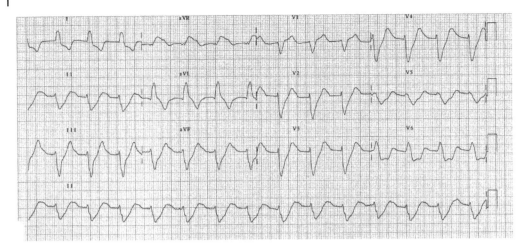

Figure 1.1.9 Hyperkalemia. Potassium increasing with progression of QRS widening. *Source:* Image obtained with permission from http://Lifeinthefastlane.com.

depression, and PR interval prolongation are all noted, the most commonly cited abnormality is the presence of a U wave corresponding to prolonged repolarization of the ventricular Purkinje fibers [3]. The presence of a U wave on the ECG is a signal to obtain an emergent potassium level so that repletion can be initiated in a timely fashion to avoid the development of fatal arrhythmias (Figure 1.1.9).

Levels of calcium, a predominantly extracellular cation, are also tightly regulated by cellular processes, and hypocalcemia can lead to neuromuscular irritability, seizures, and arrhythmias. Hypocalcemia is most often noted in association with hypoparathyroidism, vitamin D deficiency, and chronic kidney disease. The characteristic ECG finding of intermittent QT interval prolongation predisposes to life-threatening cardiac arrhythmia, including torsades de pointes, and its detection on ECG indicates emergent repletion [3].

Pacemakers

As the population ages, pacemakers are becoming more prevalent. Physicians may encounter complications ranging from nonfunctioning batteries, poor capture, lead dislodgement, and abnormalities in sensing. When patients with pacemakers present to the ED with a cardiac-related complaint, it is of the utmost importance to ensure that their pacemaker is functioning properly, with the ECG being an essential component of the diagnostic process. The absence of pacer spikes on an ECG can alert the ED physician of the need to involve cardiology early in the course of the patient's care.

Conclusion

Electrocardiography is an essential clinical tool within the practice of medicine, allowing for the detection of life-threatening pathology with an easily obtained bedside study. Its use provides invaluable information that physicians will consistently rely on for medical decision making. With continued developments and evolving technology, its diagnostic properties will only continue to evolve and expand. While it is important to recognize that a single ECG in the ED captures a brief moment in time, its diagnostic implications are limitless. The more clinicians study and use this test, the more they will obtain an increased level of confidence in its interpretation and applications.

References

1 Grosgurin, O., Plojoux, J., Keller, P.F. et al. (2010 Apr 17). Prehospital emergency physician activation of interventional cardiology team reduces door-to-balloon time in ST-segment elevation myocardial infarction. *Swiss Med. Wkly.* 140 (15–16): 228–232.

2 Brady, W.J., Adams, M., Burry, S.D., and Perron, A.D. (2002). The impact of the 12-lead ECG on ED evaluation and management. *Acad. Emerg. Med.* 40: S47.

3 Tintinalli, J. (2011). *Tintinalli's Emergency Medicine, a Comprehensive Study Guide*, 7e. Mcgraw Hill Companies, Inc.

4 O'Gara, P.T., Kushner, F.G., Ascheim, D.D. et al. (2013). ACCF/AHA guideline for the management of ST-elevation myocardial infarction: a report of the American College of Cardiology Foundation/American Heart Association Task Force on practice guidelines. *J. Am. Coll. Cardiol.* 61 (4): e78–e140.

5 Forest, R.S., Shofer, F.S., Sease, K.L., and Hollander, J.E. (2004). Assessment of the standardized reporting guidelines ECG classification system: the presenting ECG predicts 30-day outcomes. *Ann. Emerg. Med.* 44 (3): 206–212.

6 Panos, R.J., Barish, R.A., Depriest, W.W., and Groleau, G. (1988). The electrocardiographic manifestations of pulmonary embolism. *J. Emerg. Med.* 6: 301–307.

7 McGinn, S. and White, P.D. (1935). Acute cor pulmonale resulting from pulmonary embolism. *JAMA* 104 (17): 1473–1480.

8 Martin, T.P., Hanusa, B.H., and Kapoor, W.N. (1997). Risk stratification of patients with syncope. *Ann. Emerg. Med.* 29 (4): 459–466.

9 Sarasin, F.P., Hanusa, B.H., Perneger, T. et al. (2003). A risk score to predict arrhythmias in patients with unexplained syncope. *Acad. Emerg. Med.* 10 (12): 1312–1317.

10 Quinn, J.V., Stiell, I.G., McDermott, D.A. et al. (2004 Feb). Derivation of the San Francisco Syncope Rule to predict patients with short-term serious outcomes. *Ann. Emerg. Med.* 43 (2): 224–232.

11 Homer, A., Brady, W.J., and Holstege, C. (2005). *The Association of Toxins and ECG Abnormalities in Poisoned Patients*. Nice, France: Mediterranean Emergency Medicine Congress September.

12 Leibelt, E.L. and Francis, P.D. (1995). Woolf AD. ECG lead aVr versus QRS complex interval in predicting seizures and arrhythmias in acute tricyclic antidepressant toxicity. *Ann. Emerg. Med.* 26: 195–201.

2

History of the Electrocardiogram

Trale Permar[1] and Kelly Williamson[2,3]

[1] Yavapai Regional Medical Center, Prescott, AZ, USA
[2] Advocate Christ Medical Center Emergency Medicine Residency, Chicago, IL, USA
[3] Department of Emergency Medicine, University of Illinois at Chicago, Chicago, IL, USA

> *I do not imagine that electrocardiography is likely to find very extensive use in the hospital.... It can at most be of rare and occasional use to afford a record of some anomaly of cardiac action.*
> —Augustus D. Waller, 1911 [1, 2]

Since its inception as a scientific tool, the electrocardiogram (ECG) has rapidly evolved into one of the most frequently obtained studies in clinical medicine [3]. The advent of the ECG was the culmination of several branches of science converging to create a practical device that provides valuable information to healthcare providers in multiple realms of practice.

The ECG, readily available in today's medical practice, has a storied history beginning in the 1780s. It was initially postulated that mysterious fluids referred to as "animal spirits" controlled bodily functioning. Luigi Galvani, an Italian physician and physicist, discovered quite by chance that an electrical current can lead to muscle contraction when his laboratory assistant inadvertently touched a scalpel that was in contact with an electrical current to a partially dissected frog's leg, resulting in muscle contraction of the frog's leg (Figure 1.2.1) [4, 5]. This finding, one of the first discoveries in bioelectricity, laid the foundation for our current knowledge surrounding the electrical activity of muscles, action potentials, and ultimately its application to the heart.

The galvanometer, one of the first instruments used to measure electrical current, was ultimately named in honor of Dr. Galvani's findings. Invented in 1820 when the Danish physicist Hans Christian Oersted discovered electromagnetism, galvanometers were constructed by suspending a coiled wire within a magnetic field. As current passed through the wire, the wire would move according to the amount of current sensed [3, 6].

In 1856, nearly a century after Galvani's discoveries surrounding the electric activity within muscles, Albert von Koelliker, a Swiss anatomist and physicist, and Heinrich Mueller, a German anatomist, used the galvanometer to make the revolutionary discovery that an electrical current accompanies each heartbeat. Von Koelliker and Mueller attached a galvanometer to the base of a frog's ventricle and observed that the galvanometer sensed an electrical current with each myocardial contraction [4, 7]. The two scientists then discovered that placing a motor nerve isolated from a dissected frog's limb over the pulsing heart of a frog would lead to muscle contractions in the isolated frog's leg. They demonstrated that the frog limb contracted at the beginning of systole and again, though slightly weaker, at the start of diastole. This frog limb acted as the first device to measure the electrical activity of the heart, and these two contractions would later correspond to the QRS complex and the T wave of modern ECGs [1, 8].

In 1869, Alexander Muirhead, studying for a doctorate of science in electricity, was likely the first person to have recorded the actual electrical rhythm of the heart using a galvanometer. Unfortunately, the validity of this historical information is controversial, as he did not publish his findings at the time, and it was only later that the discovery was reported in a biography written by his wife [3].

The initial cardiac recordings published from the 1870s were crude and insensitive; curves extracted from multiple data points and plotted over time represent the first documentation of ventricular depolarization and repolarization (Figure 1.2.2) [6].

Great advancements in the study of cardiac electrical activity came in 1872–1873 when Gabriel Lippmann, a Luxembourg physicist and 1908 Noble Prize laureate in Physics, devised the capillary electrometer, a device consisting of a glass capillary tube containing mercury that would move with changes in electrical current (Figure 1.2.3). The advent of this device allowed the study and visualization of the electrical activity of the heart without plotting points on a graph. Shortly thereafter, a method was devised in which the readings from Lippmann's capillary electrometer could be recorded onto moving photosensitized paper, allowing for the creation of a permanent record [3, 7].

While previous studies had focused primarily on dissected animal hearts, Augustus Waller, a London physiologist and physician, discovered that the electrical potential of the heart could be recorded over the chest wall without the

need for direct contact with an exposed heart [3]. Waller is credited with the first recording of an "electrogram" from a human heart using the Lippmann capillary electrometer in 1887 (Figure 1.2.3). A year later, Waller would rename his recordings *cardiograms*. He also named the two deflections that corresponded to ventricular depolarization and repolarization "V1 and V2," which then became known in modern electrocardiography as the QRS and T waves [1]. Despite his extensive work and contributions, Waller certainly could not have predicted the impact electrocardiography would have on medicine, stating at the time that the ECG would "at most be of rare and occasional use to afford a record of some rare anomaly of cardiac action" [1].

Willem Einthoven, a Dutch physician and physiologist, continued the great advancements in electrocardiography in the late 1800s and is considered the "father" of modern day electrocardiography. His work led to the evolution of the ECG becoming the invaluable clinical tool that it is today.

In truth, Einthoven was not initially drawn to the study of electrocardiography. Early in his career he studied the musculoskeletal system, publishing his first paper on the mechanics of the elbow joint as a medical student in 1882. He next studied the eye before spending four years focused on the vagus nerve's control of respiration [6]. It was not until 1889, when Einthoven witnessed Augustus Waller record a human ECG with the capillary electrometer while attending the First International Congress of Physiology in Basel, Switzerland, that he became drawn to the study of electrocardiography [3]. The remainder of Einthoven's career would be dedicated to understanding the heart's electrical activity and methods with which to record it.

Initially, Einthoven devoted his work to the use of the capillary electrometer. He made numerous improvements on the device that led to enhanced function, resolution, and detail in the cardiograms produced (Figure 1.2.4).

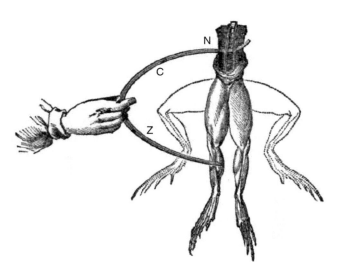

Figure 1.2.1 Galvani's frog leg, the first galvanometer. Image used with permission from Wells DA. The science of common things: a familiar explanation for the first principles of physical science. For schools, families, and young students. *Source:* Public domain [9].

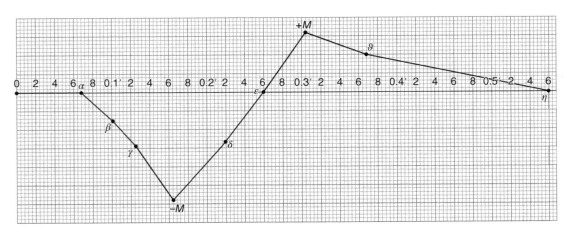

Figure 1.2.2 Initial Cardiac Recordings Plotted to Graph: Time course of variations in electric potential of the heart recorded by Englemann in 1878 using the differential rheotome. *Source:* With permission from Burch [10, p. 25].

Figure 1.2.3 Above: The Lippmann Capillary Electrometer, 1872. Below: ECG recorded in 1887 by Waller; "e" represents the electrocardiogram, "h" represents chest wall motion, "t" represents time in 0.05 s intervals. *Source:* With permission from Fisch [7, p. 1738], Copyright Elsevier and Waller [11].

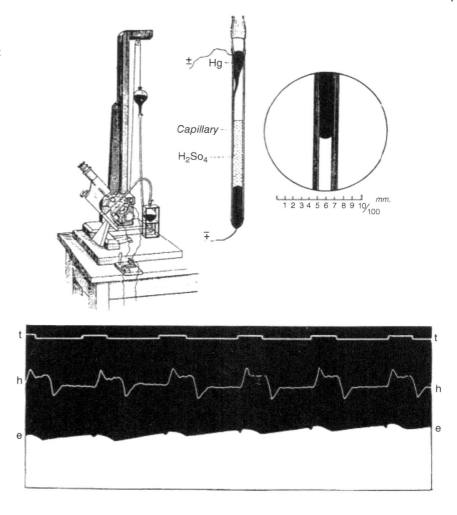

Einthoven was reportedly not satisfied with the capabilities of the capillary device, however, and began to work again with the galvanometer. Einthoven discovered that the sensitivity of the galvanometer was greatly increased by using fewer coils, which eventually lead to the creation of the string galvanometer in 1901. Rather than the coiled wire contraptions of previous galvanometers, Einthoven's string galvanometer consisted of a thin, silver-coated, quartz filament passing between two electromagnets. As current passed through the wire, movement was produced that was projected, magnified, and registered. This new device provided superior detail and sensitivity compared to its precursor, and a new field of medicine and industry was born, as the string galvanometer would soon become known as the electrocardiograph [3].

Einthoven is also responsible for the electrocardiography nomenclature that is still in use today. When Einthoven was initially using a Lippman capillary electrometer, he named the two resultant deflections "A" and "B." As device sensitivity improved, he detected a third wave, which he labeled "P"; this designation is hypothesized to be chosen based on prior work by Descartes, who used the letters "P" and "Q" to designate points on a curve in his law of refraction. As more waves were subsequently discovered, Einthoven changed his naming system to "ABCD." The advent of the string galvanometer led to continued improvement in wave detection, and Einthoven published a paper comparing the previous ECG waves with his most recently detected waves. Since he used the "ABCD" on the old tracings and these new waves were superimposed on one another, he was forced to choose a new naming system (Figure 1.2.5). He chose the designation "PQRST," likely because Descartes had used these same letters to classify consecutive points on a curve in his geometry discoveries (Figure 1.2.6). Some scholars also hypothesize that Einthoven assumed that new, as yet unseen, waves would be discovered, and leaving an open-ended labeling system would allow flexibility to designate additional waves in the future. Regardless of his underlying reasons, Einthoven continued to use the "PQRST" naming system in his subsequent publications, and this naming system remains in use today [12].

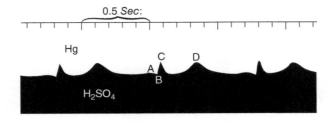

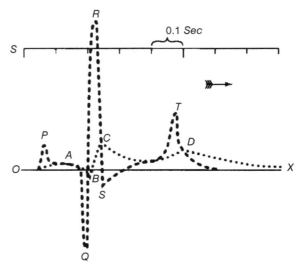

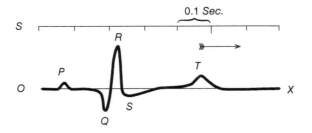

Figure 1.2.4 Above: ECG from Einthoven's capillary manometer. Below: Mathematically reconstructed ECG based on capillary manometer. *Source:* Image and caption obtained with kind permission from Springer Science and Business Media: Einthoven [13].

Figure 1.2.5 Two ECGs are shown, one superimposed on the other. Einthoven wanted to show the difference in the two curves. He labeled the uncorrected curve ABCD. This tracing was made with his refined Lippmann capillary electrometer. The other curve was mathematically corrected by Einthoven to allow for inertia and friction in the capillary tube. He chose the letters PQRST to separate the tracing from the uncorrected curve labeled ABCD. He continued to use these letters with the improved tracings from the string galvanometer. *Source:* With kind permission from Springer Science+Business Media: Einthoven [14].

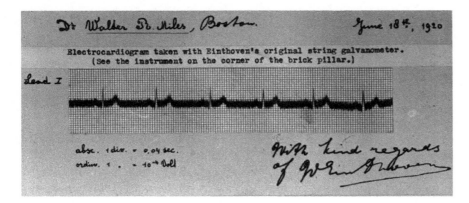

Figure 1.2.6 ECG strip from Einthoven's original string galvanometer, approx. 1903. With permission from Images from the History of Medicine, United States National Library of Medicine. *Source:* Public domain. http://ihm.nlm.nih.gov/images/A29515.

Einthoven also initially introduced three standard limb leads. Deemed *Einthoven's triangle*, this addition allowed for the ability to determine the electrical axis of the heart. Willem Einthoven ultimately won the Nobel Prize in Medicine in 1924 for his discovery of the electrocardiograph (Figure 1.2.7) [12].

Following on the contributions of Einthoven, Dr. Frank Wilson would pioneer work on precordial leads and also add discoveries such as wave form irregularities as well as arrhythmias [7]. In the 1930s, additional precordial leads were tested, and, in 1938, the American Heart Association and the Cardiac Society of Great Britain recommended use of the six precordial leads: V1–V6. In 1942, the augmented limb leads were added and the 12-lead ECG became the standard for recording ECGs.

Dr. Thomas Lewis, inspired by a meeting with Einthoven, bought a string galvanometer to use in London for further research. From 1908 to 1920, Lewis devoted his research to arrhythmias [7]. Lewis is largely credited with transforming electrocardiography into a clinical tool, rather than simply a means of conducting research on the heart. In addition to discovering numerous arrhythmias, he is

Figure 1.2.7 The first table-model Einthoven electrocardiograph manufactured by the Cambridge Scientific Instrument Company of London in 1911. *Source:* With permission from Burch [10, p. 33].

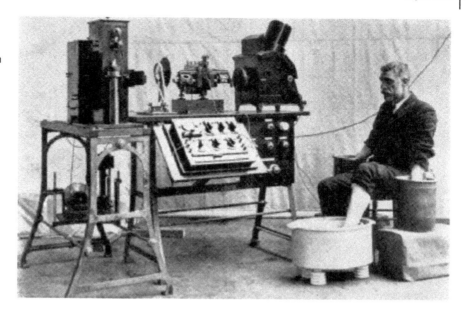

responsible for many terms that remain in use today, including *pacemaker, premature contractions,* and *auricular fibrillation* (now atrial fibrillation) [15].

Einthoven's initial electrocardiograph weighed approximately 600 pounds, occupied two rooms, and was found only in select hospitals. As industry and technology expanded, the size of the machines was reduced and portability was increased (Figure 1.2.7). By 1935, an ECG machine weighing a mere 25 pounds was introduced, and by the end of World War II, ECG machines were being produced that were compact enough to be utilized at the bedside of a hospitalized patient. In current medical

practice, nearly every emergency department in the country has a small, portable ECG machine that can be wheeled from room to room with tracings printed instantly [3].

The evolution of the ECG has been quite significant, from its inception in the late 1800s to its current use in clinical medicine, representing the integration of medicine with advancements in technology and industry. It has found utilizations well beyond its initial research confines of laboratories and is now an invaluable tool to quickly ascertain cardiac function and diagnose life-threatening arrhythmias by EMS providers, emergency physicians, and critical care physicians.

References

1 Zywietz, C. ((n.d.)). *A Brief History of Electrocardiography – Progress Through Technology.* Hannover, Germany: Biosignia Institute for Biosignal Processing and Systems Research.

2 Liebson, P.R. (2013). Willem Einthoven and the string galvanometer. *Hektoen International, A Journal of Medical Humanities* 5 (2).

3 Rivera-Ruiz, M., Cajavilca, C., and Varon, J. (2008). Einthoven's string galvanometer, the first electrocardiograph. *Tex. Heart Inst. J.* 35 (2): 174–178.

4 Dubin, D. (2000). *Rapid interpretation of EKGs.* Cover Inc.

5 Piccolino, M. (1998 Jul 15). Animal electricity and the birth of electrophysiology: the legacy of Luigi Galvani. *Brain Res. Bull.* 46 (5): 381–407.

6 Burch, G.E. and NP, D.P. (1964). *A History of Electrocardiography*, 20–30. Chicago: Year Book Medical Publishers, Inc., 56–66.

7 Fisch, C. (2000). Centennial of the string galvanometer and the electrocardiogram. *J. Am. Coll. Cardiol.* 36 (6): 1737–1745.

8 Fye, B. (1999). Profiles in cardiology: Rudolf Albert von Koelliker. *Clin. Cardiol.* 22: 376–377.

9 Wells, D.A. (1859). *The Science of Common Things: A Familiar Explanation of the First Principles of Physical Science for Schools, Families, and Young Students.*, 290. New York: Ivison, Phinney, Blakeman.

10 Burch, G.E. and DePasquale, N.P. (1990). *A History of Electrocardiography*, 2e. Norman Publishing.

11 Waller, A.D. (1887). A demonstration on man of electromotive changes accompanying the heart's beat. *J. Physiol.* 8: 229.

12 Hurst, J.W. (1998). Naming of the waves in the ECG, with a brief account of their genesis. *Circulation* 98: 1937–1942.

13 Einthoven, W. (1903). Die Galvanometrische Registerung des menschlichen Elektrocardigramms, zugleich eine Beurtheilung der Anwedung des Kapillar-Electrometers in Physiologie. *Pflugers Arch.* 99: 472.

14 Einthoven, W. (1895). Uber die Form des menschlichen Electrocardiogramms. *Pflüger's Archiv für die gesamte Physiologie des Menschen und der Tiere* 60 (30): 101–123.

15 Krikler, D.M. and Lewis, T. (1997, 2). A father of modern cardiology. *Heart* 77: 102–103.

Section II

ECG Changes in Myocardial Ischemia

1

The Cardiac Action Potential and Changes in the Setting of Acute Coronary Syndrome

How Ischemia and Infarction Impacts the ECG

Kirsti A. Campbell[1] and Michael J. Lipinski[2]

[1] *Harvard Medical School, Boston, MA, USA*
[2] *Cardiovascular Associates of Charlottesville, Charlottesville, VA, USA*

Introduction

Since 1901, the electrocardiogram (ECG) has enabled clinicians the ability to assess the electrical activity of myocardium and identify how specific alterations can be associated with pathologic changes. During the intervening years, clinicians and scientists have deconstructed the ECG so the characteristic waveform can be explained at the molecular level by shifting of sodium (Na^+), potassium (K^+), calcium (Ca^{++}), and chloride (Cl^-) ions through ion channels in the cardiomyocyte. Prior to a detailed evaluation of how ischemia can modify the "normal" ECG, it is first important to briefly review the biological processes underpinning the normal electrocardiographic tracing. Through understanding the pathophysiological changes accompanying acute or prolonged ischemia, one can anticipated how these changes may modify the normal ECG and be better prepared to identify even subtle changes on the ECG expected in the setting of ischemia. Thus, we plan to first review basic electrophysiology, the normal ECG, changes in cellular physiology associated with ischemia, and then how these changes result in characteristic signs of ischemia on the ECG.

Basic Electrophysiology

In the resting state, the interior of the cardiomyocyte has a negative charge. At the beginning of the cardiac cycle, specialized sinoatrial (SA) node cells spontaneously depolarize, beginning a wave of ionic depolarization that spreads from atria to ventricles, aided by intercellular gap junctions that allow for the quick movement of charge from cell to cell. Depolarization results in the interior of the cell becoming positively charged and enables contraction of the myocyte. It is critical to understand that as a wave of depolarization moves in the direction of an electrode on the skin surface, there is a resulting upward deflection recorded on the ECG. Alternatively, when the depolarization wave moves away from an electrode, there is a resulting downward deflection on the ECG. By mapping the electromotive force generated by the heart based on the multiple unipolar electrodes, we can generate vectors of myocardial depolarization and determine the path by which the depolarization wave spread through the heart. The myocytes then undergo repolarization, which returns the interior of the cells to a negatively charged resting state.

The depolarization of individual cardiac myocytes is typically depicted by five phases, 0–4, each distinguished by the opening, closing, and inactivation of the various sodium ion (Na^+), potassium ion (K^+), and calcium (Ca^{++}) channels. We will discuss each phase individually for both myocytes that rely predominantly on Na^+ for phase 0 depolarization and those that rely on Ca^{++}.

Action Potentials in Sodium-Dependent Depolarizers

Figure 2.1.1 illustrates the components of the action potential in correspondence with the ECG, and Figure 2.1.2 illustrates the ion channels of the cardiomyocyte corresponding to the different components of the action potential.

Electrocardiogram in Clinical Medicine, First Edition. Edited by William J. Brady, Michael J. Lipinski, Andrew E. Darby, Michael C. Bond, Nathan P. Charlton, Korin Hudson, and Kelly Williamson.
© 2021 John Wiley & Sons Ltd. Published 2021 by John Wiley & Sons Ltd.

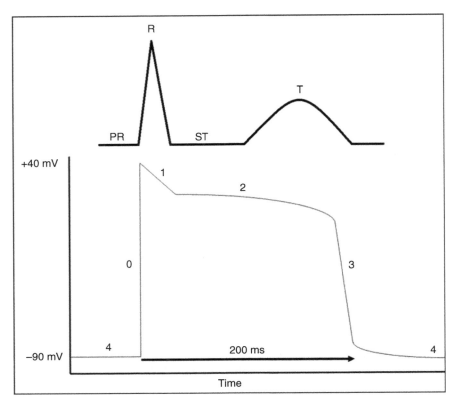

Figure 2.1.1 Timing of the action potential and its different components. The morphology and timing of the action potential is different for the atria, conduction system, and the ventricular myocardium. The included morphology of the action potential is similar to that of the ventricular myocardium and conduction system.

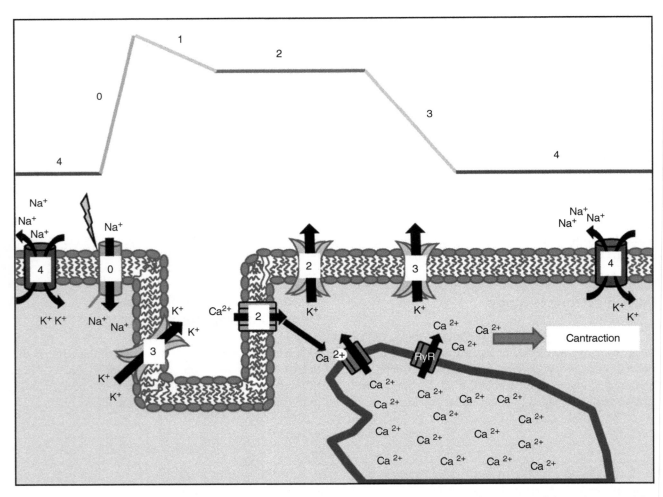

Figure 2.1.2 Cellular electrophysiology with the specific channels shown that correlate with different parts of the action potential. The specifics ion channels involved in each of the phases of the action potential are discussed throughout the chapter.

Phase 0: The Upstroke

In contractile cardiomyocytes, an inward sodium current (I_{Na}) is responsible for depolarization. It is important to note that very low Na^+ levels within the cell are maintained via Na^+/K^+ adenosine triphosphate (ATP) pumps. As a depolarizing current passes into the cardiomyocyte from adjacent cells through specialized gap junctions, the membrane potential becomes more positive than its resting potential at approximately -85 to $-96\,mV$. At a threshold potential, the voltage-gated sodium channel opens, enabling Na^+ to rush inside the cell down its concentration gradient toward its expected equilibrium potential. A rapid upstroke in membrane potential results.

As the membrane potential becomes more positive, many of the sodium channels become inactivated. It is this inactivation that leads to the refractory period for the cardiomyocyte. Importantly, although the majority of sodium channels will inactivate near the end of phase 0, a small number will remain open or spontaneously reopen before phase 4. These channels are responsible for a late inward sodium current (I_{NaL}), which acts to slow repolarization carried mostly by K^+ during the middle phases of the cardiac action potential. The importance of this I_{NaL} can be increased in pathophysiologic states.

Phase 1: Early Repolarization

As the inward sodium current brings the membrane potential close to $30\,mV$, voltage-gated potassium channels open, establishing a transient outward potassium current (I_{to}). Along with the inactivation of the phase 0 sodium channels, this leads to a quick dip in the membrane potential after the upstroke of phase 0. Furthermore, there is also outward flux of Cl^-. Two main potassium channels contribute to this rapid repolarization, which generate two potassium currents respectively known as $I_{to,fast}$ and $I_{to,slow}$. "Fast" and "slow" refer to the speed with which the channels respond to inactivation. At the end of phase 1, the myocyte membrane potential is still positive.

Phase 2: The Plateau

In phase 2, slow L-type Ca^{++} channels generate an inward calcium current ($I_{Ca,L}$) that balances the outward potassium-based I_{to} current of phase 1. These L-type channels are voltage-gated and are rapidly activated by the positive potentials achieved during phase 0 depolarization while rapidly inactivated by the characteristic dip of phase 1. I_{to} is also replaced in this phase by three potassium-rectifying currents, the ultra-rapidly activating delayed outward rectifying current (I_{Kur}, only relevant in atrial myocytes), the rapidly activating delayed outward rectifying current (I_{Kr}), and the slowly activating delayed outward rectifying current (I_{Ks}) [1, 2]. Together, these three potassium currents counteract the inward flow of Ca^{++}, and phase 2 is characterized by a plateau in the membrane potential. Although phase 2 does not actively contribute to the repolarization of the membrane potential, it subsequently provides the Ca^{++} flux necessary for triggering calcium release from the sarcoplasmic reticulum and subsequent excitation-contraction coupling.

Phase 3: Rapid Repolarization

The influx of Ca^{++} into the cell through the L-type calcium channels ultimately leads to the inactivation of those same channels, similar to the manner in which the sodium channels inactivate near the end of phase 0. With the outward flow of K^+ now mostly unopposed, the membrane potential rapidly returns toward the negative resting membrane potential. Toward the end of phase 3, inward rectifier channels (I_{k1}) that maintain the stable membrane potential of phase 4 open, bringing the potential closer to the resting membrane potential as more K^+ flows into the cell. The alpha subunit of these channels is Kir2.1, which is dependent on intracellular magnesium for its voltage-dependence.

Phase 4: Maintenance and Transition

During phase 4, the membrane potential is maintained at the resting potential as K^+ moves down its concentration gradient through the inward rectifier channel (I_{K1} channel). Since intracellular proteins carry a net negative charge and cannot move through the sarcolemma, the loss of positive charge from potassium moving out of the cell draws them toward the cell surface, making the cytoplasm at the cell surface more negative than the extracellular space. At this time, there is a small amount of sodium that enters the cell down its concentration gradient, but the membrane is largely impermeable to sodium at its resting potential. The Na^+/K^+ ATPase pump is crucial for maintaining the gradients of potassium and sodium across the sarcolemma in phase 4, an important point to remember in considering the cellular pathophysiology of ischemic damage and energy depletion. Additionally, at the more negative membrane potential, the $Na_{v1.5}$ channels previously inactivated at the depolarized potential slowly transition to a closed confirmation from which they can again open when another depolarizing current is received from another cell.

Excitation-Contraction Coupling

Beginning near the end of phase 0, the influx of calcium starts to initiate contraction of the individual myocyte. The sarcolemma contains invaginations called T tubules, which allow local interactions known as dyads between the specialized cell membrane and the large intracellular stores of calcium within the sarcoplasmic reticulum. As calcium flows into the dyad through the voltage-gated L-type channels, it binds to the ryanodine receptor (RyR2) on the sarcoplasmic reticulum, leading to the opening of these receptor-channels and amplified release of calcium into the cytoplasm from the sarcoplasmic reticulum. This process of initial calcium influx from the cell membrane leading to amplified release from the sarcoplasmic reticulum is known as calcium-induced calcium release.

The subsequent rapid rise in intracellular Ca^{++} concentration is crucial for activating the contractile machinery of the cell. Ca^{++} bind to troponin-C, exposing myosin-binding sites on actin filaments and subsequently allowing actin-myosin cross-bridge formation. The ATP-dependent cycling of cross-bridge formation and release allows for the contraction of the individual myocyte.

Action Potential in Calcium-Dependent Depolarizers

The ability of the heart to contract in a sequential and coordinated manner depends on specialized pacemaker cells in the SA node generating spontaneous action potentials. Based on their underlying cellular physiology, these cells generate action potentials typically at a rate of 60 times per minute or greater. The wave of depolarization begins at the top of the right atrium near the insertion of the superior vena cava and travels through the atria toward the atrioventricular (AV) node. While the AV node, bundle branches, and purkinje fibers of the conduction system also display automaticity, their intrinsic rate of depolarization is often only 40–50 action potentials per minute, allowing the faster SA node to control heart rate. In the setting of SA node dysfunction, the slower AV node pacemaker cells can take over, slowing the rate of contraction. The cellular physiology of contraction in these pacemaker cells is markedly different from that in contractile cardiac myoctyes.

Phase 0

The upstroke of the pacemaker cell action potential, in contrast to that of the contractile atrial-ventricular cell, is dependent on the influx of calcium and not sodium. Beginning at around −40 mV, voltage-dependent calcium channels open, allowing the influx of calcium into the cell and an increase in membrane potential. These L-type calcium channels generate a more gradual phase 0 upstroke than the $Na_{v1.5}$ channels responsible for contractile myocyte phase 0 depolarization, and they inactivate near the end of phase 0.

Phase 3

As in non-pacemaker myocytes, phase 3 repolarization is characterized by potassium influx and the absence of calcium influx after calcium channel inactivation, leading to a rapid decrease in the membrane potential.

Phase 4

The major contributor to pacemaker cell automaticity is the funny current, I_f. Near the end of phase 3, as the membrane potential dips below −40 mV, the funny current activates, allowing a mixed current of sodium and potassium to enter the cell and raise the membrane potential. The major functional component of the I_f channel is the hyperpolarization-activated, cyclic nucleotide-gated 4 channel (HCN4). While several channels involved in cellular depolarization display voltage-dependent activation, I_f channel is distinguished by two important differences. The first is that it becomes active at more negative membrane potentials, allowing it to trigger spontaneous membrane depolarization at the negative membrane potentials near the end of phase 3. The second is that its activation is dependent on intracellular concentrations of the cyclic nucleotide cAMP. Upon sympathetic-mediated increases in intracellular cAMP or muscarinic (m2) receptor-dependent decreases in cAMP, the channel becomes more or less active, respectively. This cAMP dependence contributes to autonomic effects on heart rate.

There is controversy over the relative contribution of another potential initiator of pacemaker cell depolarization: spontaneous calcium release from the sarcoplasmic reticulum through the ryanodine receptor. Following release from the sarcoplasmic reticulum, the rising intracellular calcium is pumped out of the cell through a Na^+/Ca^{++} exchanger (NCX1), with three sodium moving into the cell for every calcium ion extruded [3]. This creates a net inward positive current, further helping to depolarize the cell. The importance of this "calcium clock" in regulating pacemaker automaticity is still being elucidated.

Anatomy of the Electrical Conduction System

The sequential timing of atrial and ventricular excitation and contraction is of utmost importance in maintaining cardiac output. The structure and function of the electrical conduction system of the heart underlies the ordered and directional flow of electric current and subsequent contraction. The SA node is located in the right atrium near the crista terminalis. As already described, specialized pacemaker cells in this node are dependent on calcium for depolarization and display automaticity, generating action potentials at a rate of typically 60 beats per minute or greater. The specialized P cells are surrounded by T cells, which further intercalate into contractile myocytes within the atria. As potentials are generated by the P cells, the signal passes to the T cells and subsequently spreads throughout both atria, stimulating atrial contraction. Although the pathways through which the bulk of electrical current flows through the atria are not anatomically distinct from surrounding tissue, the cells do display functional specifications that promote efficient conduction of charge, including wide diameter and terminal placement of gap junctions to allow unidirectional flow of current. The wave of depolarization then reaches the AV node and is slowly conducted through this complex node of cells. The AV node typically provides the only means of electrical communication between the atria and ventricle. This is very important to maintain cardiac function by separating the time between atrial and ventricular contraction. It also helps prevent worrisome arrhythmias from conducting rapidly from the atria to the ventricle and vice versa. The wave of depolarization then rapidly conducts from the AV node to the bundle of His and down the bundle branches, which spread the wave of depolarization to the ventricle in an organized fashion through the purkinje fibers. Integral in this discussion are the different components of the ECG waveform. The P wave represents the depolarization of the atria, the PR interval represents the time in which electrical depolarization travels through the AV node, the QRS represents depolarization of the ventricle, and the T wave represents repolarization of the ventricle.

Biochemical Impact of Ischemia

The function of cardiac myocytes is dependent on blood supply from the coronary arteries to meet the cellular and metabolic demand of individual cells. Acute ischemic events, which often result from rupture or erosion of atherosclerotic plaque, initiate a number of changes at the biochemical level that ultimately affect the electrical conduction and contractile properties of the heart. Importantly, both the supply of oxygen and metabolic substrates and the removal of toxic cellular metabolites is impaired in the setting of ischemia.

Soon after the onset of ischemia, cardiac myocytes transition from depending on mitochondrial-based oxidative phosphorylation to anaerobic glycolysis for the generation of ATP and maintenance of cellular homeostasis. Anaerobic glycolysis is a less efficient means of producing ATP, and in the setting of reduced cellular energy, the Na^+/K^+ ATPase is impaired. Subsequently, the critical ionic gradients of

sodium and potassium across the sarcolemma diminish, limiting the ability of the myocyte to generate a physiologic action potential due to the loss of hyperpolarizing effects of the Na^+/K^+ ATPase activity. This loss of pump activity prevents K^+ from being pumped back into the cell with decreased intracellular K^+ levels. Decreased ATP levels can also lead to further extracellular flux of K^+ from cells through opening of K_{ATP} channels due to low ATP levels. This outward flux of K^+ can ultimately lead to membrane depolarization. This depolarization can inhibit fast $Na+$ channels and severely limit the upstroke velocity of the action potential. This can impact conduction velocity and contribute to the development of arrhythmias such as ventricular tachycardia and ventricular fibrillation.

The accumulation of sodium within the cell leads to increased osmotic pressure and cellular swelling. Furthermore, the dependence on anaerobic glycolysis leads to the buildup of acidic metabolites, lowering the cellular pH and contributing to the osmotic cellular swelling. The drop in cellular pH leads to further disturbances in intracellular and extracellular K^+ levels. These changes in cellular energy state and acidity have profound effects on protein synthesis and subsequently sarcomeric function. The loss of cellular function resulting from ischemia leads to several important and temporally varying changes in multiple components of the ECG complex. Understanding the generation and relative sequence of these changes can provide useful clinical hints about appropriate treatment modalities and prognosis.

ST-Segment Deviation

Injury currents flowing from the depolarized ischemic regions to normal regions results in alteration of the ST segment. Subendocardial ischemia results in ST-segment depression while transmural injury/ischemia typically results in ST-segment elevation. Abnormal ST-segment elevation in two adjacent leads with the exclusion of aVR is known as *acute injury pattern*. Injury currents can be generated from coronary thrombotic or spastic occlusion or result from pressure on the myocardium generated by pericardial fluid in acute pericarditis, fibrotic material in chronic pericarditis, cardiac tumor, or myocardial dyskinesis in the setting of ventricular aneurysm. Myocardial ischemia can result in shortening and decreased amplitude of the action potential and depolarization in which the resting membrane potential of the cardiomyocytes is less negative. The shortening and decreased amplitude of the ventricular action potential generates a systolic current of injury. A diastolic current of injury is generated through the depolarization with a less negative resting membrane

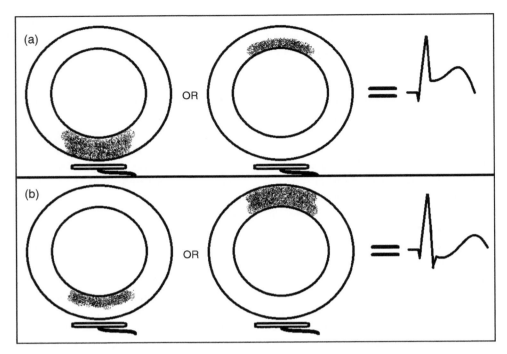

Figure 2.1.3 In part A, we see how subepicardial injury in the anterior wall (closest to the ECG lead on the bottom) or subendocardial ischemia in the posterior wall can result in ST-segment elevation in the ECG lead. In part B, we see how subendocardial ischemia in the anterior wall (closest to the ECG lead) or subepicardial injury of the posterior wall can result in ST-segment depression in the ECG lead. Ischemia or injury is denoted by the shaded portion of the myocardium.

potential. These diastolic injury currents lead to changes in the baseline on ECG while the systolic injury currents lead to changes in the ST segment. Epicardial injury typically leads to ST-segment elevation and baseline depression while endocardial injury leads to ST-segment depression and baseline elevation. However, the ECG only reveals changes to the ST-segment as alternating current (AC)-coupled amplifiers adjust the ECG to the current baseline and therefore do not show changes to the baseline.

ST segment deviation is directed toward the site of ischemia. As seen in Figure 2.1.3, this is critical because ST-segment elevation seen in one lead may represent acute subepicardial injury in the myocardial wall closest to the ECG lead but could also represent subendocardial ischemia in the myocardial wall on the opposite side of the heart. The classic example is reciprocal ST-segment depression in the case of acute myocardial infarction. Anteroseptal, anterior, inferior, and lateral ST-segment elevation myocardial infarction (STEMI) are typically associated with reciprocal changes in other leads. In the case of posterior myocardial infarction, the posterior wall of the heart can be seen best in leads V1–V3. Acute epicardial injury of the posterior wall, therefore, produces ST-segment depression in leads V1–V3. Figures 2.1.4 and 2.1.5 serve as examples of posterior myocardial infarction with ST depression seen in the precordial leads. It is important not to mistake this finding

as simply endocardial ischemia in the anterior wall, as epicardial injury represents transmural injury consistent with a large infarction.

Acute myocardial injury with pathologic ST-segment elevation in two adjacent leads represents a medical emergency and is typically associated with acute closure of one of the major epicardial coronary arteries. As will be discussed in later chapters, ST-segment elevation myocardial infarction, or STEMI, is associated with a poor prognosis if not immediately treated and may progress to develop pathologic Q-waves in the involved leads. These Q waves may develop after as little as six hours of symptoms and represents myocardial necrosis with failure of the regional myocardium to depolarize [4].

The morphology of the ST segment is also important in the assessment of ischemia. As a patient becomes tachycardic with either exercise or other stimuli such as pain, the ST segment may have an upslope to the isoelectric line. While this may technically represent ST depression, upsloping ST-segment depression is often nonspecific. However, horizontal or downsloping ST depression, especially involving T-wave inversion, is strongly associated with myocardial ischemia. An excellent example of dynamic ECG changes with downsloping ST-segment depression and T-wave abnormalities consistent with ischemia can be found in Figure 2.1.6. While correlation

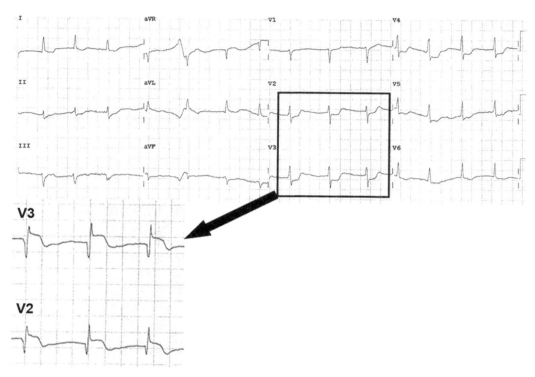

Figure 2.1.4 A 66-year-old male with longstanding hypertension, hyperlipidemia, diabetes mellitus, and known coronary disease with chronic occlusion of the left anterior descending coronary artery developed acute shortness of breath and then cardiac arrest. He was found by rescue squad in ventricular fibrillation and was defibrillated and with return of circulation developed severe bradycardia requiring external pacing. Upon arrival, external pacing was held and an ECG was performed which demonstrated a junctional rhythm with significant ST-segment depression in leads I, II, aVL, and V2–V6. The shape of the ST depression in V2–V4 was consistent with a posterior ST elevation myocardial infarction. He was taken emergently to coronary angiography and was found to now also have occlusion of a dominant left circumflex artery that supplied the posterior descending artery. When these anterior leads are rotated 180° (and thus are posterior leads) to reflect the reciprocal changes on the ECG, the characteristic shape of ST elevation MI is clearly visible.

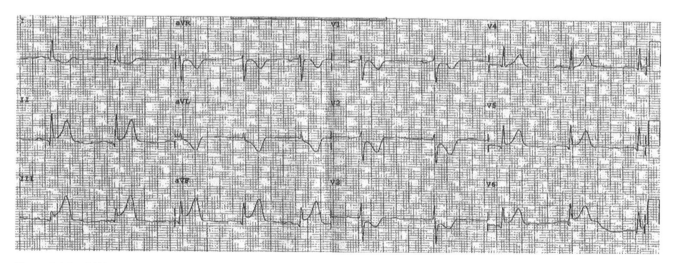

Figure 2.1.5 A 77-year-old female with hypertension, diabetes mellitus, and hyperlipidemia presented with shortness of breath and a feeling of indigestion. ECG upon presentation demonstrated sinus arrhythmia with ST elevation in leads II, III, aVF, V5, and V6 with reciprocal ST and T wave changes in I and aVL. There is also ST depression with T-wave inversion in V1–V3 consistent with posterior wall injury. Q waves appear to be forming in leads II, aVF, V5, and V6 suggesting transition from myocardial injury to myocardial infarction. The patient underwent emergent coronary angiography demonstrating total occlusion of a dominant right coronary artery.

(a)

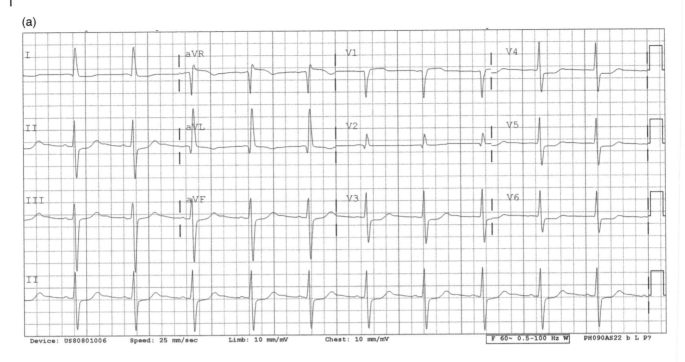

Device: US80801006   Speed: 25 mm/sec   Limb: 10 mm/mV   Chest: 10 mm/mV   F 60~ 0.5–100 Hz W   PH090AS22 b L P?

(b)

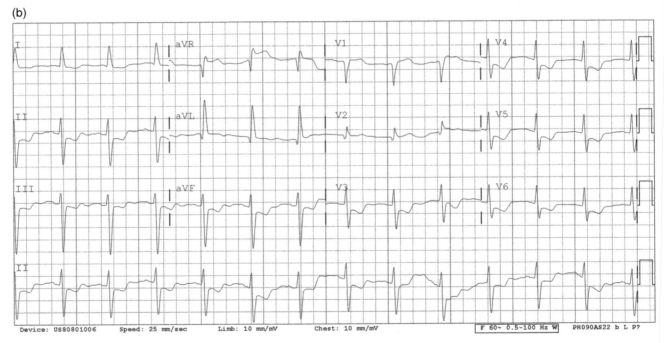

Device: US80801006   Speed: 25 mm/sec   Limb: 10 mm/mV   Chest: 10 mm/mV   F 60~ 0.5–100 Hz W   PH090AS22 b L P?

Figure 2.1.6   A 63-year-old male with longstanding hypertension presents to the emergency department following an episode of chest pain. His initial ECG (a) demonstrates normal sinus rhythm with left ventricular hypertrophy (R wave in aVL >11 mm) with diffuse ST depression and T-wave abnormalities and slight ST elevation in aVR, concerning for myocardial ischemia versus left ventricular hypertrophy with strain pattern leading to the ST and T-wave changes. The patient then developed recurrent chest pain and a repeat ECG (b) demonstrated significant worsening of ST depression with downsloping ST depression and significant T-wave abnormalities suggestive of ischemia and underwent urgent coronary angiography demonstrating a severe stenosis of the proximal left anterior descending coronary artery.

(a)

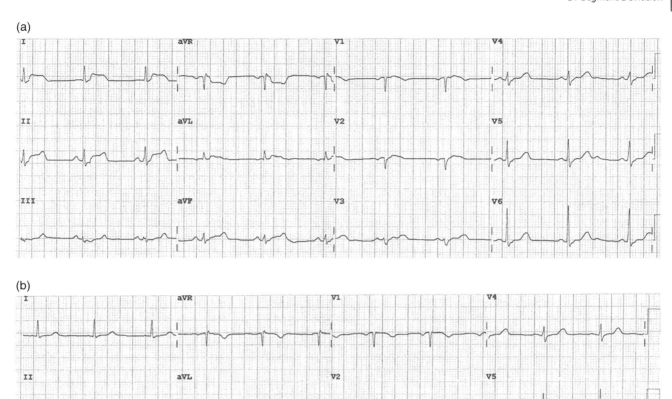

(b)

Figure 2.1.7 A 83-year-old female presented to the emergency department via rescue squad. She had symptoms of profound fatigue and fell, resulting in bilateral ankle fractures. She denied any symptoms of chest pain or shortness of breath. Initial ECG (a) demonstrated normal sinus rhythm with a bizarre ST-elevation morphology in leads I, aVL, and II and reciprocal depression in aVR. The ST segment in these leads appears "notched" with initially a normal J point and then significant rise after in the ST segment (best seen in lead II). As will be discussed in the next chapter, the ST-segment elevation does not also seem to correlate well with a coronary territory as the reciprocal ST depression does not really match the pattern of inferolateral myocardial injury. Given the unusual ECG and lack of concerning symptoms, an ECG was repeated 20 minutes later using identical lead placement and the ECG changes resolved (b). Serial troponins were negative for evidence of myocardial injury.

with patient symptoms and prior ECG is critical in the setting of horizontal or downsloping ST-segment depression, it is likely prudent to strongly consider myocardial ischemia until proven otherwise. Clinical history is also important, as hypokalemia and digitalis toxicity can also generate ST depression that may be confused with ischemia.

Recognition of pathologic ST-segment elevation is an important skill as ST-segment elevation can arise from multiple etiologies other than ischemia. ST-segment elevation is considered significant if greater than or equal to 0.1 mV or 1 mm above the isoelectric line measured at 0.04–0.08 seconds after the J-junction. As other etiologies

can lead to ST elevation, it is very important to consider the clinical context when evaluating a patient with ST-segment elevation. For example, a patient with ongoing chest pain but only with minimal ST elevation that does not meet criteria for STEMI may still require urgent coronary angiography. Alternatively, a patient with hypertension and accompanying left ventricular hypertrophy who does not have chest pain likely has ST elevation secondary to left ventricular hypertrophy. This can be challenging in patients with benign early repolarization who present with chest pain. The importance of clinical context can be seen in Figure 2.1.7 in which a patient presented with ankle fractures and no symptoms of chest pain or shortness of breath but was found to have unusual ST-segment elevation. STEMI mimics will be covered in depth in a later chapter. Another important caveat is the presence of ST-segment elevation in leads with Q waves. In patients with prior Q wave myocardial infarction, ventricular aneurysm may result in persistent ST-segment elevation and it is therefore important to assess symptoms and compare the current ECG with a previous ECG when available.

QRS Complex

The presence of pathologic Q waves can help identify the presence of myocardial infarction and remains a critical component of separating acute injury pattern from acute myocardial infarction. Q waves can be explained by loss of voltage in the region of myocardium due to infarction with the depolarization wave and resulting electrical forces headed away from the region toward noninfarcted myocardium. An example of anteroseptal Q waves with T-wave inversions consistent with evolving myocardial infarction seen with T-wave inversion can be seen in Figure 2.1.8. Pathologic Q-waves are defined as 40 ms or greater in duration and exceed 25% of the following R wave and typically develop after 6–14 hours of ischemia [4]. Q waves correlate with the site of infarction with anteroseptal (V1–V3), anterior (V2–V4), anterolateral (V4–V6), lateral (I and aVL), inferior (II, III, and aVF), and posterior MI, which presents as tall R waves in V1 and V2 (reciprocal view of Q waves for the posterior wall).

(a)

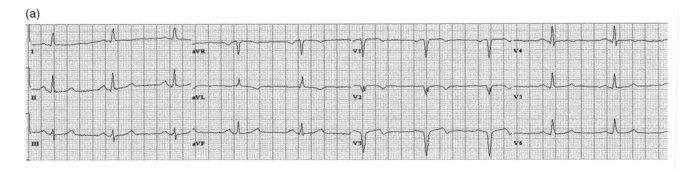

(b)

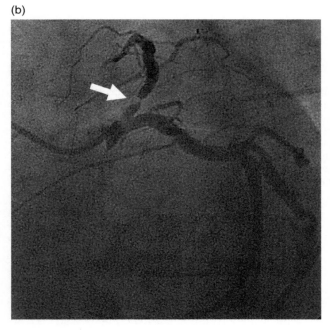

Figure 2.1.8 A 66-year-old female with diabetes mellitus, obesity, and severe left hip pain presents for evaluation for preoperative cardiovascular risk assessment prior to undergoing left hip replacement. Her ECG (a) demonstrated normal sinus rhythm with Q waves in leads V1–V3 and residual T-wave inversion/abnormalities in V1–V4 consistent with recent anteroseptal myocardial infarction. Given the morphology of the T waves, the myocardial infarction likely occurred within the last two weeks and there may still be residual ischemia. Due to the ECG, the patient underwent coronary angiography, (b) demonstrating subtotal occlusion of the proximal left anterior descending coronary artery (white arrow) best seen in the left anterior oblique caudal projection.

During myocardial infarction and severe ischemia, the R wave amplitude has been shown to increase, and the presence of "giant R waves" in the setting of chest pain has transiently been seen in the hyperacute phase of myocardial infarction [5]. The cause has been thought to be due to altered conduction [5], as experiments have shown that the increased R wave amplitude is not due to ventricular dilation. This may also be associated with a decrease in the S-wave amplitude.

Widening of the QRS complex may also suggest significant myocardial ischemia. The development of a new bundle branch block may imply severe myocardial ischemia or injury involving the myocardial septum. In patients with chest pain and new-onset left bundle branch block (LBBB), the patient is often taken emergently for coronary angiography as this finding is considered a *STEMI equivalent* and can be associated with acute occlusion of the left anterior descending coronary artery. The left anterior descending artery gives rise to the septal perforator arteries that supply blood to the left bundle branch in the interventricular septum. As the cells of the left bundle branch become ischemic, they fail to propagate the depolarization wave, and this leads to the development of a left bundle branch morphology on ECG.

In the setting of acute ischemia, the development of ventricular ectopy can be an ominous sign. In patients with ST-segment elevation, it is common to have accompanying premature ventricular contractions. If these occur during ventricular repolarization (R on T phenomenon), the rhythm may degenerate into ventricular fibrillation. Additionally, ventricular tachycardia that develops in the setting of ischemia tends to be polymorphic rather than monomorphic, unless a premature ventricular contraction in the setting of ischemia can induce monomorphic ventricular tachycardia in an individual with scar due to earlier myocardial infarction. Following reperfusion of an occluded artery, ventricular ectopy, and accelerated ventricular rhythms are common and are often not malignant [6].

T Waves

In patients with acute ischemia and development of myocardial injury, the T-wave morphology undergoes several important changes. The typical order of ECG changes are that (i) the patient develops "hyperacute peaked" T waves; (ii) ST-segment elevation; (iii) development of a Q wave; (iv) a decrease in the ST-segment elevation with flattening of the T wave (*pseudonormalization* in which physicians may not appreciate that a patient is experiencing acute myocardial infarction); (v) normal ST segment with symmetric inversion of the T waves and a prolonged QT interval. The characteristic finding on ECG associated with acute onset of ischemia is the development of *hyperacute T waves* in which there is a significant increase in T-wave amplitude and change in the morphology with "peaking" of the T waves. Figure 2.1.9 shows a classic example of hyperacute T waves in a patient who progressed to develop ST elevation. Figure 2.1.10 shows an example of dynamic ischemic changes with peaked T waves in a woman with chest pain. It is believed that these changes in T-wave morphology are due to prolongation of activity in the region of the ventricle immediately adjoining the area of infarction [7]. The T wave can also develop a "tombstone" appearance in the case of severe ST-segment elevation in which the elevated ST segment merges into the T wave and obviously portends a poor prognosis. Figures 2.1.11 and 2.1.12 serve as excellent examples of tombstones on ECG in a patient with STEMI. Another classic finding is deep T-wave inversion in the precordial leads, or Wellen's T waves, which is often associated with severe ischemia in the anterior wall, but it is important to correlate clinically as this can also be associated with intracranial bleeding. An example of Wellen's T waves can be seen in Figure 2.1.13. The presence of Q waves may help distinguish Wellen's T waves from the symmetrical inverted T waves seen in an evolving myocardial infarction. An example of evolving myocardial infarction with T-wave inversion can be seen in Figure 2.1.14. Following acute myocardial infarction with the development of Q waves, T-wave inversion will often remain for two weeks or longer following the onset of symptoms.

P Waves

Alterations in P-wave morphology in the setting of myocardial ischemia are very rare. However, changes in heart rate are very common in the setting of myocardial ischemia and can lead to either tachycardia or bradycardia. Myocardial ischemia and the resulting anginal chest pain can result in a surge of the sympathetic nervous system with resulting tachycardia. Additionally, myocardial dysfunction secondary to ischemia can decrease stroke volume, which may require an increase in heart rate to maintain cardiac output. Bradycardia is also seen during myocardial ischemia and frequently is associated with either occlusion or a severe stenosis of the proximal right coronary artery. The proximal branches of the right coronary artery supply blood to the SA node and ischemia can result in reduced automaticity. Furthermore, myocardial ischemia can result in significant disturbances of the conduction system. This can range from the development of bundle branch blocks

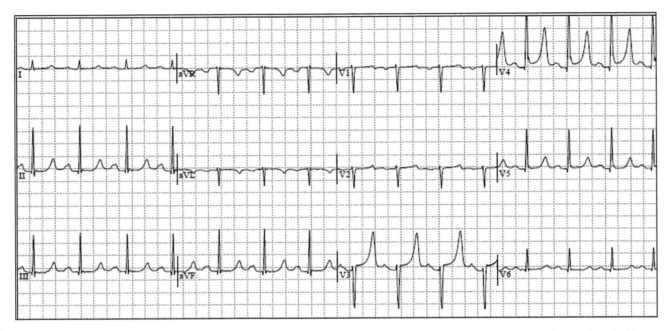

Figure 2.1.9 A 58-year-old male with hypertension, diabetes mellitus, and previously normal ECG was admitted to the hospital for chest pain. He developed acute onset of severe chest pain while in the hospital and ECG demonstrated normal sinus rhythm with peaked T waves in leads V3–V5. The patient was taken urgently for coronary angiography and progressed to develop anterior ST-segment elevation consistent with myocardial injury pattern and was found to have a subtotal occlusion of the left anterior descending coronary artery. Given the clinical context of chest pain and previously normal ECG and potassium levels, the peaked T waves represent the onset of severe ischemia, which often progresses to an injury pattern with ST-segment elevation and is unlikely to represent hyperkalemia.

(a)

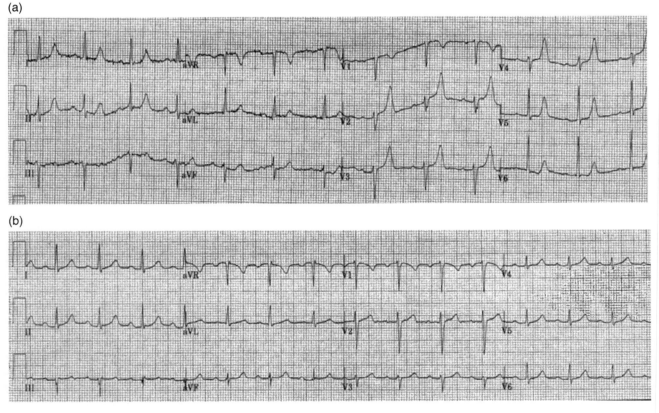

(b)

Figure 2.1.10 A 57-year-old female smoker presented with chest pain to the emergency department. Her initial ECG (a) demonstrated sinus rhythm with hyperacute T waves and poor R wave progression The peaked T waves with ST-segment abnormalities were very suggestive of myocardial ischemia. The patient had a repeat ECG (b) following administration of nitroglycerin that demonstrated resolution of the ST and T-wave abnormalities. She underwent coronary angiography, demonstrating a severe stenosis in the mid-left anterior descending coronary artery.

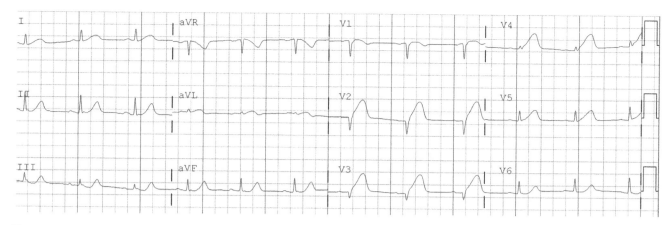

Figure 2.1.11 A 57-year-old female with no significant medical history presents with shortness of breath and back, neck, and jaw discomfort for seven hours. An ECG on presentation demonstrated normal sinus rhythm with Q waves in leads V1–V3 and ST-segment elevation in V2–V5 consistent with an acute anteroseptal myocardial infarction. The duration of chest pain was adequate (>6 hours) to develop Q waves, and the steep rise of the ST segment into the "tombstone-shaped" T wave is classic for acute ST-segment elevation myocardial infarction. This case also raises the important point that women often present with very different symptoms from men and may not have "classical symptoms" such as chest pain or pressure with radiation to the left arm.

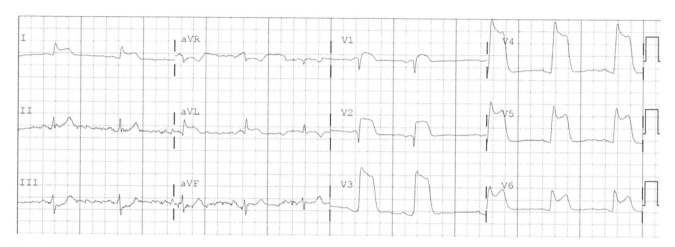

Figure 2.1.12 A 54-year-old male with hypertension and tobacco abuse presents two hours after the onset of crushing chest pain. His ECG demonstrated sinus arrhythmia with profound ST-segment elevation in leads I, aVL, and V1–V6 with reciprocal depression in aVR and III. The lack of pathologic Q waves with presence of ST-segment elevation is consistent with myocardial injury pattern that transitions to acute myocardial infarction when pathologic Q waves become present.

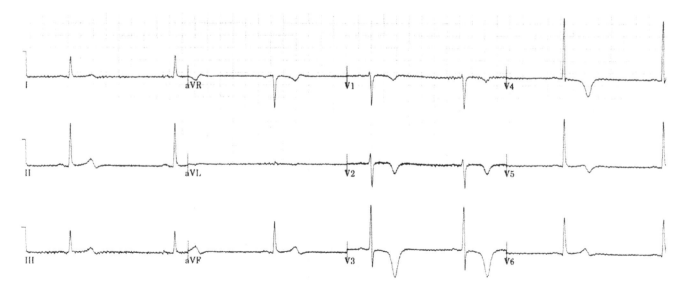

Figure 2.1.13 A 48-year-old male with hypertension and tobacco abuse presented to the emergency department with chest pain and shortness of breath for two days. His ECG demonstrated sinus bradycardia with borderline criteria for left ventricular hypertrophy and deep T-wave inversions in leads V1–V5 and diffuse T-wave abnormalities in the other leads consistent with myocardial ischemia. Given the Wellen's T waves, bradycardia, and chest pain, the patient was taken for coronary angiography, which demonstrated a severe stenosis in the proximal left anterior descending coronary artery.

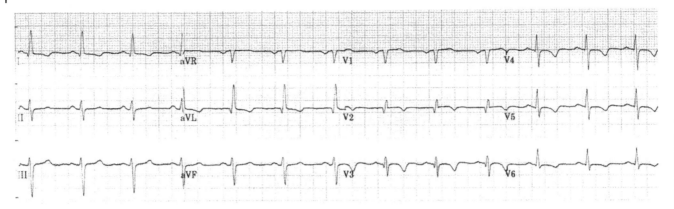

Figure 2.1.14 A 64-year-old female presented with worsening shortness of breath after experiencing what she thought was severe indigestion three days ago. The ECG demonstrates normal sinus rhythm with left anterior fascicular block, anteroseptal Q-waves seen in leads V1–V3, and diffuse anterior and lateral T-wave inversion seen in leads V2–V6 along with I and aVL suggesting recent anterior myocardial infarction. The patient underwent coronary angiography which demonstrated a subtotal occlusion of the proximal left anterior descending coronary artery.

or atrioventricular dissociation with heart block. In the case of complete AV block, ischemia in the basal aspect of the septal wall may lead to AV node dysfunction with a resulting junctional escape rhythm while ischemia in the mid septal wall may result in complete heart block through ischemia in the bundle branches with a resultant ventricular escape rhythm.

Another point of interest is the PQ or PR segment. Atrial infarction is associated with elevation of the PQ segment while PR depression can be associated with acute anterior or inferior MI in a minority of patients. PQ depression is typically associated with acute pericarditis or large myocardial infarction.

U Waves

Characteristically, the presence of inverted or negative U waves in the right precordial leads is suggestive of left anterior descending coronary artery occlusion. This tends to occur in the early stages of myocardial infarction. Furthermore, an increased U-wave amplitude or inversion of the U wave may be associated with significant blood pressure elevation.

Myocardial Ischemia: Causes Other than Acute Coronary Syndrome

The ECG plays a vital role in the identification of myocardial ischemia and may be strongly suggestive of underlying obstructive coronary artery disease. However,

the importance of clinical context cannot be overstressed. Clinicians and healthcare providers frequently encounter situations in which signs of ischemia may be present on the ECG. However, it is important to remember that ischemia results when oxygen demands of the heart outstrip the oxygen supply to the heart. While a patient may have evidence of myocardial necrosis with elevated troponins and ECG concerning for ischemia, this may be the result of severe tachycardia, anemia, left ventricular hypertrophy, decompensated heart failure, or a host of other causes. An example of this can be seen in Figure 2.1.15, in which a patient developed ECG changes of ischemia after prolonged ventricular tachycardia despite only having mild coronary artery disease.

Conclusion

The ECG plays an integral role in the evaluation for myocardial ischemia and it remains critical for all medical professions to have a basic understanding of what changes on the ECG may signal ongoing myocardial ischemia. Correct identification of myocardial ischemia or injury by emergency medical first responders in the field has led to major improvements in door-to-balloon time and led to earlier administration of life-saving medications. Regardless of your role in the medical field, the ability to identify myocardial ischemia on the ECG may make a major difference in the outcomes of your patients. Throughout the remainder of this section, we will apply the basics learned in this chapter to more specific aspects of ECG interpretation of myocardial ischemia.

(a)

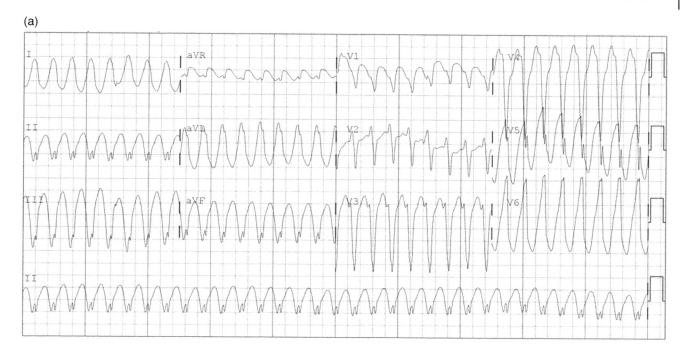

(b)

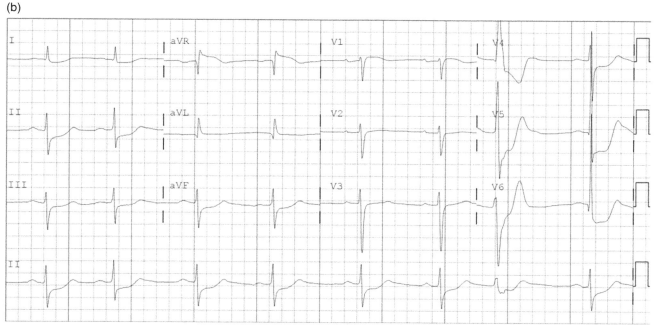

Figure 2.1.15 A 66-year-old male with history of mitral valve prolapse presented after one hour of acute onset of palpitations, lightheadedness, and shortness of breath and was found to be tachycardic and hypotensive. His ECG on presentation demonstrated a heart rate of 220 beats per minutes with wide complex tachycardia consistent with monomorphic ventricular tachycardia. Following electrical cardioversion, his ECG demonstrated sinus bradycardia, a fusion beat seen in V4–V6, and diffuse and deep ST-segment depression with ST-segment elevation in aVR, raising concern for left main coronary artery disease. However, coronary angiography only demonstrated a mild 50% stenosis in the left anterior descending (LAD). The fourth generation cardiac troponin I peaked at 17 mg/dl, revealing how ventricular tachycardia for a long duration can induce significant myocardial ischemia through demand mismatch.

References

1 Tamargo, J., Caballero, R., Gomez, R. et al. (2004). Pharmacology of cardiac potassium channels. *Cardiovasc. Res.* 62: 9–33.

2 Amin, A.S., Tan, H.L., and Wilde, A.A. (2010). Cardiac ion channels in health and disease. *Heart Rhythm* 7: 117–126.

3 Bogdanov, K.Y., Vinogradova, T.M., and Lakatta, E.G. (2001). Sinoatrial nodal cell ryanodine receptor and Na(+)-Ca(2+) exchanger: molecular partners in pacemaker regulation. *Circ. Res.* 88: 1254–1258.

4 Essen, R., Merx, W., and Effert, S. (1979). Spontaneous course of ST-segment elevation in acute anterior myocardial infarction. *Circulation* 59: 105–112.

5 Madias, J.E., Attari, M., and Bravidis, D. (2001). Giant R-waves in a patient with an acute inferior myocardial infarction. *J. Electrocardiol.* 34: 173–177.

6 Zehender, M., Utzolino, S., Furtwangler, A. et al. (1991). Just H. time course and interrelation of reperfusion-induced ST changes and ventricular arrhythmias in acute myocardial infarction. *Am. J. Cardiol.* 68: 1138–1142.

7 Kleber, A.G., Janse, M.J., van Capelle, F.J., and Durrer, D. (1978). Mechanism and time course of S-T and T-Q segment changes during acute regional myocardial ischemia in the pig heart determined by extracellular and intracellular recordings. *Circ. Res.* 42: 603–613.

2

Ischemic Electrocardiographic Changes and Correlation with Regions of the Myocardium

Thibault Lhermusier[1] and Michael J. Lipinski[2]

[1] *Division of Cardiology, Centre Hospitalo Universitaire de Toulouse Rangueil, Toulouse, France*
[2] *Cardiovascular Associates of Charlottesville, Charlottesville, VA, USA*

Introduction

The electrocardiogram (ECG) remains the single most important tool for the assessment of myocardial ischemia in patients with chest pain. As the presence of dynamic and sometimes very subtle changes in the ECG can have a profound impact on clinical management of patients, it is critical that healthcare providers be able to recognize electrocardiographic signs of ischemia. The ability to promptly identify signs of myocardial ischemia on the ECG can help initiate early life-saving therapy. As we discussed in the previous chapter, the presence of myocardial ischemia can lead to characteristic changes in the electrocardiographic waveform. While these changes may be important in differentiating between ischemia and myocardial injury, the ability to recognize which region of the myocardium is ischemic and identify the corresponding coronary territory can also impact patient care. For example, ischemia corresponding with certain coronary territories may change whether a patient should be given certain medications such as nitrates or anti-platelet therapy like thienopyridines. While exhaustive knowledge of coronary anatomy is not necessary, healthcare providers should understand some fundamental basics to help identify which electrocardiographic findings correlate with certain vascular territories. Table 2.2.1 summarizes the relationships between ECG territories and the different segments of the myocardium.

Coronary Anatomy

Though there are coronary anomalies in a small minority of patients, the anterior, lateral, and much of the septal walls of the left ventricle (LV) are supplied with blood from the left main coronary artery (LM), which arises from the left coronary sinus of the ascending aorta. The left main coronary artery typically bifurcates into the left anterior descending (LAD) artery and the left circumflex (LCX) artery. In approximately 30% of individuals, the LM trifurcates into the LAD, LCX, and ramus intermedius artery. The LAD supplies the anterior wall, anteroseptal wall via septal branches, some of the anterolateral wall via the diagonal branches, and the apex of the LV. Anteroseptal and anterior MIs are nearly always caused by occlusion of the LAD coronary artery, which is also often responsible for apical infarction and sometimes lateral infarction. The LCX supplies the posterolateral walls and the obtuse marginal branches of the LCX supply the lateral and some of the anterolateral wall of the LV. Occlusion of this artery causes posterior and lateral infarctions. When the LCX artery is dominant, it gives the posterior descending artery. Its occlusion can result in large inferoposterior and posterolateral infarctions. The right coronary artery (RCA) typically arises from the right coronary cusp and provides blood to the right ventricle (RV), inferior and posterior walls of the LV along with the inferior septum. Occlusion of the RCA causes inferior, posterior, inferoposterior, inferolateral, and RV MI. The RCA also frequently gives rise to the atrioventricular (AV) nodal

Electrocardiogram in Clinical Medicine, First Edition. Edited by William J. Brady, Michael J. Lipinski, Andrew E. Darby, Michael C. Bond, Nathan P. Charlton, Korin Hudson, and Kelly Williamson.

artery while the left bundle branches are often supplied via septal branches of the LAD. Thus, the conduction system of the heart is largely supplied by these two arteries. The posterior descending artery is supplied by the RCA in approximately 85% of individuals (right dominant), LCX in 10% of individuals (left dominant), and by both the LCX and RCA in 5% of individuals (co-dominant). The typical coronary artery distribution is shown in Figure 2.2.1. Throughout this chapter, we will also refer to specific electrocardiographic regions that correlate with the myocardium. The leads that correspond with particular regions of the myocardium can be found in Table 2.2.1.

Table 2.2.1 Relation between myocardial walls territories and ECG leads.

Cardiac Segment	ECG Leads
Anteroseptal	V1–V3
Apical	V4
Inferior	II, III, aVF
High lateral	I, aVL
Low lateral	V5, V6
Posterior	V7, V8, V9
Right ventricle	V1, V3R, and V4R

Definitions of STEMI and Non-ST Elevation ACS

The term *acute coronary syndrome* (ACS) refers to any group of clinical symptoms compatible with acute myocardial ischemia and includes unstable angina (UA), non ST-segment elevation myocardial infarction (NSTEMI), and ST-segment elevation myocardial infarction (STEMI). The terms *transmural, nontransmural, Q wave MI,* and *non-Q wave MI* were historically used to describe STEMI but are no longer recommended. The symptoms of UA/NSTEMI and STEMI are similar, and differentiating the

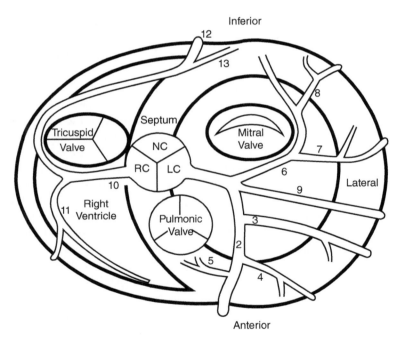

Figure 2.2.1 The included illustration shows the typical coronary anatomy from a coronal superior view of the heart demonstrating the regions of the myocardium supplied by the different coronary arteries. The figure shows the mitral valve, tricuspid valve, pulmonary valve, and aortic valve, which is divided in the noncoronary cusp (NC), left cusp, and right cusp. The aortic wall overlies the septal myocardial wall which separates the right and left ventricle. The inferior wall is at the top of the picture, the anterior wall at the bottom and the lateral wall to the right. The left cusp typically gives rise to the left main coronary artery [1], which then typically bifurcates into the left anterior descending (LAD) coronary artery [2] and the left circumflex (LCX) artery [3], but may also give rise to a ramus intermedius artery [4]. Diagonals branches [5, 6] of the LAD supply the lateral wall, the septal branches [7] of the LAD supply the septal wall, and the LAD supplies the anterior wall of the left ventricle. The obtuse marginal branches of the LCX also supply the lateral wall [8, 9] and the circumflex can occasionally supply the posterior or inferior lateral wall if a dominant vessel. The right coronary artery (RCA) [10] typically arises from the right aortic cusp and gives rise to the right marginal branch [11] that supplies the right ventricle. The RCA may then course to the inferior wall and divide into the right posterior descending artery [12] if the RCA is a dominant vessel and the posterior lateral branch [13] of the RCA.

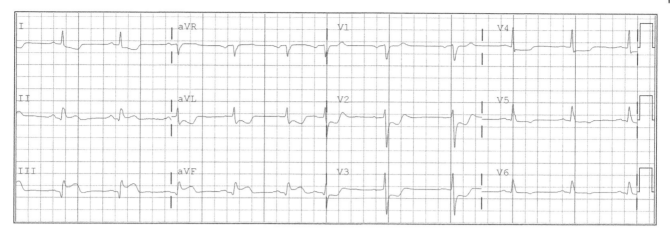

Figure 2.2.2 A 67-year-old male with known coronary artery disease with prior coronary artery bypass surgery, hypertension, and hyperlipidemia presents to the emergency department with three hours of chest pain. His ECG demonstrated normal sinus rhythm with inferior Q waves and inferior ST-segment elevation with reciprocal ST-segment depression consistent with an inferoposterior ST-segment elevation myocardial infarction. Emergent coronary angiography demonstrated severe native disease with an occluded proximal left anterior descending artery, a 99% subtotal occlusion of a large left circumflex coronary artery providing a posterior lateral branch, and an occluded right coronary artery. The left internal mammary artery to the mid-left anterior descending coronary artery was widely patent and provided collaterals to the right posterior descending coronary artery. The saphenous vein graft to the right coronary artery was totally occluded at the aorta and the saphenous vein graft to the obtuse marginal artery of the left circumflex was also occluded. Given the presence of established collaterals to the right posterior descending artery, the left circumflex system was considered the infarct related artery. While it remains unclear whether the ST elevation myocardial infarction was due to acute closure of the saphenous vein graft or progression of the left circumflex lesion, the native left circumflex lesion underwent percutaneous coronary intervention with stenting, and the ST-segment elevation and pain resolved.

two requires only clinical evaluation and ECG. Importantly, management of non ST elevation ACS and STEMI differ considerably regarding timing of revascularization and antithrombotic regimen. STEMI most commonly occurs when thrombus formation results in complete occlusion of a major epicardial coronary vessel. This form of ACS is a life-threatening, time-sensitive emergency that must be diagnosed and treated promptly via coronary revascularization by percutaneous coronary intervention or thrombolytic therapy. Unlike UA and NSTEMI, during STEMI the 12-lead ECG will show significant ST elevation (STE), as the name implies. ST elevation in the absence of left ventricular (LV) hypertrophy or left bundle branch block (LBBB) is defined by the European Society of Cardiology/ACCF/AHA/World Heart Federation Task Force for the Universal Definition of Myocardial Infarction as new STE at the J point in at least two contiguous leads of ≥2 mm (0.2 mV) in men or ≥1.5 mm (0.15 mV) in women in leads V2–V3 and/or of ≥1 mm (0.1 mV) in other contiguous chest leads or the limb leads [1]. The majority of patients will evolve ECG evidence of Q-wave infarction. New or presumably new LBBB has been considered a STEMI equivalent. The correlation between the site of coronary occlusion and the localization of the MI is generally good. However, in the presence of chronic coronary artery disease, particularly in patients with history of revascularization, the ECG at rest may not have significant anomalies. In fact the ECG is frequently normal in patients with complete obstruction of one or more coronary arteries due to the presence of a collateral circulation. As seen in Figure 2.2.2, the identification of the culprit lesion can be challenging in these patients during an ACS.

Left Main Coronary Ischemia

As the LM coronary artery supplies approximately 65–70% of myocardial blood supply, recognition of electrocardiographic changes consistent with LM ischemia is critical. LM ischemia typically presents with diffuse ST-segment depression and ST-segment elevation in lead AVR. These electrocardiographic findings are rarely isolated and often are accompanied by hypotension and symptoms of ischemia including chest discomfort and shortness of breath. While these electrocardiographic changes are most commonly associated with an atherosclerotic lesions of the LM coronary artery, it is important to recognize this pattern can be seen in other scenarios. LM ischemia can arise in the setting of aortic dissection if the dissection propagates into the LM coronary artery. An example of this can be seen in Figure 2.2.3 and is typically catastrophic for patients. Another clinical scenario where recognition of this pattern is essential is referral of young individuals for exercise stress testing following chest pain or syncope.

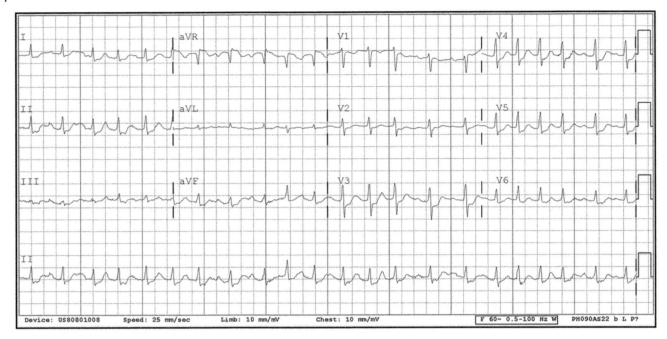

Figure 2.2.3 A 64-year-old male with past medical history of hypertension and hypercholesterolemia presented to the emergency department with excruciating chest pain and shortness of breath for two hours duration. He had tachycardia with significant hypotension (70s/30s) on presentation and soon after developed respiratory distress requiring emergent intubation and vasopressors. His ECG prior to intubation is shown below and demonstrates sinus tachycardia with frequent premature atrial complexes and diffuse ST-segment depression with ST-segment elevation in lead aVR, which raised significant concern for left main occlusion given his clinical presentation. The patient was taken emergently to the cardiac catheterization lab and coronary angiography demonstrated total occlusion of the left main coronary artery with a blunt stump and a large patent right coronary artery with no collateral blood flow to the left system. The left main artery could not be wired successfully and aortography demonstrated aortic dissection with propagation into the left cusp, which occluded the left main artery. The patient went into cardiac arrest during the procedure and did not survive.

LM ischemic pattern may develop during exercise in individuals with an anomalous LM coronary artery that arises from the right coronary cusp and courses between the aorta and pulmonary artery. As cardiac output increases, the aorta and pulmonary artery may compress the LM coronary artery and induce ischemia in these individuals, which increases the risk of sudden cardiac death and may require referral for coronary artery bypass surgery.

wrapped around the apex can be recognized by the presence of ST segment elevation in the inferior leads as well as the typical ECG modifications in the anterior leads [6, 7] (Figures 2.2.5 and 2.2.6). It is critical not to mistakenly diagnose pericarditis in these patients due to the diffuse ST-segment elevations. The morphology of ST-segment elevation is typically different in pericarditis and is discussed in a later chapter.

Anterior STEMI

The typical ECG pattern of acute anteroseptal infarction with ST-segment elevation in leads V1−V3 is highly reliable for predicting that the LAD is the infarct related artery with a specificity of 95% and sensitivity of 60–90% [2, 5]. When the ST segment is not only elevated in the anterior precordial leads but also in leads I and aVL, a proximal lesion of the LAD is suspected. The presence of reciprocal ST segment depression in the inferior leads is also suggestive of a proximal lesion. Figure 2.2.4 illustrates ECG changes in an anterior MI. Occlusion of the LAD artery

Wellens Syndrome

This syndrome is an electrocardiographic manifestation of critical proximal LAD coronary artery stenosis in patients with ACS. It is characterized by symmetrical, often deep (>2 mm), T-wave inversions in the anterior precordial leads, as illustrated in Figure 2.2.7. A less common variant is biphasic T-wave inversions in the same leads [3]. The presence of Wellens syndrome carries significant diagnostic and prognostic value. Sensitivity and specificity for significant (≥70%) stenosis of the LAD artery was found to be 69% and 89%, respectively, with a positive predictive value

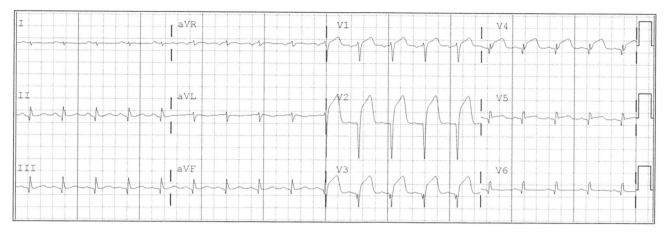

Figure 2.2.4 A 56-year-old male with history of tobacco abuse presents to the emergency department after acute onset of chest pain six hours ago. The ECG demonstrated sinus tachycardia, borderline Q-waves in the inferior leads, Q-waves in V2–V6, and impressive ST-segment elevation in leads V1–V5 consistent with acute anterior ST-segment elevation myocardial infarction. Emergent coronary angiography demonstrated total occlusion of the proximal LAD, which was treated with percutaneous coronary intervention with stenting. The presence of ST-elevation implies myocardial injury but the presence of Q-waves denotes myocardial infarction, consistent with six hours of pain.

of 86%. Again, clinical context is essential as pseudo-Wellens T waves can also occur in patients with intracranial hemorrhage, LV hypertrophy, or in patients following cocaine use. In the case of cocaine and intracranial hemorrhage, the cause of the pseudo-Wellens T waves may be the result of coronary spasm involving the proximal LAD.

Inferior STEMI

Inferior STEMI may be due to RCA or LCX occlusion (and occasionally due to a "wrap around" LAD, with concomitant anterior MI). An example of a classic inferior STEMI can be found in Figure 2.2.8. Predicting the infarct-related artery has some importance. If inferior STEMI is due to RCA occlusion, then the RV may be involved, and a right-sided ECG is indicated. If due to LCX occlusion, the RV is usually not involved. In addition, the interventional cardiologist likes to know which artery is involved before the angiogram, as this may significantly impact the how the procedure is performed.

The same pattern of Q-wave changes appears to result from either myocardial infarction caused by occlusion of a dominant RCA or a dominant LCX, but the pattern of ST segment elevation may be helpful in differentiating which artery is involved. In patients with inferior MI (STE in leads II, III, and aVF), the presence of ST-segment elevation in one or more leads related to the lateral wall (leads I, AVL, V5, and V6) is highly suggestive of LCX occlusion [8].

In practice, three criteria are highly correlated with LCX occlusion: absence of reciprocal ST depression (STD) in lead I, STE in leads V5 and V6, and ST elevation in lead II

is at least as high as that in lead III. RCA occlusion usually has reciprocal STD in lead I and STE is higher in lead III than in lead II. The combination of lead III having greater STE than lead II and STE in V1 is very suggestive of RCA occlusion [4, 9]. Identification of the culprit artery in the setting of inferior MI is highlighted in Figure 2.2.9.

Right Ventricular Infarction

RV infarction is rarely isolated and often associated with inferior MI. In nearly all cases, RV infarction is associated with proximal occlusion of the RCA. The best leads for RV infarction diagnosis are leads V3R and V4R, with an STE cutoff of 0.5 mm at the J-point, except for males under age 30, for whom a cutoff of 1 mm is more accurate. In inferior STEMI, V1 should be scrutinized for any STE and RV MI should be highly suspected if there is STE, especially if there is posterior injury. Indeed. when there is RV MI, there is usually some STE in lead V1 that prompts recording of a right sided ECG. It is recommended to record a right-sided ECG, as leads V3R and V4R have the best sensitivity and specificity for RV MI. ECG criteria for RV MI and its clinical impact has previously been reviewed in detail [10]. An example of isolated RV infarct with prominent R waves in V1 and V2 can be seen in Figure 2.2.10. In addition to RV or posterior MI, prominent R waves in V1 and V2 can also be seen with right bundle branch block (RBBB), right ventricular hypertrophy, right-sided strain (seen with large pulmonary embolism), Wolff-Parkinson-White syndrome, dextrocardia (heart on the right side of the chest), lead misplacement, normal variant, and Duchenne's muscular dystrophy [11].

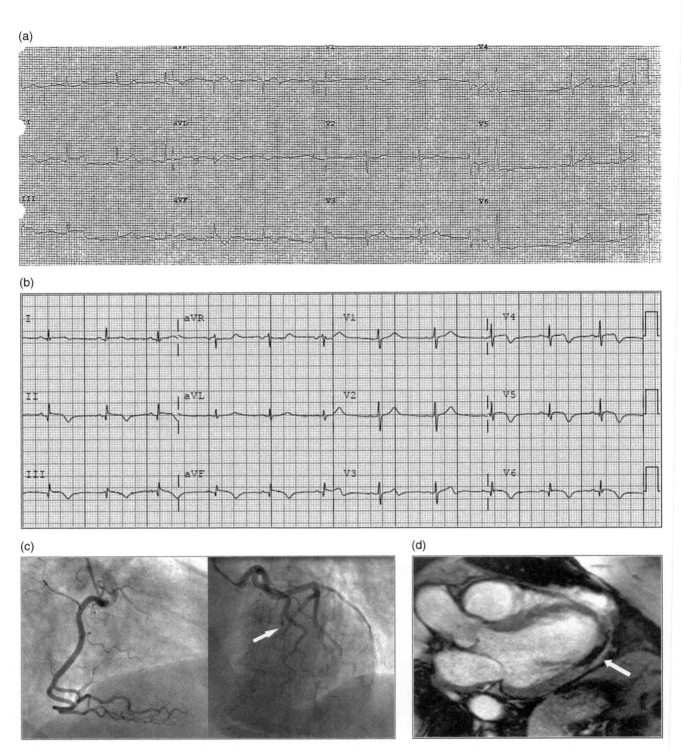

Figure 2.2.5 A 57-year-old female with no significant cardiovascular risk factors presented with two hours of sharp left-sided chest pain and shortness of breath. The initial electrocardiogram (a) demonstrated normal sinus rhythm with a premature ventricular contraction with compensatory pause with ST elevations in the inferior (II, III, and aVF) and anterolateral leads (V4–V6) with reciprocal ST depression in Leads I, aVL, V1, and V2 suggesting ST elevation myocardial infarction. The patient was taken emergently for coronary angiography but an infarct-related artery could not be identified and it was felt that the patient had pericarditis. However, the cardiac troponins continued to rise significantly to 60 mg/dL. The patient was transferred to a tertiary care facility and repeat electrocardiogram (b) demonstrated changes consistent with evolving myocardial infarction with T wave inversions in II, III, aVF, and V3–V6 raising suspicion for an acute myocardial infarction involving the anterior and inferior territory, which could be explained by a "wrap-around" left anterior descending coronary artery that courses around the apex and supplies a portion of the inferior wall. The patient underwent repeat coronary angiography three days after her initial presentation which demonstrated a patent right coronary artery and occlusion of the mid left anterior descending coronary artery (arrow) seen in the shallow left cranial orientation, which was missed during the initial angiography due to overlap with the nearby diagonal artery (c). Cardiac magnetic resonance imaging with delayed gadolinium enhancement (d) demonstrated an area of gadolinium retention in the apical inferior wall consistent with myocardial infarction (arrow) with a region of microvascular obstruction lacking gadolinium uptake with a resultant black or dark region in the myocardium. This case demonstrates the importance of utilizing the ECG to identify the likely myocardial wall experiencing injury and then taking multiple images during coronary angiography to help identify the infarct-related artery that may be missed if angiography is rushed.

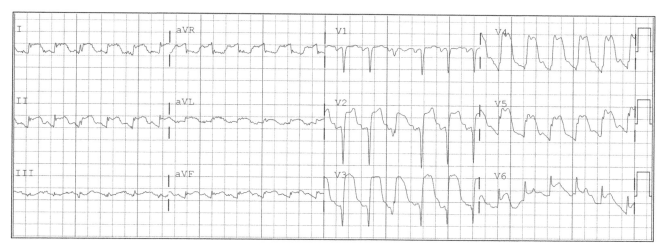

Figure 2.2.6 A 55-year-old male with no significant past medical history presents with crushing chest pressure, respiratory distress, tachycardia, and hypotension that progressively worsened over a seven-hour period. His ECG shows sinus tachycardia with a premature ventricular complex with Q waves in leads V1–V4 and what may also be Q waves in the inferior leads with profound ST-segment elevation in all leads except V1 with reciprocal changes in aVR. Emergent coronary angiography demonstrated an occluded ostial left anterior descending coronary artery, which when opened with stenting revealed a large wrap-around vessel that supplied much of the inferior wall. Left ventriculography demonstrated severely reduced left ventricular systolic function with a left ventricular ejection fraction of 15–20% and akinesis of the anterior, anteroseptal, apical, and inferoapical walls. Given persistent cardiogenic shock, the patient eventually required surgical placement of a left ventricular assist device.

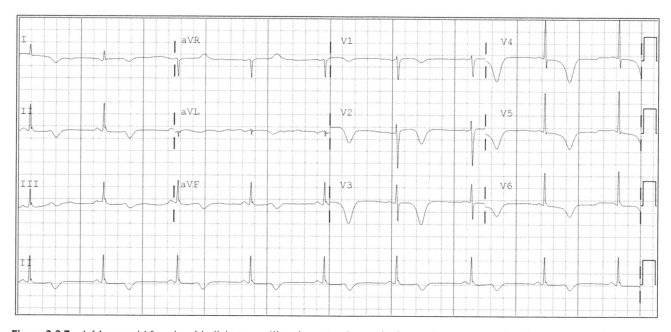

Figure 2.2.7 A 64-year-old female with diabetes mellitus, hypertension, and tobacco abuse presented to the emergency department with chest pain and developed acute respiratory distress requiring emergent intubation. Her ECG shown below demonstrated normal sinus rhythm with diffuse T-wave inversion with deep T-wave inversion in leads V2–V6 consistent with Wellens T waves. The patient underwent urgent coronary angiography after stabilization and a hazy 95% stenosis was present in the proximal LAD consistent with acute plaque rupture with thrombus.

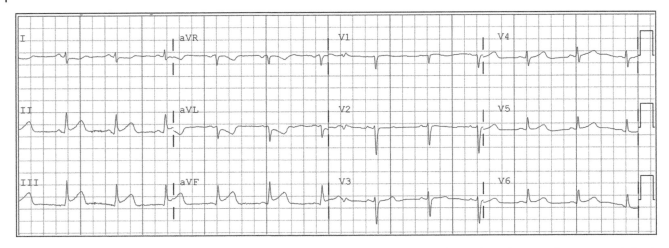

Figure 2.2.8 A 72-year-old female with hypertension, prior tobacco abuse, and chronic obstructive pulmonary disease was admitted with community acquired pneumonia and while in the hospital developed acute onset of chest pain. Her ECG demonstrated normal sinus rhythm with borderline right axis deviation with ST-segment elevation in leads II, III, aVF, V5, and V6 consistent with acute myocardial injury pattern. The lack of Q waves suggests there is not yet ECG evidence of myocardial infarction. The patient was taken for emergent coronary angiography and found to have subtotal occlusion of the right coronary artery.

RV MI usually occurs with RCA occlusion, as the RV marginal branches are coming from the RCA. As 85% of inferior STEMI are due to RCA occlusion (the rest is due to occlusion of a "dominant" circumflex), one must always consider RV MI in inferior MI. Right ventricular infarct is associated with right sided heart failure, hypotension, higher mortality, and particular sensitivity to the hypotensive effects of nitroglycerine because the ischemic RV needs higher filling pressures to maintain cardiac output. Fluids are often necessary to maintain blood pressure.

It should be suspected in the presence of reciprocal ST depression in leads II, III, aVF. In fact, this ST depression is usually the most obvious finding on the ECG because ST elevation in aVL is rarely pronounced and does not meet the actual definition of 1 mm STE for STEMI (because the QRS voltage in aVL is usually very low and ST voltage cannot exceed QRS voltage). Importantly, assuming STD in leads III and aVF is reciprocal to high lateral STE, these patients should be managed as a STEMI equivalent.

Lateral STEMI

Isolated lateral STEMI are usually due to diagonal or circumflex branch occlusions. Only about 50% of lateral MI due to coronary occlusion have significant STE, and for this reason the lateral wall is often called *electrocardiographically silent*. This is due to low QRS voltage in lateral leads, and because ST elevation is always proportional to the QRS, the STE is low voltage. In one study, 56% of patients with the LCX as the infarct-related artery had a non-diagnostic ECG [5]. However, over 95% of patients with isolated LCX occlusion have signs of ischemia on ECG [12]. The presence of ST-segment elevation in lead aVL is highly suggestive of a severe lesion in the proximal LCX [13]. An example ECG of isolated LCX artery occlusion can be seen in Figure 2.2.11. Isolated high lateral STEMI can be difficult to detect as the presence of ST elevation isolated only to leads I and aVL is very uncommon.

Posterior STEMI

ST elevation is not a perfect surrogate for complete acute persistent occlusion of an epicardial coronary artery without collateral circulation. It is neither fully sensitive nor specific. Posterior STEMI is the perfect illustration that even though the patient's ECG does not meet criteria for STEMI, he can have all the pathology of a STEMI. Most posterior STEMI are associated with either inferior STEMI, lateral STEMI, or both. A classic example of an inferoposterior STEMI due to acute occlusion of the LCX artery can be found in Figure 2.2.12. Only 3–11% of all MI are isolated posterior. In this specific case, there is possibly no ST elevation on the ECG and LCX occlusion may be subtle or invisible on the ECG. Marked isolated ST depression and tall R waves in the right precordial leads (V1–V3) in a clinical scenario consistent with STEMI is usually posterior STEMI. An example of posterior STEMI presenting with ST

(a)

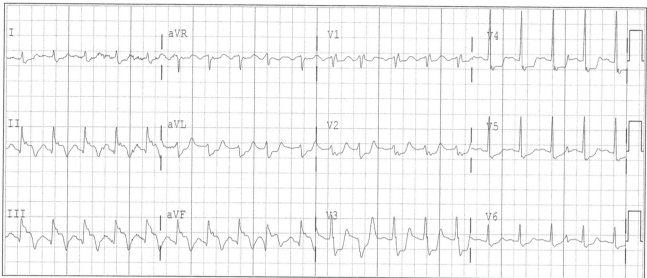

(b)

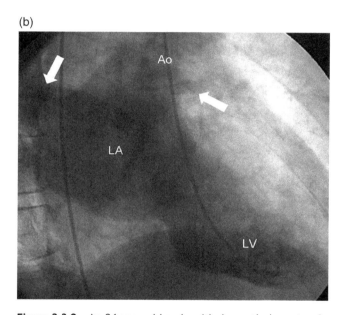

Figure 2.2.9 An 84-year-old male with dementia, hypertension, and hypercholesterolemia developed sudden onset of shortness of breath and hypotension. ECG in the emergency department demonstrated sinus tachycardia, incomplete RBBB with RSR' in V1 with ST-segment elevation in leads II, III, and aVF with significant ST-segment depression throughout all other leads. While the ECG is concerning for inferoposterior ST elevation myocardial infarction with cardiogenic shock, the diffuse ST depression was very worrisome for profound ischemia. Importantly, exam demonstrated a short blowing systolic murmur at the apex and bilateral crackles in all lung fields. The patient was taken for emergent coronary angiography, which demonstrated a chronic total occlusion of the mid-left circumflex artery and total occlusion of the mid-right coronary artery. The LCX was deemed to be a chronic occlusion given the presence of collaterals to the occluded LCX via the proximal obtuse marginal artery. However, the left ventriculography was performed, given the severity of the presentation and revealed severe mitral regurgitation with complete opacification of the left atrium (LA) and pulmonary veins (arrows) rather than complete filling of the left ventricle (LV) and aorta (Ao). An intraaortic balloon pump was placed and echocardiography demonstrated a ruptured papillary muscle, confirming the diagnosis. Given the grim prognosis and underlying dementia, comfort measures were instituted and the patient died shortly thereafter.

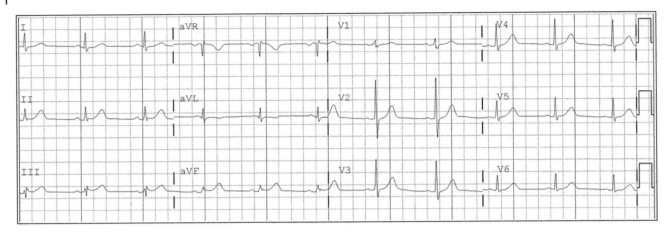

Figure 2.2.10 A 69-year-old male with hypertension presented with chest discomfort for eight hours duration. An ECG in the emergency department demonstrated normal sinus rhythm with minimal ST-segment elevation in leads III and aVF and a prominent or tall R wave in leads V1 and V2. While the minimal ST elevation raises concern for ischemia but does not meet criteria for ST-segment elevation myocardial infarction, the tall R waves in leads V1 and V2 are consistent with right ventricular infarction. The patient received sublingual nitroglycerin and developed severe hypotension requiring rapid administration of intravenous fluids. Interestingly, the patient was taken for coronary angiography demonstrated a 90% high-grade stenosis in the mid-right coronary with subtotal occlusion of a large right ventricular marginal branch.

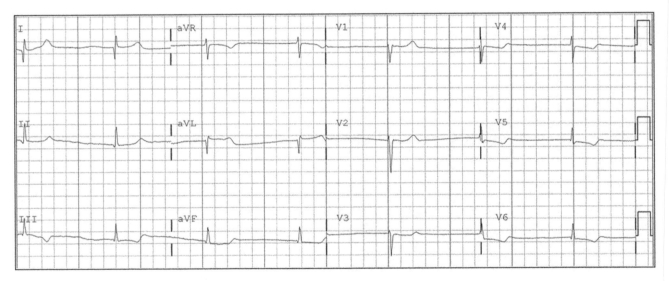

Figure 2.2.11 A 62-year-old male with hypertension, hyperlipidemia, and ongoing tobacco abuse presents to the emergency department with one day of chest discomfort and indigestion. His initial electrocardiogram shown below demonstrates bradycardia with a junctional escape rhythm, poor R-wave progression in the anterior precordial leads, lateral Q waves in leads I and aVL with borderline ST elevation especially in aVL, along with nonspecific ST depression and T-wave abnormalities in leads V3–V6, III, and aVF. Given the symptoms of chest pain and ECG findings concerning for a lateral myocardial infarction, the patient was taken urgently for coronary angiography, which demonstrated a proximal occlusion of the left circumflex artery which was treated with percutaneous coronary intervention and stenting. The left circumflex artery can frequently provide nonspecific ischemic changes or borderline ECG changes for ST elevation myocardial infarction and clinical suspicion, and cardiac biomarkers can often help guide decisions on whether to proceed with cardiac catheterization.

depression in leads V1–V3 can be seen in Figure 2.2.13. Three modalities can help to confirm the diagnosis before sending the patient for coronary revascularization: repeating the ECG within 30 minutes looking for dynamic changes, recording posterior leads (V7–V9), and echocardiography looking for posterior wall motion abnormality.

Conduction Abnormalities in the Setting of Ischemia

Atrioventricular blocks can complicate the course of MI. AV block can result from ischemia in separate locations and can significantly impact prognosis and treatment. An

(a)

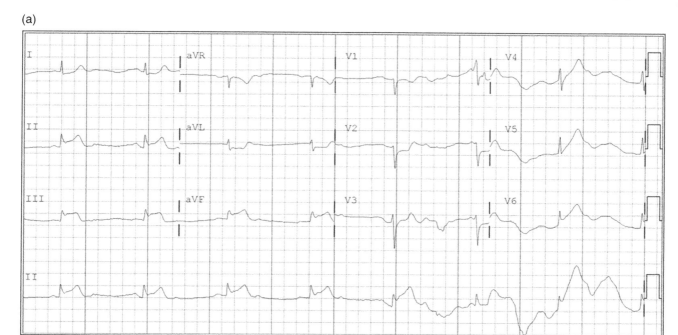

(b)

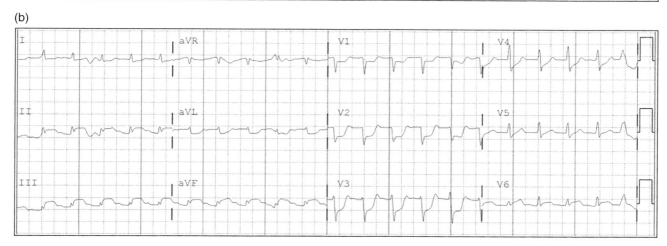

Figure 2.2.12 A 48-year-old female with longstanding diabetes mellitus, hypertension, hyperlipidemia, obesity, and tobacco abuse presents with chest pain, syncope, and cardiogenic shock. Her initial ECG (a) demonstrated sinus rhythm with 2 : 1 atrioventricular block with inferior ST-segment elevation in leads II, III, and aVF with reciprocal ST depression in V2, I, and aVL consistent with acute inferior myocardial injury pattern. The patient was taken for emergent coronary angiography and was found to have a proximally occluded dominant left circumflex artery, which was treated with percutaneous coronary intervention with stenting. Following stent placement, the patient had no reflow in the circumflex artery, which did not resolve despite multiple injections of vasodilator agents and administration of antithrombotic agents. No coronary reflow following coronary stenting is consistent with microvascular obstruction from downstream embolization of thrombus. Her ECG after PCI (b) demonstrated tachycardia with persistent ST elevation, which is associated with a poor prognosis. She remained in cardiogenic shock requiring intraaortic balloon pump and pressors and developed a myocardial-free wall rupture five days after presentation and passed away.

intranodal block is due to increase vagal tone or direct ischemia of the AV node and occurs in case of occlusion of the RCA, particularly in inferior MI. This can result in decreased blood flow to the AV node when the origin of the AV nodal artery is distal or downstream from the occlusion in the RCA. A classic example of complete AV block in the setting of inferoposterior MI can be seen in Figure 2.2.14.

The ECG usually shows incomplete block (first-degree or second-degree Mobitz Type II) or a complete block with AV dissociation (third degree) and a narrow QRS complex as there is a junctional rhythm arising from the bundle of His.

This intranodal block is usually sensitive to atropine and temporary, improving almost immediately with revascularization. The His bundle is supplied by both the AV node

(a)

(b)

(c)

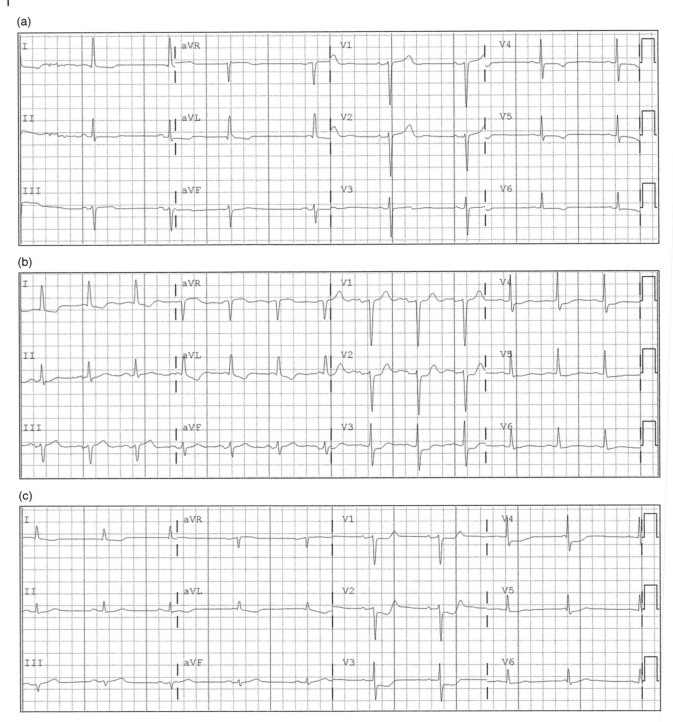

Figure 2.2.13 A 58-year-old female with longstanding diabetes mellitus, hyperlipidemia, chronic obstructive pulmonary disease, and tobacco abuse presented with shortness of breath and chest discomfort and was admitted to the hospital. The ECG on admission (a) demonstrated sinus bradycardia with a premature atrial complex and nonspecific ST-segment and T-wave changes. While in the hospital, she develops severe shortness of breath and a repeat ECG (b) revealed sinus rhythm with ST-segment depression in leads V2–V4 and deepening of ST depression and T wave inversion in I and aVL. In this context, the ECG is concerning for acute posterior myocardial infarction but was thought to represent an exacerbation of chronic obstructive pulmonary disease with ischemic or nonspecific changes on ECG related to acute respiratory failure. Over the next five hours, her symptoms progressed and required bilevel positive pressure ventilation. A repeat ECG (c) demonstrated more prominent ischemic changes and the posterior myocardial infarction was recognized. The patient underwent emergent coronary angiography which demonstrated an occluded left circumflex artery.

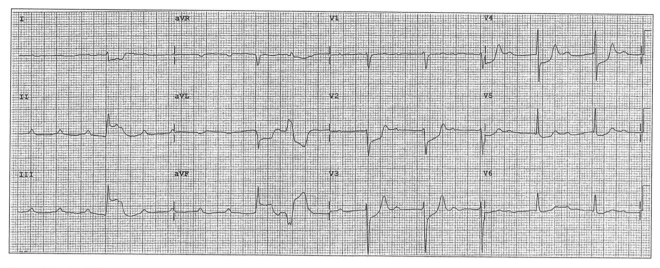

Figure 2.2.14 A 75-year-old male with hypertension presented with acute onset of chest pain, nausea, and vomiting. In route to the emergency department, the patient received sublingual nitroglycerin and developed profound hypotension requiring intravenous fluids. The ECG upon presentation demonstrated sinus atrial tachycardia with third degree atrioventricular block and a junctional escape rhythm with a ventricular escape beat and significant ST-segment elevation in leads II, III, and aVF with reciprocal ST-segment depression in V2–V5, I, and aVL consistent with acute inferoposterior myocardial injury. Emergent coronary angiography revealed an occluded proximal right coronary artery, which was opened with coronary stenting with return to normal sinus rhythm. However, the patient remained in cardiogenic shock requiring aggressive intravenous fluid administration and an echocardiogram demonstrated severe right ventricular dysfunction. Right ventricular infarction in the setting of inferoposterior myocardial infarction is an important clinical entity to recognize as nitroglycerin should be avoided as peripheral venodilation can result in a severe drop in cardiac output and aggressive intravascular fluid administration may be necessary for maintenance of blood pressure. Heart block may also result with occlusion of the right coronary artery as the atrioventricular branch typically arises from the right coronary artery.

artery from the RCA and first septal perforator branch of the LAD in 90% of patients and from the AV nodal artery of the RCA alone in 10% of patients [5]. An infranodal block is due to ischemia of His bundle or its branches in the case of occlusion of the LAD, during an anterior MI. An incomplete block is observed (isolated left anterior fascicular block, RBBB, LBBB, left posterior fascicular block, or associated with first- or second-degree AV block) or a complete block with large QRS complex. This block is not sensitive to atropine or isoproterenol and is associated with poor short-term prognosis. Temporary pacemaker or transcutaneous pacemaker should be considered emergently. Finally, occlusion of the sinoatrial artery can occur in the setting of very proximal or ostial RCA occlusion and result in loss of the P wave. This may lead to the development of a junctional escape rhythm with heart rate typically around 40–45 bpm. However, this most typically occurs in the setting of percutaneous coronary intervention when a coronary stent occludes the sinoatrial artery when treating an ostial or proximal lesion in the RCA.

Aneurysm of the Left Ventricle

A ventricular aneurysm is defined by a segmental dilatation of the LV generally due to a transmural myocardial infarction. Aneurysms may be responsible for heart failure,

peripheral embolism, ventricular arrhythmias, and ventricular rupture.

Persistent ST elevation on the ECG more than three weeks after the index event is diagnostic of LV aneurysm. The ST-segment elevation is stable over time and there are typically Q waves present. Interestingly, the extent or amplitude of ST elevation is not proportional to the size of the aneurysm. Notably, T waves have low amplitude or are even reversed in the infarct territory.

ECG in Pharmacological and Mechanical Reperfusion

The ECG can be considered as the most useful tool to identify epicardial reperfusion. Resolution of ST-segment elevation of more than 70% of the initial value at 60–90 minutes after the initiation of thrombolytic therapy is a strong predictor of successful myocardial reperfusion and is therefore associated with enhanced recovery of LV function, reduced infarct size, and improved prognosis [14]. It has to be remembered that ST-segment changes integrate both epicardial and myocardial reperfusion. Thus, patients with complete ST-resolution at 90 minutes after fibrinolysis have a 90% probability of a patent infarct-related artery associated with a successful reperfusion at the microvascular level.

However, many patients with no ST-segment resolution after fibrinolysis or primary percutaneous coronary intervention still show a patent epicardial infarct artery. In fact, in these patients the lack of ST resolution is caused by the failure of reperfusion at the level of microvasculature rather than at the epicardial vessel as illustrated in Figure 2.2.12. Thus, while ST resolution represents a powerful predictor of infarct-related artery patency, it is less accurate at predicting the persistence of epicardial vessel occlusion after reperfusion.

Therefore, in order to judge the need for adjunctive mechanical reopening of the infarct-related artery after failed fibrinolysis, by means of *rescue angioplasty*, it is important to integrate clinical and ECG data. It is reasonable to monitor the pattern of ST-segment elevation, cardiac rhythm, and clinical symptoms during the 60–90 minutes after the initiation of fibrinolytic therapy. Noninvasive findings suggesting successful reperfusion include relief of symptoms, maintenance, or restoration of hemodynamic and electrical stability, and a reduction of at least 50% in the initial ST-segment elevation. In this scenario, the presence of particular arrhythmias, such as not rapid ventricular tachycardia, idioventricular rhythm, or nonsustained bradycardia, early after fibrinolytic administration, represent highly specific markers of reperfusion. Otherwise, persistence of ischemic chest pain, absence of resolution of the qualifying ST-segment elevation, and hemodynamic or electrical instability are generally predictors of failed pharmacological reperfusion, necessitating rescue angioplasty.

Conclusion

Changes due to myocardial ischemia on the ECG can help medical providers identify the culprit artery and involved myocardial territory. In the case of the interventional cardiologist, this information is very important as it may guide the approach taken during coronary angiography and determine whether the operator quickly assesses the non-culprit vessel prior to treating the infarct-related artery. It may also help determine which medications should be utilized prior to coronary angiography. For example, in patients with inferior STEMI, especially those with reciprocal changes in V1−V3 consistent with inferoposterior MI, we avoid nitrates prior to entering the cardiac cath lab given concern for RV involvement as this may lead to severe hypotension. Additionally, avoidance of beta-blockade in these patients unless tachycardic may be prudent as AV nodal blockade may precipitate heart block. In the case of STEMI, the emphasis should be on minimizing door to balloon time as time is muscle. Through understanding subtle changes in the ECG, one can often identify the infarct-related artery prior to coronary angiography and therefore plan accordingly.

References

1 Thygesen, K., Alpert, J.S., Jaffe, A.S. et al. (2012). Third universal definition of myocardial infarction. *J. Am. Coll. Cardiol.* 60: 1581–1598.

2 Taglieri, N., Saia, F., Alessi, L. et al. (2014). Diagnostic performance of standard electrocardiogram for prediction of infarct related artery and site of coronary occlusion in unselected STEMI patients undergoing primary percutaneous coronary intervention. *Eur. Heart J. Acute Cardiovasc. Care* 3 (4): 326–339.

3 de Zwaan, C., Bar, F.W., and Wellens, H.J. (1982). Characteristic electrocardiographic pattern indicating a critical stenosis high in left anterior descending coronary artery in patients admitted because of impending myocardial infarction. *Am. Heart J.* 103: 730–736.

4 Herz, I., Assali, A.R., Adler, Y. et al. (1997). New electrocardiographic criteria for predicting either the right or left circumflex artery as the culprit coronary artery in inferior wall acute myocardial infarction. *Am. J. Cardiol.* 80: 1343–1345.

5 Frink, R.J. and James, T.N. (1973). Normal blood supply to the human His bundle and proximal bundle branches. *Circulation* 47: 8–18.

6 Sapin, P.M., Musselman, D.R., Dehmer, G.J., and Cascio, W.E. (1992). Implications of inferior ST-segment elevation accompanying anterior wall acute myocardial infarction for the angiographic morphology of the left anterior descending coronary artery morphology and site of occlusion. *Am. J. Cardiol.* 69: 860–865.

7 Porter, A., Sclarovsky, S., Ben-Gal, T. et al. (1998). Value of T-wave direction with lead III ST-segment depression in acute anterior wall myocardial infarction: electrocardiographic prediction of a "wrapped" left anterior descending artery. *Clin. Cardiol.* 21: 562–566.

8 Huey, B.L., Beller, G.A., Kaiser, D.L., and Gibson, R.S. (1988). A comprehensive analysis of myocardial infarction due to left circumflex artery occlusion: comparison with infarction due to right coronary artery and left anterior descending artery occlusion. *J. Am. Coll. Cardiol.* 12: 1156–1166.

9 Zimetbaum, P.J., Krishnan, S., Gold, A. et al. (1998). Usefulness of ST-segment elevation in lead III exceeding that of lead II for identifying the location of the totally occluded coronary artery in inferior wall myocardial infarction. *Am. J. Cardiol.* 81: 918–919.

10 Moye, S., Carney, M.F., Holstege, C. et al. (2005). The electrocardiogram in right ventricular myocardial infarction. *Am. J. Emerg. Med.* 23: 793–799.

11 Mattu, A., Brady, W.J., Perron, A.D., and Robinson, D.A. (2001). Prominent R wave in lead V1: electrocardiographic differential diagnosis. *Am. J. Emerg. Med.* 19: 504–513.

12 Dunn, R.F., Newman, H.N., Bernstein, L. et al. (1984). The clinical features of isolated left circumflex coronary artery disease. *Circulation* 69: 477–484.

13 Kim, T.Y., Alturk, N., Shaikh, N. et al. (1999). An electrocardiographic algorithm for the prediction of the culprit lesion site in acute anterior myocardial infarction. *Clin. Cardiol.* 22: 77–83.

14 Schroder, R. (2004). Prognostic impact of early ST-segment resolution in acute ST-elevation myocardial infarction. *Circulation* 110: e506–e510.

3

STEMI Mimics

Peter M. Pollak

Division of Cardiovascular Medicine, Mayo Clinic Florida, Jacksonville, FL, USA

Introduction

Cardiovascular disease remains the leading cause of death worldwide, and chest pain is one of the most common presenting complaints among emergency department patients accounting for over 7 million visits annually [1]. Reperfusion therapy in patients with ST-elevation myocardial infarction (STEMI) in the form of primary PCI or thrombolytic therapy can drastically improve mortality and morbidity by opening a closed coronary artery. The benefit of reperfusion therapy is exquisitely time sensitive and wanes quickly making the swift and accurate recognition of STEMI imperative [2]. National and local organizations have dramatically improved clinical outcomes for STEMI patients through the development of networks and systems to facilitate access to reperfusion therapy primarily focused on primary percutaneous coronary intervention (PCI) because of its superiority over thrombolysis [3]. These "door-to-balloon" initiatives, such as the American Heart Association's *Mission: Lifeline*, are effective through rapid activation of a large group of resources to bring a patient with a closed artery swiftly into a capable cardiac catheterization laboratory [4].

The keystone of prompt STEMI recognition remains the 12-lead surface electrocardiogram (ECG). It is inexpensive, nearly harmless, and fast, and data can be easily transmitted, allowing STEMI detection and treatment to move into the patient's home. Nevertheless, the backbone of STEMI diagnosis, the 12-lead ECG, is imperfect. Patients may present with ST elevation (STE) yet have a diagnosis other than an occluded coronary artery. These so-called *STEMI mimics* pose a clinical dilemma and real risk of patient harm. Inappropriate use of thrombolytic therapy exposes the patient to risk of cerebral hemorrhage. Complications from unnecessary coronary angiography as well as delay in

diagnosis and initiation of appropriate therapy are also possible. Improper activation of the STEMI network also causes substantial fiscal waste.

The astute physician familiar with STEMI mimics can avoid these pitfalls with greater accuracy of ECG interpretation. The ultimate goal remains to maximize swift and accurate diagnosis of true STEMI patients while simultaneously avoiding delays in treatment. The most powerful tool in these difficult situations remains the physician's clinical acumen and assessment of the patient's clinical history to determine the clinical context and then interpret the ECG in that context – in other words, does the patient look like he or she is experiencing a STEMI? STEMI mimics all involve some degree of ST-segment elevation, yet less commonly involve an acute chest pain syndrome. In other words, the patient *with* ST-segment elevation but *without* a convincingly clinical picture of STEMI should prompt the provider to suspect a nonacute myocardial infarction presentation. Table 2.3.1 provides a list of STEMI mimics and STEMI confounders while Table 2.3.2 provides a list of STEMI mimics with ECG features and distinguishing characteristics.

Myocarditis and Myopericarditis

Inflammation of the pericardium and underlying heart muscle causes chest pain with ST-segment elevation in three-quarters of cases [5]. Alternately, nearly half of patients with presumed acute coronary syndrome but no identified coronary lesion on angiography demonstrate evidence of myocarditis by cardiac MRI [6].

Myocarditis and myopericarditis can affect people of all ages and present across a broad continuum of clinical severity, ranging from mild chest discomfort to cardiogenic

Electrocardiogram in Clinical Medicine, First Edition. Edited by William J. Brady, Michael J. Lipinski, Andrew E. Darby, Michael C. Bond, Nathan P. Charlton, Korin Hudson, and Kelly Williamson.
© 2021 John Wiley & Sons Ltd. Published 2021 by John Wiley & Sons Ltd.

Table 2.3.1 STEMI mimics versus confounders.

STEMI Mimic	STEMI Confounder
Definition: Clinical condition with ECG characteristics similar to AMI but not due to acute thrombotic coronary vessel occlusion.	Definition: Clinical conditions with ECG characteristics that obscure the diagnosis of acute myocardial infarction
Examples:	Examples:
Myocarditis and myopericarditis	Ventricular paced rhythm
Benign early repolarization	Left bundle branch block
Left ventricular hypertrophy	Right bundle branch block
Post-infarction ventricular aneurysm	Left ventricular hypertrophy
Coronary vasospasm	
Apical ballooning syndrome	
Brugada pattern	
Hyperkalemia	
Post-cardioversion/defibrillation	
Hypothermia/Osborne waves	
Pulmonary embolism	
Pneumothorax	
Small bowel obstruction	
Pancreatitis	

Table 2.3.2 STEMI mimics – distinguishing characteristics.

STEMI Mimic	ECG Characteristic	Clinical characteristic
Myocarditis and myopericarditis	STE in multiple coronary distributions, PR depression, PR elevation in aVR.	Positional pain, audible friction rub.
Benign early repolarization	Concave ST segments with peaked symmetrical T waves.	Atypical or no chest pain. May be incidental finding. Young and male.
Left ventricular hypertrophy and HCM	Stable STE. Deep TWI. Most often anterior. High accompanying QRS voltage.	S4 gallop. Longstanding hypertension.
Post-infarction ventricular aneurysm	Stable STE. Accompanying Q waves.	History of prior infarct. S3 gallop.
Coronary vasospasm	Highly variable ST elevation. May come and go within minutes.	Abrupt response or resolution with nitrates. Mercurial presentation.
Apical ballooning syndrome	Can be difficult to distinguish by ECG.	Recent emotional shock or trauma. Female more commonly.
Brugada pattern	Coved ST segment appearance atypical for AMI.	More often incidental finding. Sodium channel blockers can accentuate.
Hyperkalemia	Variable and "odd-looking" ST elevation. QRS widening.	Resolves quickly with treatment of potassium level.
Post-cardioversion/ shock	Can be difficult to distinguish. Rarely with reciprocal ST depression.	History of recent cardioversion or defibrillation. Rare with ICD.
Hypothermia/Osborne waves	J-point elevation is most prominent portion of ST segment elevation.	Patient is cold, usually <35°C. Can be therapeutic or environmental hypothermia.
Pulmonary embolism	Sinus tachycardia may be dramatic.	Generally massive PE required to cause STE, so patient very ill and hypoxic. Hemodynamically unstable. McConnell's sign on echo.
Pneumothorax	Axis shift. Atypical STE appearance.	Decreased breath sounds. CXR diagnostic.
Small bowel obstruction	Atypical STE appearance.	Abdominal X-ray. Tenderness on exam.
Pancreatitis	Atypical STE appearance.	Elevated lipase. Tenderness on exam.

shock. The term *myocarditis* refers to an inflammatory process of the heart muscle, while *pericarditis* refers to inflammation of the serous lining surrounding the heart. Because the pericardium is electrically silent, the presence of ST-segment changes implies adjacent myocardial involvement and the term *myopericarditis* is used.

Most often the etiology of inflammation is unknown; however, viral and autoimmune causes of pericarditis are felt to be the most common. With prompting, a patient may recall a viral prodrome or exposure though the source of viral exposure rarely would also have myocarditis or myopericarditis. Tuberculosis is a more common offender in immunocompromised patients and in locations with high rates of endemic tuberculosis.

The pain of pericarditis is classically worse with inspiration and lying down. A friction rub may be present on exam. Troponin and creatinine kinase can be positive in the setting of inflammatory myocardial injury and may be negative in the setting of isolated pericardial inflammation. A rub on cardiac auscultation is a highly specific but very insensitive physical exam finding, and is frequently absent when even a small effusion is present [7]. While a small pericardial effusion is not uncommon, it is rare for pericarditis to present with cardiac tamponade.

The classic distinguishing features of myopericarditis on ECG include PR-segment depression, ST-segment elevation in more than one coronary distribution, and PR-segment elevation in lead aVR. Serial ECGs can be helpful in distinguishing myopericarditis from STEMI because the evolution of change with STEMI is more rapid than with

inflammation. Additionally a second ECG may include features more characteristic of one diagnosis. ST-segment elevation in multiple coronary distributions, especially in a stable patient, strongly favors inflammation over STEMI. Patients with multiple simultaneous occluded arteries typically present with shock or death [8]. Pericardial effusion when present can muffle the presence of a pericardial friction rub, reduce voltage obscuring subtle PR and ST changes, and when massive reveal *electrical alternans* from the heart swinging within the pericardial sac. While aspirin and angiography are unlikely to be harmful, hemorrhagic pericarditis can occur in the setting of thrombolysis and carries a dire prognosis. Finally, complicating matters is the occasional incidence of pericardial inflammation due to myonecrosis in acute myocardial infarction. Figures 2.3.1 and 2.3.2 provide examples of patients with ST-segment elevation who were diagnosed with myopericarditis.

Early Repolarization

Benign early repolarization (BER) is a normal variant found in approximately 1% of the overall population but more commonly in younger male patients. It has also been called "young male pattern" ECG. BER is recognized by ST-segment elevation beginning at the J point, predominantly in the left precordial leads. As the name suggests, BER is not itself a pathologic finding and has not been tied to a disease process. For unknown reasons, BER is seen more frequently in chest pain patients who have used cocaine.

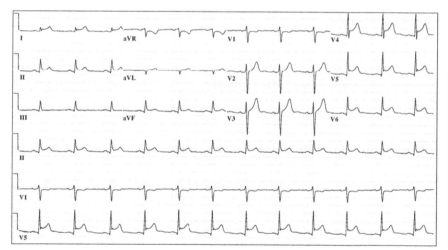
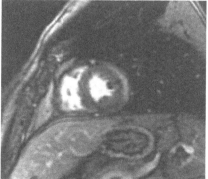

Figure 2.3.1 ST elevation in myocarditis. A 58-year-old man presented to the emergency department with new severe chest pain. His ECG (above) revealed ST elevation and he was sent for an emergent angiogram which revealed no culprit lesion. His chest pain persisted and his biomarkers (troponin T) rose. There was no rub by physical exam. A cardiac MRI was performed revealing subepicardial late gadolinium enhancement consistent with myopericarditis. He was treated with NSAIDs and Colchicine with resolution of his symptoms. On his ECG, note the presence of diffuse ST elevation covering multiple coronary distributions. Also note the subtle depression (or downsloping) of the PR-segment, seen best in the anterior precordial leads and the elevation of the PR segment in aVR.

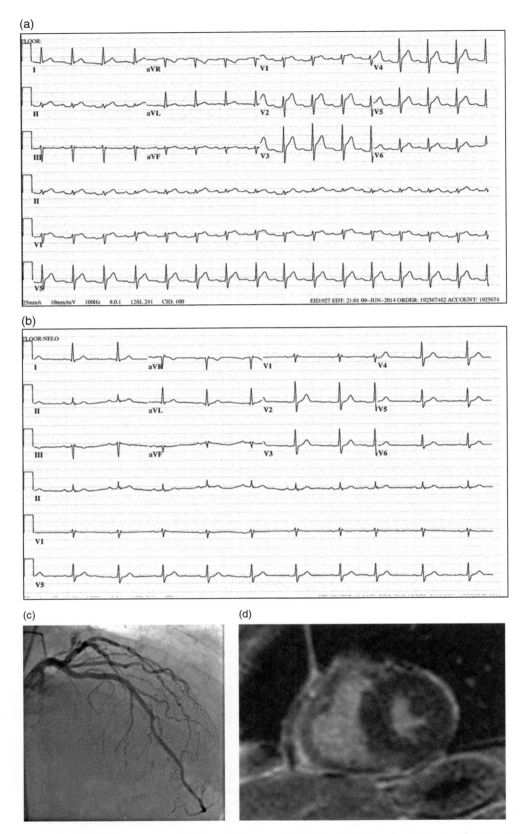

(a)

(b)

(c)

(d)

Figure 2.3.2 STE in myopericarditis #2. An 82-year-old male presented to the emergency department with new severe chest pain. His ECG (a) was compared to his baseline (b), which revealed new anterolateral ST elevation, and a STEMI alert was called. Emergent coronary angiography (c) revealed no culprit lesion. His troponin rose and cardiac MRI (d) revealed subepicardial late gadolinium enhancement consistent with myopericarditis. Notably his ECG shows PR-segment depression in the area of ST elevation; however, his STE is not as diffuse as the last patient, illustrating how inflammation can be regional and overlap with a coronary distribution. He was treated with NSAIDs and colchicine with resolution of his pain and symptoms.

The electrocardiographic characteristics of BER focus on ST-segment elevation with the following features [1]: concave ST-segment elevation (meaning the ST segment remains below an imaginary line connecting the J point to the peak of the T wave) [2], notching or slurring of the J point [3], accentuated, symmetric, and concordant T waves [4], temporal stability. ST-segment elevation is generally less than 3.0 mm with a range of 0.5–5.0 mm. Conceptually the appearance is as if the ST-segment has been evenly lifted upwards from the isoelectric baseline at the J point. When J point itself is notched or irregular, this is highly suggestive of BER. The ST-segment and T-wave abnormalities of BER are most often seen in the anterior precordium (leads V1–V4). At times, coexistent changes may also exist in the inferior or lateral leads; however, BER-related changes noted only in the limb leads are unusual. An example of BER can be found in Figure 2.3.3.

In a chest pain patient with a concerning history and BER pattern, a prior ECG and repeat ECG can be very helpful because the ECG pattern is typically stable over time with changes occurring over decades while STEMI-related changes, on the other hand, evolve over minutes to hours. In addition, rapid bedside echocardiography has adequate performance characteristics to determine whether a large anterior wall motion abnormality is present. In a young, otherwise healthy patient with chest pain where BER is suspected, the bedside echo can save an unnecessary trip to the cath lab.

Left Ventricular Hypertrophy

Increased heart muscle mass increases the current passing through the cells and is reflected as higher voltage on surface ECG. The left ventricular hypertrophy (LVH) ECG pattern can present a vexing challenge to the provider. It is one of the most common pathologic findings on ECG and is strongly associated with hypertension, which itself identifies patients at higher risk for cardiac events. It is important to bear in mind that while 50% of the adult population diagnosed with hypertension will have LVH by echocardiogram, only 20% of those will have characteristic ECG findings of LVH. Moreover, the presence of concomitant downsloping ST segment depression, the so-called "strain" appearance, further degrades prognosis and is present in up to 80% of patients [9].

There are many criteria for determining LVH by ECG, all of which rely on the increase in voltage reflected by the increased myocardial mass along with either leftward axis or left atrial abnormality. Unfortunately, all ECG criteria suffer from relatively poor performance characteristics (sensitivity ~50% and specificity ~80%) when validated against LV mass calculated by echo or cardiac CT [10]. While the detection of underlying, anatomic LVH is important with respect to patient management, in this particular instance, we are addressing only the secondary repolarization

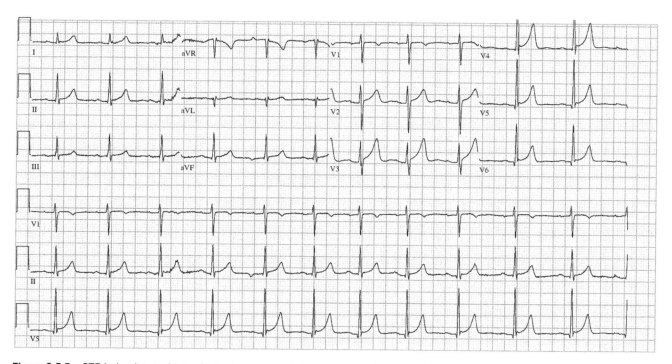

Figure 2.3.3 STE in benign early repolarization pattern. A 32-year-old male presented to the emergency department with new severe chest pain. His ECG is shown. On exam he was noted to be tender over the lateral precordium with point tenderness over the fifth rib. A diagnosis of costochondritis was made and he was discharged to home. This ECG illustrates the STE often seen in young males. Note the concave (inward) curve of the upsloping ST segment.

abnormalities due to LVH – in essence, the ST segment deviations (both elevation and depression) as well as T-wave inversions. In the setting of extreme forms of LVH such as hypertrophic cardiomyopathy (HCM), these changes can be dramatic classically with large QRS voltage and deep biphasic T waves, which can be confused with Wellens waves. While the ECG of patients with HCM can evolve over years, changes are rarely dramatic and sudden.

ST segment elevation in the setting of LVH is most often seen in the anterior distribution (leads V1–V4), frequently seen with prominent T waves, and can be up to 5 mm in height. The lateral leads, leads I, aVL, V5, and V6, demonstrate large, prominent, positively oriented QRS complexes with marked ST segment depression and T-wave inversion. Inferior ST segment elevation should not quickly be ascribed to LVH. The LVH with pattern is associated with poor R wave progression, most commonly producing a QS pattern anteriorly. Leftward axis and left atrial abnormality add credence to ST segment elevation stemming from LVH. The ST segment elevation associated with LVH is generally unchanging over time, making a previous ECG for comparison particularly useful as well as serial ECGs – in both instances, the lack of change (likely LVH) or evolving ST segments (likely STEMI) will assist with the correct diagnosis. Reciprocal ST depression, seen in AMI, is generally not seen in LVH. An example of ST elevation on ECG in a patient with LV hypertrophy can be seen in Figure 2.3.4.

Important clinical clues help distinguish the patient with LVH from STEMI. Most patients with LVH and baseline STE have had severe hypertension requiring multiple antihypertensive medicines for a protracted time; however, patients may present to the ED with previously undiagnosed hypertension. Patients with significant LVH due to long-standing hypertension also frequently have supranormal ejection fractions making a new anterior wall motion abnormality more obvious by bedside echocardiogram. It is not uncommon (nor incorrect) to make the diagnosis of a STEMI mimic in such patients in the cardiac catheterization lab. Because hypertensive crisis raises the risk of intra-cerebral hemorrhage with thrombolysis, systolic blood pressures greater than 180 mm Hg are a relative contra-indication to lytics. Finally, the absence of chest pain should always raise the scepter of a STEMI mimic and prompt further consideration.

Prior Infarction and Ventricular Aneurysm

ST-segment elevation on an ECG in the setting of known previous myocardial infarction may be due to the presence of ventricular aneurysm. A diagnostic challenge exists because the patient has established coronary disease and, thus, increased risk of acute MI. In the pre-reperfusion era, rates of LV aneurysm approached 10%, but they have decreased dramatically since the introduction of fibrinolysis and mechanical reperfusion. Approximately one quarter of patients with persistent ST-segment elevation following STEMI will have an LV aneurysm as determined by echocardiography [11].

The patient's history of present illness, past medical history, and prior ECG – when considered together – are the most useful tools to identify LV aneurysm and distinguish the ST-segment elevation from that of STEMI. The patient should be able to clarify whether he or she had a prior heart attack, and to what degree their current presentation is similar or dissimilar. The bedside echocardiogram in this case is generally unhelpful because the preexisting wall motion abnormality is difficult to distinguish from a new one.

When present, the ECG in the setting of ventricular aneurysm contains ST-segment elevation of varying morphologies and magnitudes, ranging from obvious, convex ST-segment elevation to minimal, concave elevations. Pathologic Q waves are almost always present in the leads with ST-segment elevation and provide a valuable clue to the underlying diagnosis. Inverted T waves of minimal magnitude can be seen. Serial ECGs can be invaluable with dynamic changes suggesting STEMI and the absence of evolution suggesting aneurysm. Prior ECGs are less reliable because the ventricular aneurysm and accompanying STE may have arisen during post-infarction remodeling since the last ECG was performed. Similarly, bedside echocardiography may be less useful because it will be difficult to determine the acuity of a wall-motion abnormality.

Vasospasm (Prinzmetal or Variant Angina)

Coronary vasospasm may present with a wide range of symptoms and severities depending on the amount of myocardium affected and degree of ischemia. Milder vasospasm can cause chest pain or shortness of breath while more diffuse or severe coronary vasospasm can lead to severe STEMI equivalents with concomitant heart failure and ventricular fibrillation.

Vasospasm is common among patients presenting to emergency departments with chest pain syndromes. The Clopidogrel and Acetyl Salicylic Acid in Bypass Surgery for Peripheral ARterial Disease (CASPAR) trial found 49% of patients presenting with acute chest pain who did not have a culprit lesion by angiography did

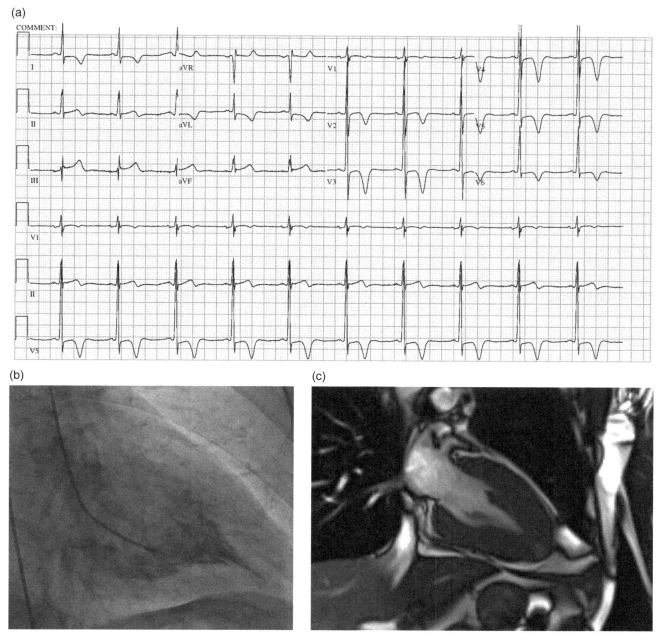

Figure 2.3.4 STE with LV hypertrophy. A 59-year-old male presented to the emergency department with chest pain and shortness of breath. ECG (a) revealed inferior ST elevation and anterior and lateral deep T-wave inversions. A STEMI alert was called and emergent cardiac catheterization performed, which revealed no culprit coronary lesion. His left ventriculogram (b) demonstrated cavity obliteration in the apex consistent with apical-variant hypertrophic cardiomyopathy. This was confirmed by ECG and cardiac MRI (c). His ECG is notably consistent with his baseline, and the pattern of deep T-wave inversions across the precordium is typical for this condition which often manifests with chest pain and shortness of breath.

have coronary vasospasm by acetylcholine challenge [12]. Coronary vasospasm has no clear demographic and occurs along the length of any of the coronary arteries. Tobacco, cocaine, and ergonovine derivatives, are all associated with coronary spasm, and vasospasm occurs in both atherosclerotic as well as angiographically normal vessels. Kounis syndrome is the term for a form of coronary vasospasm caused by allergic histamine release [13]. The final diagnosis of coronary vasospasm is often challenging to make conclusively, and

(a)

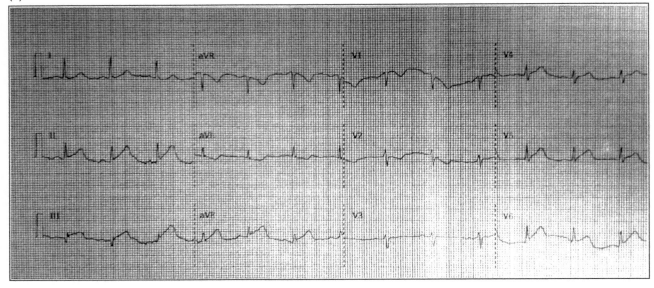

(b)

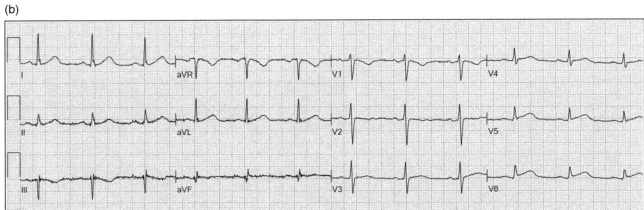

(c)

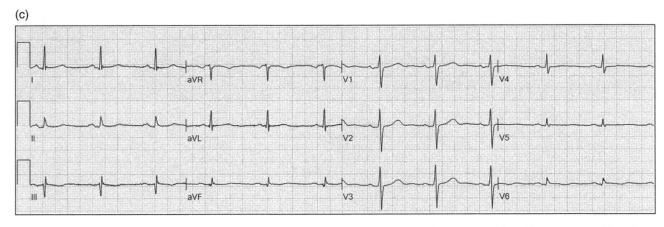

Figure 2.3.5 STE with vasospasm. A 55 year old woman presented to the emergency department with sudden severe crushing chest pain and shortness of breath. Her initial ECG (a) demonstrated inferior STE and a STEMI alert was activated. A repeat ECG (b, #2) performed five minutes later revealed resolution of her inferior ST segment changes and new lateral changes. Emergent cardiac catheterization was initially deferred, however with a rising troponin, it was performed and showed no culprit lesion. Catheter-induced coronary spasm was not noted, but significant coronary dilation with nitroglycerin administration was seen. With vasodilator treatment, her ECG returned to baseline (c, #3). She was discharged on long-acting nitrates and calcium channel blocking agents. Coronary vasospasm can be profound causing acute ischemia and infarction. Typically vasospasm responds well to nitrates and leads to a mercurial ECG findings.

may require acetylcholine or methergine challenge in the cardiac catheterization lab although these provocation tests have generally fallen out of favor. An example of STE on ECG in a patient with vasospasm can be seen in Figure 2.3.5.

Because acute coronary vasospasm can lead to near complete cessation of blood flow in the affected coronary artery, its presentation and pathophysiology parallels STEMI with the important distinction of absent vessel thrombosis. Rapid response to nitrates is characteristic of coronary vasospasm and can be a discriminating clinical tool.

The association of coronary vasospasm with cocaine (or other amphetamine) ingestion presents additional challenges. Cocaine is both vasospastic as well as thrombogenic, leaving users at increased risk for both. In a patient with a clear amphetamine toxidrome (i.e. hypertension, agitation, etc.) as well as ST segment elevation, it is prudent to treat the patient with intravenous benzodiazepines as well as nitrates and then repeat the ECG to determine persistence of ST-segment elevation. STEMI must remain in the working diagnosis and, if unable to demonstrate resolution of the ST-segment elevation within a short period of time, reperfusion therapy should follow.

Apical Ballooning Syndrome (Takotsubo Cardiomyopathy)

Apical ballooning syndrome (ABS) is a form of stress-induced cardiomyopathy and has had multiple names including Takotsubo cardiomyopathy and "broken heart syndrome." While the original description involves dyskinesis of the LV apex, multiple variations, including basal and mid-cavitary dyskinesis, have also been reported. The clinical presentation of ABS is frequently indistinguishable from acute coronary syndrome and may mimic STEMI both clinically and on ECG [14].

Patients can present with the full spectrum of chest pain equivalents from vague atypical chest pain to severe chest pain with acute heart failure and malignant dysrhythmia. The spectrum of ECG findings also varies, from subtle changes to profound anterior ST segment elevation. In its most common apical form, the ECG changes are limited to the anterior precordial leads, reflecting apical location of injury; however, the inferior leads can also be involved. Because the history and ECG and even echocardiogram can be indistinguishable from true AMI, the diagnosis of ABS is most often made in the heart catheterization lab following diagnostic angiography. An example of STE in Takotsubo cardiomyopathy can be seen in Figure 2.3.6.

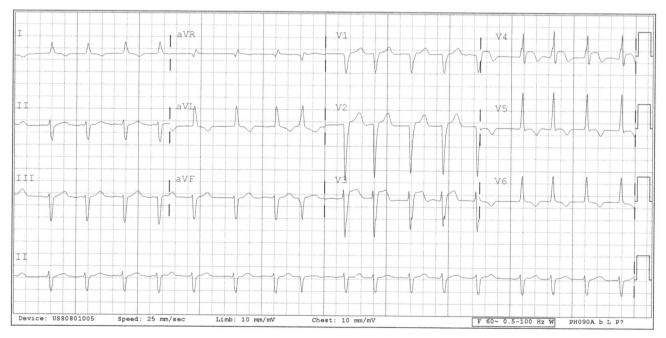

Figure 2.3.6 STE in apical ballooning syndrome (Takotsubo cardiomyopathy). A 59-year-old male presented to the emergency department with sudden severe chest pain and shortness of breath. The ECG shown was obtained and he was sent for emergent coronary angiography. No culprit lesion was found, and his apex was noted to be dyskinetic on left ventriculogram. A diagnosis of apical ballooning syndrome was made, and he was discharged home on a beta blocker and ACE-inhibitor. On three month follow-up, his echocardiogram had returned to normal.

Brugada Pattern and Idiopathic Ventricular Fibrillation

Brugada and Brugada first described their eponymous syndrome in 1992 as the coincidence of right bundle branch block (complete or incomplete) with anterior ST elevation (V1–3) and associated sudden cardiac death despite structurally normal hearts [15]. Since then, much has been learned about this rare inherited disease. It occurs in approximately 5 out of 100 000 people across all nationalities, has an autosomal dominant inheritance pattern, and a male predominance (~70%) [16]. Three subtypes have been described, with subtle variations in the shape of the ST segment. The underlying mechanism, resulting from a gene mutation, is a sodium channel loss of function [17].

Clinically, the disease can present at any age, but the mean age of sudden death is 41 years. The characteristic ECG findings are dynamic and may vary from one ECG to the next. Chest pain is not part of the Brugada syndrome. Patients may present for evaluation following syncope, which in this setting likely represents aborted sudden death and is a poor prognostic marker. The disease and ECG findings can be exacerbated by multiple medications as well as conditions that alter myocardial membrane electrical stability (e.g. fever, hypokalemia, ischemia, bradycardia, and increased autonomic tone). Vaughan Williams class Ic antiarrhythmic medications (e.g. flecainide and procainamide) are potent sodium channel blockers and can elicit the Brugada pattern in suspected cases. Moving the anterior leads superior one rib space may elucidate the pattern in suspicious cases. A large number of medications in addition to sodium channel blockers have been reported to elicit a Brugada-like pattern on ECG, yet the significance of these findings remains unknown.

The diagnostic challenge could present to the emergency department as a 41yo male resuscitated VF arrest who is noted to have STE in leads V1–V3. Accurately distinguishing a previously undiagnosed patient with Brugada syndrome from a patient with VF due to occlusion of the left anterior descending (LAD) can require angiography. Brugada syndrome is much less common than acute MI as a cause of VF arrest overall; however, Brugada syndrome by definition occurs in patients with structurally normal hearts, so a rapid bedside echocardiogram revealing normal wall motion should significantly decrease the likelihood of AMI. A prior ECG with Brugada pattern can be confirmatory, but as the ECG findings can vary in presentation, their absence does not rule out Brugada.

Hyperkalemia

As the serum potassium concentration rises, ECG changes develop that can mimic AMI [18]. The elevation of the ST-segment occurs following peaking of the T wave and widening of the QRS complex, both of which suggest high serum potassium concentrations. Though the accompanying ST-segment elevation may be most impressive in a single region, the ECG changes of hyperkalemia are present throughout the limb and precordial leads. A STEMI mimic following cardiac arrest in a patient with hyperkalemia is shown in Figure 2.3.7.

High clinical suspicion and awareness of clinical context is key to this diagnosis, as the ECG changes will resolve quickly with appropriate treatment of the potassium level, which may be more life-threatening than the potential infarction. Because pseudoinfarction from hyperkalemia has only been described in patients with diabetic ketoacidosis or renal failure, the chest pain is uncommon but dyspnea from volume overload and acidosis may occur.

Post-Cardioversion/Shock

ST elevation may occur following transthoracic electrical cardioversion or defibrillation in up to 20% of patients. ST-segment deviation following countershock by internal cardioverter-defibrillator may be seen in 25% of patients [19]. The ST-segment elevation is transient and resolves within minutes but can be up to 5 mm [20]. While impressive and alarming, this finding has not been associated with evidence of ongoing myocardial injury [21].

The clinical challenge is determining whether the arrhythmia requiring electrical shock was precipitated by STEMI or whether the STE merely reflects the shock itself. Once again, a repeat ECG and rapid bedside echocardiogram can provide valuable information. If normal wall motion is seen by echo, the likelihood of STEMI becomes very small. Moreover, the ST elevations following electrical shock resolve within minutes whereas those from STEMI will tend to persist and evolve.

Hypothermia and Osborn Waves

Prominent J point elevations, also known as Osborn waves, are a common finding in the hypothermic patient [22]. When profound, the ST-segment can be elevated potentially mimicking STEMI. Aside from the patient's temperature, other clues on ECG include bradycardia and motion artifact from shivering. The mechanism and clinical implications of the Osborn wave remain unclear, but it is a transient finding that resolves with normothermia. Osborn waves can occur with either therapeutic hypothermia or environmental hypothermia [23].

(a)

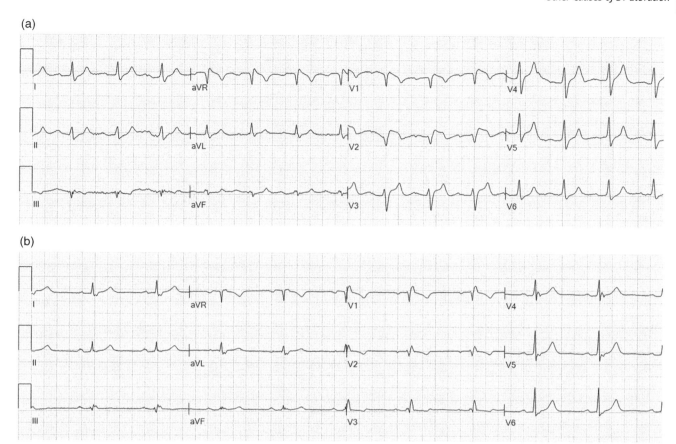

(b)

Figure 2.3.7 (a) STE with hyperkalemia following defibrillation. (b) ECG of same patient following administration of insulin and D50. A 56-year-old male was brought to the emergency department following cardiac arrest at home. He received bystander cardiopulmonary resuscitation and two shocks from an automated external defibrillator. Upon seeing his initial ECG (a), a STEMI alert was called; however, a bedside echocardiogram revealed no wall motion abnormality, and his potassium was noted to be 7.3 mmol/dL. He was treated with insulin and D50, and his ECG was repeated (b) which revealed resolution of his STE. Note the widened QRS, the appearance of the ST segment on the initial ECG not typical of ST elevation in myocardial infarction, and the absence of reciprocal depression. Though none of those features can guarantee the absence of accompanying myocardial infarction, the resolution of ST changes on repeat ECG illustrate the high value of serial electrocardiograms in questionable cases. Also worth noting is the similarity of mechanism at the cellular level, where the injury current during infarction is mediated by localized hyperkalemia.

Pulmonary Embolism

Pulmonary embolism (PE) is common in patients presenting to the ED and must always be considered in the differential diagnosis of acute chest pain. The distinction between acute coronary syndrome and PE can be challenging. Both can cause ST changes and troponin elevation, yet very few patients with PE have ECGs which mimic AMI [24]. All reported cases of STE with PE were in the anterior leads, occurred in cases of massive emboli, and were associated with hemodynamic instability. The presenting symptom in such cases is frequently syncope representing brief cessation of circulation, and the sudden profound increase in pulmonary vascular resistance is more likely to cause significant right ventricular (RV) strain that will be visible on echocardiogram. While echocardiogram is not useful for making the diagnosis of PE, it is indicated to identify RV dysfunction in the hemodynamically unstable patient with suspected massive PE. In contrast to every other STEMI mimic, the use of thrombolytics in the case of massive PE causing hemodynamic compromise is most likely helpful [25]. Moreover, activation of the STEMI network and emergent angiography can cause a life-threatening delay in appropriate treatment and increase the risk of bleeding with thrombolysis due to arterial puncture. In Figure 2.3.8, a patient presents with PE and STE on ECG.

Other Causes of ST Elevation

Processes that mechanically affect the heart will cause ECG changes and can mimic acute MI. Tension pneumothorax, particularly left sided, can mimic anterior MI and has been reported [26]. Cardiac contusion causes myocardial injury and

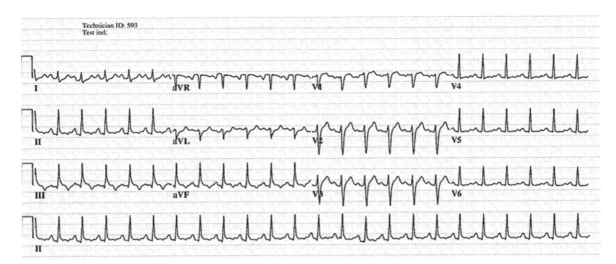

Technician ID: 593
Test ind:

Figure 2.3.8 STE in acute pulmonary embolism. A 23-year-old woman presented to the emergency department with sudden severe chest pain and shortness of breath. She was noted to be tachycardic, hypotensive, and hypoxic. The above ECG was performed and a STEMI alert called. She was diverted from the cath lab to the CT scanner where she was found to have massive bilateral pulmonary emboli. She was treated with thrombolytic therapy. This ECG demonstrates the most common electrocardiographic finding in acute PE – tachycardia. Also notably, though relatively uncommon, this ECG illustrates the S1Q3T3 pattern that can be associated with sudden severe RV strain. This patient had the echocardiographic correlate known as McConnell's sign, where a dilated hypocontracile right ventricle has preserved apical contractility in the setting of sudden afterload increase as in large PE.

(a)

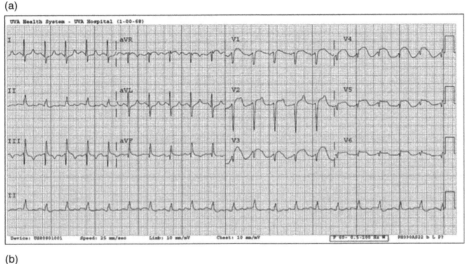

(b)

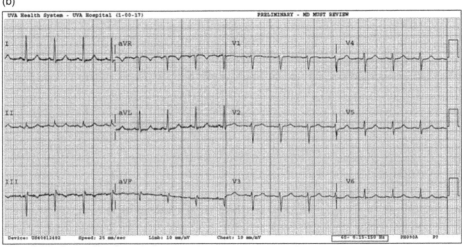

Figure 2.3.9 STE associated with small bowel obstruction. A 45-year-old woman on postoperative day #5 recovering from total abdominal hysterectomy for fibroids developed severe shortness of breath. She had been on typical DVT prophylaxis. She was taken to the cardiac catheterization laboratory for emergent angiography which revealed no culprit lesion. A CT scan showed evidence of acute small bowel obstruction and she was taken for exploratory laparotomy and lysis of adhesions with resection of a small section of necrotic bowel. The ECG (a) obtained during initial evaluation of the dyspnea shows clear ST-segment changes with tachycardia when compared to the patient's baseline electrocardiogram (b).

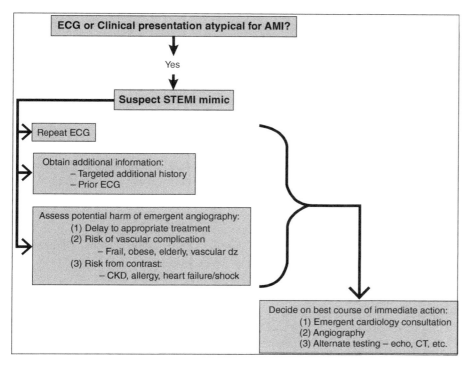

Figure 2.3.10 STEMI mimic evaluation algorithm.

results in injury currents. Small bowel obstruction has also been reported to mimic STEMI [27]. An example of STE in a patient with small bowel obstruction can be seen in Figure 2.3.9. Inflammation close to the heart can likewise cause ECG changes akin to pericarditis. This has been reported with pancreatitis as well as cholecystitis and pneumonia [28] [29].

Conclusion

Swift and accurate diagnosis of STEMI is the foundation of the STEMI network and vital to bringing rapid life-saving reperfusion therapy to patients with acute myocardial infarction. Invoking the mobilization of considerable resource, the use of potentially harmful drugs, and the potential for delay in appropriate treatment all underscore the importance of arriving at the correct diagnosis. The astute clinician with greater awareness of the array of STEMI mimics and their subtleties is more likely to arrive at the correct diagnosis and avoid potential waste and harm.

In the time-sensitive setting of emergency evaluation and triage, and algorithmic approach can facilitate rapid and accurate decision-making. One such algorithm is shown in Figure 2.3.10 and summarizes the available tools for distinguishing a STEMI mimic from a true STEMI and moving toward the most appropriate disposition. Whenever the clinical context or ECG or both are atypical for AMI, consider a STEMI mimic. Targeted additional history including prior ECG and then repeat ECG can add tremendously to the available information and require only minutes to obtain. When considering a STEMI activation in the setting of a possible mimic, bear in mind the risks to the patient of delay in alternate diagnosis or treatment (e.g. PE) as well as that from emergent angiography (e.g. vascular complication, nephrotoxicity, and allergy). Frequently, a STEMI mimic can only be safely diagnosed after AMI has been ruled out with angiography.

References

1 Niska, R., Bhuiya, F., and Xu, J. (2010). National Hospital Ambulatory Medical Care Survey: 2007 emergency department summary. *National Health Statistics Reports*: 1–31.

2 Maeng, M., Nielsen, P.H., Busk, M. et al. (2010). Time to treatment and three-year mortality after primary percutaneous coronary intervention for ST-segment elevation myocardial infarction-a DANish trial in acute myocardial Infarction-2 (DANAMI-2) substudy. *The American Journal of Cardiology* 105: 1528–1534.

3 Keeley, E.C., Boura, J.A., and Grines, C.L. (2003). Primary angioplasty versus intravenous thrombolytic therapy for acute myocardial infarction: a quantitative review of 23 randomised trials. *Lancet* 361: 13–20.

4 Jollis, J.G., Granger, C.B., Henry, T.D. et al. (2012). Systems of care for ST-segment-elevation myocardial infarction: a report from the American Heart Association's Mission: lifeline. *Circulation. Cardiovascular Quality and Outcomes* 5: 423–428.

5 Bruce, M.A. and Spodick, D.H. (1980). Atypical electrocardiogram in acute pericarditis: characteristics and prevalence. *Journal of Electrocardiology* 13: 61–66.

6 Codreanu, A., Djaballah, W., Angioi, M. et al. (2007). Detection of myocarditis by contrast-enhanced MRI in patients presenting with acute coronary syndrome but no coronary stenosis. *Journal of magnetic resonance imaging* 25: 957–964.

7 Spodick, DH. (2003). Acute pericarditis: current concepts and practice. *JAMA: The Journal of the American Medical Association* 289: 1150–1153.

8 Pollak, P.M., Parikh, S.V., Kizilgul, M., and Keeley, E.C. (2009). Multiple culprit arteries in patients with ST segment elevation myocardial infarction referred for primary percutaneous coronary intervention. *The American Journal of Cardiology* 104: 619–623.

9 Sullivan, J.M., Vander Zwaag, R.V., el-Zeky, F. et al. (1993). Left ventricular hypertrophy: effect on survival. *Journal of the American College of Cardiology* 22: 508–513.

10 Hancock, E.W., Deal, B.J., Mirvis, D.M. et al. (2009). AHA/ACCF/HRS recommendations for the standardization and interpretation of the electrocardiogram: part V: electrocardiogram changes associated with cardiac chamber hypertrophy: a scientific statement from the American heart Association Electrocardiography and Arrhythmias Committee, Council on Clinical Cardiology; the American College of Cardiology Foundation; and the Heart Rhythm Society: endorsed by the International Society for Computerized Electrocardiology. *Circulation* 119: e251–e261.

11 Galiuto, L., Barchetta, S., Paladini, S. et al. (2007). Functional and structural correlates of persistent ST elevation after acute myocardial infarction successfully treated by percutaneous coronary intervention. *Heart* 93: 1376–1380.

12 Ong, P., Athanasiadis, A., Hill, S. et al. (2008). Coronary artery spasm as a frequent cause of acute coronary syndrome: the CASPAR (Coronary Artery Spasm in Patients With Acute Coronary Syndrome)

study. *Journal of the American College of Cardiology* 52: 523–527.

13 Kounis, N.G. and Zavras, G.M. (1991). Histamine-induced coronary artery spasm: the concept of allergic angina. *The British Journal of Clinical Practice* 45: 121–128.

14 Prasad, A., Lerman, A., and Rihal, C.S. (2008). Apical ballooning syndrome (Tako-Tsubo or stress cardiomyopathy): a mimic of acute myocardial infarction. *American Heart Journal* 155: 408–417.

15 Brugada, P. and Brugada, J. (1992). Right bundle branch block, persistent ST segment elevation and sudden cardiac death: a distinct clinical and electrocardiographic syndrome. A multicenter report. *Journal of the American College of Cardiology* 20: 1391–1396.

16 Benito, B., Sarkozy, A., Mont, L. et al. (2008). Gender differences in clinical manifestations of Brugada syndrome. *Journal of the American College of Cardiology* 52: 1567–1573.

17 Antzelevitch, C., Brugada, P., Borggrefe, M. et al. (2005). Brugada syndrome: report of the second consensus conference: endorsed by the Heart Rhythm Society and the European Heart Rhythm Association. *Circulation* 111: 659–670.

18 Simon, B.C. (1988). Pseudomyocardial infarction and hyperkalemia: a case report and subject review. *The Journal of Emergency Medicine* 6: 511–515.

19 Gurevitz, O., Lipchenca, I., Yaacoby, E. et al. (2002). ST-segment deviation following implantable cardioverter defibrillator shocks: incidence, timing, and clinical significance. *Pacing and Clinical Electrophysiology* 25: 1429–1432.

20 Van Gelder, I.C., Crijns, H.J., Van der Laarse, A. et al. (1991). Incidence and clinical significance of ST segment elevation after electrical cardioversion of atrial fibrillation and atrial flutter. *American Heart Journal* 121: 51–56.

21 Kok, L.C., Mitchell, M.A., Haines, D.E. et al. (2000). Transient ST elevation after transthoracic cardioversion in patients with hemodynamically unstable ventricular tachyarrhythmia. *The American Journal of Cardiology* 85: 878–881, A9.

22 Antzelevitch, C. and Yan, G.X. (2010). J wave syndromes. *Heart Rhythm: The Official Journal of the Heart Rhythm Society* 7: 549–558.

23 Noda, T., Shimizu, W., Tanaka, K., and Chayama, K. (2003). Prominent J wave and ST segment elevation: serial electrocardiographic changes in accidental hypothermia. *Journal of Cardiovascular Electrophysiology* 14: 223.

24 Falterman, T.J., Martinez, J.A., Daberkow, D., and Weiss, L.D. (2001). Pulmonary embolism with ST segment elevation in leads V1 to V4: case report and review of the

literature regarding electrocardiographic changes in acute pulmonary embolism. *The Journal of Emergency Medicine* 21: 255–261.

25 Fasullo, S., Paterna, S., and Di Pasquale, P. (2009). An unusual presentation of massive pulmonary embolism mimicking septal acute myocardial infarction treated with tenecteplase. *Journal of Thrombosis and Thrombolysis* 27: 215–219.

26 Ruo, W. and Rupani, G. (1992). Left tension pneumothorax mimicking myocardial ischemia after percutaneous central venous cannulation. *Anesthesiology* 76: 306–308.

27 Mixon, T.A. and Houck, P.D. (2003). Intestinal obstruction mimicking acute myocardial infarction. *Texas Heart Institute Journal* 30: 155–157.

28 Khairy, P. and Marsolais, P. (2001). Pancreatitis with electrocardiographic changes mimicking acute myocardial infarction. *Canadian Journal of Gastroenterology* 15: 522–526.

29 Ryan, E.T., Pak, P.H., and DeSanctis, R.W. (1992). Myocardial infarction mimicked by acute cholecystitis. *Annals of Internal Medicine* 116: 218–220.

4

Confounders of ST-Elevation Myocardial Infarction

Amy West Pollak

Division of Cardiovascular Medicine, Mayo Clinic Florida, Jacksonville, FL, USA

Introduction

Difficulty in determining whether ST elevation (STE) constitutes an acute myocardial infarction typically stems from two general categories: (i) there is an underlying pathology that mimics an ischemic pattern of STE or (ii) the typical ischemic repolarization changes are confounded by the patient's baseline abnormal ECG. In this chapter, we'll discuss the ECG patterns that often cofound diagnosis of ischemic ST elevation: left bundle branch block, left ventricular hypertrophy, and ventricular paced rhythm. Additionally, considerations with right bundle branch block (RBBB) will be briefly addressed.

Left Bundle Branch Block

Typical Pattern

In a left branch bundle block (LBBB), the QRS duration is >120 ms with a predominantly negative QS or rS in lead V1, while there is a monophasic R wave in lead V6. Leads I and aVL are associated with ST depression (Figure 2.4.1). The usual appearance of ST segments with LBBB is explained by the concept of appropriate discordance, wherein the ST segment or T-wave complex is in the opposite direction from the primary terminal portion of the QRS complex. For instance, because of the monophasic R wave in lead V6, there will usually be negative ST segment deflection.

LBBB and Ischemic Heart Disease

LBBB can be a sign of underlying heart disease in a variety of settings. With acute ST elevation myocardial infarction and LBBB, patients typically present in one of three situations:

(i) a new LBBB as a STEMI equivalent, (ii) known underlying LBBB with concern for new ischemic changes, (iii) or a LBBB that is age indeterminate and may reflect chronic ischemic heart disease or underlying cardiomyopathy. In order to preserve the door-to-balloon time for acute ST elevation myocardial infarction, it is critical to focus on differentiating between a new LBBB that is a STEMI equivalent, new ischemic changes to an old LBBB, and a chronic heart condition that results in a LBBB.

The Sgarbossa criteria published in 1996 [1], still represent the best available framework in which to evaluate for acute ischemia in a patient who presents with chest pain and a known LBBB. The Sgarbossa criteria use a point-based system to determine the likelihood of an acute coronary syndrome with an underlying LBBB. However, it is helpful at the patient bedside to instead focus on the three key components of the Sgarbossa criteria: (i) Concordant ST segment elevation >1 mm, which is strongly suggestive of AMI (odds ratio of 25); (ii) Concordant ST segment depression >1 mm in leads V1–V3, which is also strongly suggestive of AMI (odds ratio of 6); and (iii) ST segment elevation >5 mm discordant from QRS complex, which is only somewhat suggestive of AMI (odds ratio of 4). Unfortunately, this third criterion of excessive discordant ST-segment elevation was subsequently shown to have both poor sensitivity and specificity.

Smith et al. [2, 3] have modified the original Sgarbossa criterion, replacing the absolute ST-elevation measurement of ≥5 mm with an ST-elevation/S wave ratio less than −0.25. In other words, this criterion is defined as positive, or abnormal, if the magnitude of ST segment elevation is ≥25% of the size of the accompanying S wave, an acute coronary occlusion is potentially indicated. This new criterion significantly improved the diagnostic utility of the Sgarbossa rule for diagnosing AMI in the presence of

Electrocardiogram in Clinical Medicine, First Edition. Edited by William J. Brady, Michael J. Lipinski, Andrew E. Darby, Michael C. Bond, Nathan P. Charlton, Korin Hudson, and Kelly Williamson.
© 2021 John Wiley & Sons Ltd. Published 2021 by John Wiley & Sons Ltd.

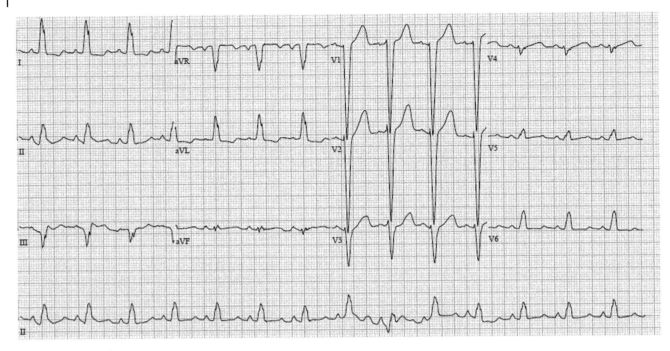

Figure 2.4.1 LBBB.

LBBB. It is important to remember that although the Sgarbossa criteria are very specific (96%), they have a very low sensitivity (36%) [1] (Case 2.4.1).

When a patient presents with chest pain and a "new" LBBB, the immediate concern is whether this represents a STEMI equivalent. In the 2013 American Heart Association/American College of Cardiology Foundation *Guideline for the Management of ST-Elevation Myocardial Infarction,* the issue of new or "presumed new" LBBB as a STEMI equivalent is addressed [4]. A new LBBB as a STEMI equivalent occurs infrequently [5] and "should not be considered diagnostic of acute myocardial infarction in isolation." Certainly patients can present with an acute LAD occlusion and new LBBB on their ECG. Remember

---

Case 2.4.1   LBBB with >5 mm ST Elevation in Leads V2

A 62-year-old male who presented with atypical chest pain was found to have >5 mm STE in lead V2, consistent with the Sgarbossa criteria that has the smallest odds ratio for STEMI. The patient was found to have nonobstructive coronary artery disease at the time of catheterization.

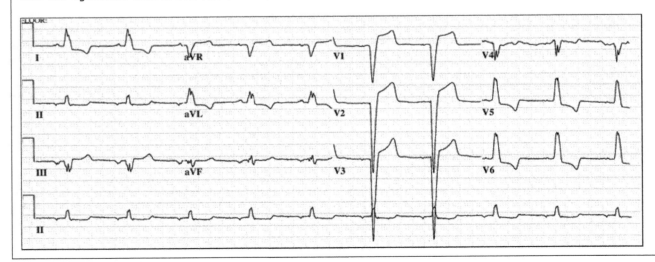

Case 2.4.2   New LBBB in the Setting of an Acute Myocardial Infarction

A 56-year-old male presented with a new LBBB and cardiogenic shock. He was stabilized with an intra-aortic balloon pump and taken for emergent cardiac catheterization, which showed a proximal LAD occlusion. Restoration of TIMI grade 3 flow in the LAD resulted in stabilization of

the blood pressure. The key to identifying this patient's new LBBB as a STEMI equivalent is his clinical presentation of acute cardiogenic shock, which can be seen with a very proximal LAD occlusion. Importantly, no ECG evidence of AMI is noted here.

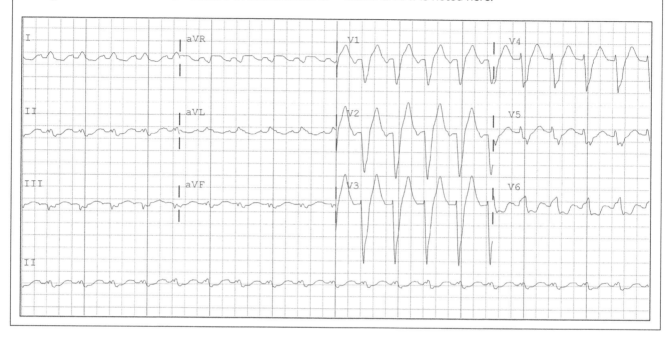

that the LAD occlusion must be proximal to the first septal perforator in order to cause ischemic injury to the conduction system resulting in a LBBB. The decision to take a patient emergently to the cardiac catheterization for a suspected coronary occlusion requires a compatible clinical scenario, in addition to the presence of new LBBB (Case 2.4.2).

Left Ventricular Hypertrophy

The presence of left ventricular hypertrophy with associated STE, in a multivariate analysis predicted the greatest number of false positive STEMI's [6]. Typically STE with LVH is concave upward in the precordial leads. However, it can be challenging to distinguish from acute ischemia. One proposed strategy to diagnose acute LAD territory ischemic changes with greater specificity is a ratio of ST segment to R-S wave height ≥25% [7] for patients with LVH. However, this has not been incorporated into the current STEMI guidelines. For patients presenting with chest pain and LVH, almost three-quarters will not have an underlying

acute coronary syndrome [8]. Rather, hypertensive heart disease or congestive heart failure are more commonly associated with LVH [8]. For some cases of LVH, there are minimal ST segment repolarization abnormalities at baseline (Case 2.4.3), which can facilitate the diagnosis of ischemic STE. Fundamentally, looking at the patient's clinical presentation and comparisons with prior ECGs can help to clarify whether there is an acute myocardial infarction.

Ventricular Paced Rhythm

A paced ventricular rhythm results in a wide QRS complex. Typically, ventricular pacing originating from a right ventricular lead will result in a LBBB (Figure 2.4.2) morphology and conversely a biventricular pacemaker with the addition of a left ventricular lead causes a RBBB morphology. Ventricular pacing can distort the underlying electrical baseline even when pacing is paused temporarily because of "t-wave memory" [9]. The Sgarbossa criteria were evaluated as possible solution to the detection of

Case 2.4.3   Pericarditis and Minimal LVH

A 57-year-old woman who presented with chest pain in the setting of known hypertension and left ventricular hypertrophy on prior ECG. Note the diffuse STE along with PR depression, consistent with pericarditis.

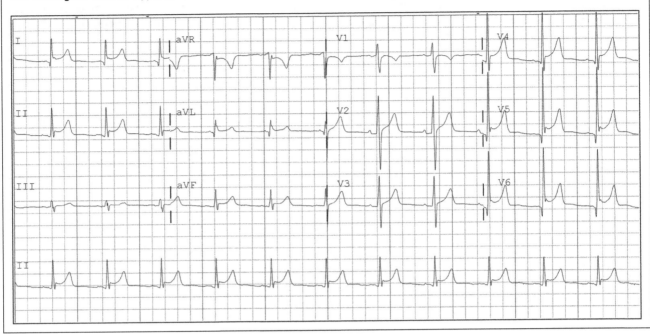

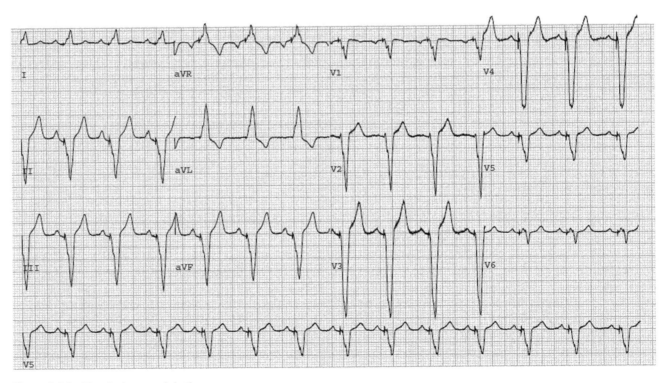

Figure 2.4.2   Ventricular paced rhythm.

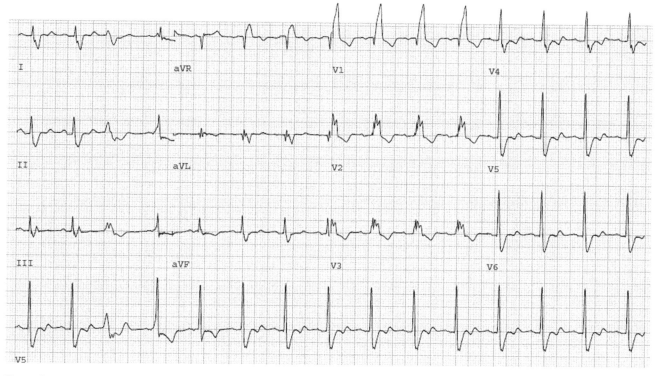

Figure 2.4.3 RBBB.

acute myocardial infarction with a ventricularly paced rhythm; however, they have only a modest specificity and a very low sensitivity [10]. Therefore, the presence of an underlying ventricularly paced rhythm is nondiagnostic for acute STE myocardial infarction.

Right Bundle Branch Block (RBBB)

The presence of a RBBB does not typically confound the detection of an ST-elevation myocardial infarction. A

RBBB has a broad, monophasic R or RSR' in lead V1 along with ST depression in the precordial leads and typically a wide S or rS in lead V6 (Figure 2.4.3). Patients with a proximal RCA STEMI may present with a new RBBB without typical STE due to the anterior T-wave inversions masking subtle ischemic ST segment changes [11]. Patients with a new RBBB and acute myocardial infarction have high mortality [11] and should be carefully considered for urgent cardiac catheterization.

References

1 Sgarbossa, E.B., Pinski, S.L., Barbagelata, A. et al. (1996). Electrocardiographic diagnosis of evolving acute myocardial infarction in the presence of left bundle-branch block. GUSTO-1 (global utilization of streptokinase and tissue plasminogen activator for occluded coronary arteries) investigators. *The New England journal of medicine* 334: 481–487.

2 Smith, S.W., Dodd, K.W., Henry, T.D. et al. (2012). Diagnosis of ST-elevation myocardial infarction in the presence of left bundle branch block with the ST-elevation to S-wave ratio in a modified Sgarbossa rule. *Ann Emerg Med.* 60: 766–776.

3 Meyers, H.P., Limkakeng, A.T., Jaffa, E.J. et al. (2015). Validation of the modified Sgarbossa criteria for acute coronary occlusion in the setting of left bundle branch block: a retrospective case-control study. *Am Heart J.* 170: 1255–1264.

4 O'Gara, P.T., Kushner, F.G., Ascheim, D.D. et al. (2013). ACCF/AHA guideline for the management of ST-elevation myocardial infarction: a report of the American college of cardiology foundation/american heart association task force on practice guidelines. *Circulation* 127: e362–e425.

5 Chang, A.M., Shofer, F.S., Tabas, J.A. et al. (2009). Lack of association between left bundle-branch block and acute myocardial infarction in symptomatic ED patients. *The American journal of emergency medicine* 27: 916–921.

6 McCabe, J.M., Armstrong, E.J., Kulkarni, A. et al. (2012). Prevalence and factors associated with false-positive ST-segment elevation myocardial infarction diagnoses at primary percutaneous coronary intervention-capable centers: a report from the activate-SF registry. *Archives of internal medicine* 172: 864–871.

7 Armstrong, E.J., Kulkarni, A.R., Bhave, P.D. et al. (2012). Electrocardiographic criteria for ST-elevation myocardial infarction in patients with left ventricular hypertrophy. *The American journal of cardiology* 110: 977–983.

8 Larsen, G.C., Griffith, J.L., Beshansky, J.R. et al. (1994). Electrocardiographic left ventricular hypertrophy in patients with suspected acute cardiac ischemia – its influence on diagnosis, triage, and short-term prognosis: a multicenter study. *Journal of General Internal Medicine* 9: 666–673.

9 Rosenbaum, M.B., Blanco, H.H., Elizari, M.V. et al. (1982). Electrotonic modulation of the T wave and cardiac memory. *The American Journal of Cardiology* 50: 213–222.

10 Sgarbossa, E.B., Pinski, S.L., Gates, K.B., and Wagner, G.S. (1996). Early electrocardiographic diagnosis of acute myocardial infarction in the presence of ventricular paced rhythm. GUSTO-I investigators. *The American Journal of Cardiology* 77: 423–424.

11 Widimsky, P., Rohac, F., Stasek, J. et al. (2012). Primary angioplasty in acute myocardial infarction with right bundle branch block: should new onset right bundle branch block be added to future guidelines as an indication for reperfusion therapy? *European Heart Journal* 33: 86–95.

5

The Prognostic Value of the Electrocardiogram in Acute Coronary Syndromes

Benjamin Shepple[1] and Robert Gibson[2]

[1]*Division of Cardiology, University of Tennessee Medical Center, Knoxville, TN, USA*
[2]*Division of Cardiovascular Medicine, University of Virginia Health System, Charlottesville, VA, USA*

Introduction

The electrocardiogram (ECG) is essential in the diagnosis and management of ischemic heart disease both in the acute and chronic setting. Coronary artery disease can be diagnosed in a wide spectrum of patients. Patients with coronary artery disease can be asymptomatic, have stable angina or angina equivalent, present as an acute coronary syndrome, or present as sudden cardiac death (SCD). Early prognostication of patients presenting with an acute coronary syndrome is necessary to guide treatment decisions and inform patients. The ECG is a valuable tool that provides prognostic information throughout the spectrum of patients with coronary artery disease – acute coronary syndromes before and after medical or reperfusion therapy, stable coronary artery disease, and in asymptomatic patients. It will be the purpose of this chapter to review ECG findings and their relationship to prognosis in the setting of acute coronary syndromes. The ECG is just one of many tools helpful in defining prognosis and should not be interpreted in isolation of other clinical findings. The treatment of acute coronary syndromes has changed rapidly, and we are now in the reperfusion and percutaneous intervention era. Multiple studies will be cited across a wide spectrum of treatment eras for myocardial infarction; therefore, it will be important to understand the presented findings in the context of the patient population being studied and the treatments received so that one can appropriately apply prognostic information of the ECG to an individual patient.

The ECG in Acute Coronary Syndromes

Acute coronary syndromes include ST-elevation myocardial infarction (STEMI), non-ST elevation myocardial infarction (NSTEMI), and unstable angina (UA). Patients presenting with chest pain or a symptom that could be due to an acute coronary syndrome should have an ECG within 10 minutes of presentation [1]. The initial ECG begins the well-defined process of determining the correct diagnosis and beginning the process of risk stratification.

ST Elevation Myocardial Infarction (STEMI)

A STEMI is diagnosed when a patient has a clinical presentation of acute coronary ischemia with diagnostic ST elevation (STE) on the ECG as defined in the third universal definition of myocardial infarction [2]. ST elevation on an ECG that meets criteria for acute myocardial injury correlates pathologically with acute thrombotic occlusion of an epicardial coronary artery. In the absence of contraindications, a STEMI is managed by emergent reperfusion therapy with either thrombolytic therapy or percutaneous intervention. A STEMI is a life-threatening condition with a wide range in prognosis depending on the patient's co-morbidities, time to presentation, time to reperfusion, and effectiveness of therapy. Prognostic value is present on the ECG during

Electrocardiogram in Clinical Medicine, First Edition. Edited by William J. Brady, Michael J. Lipinski, Andrew E. Darby, Michael C. Bond, Nathan P. Charlton, Korin Hudson, and Kelly Williamson.

myocardial injury, in the evolution of the ECG in response to therapy, and in long-term changes on the ECG.

The ECG during Myocardial Injury

There is a predictable evolution of ECG changes that begin when an epicardial coronary artery becomes occluded. This evolution of change is altered with reperfusion. Both the initial evolution and response of the ECG to reperfusion contain prognostic information. The first electrocardiographic change seen on an ECG following occlusion of a coronary artery is an increase in the amplitude of the T waves (termed hyperacute T waves). A hyperacute T wave represents a qualitative assessment and does not have a formal definition. Hyperacute T waves can also be seen in hyperkalemia and in situations where there is an increased QRS voltage – left ventricular hypertrophy. Dressler and Roesler [3] in 1947 described the initial ECG changes in acute myocardial infarction in 27 patients. In 25 of the 27 patients an increase in the amplitude of the T wave was the first electrocardiographic change (see Figure 2.5.1). An increase in T-wave amplitude is not chronic and typically within 24 the T waves had inverted. In five patients the T wave remained at an increased amplitude past 24 hours, and in these patients there was a 60% mortality compared to 14% mortality in the group with T waves regressing within the first 24 hours. The next phase of ST-T wave

changes in the setting of an occluded epicardial coronary artery is elevation of the ST segment; therefore, patients with hyperacute T waves in the setting of a possible acute coronary syndrome require serial ECGs. The degree of elevation and the number of leads involved is directly related to infarct size and patient outcome; further, patients with greater degree and number of leads with STE have a relatively greater benefit from fibrinolytic therapy [4, 5]. As an acute infarct progresses pathologic Q waves may develop in the distribution of the infarct territory (See Figure 2.5.1 where Q waves are present in V1/V2).

The pattern of ST elevation on the ECG indicates the region of myocardial injury and suggests the causative epicardial coronary artery. Anterior STE (Leads V1–V4) is due to occlusion of the left anterior descending coronary artery (see Figure 2.5.2) and is related to a worse outcome as compared to inferior ST elevation (Leads II, III, aVF) which can be caused by occlusion of either the right coronary artery or circumflex artery [6–8]. Lee et al. [6] published a multivariate analysis on the 41 021 patients enrolled in the GUSTO-I trial (randomized trial evaluating four thrombolytic strategies in patients with STEMI). The 30-day mortality for an anterior wall infarction was 9.9% compared to 5% in infarctions in the inferior wall (Odds Ratio 2.11). Similarly, Schroeder et al. [7] reported a 30-day mortality of 6.5% in anterior infarct versus 3.8% in inferior infarcts in a substudy of 2719 patients in the InTIME II Study (Intravenous nPA for treatment of infarcting myocardium

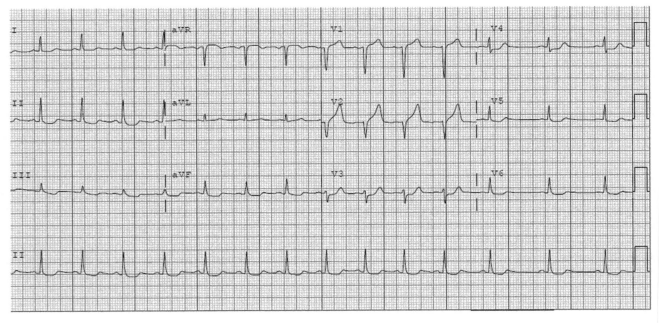

Figure 2.5.1 A 53-year-old male presenting with chest pain. ECG with a hyperacute T wave in lead V2 and diffuse ST depression. The T wave was significantly more peaked compared to his prior ECG. He had an occluded proximal LAD and had a large anterior myocardial infarction.

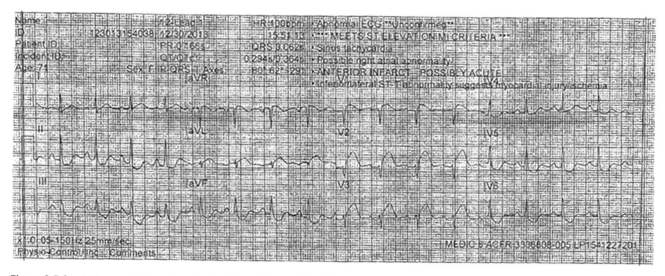

Figure 2.5.2 A 71-year-old female who developed chest pain while shopping. Pre-hospital ECG shows anterior ST elevation and inferolateral ST depression. STEMI alert was activated pre-hospital, which facilitated a rapid door to balloon time.

early). Trzeciak et al. in a substudy of patients with STEMI and cardiogenic shock in the PL-ACS registry demonstrated a significant difference in outcome based on the angiographically determined infarct related artery. Morality in hospital, at 30 days, at 6 months, and at 12 months had a similar trend between the infarct artery groups. The 30-day mortality for the left main, left anterior descending, circumflex, and right coronary artery groups respectively were 72.7%, 47.6%, 46.6%, and 36.6%. The one-year mortality for the groups were 77.7%, 58.2%, 55.1%, and 45%, respectively. Infarct size is directly related to the amount of myocardium distal to the obstructed coronary artery, time to reperfusion, extent of reperfusion, and presence or absence of any collateral circulation. Final infarct size as measured by CMR three months after an acute infarct provides independent prognostic information. An increase in infarct size is directly related to all-cause mortality and admissions for heart failure [9].

The circumflex coronary artery supplies the lateral wall of the heart and can also supply varying portions of the posterior and inferior walls of the heart; rarely, the circumflex coronary artery can provide marginal branches that supply the right ventricle. The lateral and posterior walls of the heart are not well represented on the standard 12-lead ECG, and infarcts related to the circumflex artery in general are smaller than those involving the left anterior descending (LAD) and right coronary arteries (RCA). For these reasons, occlusion of the left circumflex coronary artery may not present with ST elevation on the ECG. This understandably represents a diagnostic challenge and often delays reperfusion therapy. Studies of STEMI, therefore, underrepresent myocardial infarctions due to acute

occlusion of the left circumflex. Approximately 50% of patients presenting with acute occlusion of the left circumflex coronary artery do not have ST elevation on the ECG [10, 11], which is in contrast to >93% of patients with an acutely occluded left anterior descending artery have anterior STE on ECG at the time of presentation [10]. See Figure 2.5.3 for an example of an ECG in a patient with acute occlusion of the left circumflex coronary artery. Huey et al. followed 241 patients with acute myocardial infarction; 17% of the patients had infarction due the left circumflex coronary artery and 38% of these patients did not have ST segment elevation or depression on their ECG [11]. Despite not being recognized easily, patients with acute occlusion of the left circumflex artery would benefit from early reperfusion [12]. Kim et al. [13] using the Korea Acute Myocardial Infarction Registry sought to better define patient characteristics and outcomes in patients presenting with acute myocardial infarction due to angiographically confirmed occlusion of the circumflex coronary artery. Door-to-balloon time in patients with circumflex coronary artery occlusion averaged 143 minutes which was double the average time for occlusion of the RCA or LAD coronary arteries. Primary PCI was performed in 43.4% of patients with circumflex occlusion compared to 78.9% and 74.5% for the LAD and RCA coronary arteries. There was no statistically significant difference in hospital mortality between groups based upon infarct related artery. Stribling et al. [14] used the National Cardiovascular Data Registry to determine if there was a difference in outcome between patients with acute occlusion of the left circumflex coronary artery who presented as either a STEMI or NSTEMI. There were 27711 patients who were included that

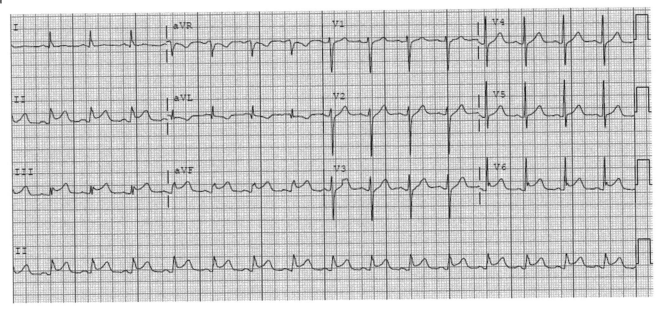

Figure 2.5.3 A 55-year-old male with inferolateral STEMI. He had an occluded left circumflex artery.

presented with an acute infarction and were found to have occlusion of the left circumflex coronary artery: 67% of the patients presented as a STEMI and 33% presented as a NSTEMI (it was possible to reclassify patients into the STEMI arm after angiography revealed occlusion). Patients with a STEMI as the clinical presentation had a worse in-hospital mortality and were more likely to have a proximal occlusion of the left circumflex as compared to patients presenting with a NSTEMI [14]. It is important to not solely rely on electrocardiographic findings to determine the need for emergent cardiac catheterization. Clinical parameters must dictate early catheterization in patients with chest pain that can't be managed medically, hemodynamic or electrical instability, or heart failure.

The degree of STE and number of leads with STE relate to patient outcome [15–17]. This correlation was evident prior to reperfusion therapies. Nielsen in 1973 demonstrated that major STE (≥5 mm in anterior leads and ≥2 mm in inferior leads) as compared to less STE was associated with increased mortality, heart failure, cardiac arrest, cardiogenic shock, and AV block [17]. Fresco et al. [15] in a substudy of the GISSI-2 trial showed in 7755 patients that in-hospital mortality increased as the number of leads with ST elevation increased in an acute MI. Schröder et al. demonstrated in 2719 patients in the InTIME II Study (compared two thrombolytic therapies for acute MI) that the degree of STE was related to mortality. Bhave et al. used the ACTIVATE-SF database of patients presenting with STEMI to look for risk factors for post infarct LVEF of <40%; ST segment elevation of >2 mm had an odds ratio of 2.78 for the development of a LVEF <40% [18]. ST-segment deviation

has been quantitatively assessed using three different methods – summed ST elevation (sum STE) [16], summed ST deviation (sum STD) [19], and maximum ST elevation (max STE) [7]. The sum STE score is obtained by adding together the degree of ST elevation 20 ms after the QRS complex in leads I, aVL, and V1–V6 for anterior infarcts and in leads II, III, aVF, V5, and V6 for inferior infarcts [16]. A large sum STE score was associated with a lower rate of successful reperfusion and an increased mortality in the ISAM study (streptokinase versus placebo in acute myocardial infarction) [16]. The sum STD adds the sum of reciprocal ST depression to the sum of the ST elevation [20]. In both anterior and inferior infarcts the sum of reciprocal ST depression is directly related to infarct size and mortality [20].

ECG findings can predict the presence of a right ventricular (RV) infarct. The RV is not well represented on the standard 12-lead ECG. The presence of ST elevation in lead V1 in the setting of inferior ST elevation (with lead III greater in amplitude than lead II) suggests RCA occlusion and RV infarction. Right-sided chest leads are more sensitive in detecting an RV infarct with STE in lead V4R being the most specific ECG finding for an RV infarct. It has been reported that in the setting of an inferior infarct due to the RCA (STE in lead III greater than in lead II) ST elevation in V1, V4R, or both has a sensitivity of 79% and a specificity of 100% for RV infarction [21]. Typically, the right ventricle is supplied by acute marginal branches from the right coronary artery. An occlusion of the RCA proximal to the marginal branches results in RV infarction. Rarely, the right ventricle can be supplied by branches of a dominant circumflex artery. As a result of the anatomy described, a RV infarction will almost always occur with an inferior LV wall infarction due to proximal occlusion of the RCA; an isolated infarction of the RV is rare. Approximately 25% of inferior STEMIs are accompanied by an RV infarct [22]. The presence of an RV infarct is prognostically important and has important implications on hemodynamic management. The clinical syndrome of an RV infarction often includes elevated jugular venous pressure, hypotension, and shock in the presence of clear lung fields. Due to the fact that an RV infarct requires a proximal occlusion of the RCA, it is associated with a larger infarct size, more SA and AV node involvement, bradycardia, and heart block with up to 50% of patients with an RV infarct having high degree AV block [23, 24]. RV infarction can result in increased RA pressure, which is the presence of an interatrial defect (PFO/ASD) and can lead to hypoxemia due to right to left shunting. There is a higher incidence of atrial fibrillation (up to one-third of patients) and ventricular arrhythmias in the setting of an RV infarct [23, 25]. Further, in-hospital mortality is increased when there is an RV infarction in the setting of an inferior STEMI as compared to an inferior STEMI alone (31% versus 6% in-hospital mortality) [26]. Unlike the left ventricle, the RV tends to recover fully following an infarction and long-term mortality based on RV infarction alone is probably not increased.

The presence of a left bundle branch block (LBBB) on the ECG during a clinical presentation that is potentially an acute coronary syndrome complicates the diagnosis and acute management. It is known that the presence of a LBBB during an acute infarction is a marker of increased risk [27]. A new LBBB in a clinical setting consistent with an acute myocardial infarction is considered a STEMI equivalent; however, most patients presenting with a possible acute coronary syndrome with a LBBB on ECG do not have an acutely occluded coronary artery [28] (see Figure 2.5.4). The third universal definition of myocardial infarction published in 2012 [2] includes a new LBBB as a criteria for acute infarction if there is a rise and fall of cardiac troponin. The 2013 AHA STEMI guidelines [29] state that a LBBB alone should not be considered in isolation to represent an acute myocardial infarction.

Jain et al. [28] published a retrospective study of a cohort of patients with presumed STEMI from a large PCI network to better define implications of a presumably new LBBB. There were 892 patients with STEMI between 2004 and 2009; 36 of these patients had a new or presumably new LBBB. A final diagnosis of an acute coronary syndrome was made in 39% of these patients with an occluded coronary artery found in five of the patients with an acute infarct (two of the five had an occluded LAD). The group of patients with a LBBB were older had a higher TIMI risk score, and if taken for cardiac catheterization had a longer door-to-balloon time. The presence of a LBBB masks many of the ischemic changes typically seen. Sgarbossa et al. [30] evaluated the 131 patients (0.5% of the total enrolled patients) in the GUSTO-1 clinical trial who presented with chest pain and an ECG showing a LBBB and compared ECG findings to control patients with known CAD and

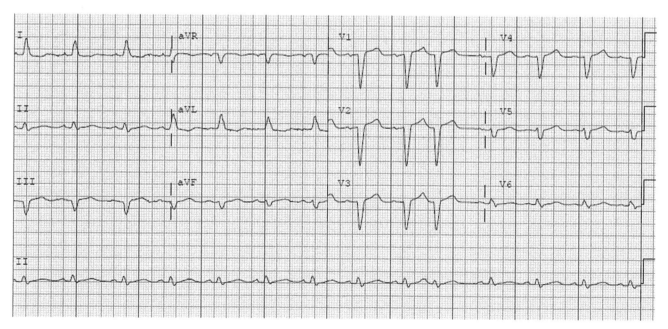

Figure 2.5.4 A 52-year-old male presented with shortness of breath. ECG showed a presumed new LBBB. He did not have an occluded coronary artery.

chronic LBBB. Three ECG criteria were found to have independent value in the diagnosis of an acute MI in patients with a LBBB. These three criteria are collectively called the Sgarbossa criteria and include: ST-segment elevation ≥1 mm concordant with the QRS complex; ST-segment depression ≥1 mm in leads V1, V2, or V3; and ST segment elevation ≥5 mm discordant with the QRS complex [30]. These findings had respective odds ratios of an acute MI of 25.2, 6, and 4.3.

The ECG in Response to Therapy

Reperfusion of myocardium is prognostically important. Time to reperfusion is inversely related to outcome. Further, the presence of absence of reperfusion often guides therapy. There are a number of features on the ECG that indicate that reperfusion has or has not occurred. These features include resolution of ST segment changes, T-wave changes, and accelerated idioventricular rhythm (AIVR).

In the fibrinolytic era, resolution of ST elevation on ECG was used as a marker of reperfusion and was a strong predictor of outcome, infarct size, and left ventricular ejection fraction [8, 16, 31, 32]. Schröder et al. [16] did a retrospective evaluation of the ISAM study group (randomized trial of streptokinase versus placebo for STEMI). ST segment resolution of >70% at 3 hours was strongly predictive of a good outcome and small infarct. In comparison, ST segment elevation resolution of <30% at 3 hours was predictive of a higher mortality and large infarct. There were 1431 patients evaluated in this study with mortality rates at 2 years of 8.1%, 13.7%, and 20.8% based on complete (>70%), partial (30–70%), and no resolution (<30%) at 3 hours, respectively. Further, anterior infarctions were associated with less ST resolution compared to inferior infarctions. Dong J et al. in 2002 [33] published a prospective evaluation of 243 patients presenting with acute STEMI treated with either coronary stenting (122 patients) or thrombolysis (121 patients). Ninety minutes after initiation of therapy an ECG was obtained and patients were grouped based on complete, partial, and no ST segment resolution. Early resolution correlated with smaller infarct size on Tc-99 m sestamibi scintigraphy and six-month mortality.

The resolution of ST segment elevation in the PCI era remains a valuable prognostic tool (see Figure 2.5.5). Wong et al. in 2010 [34] performed a systematic review to investigate the question of whether ST segment resolution following percutaneous coronary intervention had the same prognostic value as accepted following fibrinolytic therapy. Eighteen studies were included with 32 341 patients in the fibrinolytic cohort and 1913 patients in the PCI cohort. Higher ST resolution scores were equally associated with lower 30-day mortality in both the fibrinolytic and PCI groups. Claeys et al. [35] prospectively enrolled 91 patients with acute STEMI treated with PTCA. At the end of the coronary intervention, patients were separated into two groups based on resolution of ST segment elevation as

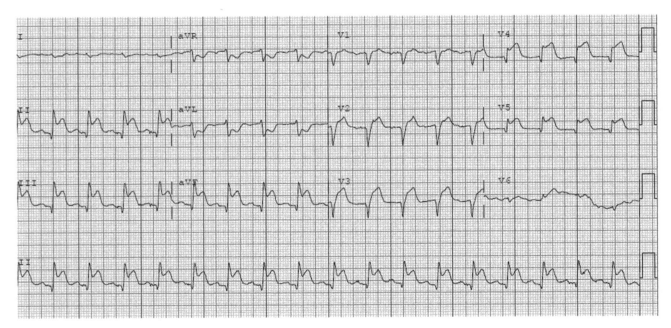

Figure 2.5.5 First ECG after RCA reperfusion in patient from Figure 2.5.1. There has been complete resolution of inferior ST elevation. Pathologic Q waves are not present.

compared to ECG on presentation (<50% or >50%). Thirty-six percent of patients had ST-segment resolution of less than 50%. The cardiac death rate was 15% at 1 year for the group with <50% ST-segment resolution, compared with a death rate of 2% at 1 year for patients with >50% ST-segment resolution. Age >55 and SBP <120 were the strongest predictors of <50% ST-segment resolution. Buller et al. evaluated the ECG 30 minutes after primary PCI in 4866 patients in the APEX-AMI trial using six different methods to quantify ST-segment resolution. Irrespective of the method used, ST-segment recovery was a strong predictor of death and heart failure.

A study by Ndrepepa et al. [36] that enrolled patients with an acute STEMI who were treated with primary PCI questioned whether ST segment resolution was associated with a better outcome in patients who were reperfused by PCI. In this study, 900 patients presenting with STEMI within first 24 hours after symptom onset were treated with primary PCI. An ECG was obtained at presentation and then at 90 and 120 minutes after first balloon inflation. Three groups were then defined – no resolution (<30%), 30–70% (partial resolution), and >70% (complete resolution). Five-year mortality was the primary endpoint and there was no difference between the three groups of ST segment resolution. Further, ST segment resolution was not related to LVEF or recurrent MI. This study had significantly different results compared to the above-mentioned trials. There were fewer patients in this trial, and the time of the ECG was 90 minutes after intervention, where Claeys et al. and Buller et al. used an ECG at 30 minutes after

intervention to determine ST segment resolution. See Figure 2.5.6 as an example of a patient with myocardial injury in both the LAD and RCA territories that after reperfusion had persistent ST elevation. This patient's course was complicated by a large infarction of both the anterior and inferior walls along with cardiogenic shock requiring placement of an intra-aortic balloon pump; he survived to hospital discharge. The majority of evidence supports that delay of ST segment elevation resolution is a marker of a poor prognosis.

AIVR is a wide complex tachycardia that is faster than a ventricular escape rhythm (30–40 bpm) but slower than ventricular tachycardia (VT) (<120 bpm). It occurs commonly in the setting of STEMI (up to 20% of patients) and has been considered a marker of reperfusion. The presence of AIVR is considered to be a positive prognostic indicator, as it suggests reperfusion. See Figures 2.5.7 and 2.5.8 for examples of AIVR.

ECG after Completion of Infarction

A Q wave is the first negative deflection of a QRS complex that is not preceded by an R wave. A pathologic Q wave was defined previously and is an electrocardiographic sign of a prior myocardial infarction (see Figure 2.5.9). A large R wave in V1/V2 can be a Q-wave equivalent secondary to a posterior myocardial infarction. A Q wave occurs due to the electrical silence of infarcted tissue, and the presence of Q waves identifies the anatomic region of a prior infarction.

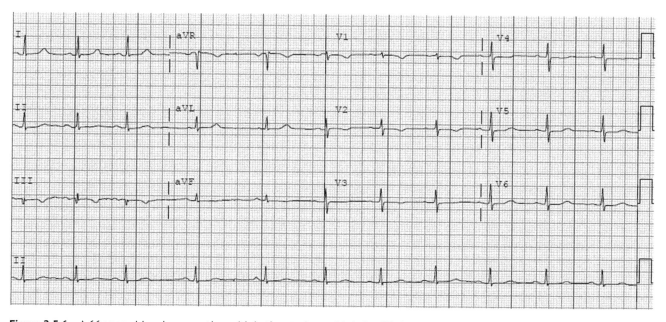

Figure 2.5.6 A 66-year-old male presenting with both anterior and inferior ST elevation; found to have an occluded LAD and severe stenosis of the proximal RCA.

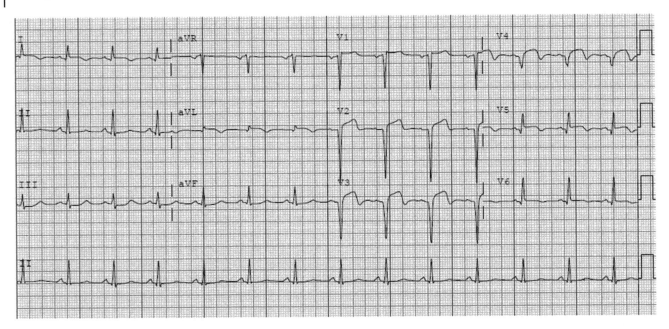

Figure 2.5.7 Two runs of accelerated idioventricular rhythm (AIVR).

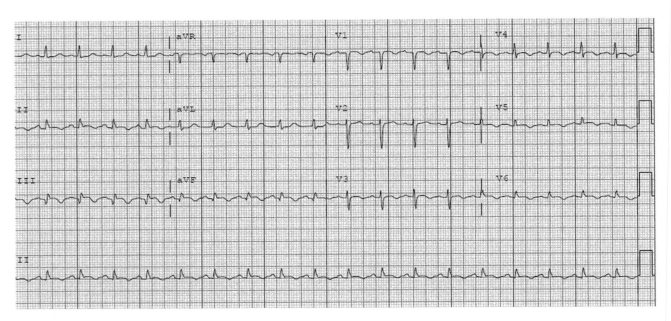

Figure 2.5.8 Accelerated idioventricular rhythm (AIVR).

A pathologic Q wave can develop on an ECG after either a transmural or subendocardial myocardial infarction. It was previously thought that only transmural infarcts could result in a Q wave; however, it has been shown subendocardial infarctions can also cause pathological Q waves and that transmural infarctions do not always result in pathologic Q wave formation [37, 38]. An infarction that results in a Q wave tends to involve more myocardium than an infarction that does not result in a Q wave [37]. An individual patient's first myocardial infarction is more likely to result in the formation of a Q wave, and subsequent infarcts in the same patient are less likely to generate a Q wave [37]. Myocardial infarctions were previously classified as either Q wave or non-Q wave; however, this classification system is no longer used. A Q wave is valuable in diagnosing the presence of an infarct, but it has limited value in terms of sensitivity, and the lack of a pathologic Q wave does not equate to the lack of prior myocardial infarction. Following

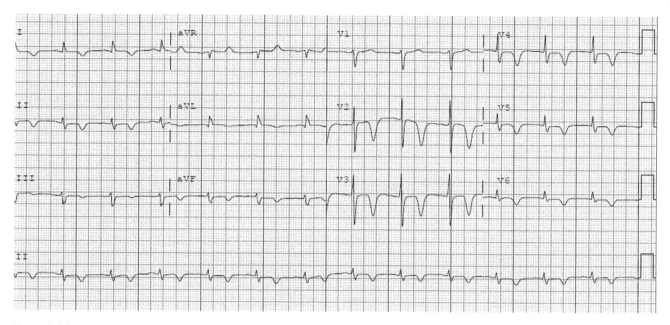

Figure 2.5.9 A 45-year-old male with anterior and lateral STEMI. He later developed an apical thrombus.

thrombolytic therapy for STEMI, patients whose infarctions do not result in a Q wave have a better prognosis than in those patients who develop a pathologic Q wave [39]. In patients presenting within six hours of symptom onset who are diagnosed with STEMI, the presence of a Q wave on the ECG in the infarct territory is a poor prognostic sign [40]. Patients with Q waves at presentation are more likely to be older, have diabetes, have higher degree of ST elevation, and have longer time to presentation, and these patients have increased risk of mortality, heart failure, and shock [40]. Also, patients with Q waves at presentation are less likely to have normal perfusion following PCI, less likely to have complete ST segment elevation resolution, and overall have increased degree of biomarker elevation [40].

The distinction between Q wave and non-Q-wave myocardial infarction may be important prognostically, both early and in the late post-discharge phase. Q-wave infarctions were previously termed *transmural*, whereas non-Q-wave infarctions were referred to as "nontransmural" or "subendocardial." Such pathologic distinctions are imprecise [37]. Confinement of the infarction to the subendocardial zone is observed in only ~ 50% of patients studied at autopsy following non-Q-wave infarct events. Q-wave infarctions are anatomically larger, resulting in lower ejection fractions and higher short-term mortality rates, especially in the pre-reperfusion era (Figure 2.5.10). Non-Q-wave infractions are best thought of as incomplete events with higher rates of recurrent infarction (usually in the same territory as the original injury), and late death. Indeed, by one to two years, mortality rates are comparable.

Non-Q-wave infarctions may initially be small or limited in their size and scope by virtue of spontaneous thrombolysis or by the presence of collateral channels subserving the infarct zone [41–43].

UA/NSTEMI

UA and NSTEMI are two similar acute coronary syndromes in which there is a decrease in myocardial oxygen supply due to an acute change of a coronary lesion that results in decreased blood flow to a region of myocardium. Among these two syndromes are a wide variety of clinical presentations and outcomes. UA can be an insidious problem that occurs over weeks while a NSTEMI can present acutely and result in a large infarction. The ECG is valuable in diagnosing the presence of myocardial ischemia and many of the ECGs findings during a presentation with either UA/NSTEMI are useful prognostically. A normal ECG is not uncommon during presentation for UA/NSTEMI, and a normal ECG does not rule out an acute coronary syndrome.

ST-Segment Depression

The hallmark of myocardial ischemia on the ECG is dynamic ST segment depression. The degree of ST segment depression is a continuous variable – any ST depression of ≥0.5 mm confers some risk and with an increase in ST segment depression there is a linear increase in specificity for

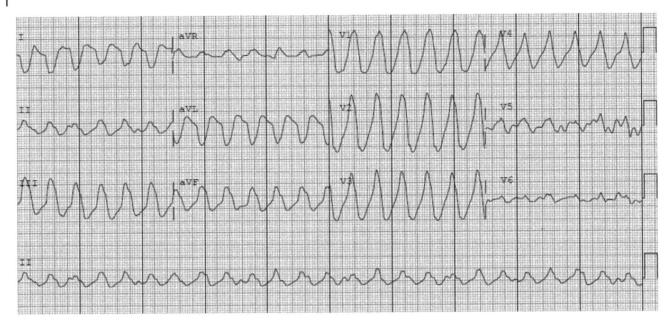

Figure 2.5.10 Thirty-five day mortality rate by percent sum of ST segment resolution. No, partial, and complete resolution were, respectively, associated with a 17.5, 4.3, and 2.5% mortality at 35 days in the INJECT trial (randomized patients to reteplase and streptokinase for acute MI). Source: Copied directly from reference [19].

myocardial ischemia and increased risk of adverse events. Diagnostic ECG stress testing attempts to create myocardial ischemia by increasing myocardial oxygen demand beyond oxygen supply due to a coronary lesion resulting in limited flow. In the setting of an acute coronary syndrome, this mismatch in myocardial oxygen balance is caused by an abrupt decrease in flow from acute narrowing or a coronary artery; thus, resulting in new myocardial ischemia either with exertion or at rest. The presence ST depression on the admission ECG in the setting of a myocardial infarction is predictive of increased 30-day and 6-month mortality. The presence of ST depression is also related to an increase risk of three-vessel disease with Savonitto et al. reporting 36% of patients with ST depression on their presenting ECG during an acute coronary syndrome being diagnosed angiographically with three-vessel disease [44]. Cannon et al. [22] analyzed the ECG at time of enrollment in the TIMI III registry to evaluate the prognostic significance of ECG changes in patients diagnosed with UA or NSTEMI. In a cohort of 1416 patients, 12.6% had ST segment depression ≥1 mm, 20.5% had T-wave inversion, and 60% had no ECG changes. Patients with ST depression were more likely to have three-vessel CAD and CAD that was treated with revascularization. At one year, the mortality for patients with ≥1 mm ST depression was 9.8% compared to 5.5% in patients without ECG changes. Anterior ST depression was associated with a higher risk of death or MI at one year compared to inferior/lateral ST depression. T-wave inversions in this study were not related to outcome.

Degree of ST segment depression has a linear relationship to risk of death. Kaul et al. in patients with an acute coronary syndrome showed the mortality at six months to be 2.9% in patients without ST segment depression, 5.3% in patients with 1 mm ST segment depression, and 11.7% in patients with 2 or more mm of ST segment depression [45]. The TIMI risk score is a well-known tool for assessing risk in patients with UA or NSTEMI. ST segment depression is one of seven clinical variables in the scoring tool [46]. The presence of ST depression (either new or persistent from admission) on an ECG at the time of discharge following an admission for NSTEMI is related to increased mortality at six months and increased risk of recurrent myocardial infarction [47]. ST depression involving eight or more leads with ST elevation in lead AVR and V1 is considered to represent global ischemia and is associated with left main or three-vessel CAD in 75% of patients [48]. A patient who has both active ischemic symptoms and these electrocardiographic findings should be considered a high-risk patient. See Figure 2.5.11 for an example of a patient presenting with an acute coronary syndrome who was found to have severe left main disease.

T-Wave Inversions

The vector of the T wave is normally in the same direction as the QRS complex. In the setting of ischemia T-wave inversions can occur. T-wave inversions can be an electrocardiographic

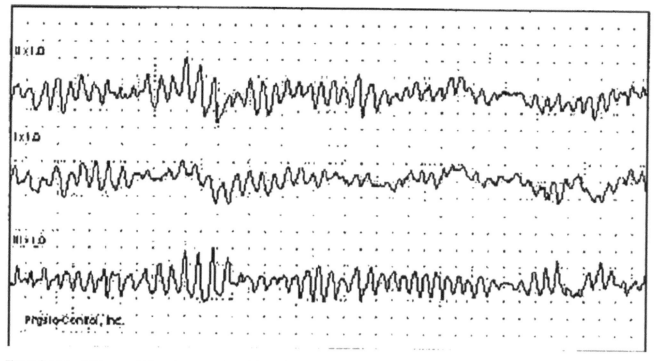

Figure 2.5.11 A 76-year-old female presenting with cardiogenic shock. Note the ST segment elevation in lead aVR. Found to have severe left main stenosis.

marker of ischemia; however, they are much less specific for ischemia than ST depression, and the differential diagnosis for T-wave inversions is broad. The inferior leads are particularly susceptible to alterations in T-wave morphology. Inverted T waves in the inferior leads can be due to patient position, hyperventilation, or acute intra-abdominal pathology in addition to ischemia. T-wave inversions do not localize ischemia to a particular myocardial region, unless they are consistent with Wellens T wave discussed in the subsequent section. Savonitto et al. performed a retrospective analysis of the presenting ECG in patients presenting with an acute coronary syndrome in the Gusto IIb trial. The 30-day rate of death or reinfarction was 5.5% in the group of patients with either T-wave inversions (or pseudonormalization), 9.4% in patients with ST elevation, 10.5% in patients with ST segment depression, and 12.4% in patients with both ST elevation and depression [44]. In this cohort, patients with T-wave inversions had a rate of angiographically normal coronary arteries of 19%. Compared to other electrocardiographic markers of ischemia, T-wave changes have the most benign prognosis.

Wellens syndrome identifies a subgroup of patients presenting with an acute coronary syndrome. Zwaan, Bär, and Wellens in 1982 published a case series of 145 patients presenting with UA; 18% of the patients in this series had symmetrical deep anterior T-wave inversions (now termed Wellens T waves) [49]. This group of patients had a high rate of significant proximal LAD obstruction and significant

risk of developing an anterior myocardial infarction. T-wave inversions do not anatomically localize ischemia except in the presence of Wellens T waves, which localizes ischemia to the LAD territory. Anterior T-wave inversions can also be caused by persistent juvenile pattern, RVH, RBBB, Takotsubo cardiomyopathy, and intracranial pathology.

A normal ECG or an ECG with minor nonspecific findings can occur in the setting of an acute coronary syndrome. The presence of dynamic ST depression can diagnose ischemia and the presence of T-wave inversions can strongly suggest ischemia, but the absence of ischemic changes does not rule out an acute coronary syndrome. The presence of a normal or nonspecific ECG in the setting of either UA/NSTEMI is prognostically valuable, as these patients have a lower risk of death. However, patients who initially present with a normal ECG but then develop ischemic changes have an increased risk of in-hospital adverse events compared to patients whose initial ECG showed the same ischemic changes [50]. This finding may be due to a delay in therapy in patients with a normal ECG. It is important to remember that though a normal ECG is prognostically valuable, it does not rule out an acute coronary syndrome. Other data including the patient's history, symptoms, physical exam, imaging, and biomarkers are necessary to either establish or rule out the diagnosis of an acute coronary syndrome.

Initial Normal ECG

A normal initial ECG has both diagnostic and prognostic value. Karlson et al. assessed the additive benefit of electrocardiography in 7157 consecutive patients with chest pain [51]. The presence of a normal ECG was associated with acute MI in only 6% of patients, while new ischemic ECG changes in the setting of typical chest pain were associated with MI in 88% of patients. Depending on the characteristics of the patient's chief complaint, the incidence of acute infarction among patients with an initially normal ECG can range from <0.6% to 26% [51, 52]. Also, the risk of a major in-hospital cardiac complication is very low in the vast majority of these patients. Indeed, in one study by Brush et al., it was shown that even among admitted patients with a > 75% probability of acute coronary syndrome, those with a normal initial and follow-up ECG had a <1% incidence of life-threatening events such as VF, sustained VT or high grade AV block [53]. Other investigators have confirmed the excellent prognosis of patients with chest pain and no ECG abnormalities, including those who are subsequently diagnosed with acute MI based on serial cardiac enzymes [54, 55].

Takotsubo Cardiomyopathy

Takotsubo cardiomyopathy, also known as stress-induced cardiomyopathy, apical ballooning syndrome, or broken heart syndrome, can mimic the presentation of an acute coronary syndrome. This cardiomyopathy results in a typical pattern of LV dysfunction in which the circumferential base of the heart is preserved and the apex is dilated an akinetic, which is how it received the name apical ballooning syndrome.

The pattern of left ventricular dysfunction in Takotsubo cardiomyopathy is not based on vascular territories. There are less common variations of this cardiomyopathy that result in which the circumferential midwall or apex are akinetic and the remainder of the myocardium is normal or hypercontractile. There are no specific diagnostic criteria, but in general the diagnosis is made when the above features are present in a patient with an acute clinical presentation (cardiac symptoms, ECG changes, positive troponin) with other etiologies of LV dysfunction ruled out – coronary artery disease, myocarditis, and pheochromocytoma. Takotsubo cardiomyopathy is usually precipitated by an acute stress event that can be emotional, physical, or medical in nature. The pathophysiology of this disease is accepted to be secondary to an abnormal myocardial response to increased circulating catecholamines. In general, the clinical course is favorable and most patients have complete normalization of left ventricular function. A small percentage of patients can present with recurrent episodes of Takotsubo cardiomyopathy. Complications of Takotsubo cardiomyopathy can include heart failure, shock, ventricular tachyarrhythmias, long QT with subsequent torsades, and LV outflow obstruction due to the hypercontractile base.

The ECG in Takotsubo cardiomyopathy can be normal or show ST segment elevation, T-wave inversions, nonspecific ST-T wave changes, or new or old LBBB. Approximately one-third of patients present with STE and one-third with T-wave inversions (see Figure 2.5.12). Electrocardiographic findings have not been shown to be related to degree of LV dysfunction or outcome [56, 57]. The majority of patients with Takotsubo cardiomyopathy develop QT prolongation that can result in the development of torsades de pointes (TdP). TdP is more likely in patients with other risk factors such as genetic long QT syndrome, medications that prolong QT, and in the setting of electrolyte abnormalities such as hypokalemia, hypocalcaemia, and hypomagnesaemia [58].

Arrhythmia and Conduction Disease

The cardiac conduction system is affected in both chronic ischemic heart disease and in acute myocardial infarction. Cardiac scar from prior infarction can create the electrical substrate needed for development of VT. The risk of conduction disease or tachyarrhythmia in the setting of an acute infarct is related to infarct size. Conduction disease and tachyarrhythmias occur more often in patients with high degrees of STE on ECG at presentation [17]. Tachyarrhythmias and conduction disease are markers of severity of disease but can also contribute to rapid clinical decline and are a mechanism of SCD and require urgent therapy. The following sections will discuss the prognostic relationship between the development of a tachyarrhythmia or conduction disease in the setting of an acute infarct.

Ventricular Arrhythmias

Myocardial ischemia creates a myocardial substrate that is prone to ventricular arrhythmias. There are many proposed mechanisms that include changes in ion currents, electrolyte changes, enhanced automaticity, and increased sympathetic activity [59]. Ventricular arrhythmias are a common mechanism of SCD. VT and ventricular fibrillation (VF) can occur during myocardial ischemia, early after infarction, or as a late consequence due to myocardial scar. VT/VF are significantly more common in STEMI as compared to NSTEMI. The incidence of sustained VT (>30 seconds in duration or having hemodynamic significance) or VF during a STEMI is approximately 5% [60] as compared

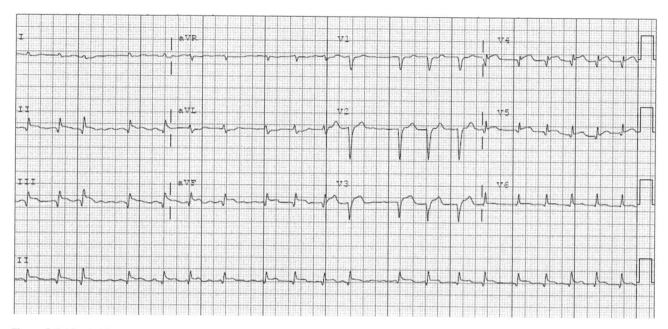

Figure 2.5.12 A 60-year-old male with two prior liver transplants admitted with chest pain and diagnosed with Takotsubo's cardiomyopathy. ECG shows Wellen's T waves; ACS with LAD occlusion and Takostsubo's were both possible. His echocardiogram showed basal hypercontractility and a dilated, akinetic LV apex. Coronary arteries were angiographically normal. His left ventricular function returned to normal.

to 2.6% in patients admitted for NSTEMI [61]. Premature ventricular contractions (PVCs), VT, and VF will be discussed. AIVR was discussed in the reperfusion section of STEMI.

Premature Ventricular Contractions

PVCs are early single ventricular beats that interrupt the underlying rhythm. PVCs are common, and when occurring occasionally are of no prognostic significance. In the setting of myocardial ischemia it was previously thought that the presence of PVCs was predictive of the development of VT/VF, and lidocaine was used to suppress PVCs. However, it was shown that this practice decreased ventricular arrhythmias at the cost of increasing mortality (via a mechanism of increased bradycardia and asystolic events) [62]. It is now known that PVCs occur just as commonly in patients who do and who do not develop VF and their treatment/suppression in the setting of a myocardial infarction is not recommended [59].

Ventricular Tachycardia

VT is a regular wide complex rhythm with a rate >120 that is dissociated from atrial activity. The underlying mechanism of monomorphic VT is usually re-entry around

myocardial scar (increased automaticity is a less common mechanism); therefore, monomorphic VT is not an arrhythmia of ischemia but rather an arrhythmia of scar. Nonsustained VT (defined as three beats in a row with a rate >120) is common early in the course of a myocardial infarction and in the setting of NSTEMI has been shown to be associated with an increased risk of SCD over the next year [63]. However, sustained VT occurs later in the course of myocardial infarction and occurs more frequently in patients with large infarction and left ventricular dysfunction; in this setting, the presence of VT is associated with increased mortality [59] (See Figure 2.5.13 for example of sustained VT). VT often results in a pulseless cardiac arrest, but irrespective of its acute hemodynamic effects, sustained VT must be treated quickly as to prevent clinical deterioration or prevent degeneration into VF.

Ventricular Fibrillation

VF is a disordered, low-amplitude ventricular arrhythmia that requires immediate treatment with defibrillation or otherwise it results in death (see Figure 2.5.14). VT can at times be tolerated hemodynamically; however, VF invariably is associated with a pulseless cardiac arrest. Most deaths in the setting of STEMI occur during the first hour and VF is thought to be the mechanism. VF in the setting of myocardial ischemia is considered either primary or secondary.

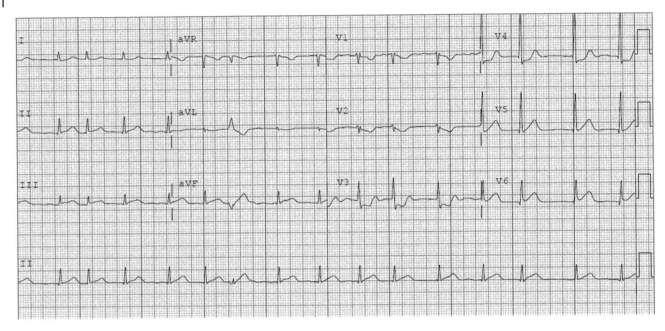

Figure 2.5.13 Ventricular tachycardia.

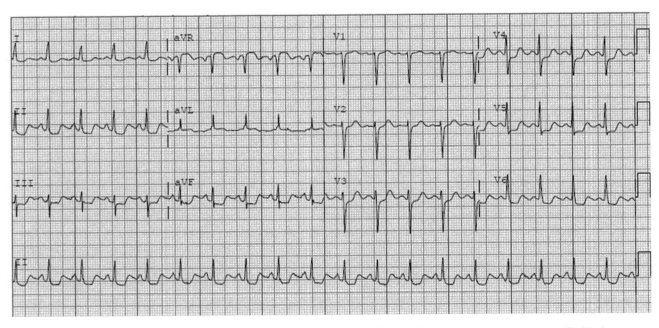

Figure 2.5.14 A 58-year-old female with new onset chest pain, anterior STEMI on ECG, complicated by ventricular fibrillation en route to the emergency department. She received immediate defibrillation and did well following PCI of the LAD.

Primary VF occurs suddenly and unpredictably. Secondary VF occurs in the setting of heart failure or cardiogenic shock. The incidence of primary VF (defined as VF not associated with heart failure or shock in the first 48 hours after myocardial infarction) has been reported to be 2.8% in the thrombolytic era and it is associated with a higher in-hospital mortality (10.8% versus 5.9% in patients without primary VF) [64]. Secondary VF is an independent predictor of in-hospital morality, but not a long term increase in mortality in patients who survive until hospital discharge. The mortality in patients with secondary VF was reported to be 56% as compared to 16% in similar patients without VF in a large study before the use of thrombolytic therapy [65]. In the percutaneous coronary intervention era of reperfusion of myocardial infarction the incidence of VT/VF is similar and is associated with a worse outcome and the risk of VT/VF is increased in patients who have poor coronary flow after intervention or failure of ST segment resolution [66].

Supraventricular Tachycardia

Sinus Tachycardia

Sinus tachycardia can be due to a number of mechanisms in the setting of an acute coronary syndrome, including pain, hypovolemia, hypoxia, heart failure, shock, or due to medications. Sinus tachycardia that persists after treatment for a myocardial infarction is concerning for significant left ventricular dysfunction, as an increased heart rate is required to maintain cardiac output in the setting of decreased stroke volume. In the setting of ischemia, tachycardia increases myocardial oxygen demand and may be a contributing factor to myocardial ischemia.

Heart rate at presentation, heart rate variability, and heart rate at discharge relate to patient prognosis. There is a linear relationship between admission heart rate and mortality in patients presenting with STEMI [67]. A study by Zhang Han et al. [67] evaluated 7249 patients with STEMI. Patients were divided into four quartiles of admission heart rate (Q1 <66 bpm, Q2 66–76 bpm, Q3 77–88 bpm, Q4 >88 bpm). The 30-day all-cause mortality in nondiabetic patients increased from 6.9% in Q1 to 17.3% in Q4 and in diabetic patients the 30-day mortality was 9.4% in Q1 versus 24.6% in Q4. Jensen et al. [68] evaluated heart rate at

discharge in patients enrolled in the BASKET-PROVE trial – a trial comparing BMS to everolimus eluting stent. This trial included about equal portions of patients with stable angina, NSTEMI, and STEMI, all of which received PCI. Heart rate at discharge was found to be significantly associated with prognosis both in terms of mortality and cardiovascular events (see Figure 2.5.15). The use of beta blockers was similar across all heart rates. All-cause mortality at two years was increased 16.9 times in patients with a discharge heart rate greater than 90 bmp as compared to patients with a discharge heart rate < 60. Resting heart rate is also an independent risk factor for cardiovascular mortality, and hospitalization due to a cardiovascular cause in patients with coronary artery disease and in heart failure of either an ischemic or nonischemic etiology [69].

Atrial Fibrillation

Atrial fibrillation is the most common cardiac arrhythmia, and it is both heterogeneous in its presentation and in the patient population in which it is diagnosed. Patients with ischemic heart disease develop atrial fibrillation at a higher incidence than patients without heart disease. Atrial fibrillation can be secondary to atrial ischemia or due to acute heart failure in the setting of a large acute myocardial infarction. RCA occlusion results in a higher incidence of atrial fibrillation than does occlusion of the LAD [17]. The incidence of new atrial fibrillation while admitted for myocardial infarction is approximately 10% [70]. The development of new atrial fibrillation in the setting of an acute

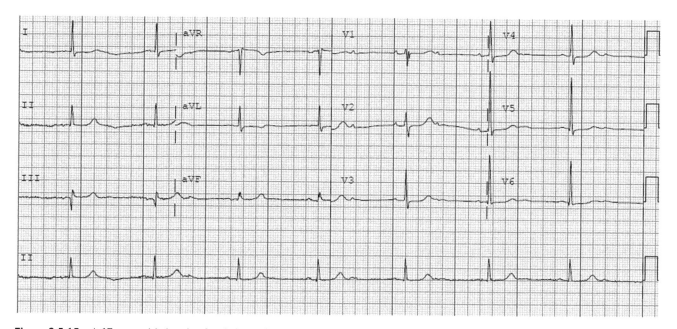

Figure 2.5.15 A 67-year-old shortly after inferior STEMI in the setting of newly discovered three-vessel CAD. He had persistent sinus tachycardia in the setting of severe LV dysfunction and cardiogenic shock.

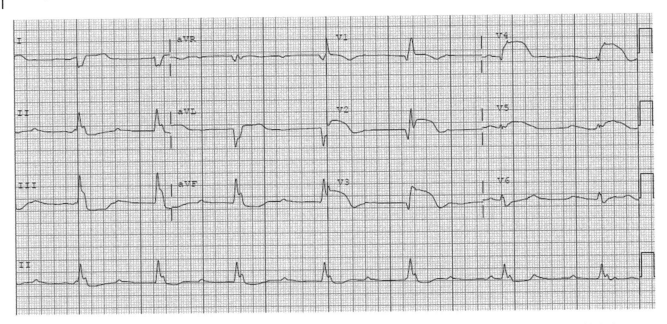

Figure 2.5.16 A 66-year-old male with recent anterior and inferior infarction; Q waves are present in the anterior and inferior leads. Atrial fibrillation is present.

myocardial infarction has been shown in a number of trials to be an independent risk factor for in hospital and long term mortality [70, 71]. Atrial fibrillation occurs more often in patients with advanced age, history of hypertension, and history of myocardial infarction, and occurs more frequently in patients who develop other complications from their myocardial infarction such as heart failure and ventricular arrhythmias; however, after correction for these differences atrial fibrillation remains an independent predictor of death [70, 71]. See Figure 2.5.16 and 2.5.17 for examples of patients with infarcts who developed atrial fibrillation.

AV Conduction Delay and Heart Block

Atrioventricular (AV) conduction refers to the time required for atrial depolarization to occur, conduct to the ventricle, and cause ventricular depolarization. AV block is categorized into first-, second-, and third-degree types. First-degree AV block is defined as a PR interval of >200 milliseconds. Second-degree AV block is either Type 1 (decremental AV conduction results in intermittent block) or Type 2 (intermittent block in setting of a consistent PR interval). Third-degree AV block, also known as complete heart block, occurs when atrial activity does not conduct to the ventricle. See Figure 2.5.18 for an example of 2:1 AV block which can either be Type 1 or Type 2. In patients with known CAD the presence of PR interval > 220 ms has been shown to be independently related to increased risk of heart failure, cardiovascular mortality, and all-cause mortality [72]. Prior to either reperfusion therapy with either thrombolytics

or PCI for the treatment of acute myocardial infarction, it was shown that 11.5% of patients develop AV conduction delay or block (2% first degree, 3% second degree, and 6.5% third degree) with an increase in mortality associated with increased degree of AV block (10%, 27%, and 45% risk of in-hospital mortality, respectively) [73]. In the PCI era, it has been shown that the risk of developing AV block has decreased. In a study of 2073 patients presenting with STEMI, 2.7% developed third-degree AV block and 0.5% developed second-degree AV block. Risk factors for developing third-degree AV block included RCA as the culprit artery, age, female gender, diabetes, hypertension, and congestive heart failure [74].

Complete heart block occurs in the setting of a myocardial infarction when there is either increased vagal tone in the AV node (early and atropine responsive) or AV nodal ischemia/infarction occurs (late and less responsive to atropine) [75]. The AV node is supplied by the right coronary artery in 90% of patients and by the left circumflex coronary artery in 10% of patients. It makes sense, then, that most patients with complete heart block present with an inferior STEMI. It is much less common to have complete heart block in the setting of an NSTEMI. Complete heart block occurs more commonly with inferior infarcts as compared to anterior infarcts [17], and complete heart block in the setting of anterior infarct is associated with a severe reduction in left ventricle function [76]. See Figure 2.5.19 for an example of complete heart block in the setting of an anterior infarct. The presence of complete heart block is predictive of both in-hospital and long-term mortality [76].

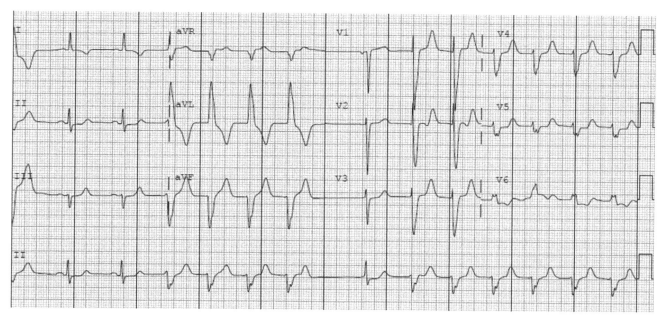

Figure 2.5.17 A 78-year-old female with an acute posterior infarct in a patient with atrial fibrillation and suspected embolic etiology of infarction. She did not survive to coronary angiography.

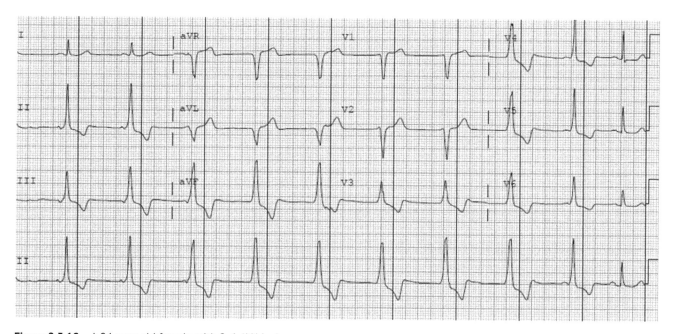

Figure 2.5.18 A 84-year-old female with 2:1 AV block.

Prolonged QTc Interval

The corrected QT interval (QTc) may be a valuable clinical tool for the identification of patients who are at high risk of developing life-threatening ventricular arrhythmias leading to SCD. This is certainly true in the congenital long QT syndromes, first described in 1957 by Jervell and Lange-Nielsen [77]. The assessment of the QTc is also useful for monitoring adverse effects of pharmacologic agents that cause QTc

prolongation and thus place patients at increased risk of SCD. Since 1981, evidence has accumulated, suggesting a prognostic role of QTc interval measurements in the setting of an acute coronary syndrome. Indeed, several investigators have shown that QTc prolongation is not only common but an early indicator of increased risk of VT and VF, in-hospital and post-discharge mortality, recurrent ischemia and infarction [78–81]. Some have postulated that QTc prolongation may be the earliest ECG manifestation of acute cardiac ischemia.

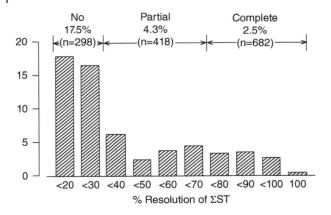

Figure 2.5.19 A 45-year-old male with an anterior STEMI complicated by complete heart block. The patient presented 24 hours after the chest pain after having an episode of syncope.

Resolution of an initially prolonged QTc has in general been correlated with a more favorable outcome. Nevertheless, additional studies are needed to determine whether QTc measurement improves risk stratification in comparison with the more-established markers of risk, such as those recommended in current clinical practice guidelines.

Conclusion

The ECG is a noninvasive tool that provides immediate diagnostic and prognostic information. The ECG is essential in the management of patients with suspected or known cardiac disease and guides therapy throughout the natural history of cardiac disease. The ECG has been clinically available for >100 years and is a tool that will never cease to be of value in the management of patients with cardiac disease.

References

1 Anderson, J.L., Adams, C.D., Antman, E.M. et al. (2007). ACC/AHA 2007 guidelines for the management of patients with unstable angina/non ST-elevation myocardial infarction executive summary. *J. Am. coll. cardiol.* 50: 652–726.

2 Thygesen, K., Alpert, J.S., Jaffe, A.S. et al. (2012). Third universal definition of myocardial infarction. *Eur. heart journal* 33: 2551–2567.

3 Dressler, W. and Rooesler, H. (1947). High T wave in the earliest stage of myocardial infarction. *Am. heart journal.* 34: 627–645.

4 Aldrich, H.R., Wagner, N.B., Boswick, J. et al. (1988). Use of the initial ST-segment deviation for prediction of final electrocardiographic size of acute myocardial infarct. *Am. J. Cardiol.* 61: 749–753.

5 Bar, F.W., Vermeer, F., de Zwaan, C. et al. (1987). Value of admission electrocardiogram in predicting outcome of thrombolytic therapy in acute myocardial infarction: a randomized trial conducted by the Netherlands Interuniversity Cardiology Institute. *Am. J. Cardiol.* 59: 6–13.

6 Lee, K.L. et al. (1995). Predictors of 30-day mortality in the era of reperfusion for acute myocardial infarction: results from an international trial of 41,021 patients. *Circulation* 91: 1659–1668.

7 Schröder, K. et al. (2001). Extent of ST-segment deviation in a single electrocardiogram lead 90 min after thrombolysis as a predictor of medium-term mortality in acute myocardial infarction. *Lancet* 358: 1479–1486.

8 Schröder, R., Dissmann, R., Brüggermann, T. et al. (1994). Extent of early ST-segment elevation resolution: a simple but strong predictor of outcome in patients with acute myocardial infarction. *J. Am. Coll. Cardiol.* 24: 384–391.

9 Lonborg, J. et al. (2013). Final infarct size measured by cardiovascular magnetic resonance in patients with ST elevation myocardial infarction predicts long term outcome: an observational study. *Eur. Heart J. Cardiovasc. Imaging* 14 (4): 387–395.

10 Blanke, H. et al. (1984). Electrocardiographic and coronary arteriographic correlations during acute myocardial infarction. *Am. J. Cardiol.* 54: 249–255.

11 Huey, B.L., Beller, G.A., Kaiser, D.L., and Gibson, R.S. (1988). A comprehensive analysis of myocardial infarction due to left circumflex artery occlusion: comparison with infarction due to right coronary artery and left anterior descending artery occlusion. *J. Am. Coll. Cardiol.* 12 (5): 1156–1166.

12 O'Keefe, J.H., Sayed-Taha, K., Gibson, W. et al. (1995). Do patients with left circumflex coronary artery-related acute myocardial infarction without ST segment elevation benefit from reperfusion therapy? *Am. J. Cardiol.* 75 (10): 718–720.

13 Kim, S.S., Choi, H.S., Jeong, M.H. et al. (2011). Clinical outcomes of acute myocardial infarction with occluded left circumflex artery. *J. Cardiol.* 57: 290–296.

14 Stribling, W.K. et al. (2011). Left circumflex occlusion in acute myocardial infarction (from the national cardiovascular data registry). *Am. J. Cardiol.* 108: 959–963.

15 Fresco, C., Maggioni, A.P., Santoro, E. et al. (1994). Predictors of in-hospital death in 7,755 patients with first MI arriving in hospital with Killip 1 class. *Circulation* 90 (4). [500-500].

16 Schröder, R., Dissmann, R., Brüggermann, T. et al. (1994). Extent of early ST-segment elevation resolution: a simple

but strong predictor of outcome in patients with acute myocardial infarction. *J. Am. Coll. Cardiol.* 24: 384–391.

17 Nielsen, B.L. (1973). ST-segment elevation in acute myocardial infarction. *Circulation* 48: 338–345.

18 Bhave, P.D., Hoffmayer, K.S., Armstrong, E.J. et al. (2012 Feb 1). Predictors of depressed left ventricular function in patients presenting with ST-elevation myocardial infarction. *The American journal of cardiology.* 109 (3): 327–331.

19 Schröder, R., Wegscheider, K., Schröder, K. et al. (1995). Extent of early ST segment elevation resolution: a strong predictor of outcome in patients with STEMI and a sensitive measure to compare thrombolytic regimens. *J. Am. Coll. Cardiol.* 26: 2657–2664.

20 Willems, J.L., Willems, R.J., Willems, G.M. et al. (1190). Significance of initial ST segment elevation and depression for the management of thrombolytic therapy in acute myocardial infarction. European cooperative study group for recombinant tissue-type plasminogen activator. *Circulation* 82: 1147–1158.

21 Zimetbaum, P.J. and Josephson, M.E. (2003). Use of the electrocardiogram in acute myocardial infarction. *NEJM* 348: 933–940.

22 Cannon, C.P., McCabe, C.H., Stone, P.H. et al. (1997, 1997). The electrocardiogram predicts one-year outcome of patients with unstable angina and non-Q wave myocardial infarction: results of the TIMI III registry ECG ancillary study. *J. Am. Coll. Cardiol.* 30: 133–140.

23 Kinch, J.W. and Ryan, T.J. (1993). Right ventricular infarction. *NEJM* 330 (17): 1211–1217.

24 Sugiura, T., Iwasaka, T., Takahashi, N. et al. (1991). Atrial fibrillation in inferior wall Q-wave acute myocardial infarction. *Am. J. Cardiol.* 67: 1135–1136.

25 Braat, S.H., de Zwaan, C., Brugada, P. et al. (1984). Right ventricular involvement with acute inferior wall myocardial infarction identifies high risk of developing atrioventricular nodal conduction disturbances. *Am. Heart J.* 107: 1183–1187.

26 Zehender, M., Kasper, W., Kauder, E. et al. (1993). Right ventricular infarction as an independent predictor of prognosis after acute myocardial infarction. *NEJM* 328: 981–988.

27 Fibrinolytic Therapy Trialists' (FTT) Collaborative Group (1994). Indications for fibrinolytic therapy in suspected acute myocardial infarction: collaborative overview of early mortality and major morbidity results from all randomized trials of more than 1000 patients. *Lancet* 343: 311–322.

28 Jain, S., Ting, H.T., Bell, M. et al. (2011). Utility of LBBB as a diagnostic criterion for acute myocardial infarction. *Am. J. Cardiol.* 107: 1111–1116.

29 O'Gara, P.T., Kushner, F.G., Ascheim, D.D. et al. (2013, 2013). ACCF/AHA STEMI guidelines. *J. Am. Coll. Cardiol.* 61 (4): e78–e140.

30 Sgarbossa, E., Pinski, S.L., and Barbagelata, A. (1996). For the GUSTO-1 investigators. Electrocardiographic diagnosis of evolving acute myocardial infarction in the presence of left bundle-branch block. *N. Engl. J. Med.* 334: 481–487.

31 Schröder, R., Wegscheider, K., Schröder, K. et al. (1995). Extent of early ST segment elevation resolution: a strong predictor of outcome in patients with acute myocardial infarction and a sensitive measure to compare thrombolytic regimens. A substudy of the international joint efficacy comparison of thrombolytics (INJECT) trial. *J. Am. Coll. Cardiol.* 26: 1657–1664.

32 Dissmann, R., Goerke, M., von Ameln, H. et al. (1993). Prediction of early reperfusion and left ventricular damage by ST segment analysis during thrombolysis in acute myocardial infarction. *Z. Kardiol.* 82: 271–278.

33 Dong, J., Ndrepapa, G., Schmitt, C. et al. (2002). Early resolution of ST segment elevation correlates with myocardial salvage assessed by Tc-99m sestamibi scintigraphy in patients with acute myocardial infarction after mechanical or thrombolytic reperfusion therapy. *Circulation* 105: 2946–2949.

34 Wong, C.K., Leon de la Barra, S., and Herbison, P. (2010). Does ST resolution achieved via different reperfusion strategies (fibrinolysis vs percutaneous coronary intervention) have different prognostic meaning in ST-elevation myocardial infarction? A systemic review. *Am. Heart J.* 160 (5): 842–848.

35 Claeys, M.J., Bosmans, J., Veenstra, L. et al. (1999). Determinants and prognostic implications of persistent ST-segment elevation after primary angioplasty for acute myocardial infarction: importance of microvascular reperfusion injury on clinical outcome. *Circulation* 99: 1972–1977.

36 Ndrepepa, G., Alger, P., Kufner, S. et al. (2012). ST-segment resolution after primary percutaneous coronary intervention in patients with acute ST segment elevation myocardial infarction. *Cardiol. J.* 19 (1): 61–69.

37 Phibbs, B., Marcus, F., Marriott, H.J.C. et al. (1999). Q-wave versus non-Q wave myocardial infarction: a meaningless distinction. *J. Am. Coll. Cardiol.* 33 (2): 576–582.

38 Savage, R.M., Wagner, G.S., Ideker, R.E. et al. (1999). Correlation of postmortem anatomic findings with electrocardiographic changes in patients with myocardial infarction: retrospective study of patient with typical anterior and posterior infarcts. *Circulation* 55: 279–285.

39 Goodman, S.G., Langer, A., Ross, A.M. et al. (1998). Non-Q-wave versus Q-wave myocardial infarction after thrombolytic therapy. *Circulation* 97: 444–450.

40 Armstrong, P.W., Fu, Y., Westerhout, C.M. et al. (2009). Baseline Q-wave surpasses time from symptom onset as a prognostic marker in ST-segment elevation myocardial

infarction in patients treated with primary percutaneous intervention. *J. Am. Coll. Cardiol.* 53 (17): 1503–1509.

41 Gibson, R.S., Beller, G.A., Gheorghiade, M. et al. (1986). The prevalence and clinical significance of residual myocardial ischemia two weeks after acute uncomplicated non-Q wave infarction: a propective natural history study. *Circulation* 73 (1): 186–198.

42 Gibson, R.S. (1987). Clinical, functional and angiographic distinctions between Q wave and non-Q wave myocardial infarction: evidence of spontaneous reperfusion and implications for interventional trials. *Circulation* 75 (suppl 5): 128–138.

43 Gibson, R.S. (1988). Non-Q wave myocardial infarction: diagnosis, prognosis and management. *Curr. Probl. Cardiol.* 13: 1–72.

44 Savonitto, S., Ardissino, D., Granger, C.B. et al. (1999, 1999). Prognostic value of the admission electrocardiogram in acute coronary syndromes. *JAMA* 281: 707–713.

45 Kaul, P. et al. (2005). Relation between baseline risk and treatment decisions in non-ST elevation acute coronary syndromes: an examination of international practice patterns. *Heart* 91: 876–881.

46 Kaul, P., Newby, L.K., Fu, Y. et al. (2005). Relation between baseline risk and treatment decisions in non-ST elevation acute coronary syndromes: an examination of international practice patterns. *Heart* 91: 876–881.

47 Hersi, J., Fu, Y., Wong, B. et al. (2004). Does the discharge ECG provide additional prognostic insight(s) in non-ST elevation ACS patients from that acquired on admission? *Eur. Heart J.* 24: 522–531.

48 Wagner, G.S., Macfarlane, P., Wellens, H. et al. (2009). AHA/ACCF/HRS recommendations for the standardization and interpretation of the electrocardiogram, part VI: acute ischemia/infarction. *J. Am. Coll. Cardiol.* 53 (11): 1003–1011.

49 Zwaan, C., Bär, F., and Wellens, H. (1982). Characteristic electrocardiographic pattern indicating a critical stenosis high in left anterior descending artery in patients admitted because of impending myocardial infarction. *Am. Heart J.* 103: 730–736.

50 Welch, R.D., Zalenski, R.J., Frederick, P.D. et al. (2001). Prognostic value of a normal or nonspecific initial electrocardiogram in acute myocardial infarction. *JAMA* 286: 1977–1984.

51 Karlson, B.W., Herlitz, J., Wiklund, O. et al. (1991). Early prediction of acute myocardial infarction from clinical history, examination and electrocardiogram in the emergency room. *Am. J. Cardiol.* 68: 171–175.

52 Rouan, G.W., Lee, T.H., Cook, L.F. et al. (1989). Clinical characteristics and outcome of acute myocardial infarction in patients with initially normal or nonspecific electrocardiograms. *Am. J. Cardiol.* 64: 1087–1092.

53 Brush, J.E., Brand, D.A., Acampora, D. et al. (1985). Use of the initial electrocardiogram to predict in-hospital complications of acute myocardial infarction. *N. Engl. J. Med.* 312: 1137–1141.

54 Stark, M.E. and Vacek, J.L. (1987). The initial electrocardiogram during admission for myocardial infarction – use as a predictor of clinical course and facility utilization. *Arch. Intern. Med.* 147: 843–846.

55 Zalenski, R.J., Sloan, E.P., Chen, E.H. et al. (1988). The emergency department ECG and immediately life-threatening complications in initially uncomplicated suspected myocardial ischemia. *Am. J. Emerg. Med.* 17: 221–226.

56 Dib, C., Asirvatham, S., Elesber, A. et al. (2009). Clinical correlates and prognostic significance of electrocardiographic abnormalities in apical ballooning syndrome. *Am. Heart J.* 157: 933–938.

57 Regnante, R.A., Zuzek, R.W., Weinsier, S.B. et al. (2009). Clinical characteristics and four-year outcomes of patients in the Rhode Island takotsubo cardiomyopathy registry. *Am. J. Cardiol.* 103 (7): 1015–1019.

58 Samuelov-Kinori, L., Kinori, M., Kogan, Y. et al. (2009). Takotsubo cardiomyopathy and QT interval prolongation: who are the patients at risk for torsades de pointes? *J. Electrocardiol.* 42: 353–357.

59 Bonow, R., Mann, Zipes, D.P., and Libby, P. (2012). *Braunwald's Heart Disease: A Textbook of Cardiovascular Medicine*, 9e. Saunders, and imprint of Elsevier Inc.

60 Mehta, R.H., Starr, A.Z., Lopes, R.D. et al. (2009). Incidence and outcomes associated with ventricular tachycardia or fibrillation in patients undergoing primary percutaneous intervention. *JAMA* 301 (17): 1779–1789.

61 Rahimi, K., Watzlawek, S., Thiele, H. et al. (2006). Incidence, time course, and predictors of early malignant ventricular arrhythmias after non-ST-segment elevation myocardial infarction in patients with early invasive treatment. *Eur. Heart J.* 27: 1706–1711.

62 MacMahon, S. (1988). Effects of prophylactic lidocaine in suspected acute myocardial infarction. An overview of results from the randomized, controlled trials. *JAMA* 260 (13): 1910–1916.

63 Scirica, B.M., Braunwald, E., Belardinelli, L. et al. (2010). Relationship between nonsustained ventricular tachycardia after non-ST elevation acute coronary syndrome and sudden cardiac death. *Circulation* 122: 455–462.

64 Volpi, A., Maggioni, A., Franzosi, M.G. et al. (1987). In-hospital prognosis of patients with acute myocardial infarction complicated by primary ventricular fibrillation. *N. Engl. J. Med.* 317: 257–261.

65 Behar, S., Reicher-Reiss, H., Shechter, M. et al. (1993). Frequency and prognostic significance of secondary ventricular fibrillation complicating acute myocardial infarction. *Am. J. Cardiol.* 71: 152–156.

66 Mehta, R.H., Starr, A.Z., Lopes, R.D. et al. (2009). Incidence of and outcomes associated with ventricular tachycardia or fibrillation in the patients undergoing primary percutaneous coronary intervention. *JAMA* 301 (17): 1779–1789.

67 Han, Z., Yan-min, Y., Jun, Z. et al. (2012). Prognostic value of admission heart rate in patients with ST segment elevation myocardial infarction: role of type 2 diabetes mellitus. *BMC Cardiovasc. Disord.* 12: 104.

68 Jensen, M.T., Kaiser, C., Sandsten, K.E. et al. (2013). Heart rate at discharge and long-term prognosis following percutaneous coronary intervention in stable and acute coronary syndromes – results from the BASKET PROVE trial. *Int. J. Cardiol.* 168: 3802–3806.

69 Diaz, A., Bourassa, M.G., Guertin, M.C., and Tardif, J.C. (2005). Long-term prognostic value of resting heart rate in patients with suspected or proven coronary artery disease. *Eur. Heart J.* 26: 967–974.

70 Wong, C.K., White, H.D., Wilcox, R.G. et al. (2000). New atrial fibrillation after acute myocardial infarction independently predicts death: the GUSTO-III experience. *Am. Heart J.* 140: 878–885.

71 Pizzetti, F., Turazza, F.M., Franzosi, M.G. et al. (2001). Incidence and prognostic significance of atrial fibrillation in acute myocardial infarction: the GISSI-3 data. *Heart* 86: 527–532.

72 Crisel, R.K., Farzaneh-Far, R., Na, B., and Whooley, M.A. (2011). First-degree atrioventricular block is associated with heart failure and death in persons with stable coronary artery disease: data from the heart and soul study. *Eur. Heart J.* 32: 1875–1880.

73 Brown, R.W., Hunt, D., and Sloman, J.G. (1969). The natural history of atrioventricular conduction defects in acute myocardial infarction. *Am. Heart J.* 78 (4): 460–466.

74 Gang, U.J.O., Hvelplund, A., Pedersen, S. et al. (2012). High-degree atrioventricular block complicating ST-segment elevation myocardial infarction in the era of primary percutaneous coronary intervention. *Europace* 14: 1639–1645.

75 Wong, C.K., White, H.D., Wilcox, R.G. et al. (2000). New atrial fibrillation after acute myocardial infarction independently predicts death: the GUSTO-III experience. *Am. Heart J.* 140: 878–885.

76 Aplin, M., Engstrom, T., Vejlstrup, N.G. et al. (2003). Prognostic importance of complete atrioventricular block complicating acute myocardial infarction. *Am. J. Cardiol.* 92 (7): 853–856.

77 Jervell, A. and Lange-Nielsen, F.P. (1957). Congenital deaf-mutism, functional heart disease with prolongation of the QT interval and sudden cardiac death. *Am. Heart J.* 54: 59–68.

78 Taylor, G.J., Crampton, R.S., Gibson, R.S. et al. (1981). Prolonged QT interval at onset of acute myocardial infarction in predicting early phase ventricular tachycardia. *Am. Heart J.* 102: 16–24.

79 Ahnve, S. (1985). QT interval prolongation in acute myocardial infarction. *Eur. Heart J.* 6: 85–95.

80 Gadaleta, F.L., Llois, S.C., and Lapuente, A.R. (2003). Prognostic value of corrected QT interval prolongation in patients with unstable angina pectoris. *Am. J. Cardiol.* 92: 203–205.

81 Gadaleta, F.L., Llois, S.C., and Sinisi, V.A. (2008). Corrected QT interval prolongation: a new predictor of cardiovascular risk in patients with non-ST-elevation acute coronary syndrome. *Rev. Esp. Cardiol.* 61: 572–578.

6

ECG Tools

Alternate Lead Placement, Serial ECGs, and ECG Monitoring

Augustus E. Mealor[1], Yasir Akhtar[2], and Michael Ragosta[2]

[1] *University of Tennessee College of Medicine, Erlanger Heart and Lung Institute, Chattanooga, TN, USA*
[2] *Division of Cardiovascular Medicine, University of Virginia Health System, Charlottesville, VA, USA*

Introduction

The interpretation of the standard 12-lead electrocardiogram (ECG) may provide valuable information regarding the presence of myocardial ischemia in patients with chest pain or symptoms concerning for angina. However, evaluation of the ECG should not be a static process. The evaluation of the ECG should also include assessment of a prior ECG for the patient if available. In addition, dynamic changes on the ECG over time may be a powerful tool in assessing for myocardial ischemia. An obvious example is repeating the ECG following administration of nitroglycerin, which leads to venodilation, reduction in cardiac preload, and therefore a decrease in myocardial wall tension in the left ventricle. The decreased wall tension leads to a reduction in the amount of oxygen necessary to support cardiac output. This reduction in myocardial oxygen demand may decrease myocardial ischemia and lead to changes on the ECG with normalization of changes consistent with myocardial ischemia. These dynamic changes on ECG can also be used to guide medical therapy. Finally, the inclusion of additional leads to the ECG may also help identify injury currents that were not identified in the standard 12-lead ECG. In this chapter, we will review various techniques that can improve the diagnostic accuracy of the ECG in patients presenting with symptoms concerning for myocardial ischemia.

Right-Sided Leads

Approximately 30% of inferior myocardial infarctions (MI) involve the right ventricle (RV) [1]. The RV receives its blood supply primarily through right ventricular marginal branches of the right coronary artery (RCA), thus RV infarction is typically seen in the setting of an acute inferior wall MI due to occlusion of the RCA proximal to the origin of the RV marginal branches. Accordingly, ST-segment changes on the inferior leads are usually seen, and it is prudent to look for RV involvement in all patients presenting with acute inferior wall ST-segment elevation MI (STEMI).

Isolated MI of the RV alone (i.e. without LV involvement) is rare, and according to a large autopsy series, accounted for only 3% of MIs [1]. The mechanisms for isolated RV MI include proximal occlusion of a nondominant RCA, proximal occlusion of a dominant RCA with collateral circulation to the posterior descending artery (PDA) and posterolateral branch, or isolated occlusion of one or more large right marginal branches. The latter is more likely to be seen iatragenically during percutaneous coronary intervention of a RCA with loss of an RV side branch at the site of RCA stenting.

Occlusion of the RCA or a large RV branch may cause RV dysfunction but does not always result in RV necrosis [2]. The RV is thin-walled in comparison to the LV with less workload and a lower oxygen demand. Furthermore, the RV receives some blood supply directly from the RV cavity contributing to its resistance to coronary occlusion. Conditions associated with a greater vulnerability to RV ischemia and higher likelihood of RV infarction include pulmonary hypertension and RV hypertrophy.

Recognition of acute RV MI is important. RV infarction produces a classic clinical triad of venous congestion with jugular venous distension (JVD), hypotension, and clear lung fields [3]. However, the clinical presentation ranges from minimal to no evidence of RV dysfunction or hemodynamic compromise and cardiogenic shock. In one study, JVD and Kussmaul's sign (inspiratory increase in JVD) carried a sensitivity of 88% and specificity of 100% for hemodynamically significant RV infarction [4].

Electrocardiogram in Clinical Medicine, First Edition. Edited by William J. Brady, Michael J. Lipinski, Andrew E. Darby, Michael C. Bond, Nathan P. Charlton, Korin Hudson, and Kelly Williamson.
© 2021 John Wiley & Sons Ltd. Published 2021 by John Wiley & Sons Ltd.

The cumulative effects of RV dysfunction include acute right ventricular dilation, decreased RV output, and a shift of the interventricular septum toward the LV, thereby compromising LV filling and compliance. This may be compounded by bradycardia or atrioventricular dyssynchrony due to associated sinus or AV nodal ischemia. Patients with associated LV dysfunction due to coexisting inferior wall infarction are particularly at risk for developing cardiogenic shock.

The electrocardiographic changes in right ventricular infarction may be subtle and fleeting. On the standard 12-lead ECG, ST-segment elevation may be apparent in V1 (Table 2.6.1). However, the clinician needs to obtain a right-sided ECG or RV leads for the greatest sensitivity and specificity (Figure 2.6.1). Examination of right ventricular leads should be performed as early as possible because right-sided ST-segment elevation is a transient phenomenon, lasting approximately 10 hours after onset of chest pain [5]. Multiple studies have shown that ST elevation >1 mm in V4R detects RV MI with a sensitivity and

specificity greater than 80% and 90%, respectively [2]. Decreasing the threshold to 0.5 mm does little to increase sensitivity though specificity suffers significantly. Other criteria have been proposed but are less well established. For instance, in one small study, a QS pattern in V3R and V4R had a 78% and 100% sensitivity and specificity [7]. Other electrocardiographic changes associated with acute RV infarction include sinus bradycardia and various types of heart block. These changes depend on the site of coronary occlusion relative to the sinoatrial nodal artery and AV nodal artery but may also occur due to the increased vagal tone associated with acute inferior wall MI.

The differential diagnosis for ST segment elevation in V4R includes antero-septal MI, prior MI with ventricular aneurysm, pericarditis, and pulmonary embolus. Anterior MI rarely extends to V5R, and typically ST depression decreases as leads progress rightward. In RV MI, ST elevation (STE) typically increases or remains the same as the leads progress rightward. Figures 2.6.2 and 2.6.3 demonstrate the use of RV leads in a patient with suspected RV infarction.

Clinically, patients with right ventricular infarction are highly dependent upon preload and therapy with diuretics and vasodilatory medications such as nitrates and morphine must be used with extreme caution. In the setting of inferior STEMI, urgent revascularization of the infarct related artery is important and, in the event of acute closure of the RCA with associated RV infarction, every effort should be made to restore patency of the RV marginal artery as well as the LV myocardial branches. The role of revascularization in patients with isolated RV infarction is less clear. Symptoms unrelieved by medical therapy or those

Table 2.6.1 Standard 12-lead ECG evidence of right ventricular MI.

ST elevation in lead III > II

ST elevation in lead V1, ST depression in lead V2

ST elevation in lead V2 > ST depression in lead aVF

New heart block [6]

New right bundle branch block [6]

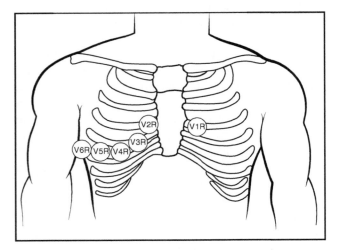

Figure 2.6.1 The right-side ECG. After obtaining a standard 12-lead ECG, the electrode wires for leads V1 and V2 are switched, and the remaining leads V3–V6 are placed laterally across the right chest in a mirror image to the standard precordial leads. V4R should fall in the fifth intercostal space in the midclavicular line. V3 is placed between V2R and V4R. V6 is placed in the anterior axillary line, and V5R is located between V4R and V5R.

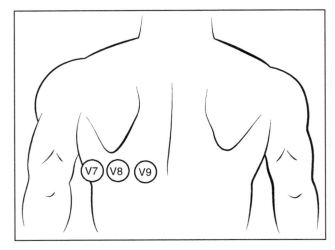

Figure 2.6.2 The posterior ECG. Leads V7–V9 are placed on the same horizontal plane as lead V6 with V7 at the posterior axillary line, V8 below the scapular angle, and V9 located medial to the left paraspinal muscle.

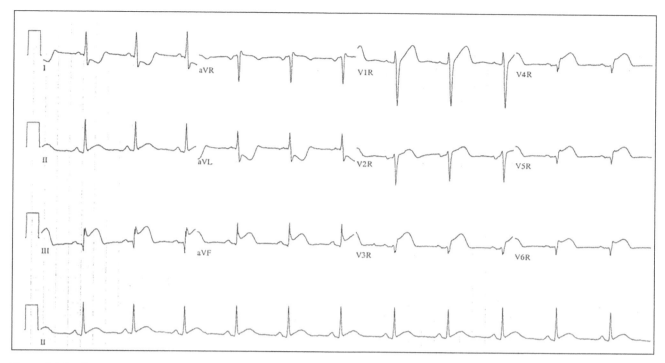

Figure 2.6.3 Right-sided ECG in a patient with acute occlusion of the proximal RCA. ST elevation with Q waves in inferior leads II, III, aVF indicated injury pattern and infarction of the inferior wall of the heart. ST elevation in the right-sided precordial leads indicates extension of injury to the right ventricle. QR pattern in V3R and V4R is specific for RV infarction.

with hemodynamic compromise may benefit from revascularization. Interestingly, despite the potential for great instability during the acute phase, the RV has a remarkable ability to recover function. Prognosis is principally determined by the degree of associated LV dysfunction.

Posterior ECG

Formerly known as the posterior LV wall, the basal inferior and inferolateral LV segments lie in a spot blind to the standard 12-lead ECG. These segments face away from the standard leads and are more distant from the anterior chest wall than other regions of the left ventricle. The result is that vectors from the inferobasal and inferolateral walls project with diminished amplitude and appear inverted when viewed from the anterior position of the standard leads.

Isolated posterior MI is uncommon (3–11% of infarctions) and usually seen in association with acute inferior wall MI. A "posterior" transmural MI classically presents with ST depression and an R wave in anteroseptal leads. This pattern is often mistaken for anterior ischemia when, in fact, it is the inverted projection of a basal inferior or inferolateral STEMI. Moreover, as many as 60% of patients with infarction of the inferobasal/inferolateral walls do not manifest reciprocal ST depression in anterior precordial leads [8]. Using standard leads alone, the extent of an infarction may be underappreciated or the diagnosis of MI missed entirely when urgent reperfusion therapy is indicated.

Obtaining additional leads V7–V9 (posterior leads), located on the posterior left hemithorax, improves the sensitivity of the ECG for basal inferior and inferolateral MI (Figure 2.6.4). Clinical guidelines for diagnosis and management of acute MI state that posterior ECG leads should be obtained if there is any clinical suspicion of basal inferior or inferolateral infarction (Table 2.6.2) [9].

ST elevation >1 mm in V7–V9 confirms the presence of inferolateral or basal inferior MI with a sensitivity as high as 90% [10]. Two studies in which the circumflex artery was occluded by a balloon angioplasty catheter during continuous ECG monitor found a minimum ST elevation of 0.5 mm to have better diagnostic value [11, 12]. In both studies, the average maximum ST elevation was less than 1 mm. Q waves are considered pathologic if wider than 0.04 second or greater in amplitude than one quarter of the following R wave [4]. The ACC/AHA guidelines have not included specific criteria for diagnosis of acute posterior MI using posterior leads.

The basal inferior and inferolateral segments are supplied by the distal RCA and the LCX coronary arteries. The inferior wall is supplied by the PDA, which, in 90% of

(a)

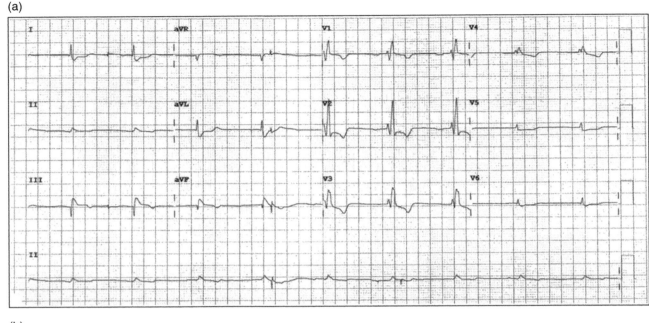

(b)

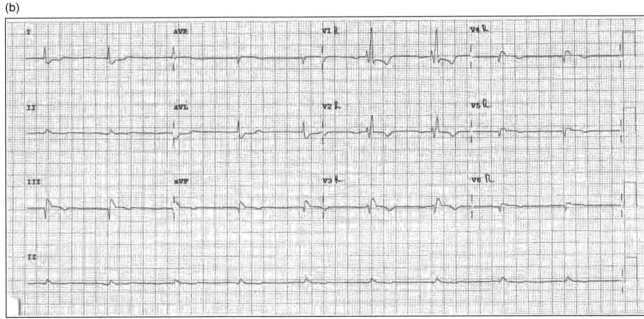

Figure 2.6.4 (a) Standard 12-lead ECG in a patient presenting more than 48 hours after onset of chest pain showing evolving inferior wall MI. (b) Right-side leads show less than 0.5 mm of ST elevation in V4R with Q waves. This patient was found to have an occlusion of his proximal RCA.

humans, arises from the RCA, and from the LCX in the remaining 10%. Occlusion of the vessel supplying the PDA causes infarction of not only the basal segment of the inferior wall but also its downstream segments, producing ST deviation in inferior leads II, III, and aVF. Hence, most basal inferior wall infarctions are identifiable on the standard 12-lead ECG. In this setting, posterior leads help to identify the additional extent of myocardium involved.

In most patients, the inferolateral wall lies in the terminal distribution of the LCX and its obtuse marginal branches. Occasionally, a large RCA system will extend posterolateral branches to supply the inferolateral wall. The inferolateral wall is vulnerable because it is not directly imaged by the standard ECG and occlusion of a vessel supplying it will often not produce changes imaged by the standard 12 leads.

Table 2.6.2 Recommendations for posterior ECG leads.

Posterior ECG leads should be obtained if any of the following changes are noted on the 12-lead ECG:

- Inferior MI
- Lateral MI
- ST depression in leads V1–V3
- ST elevation in V1, V2
- Borderline ST elevation in inferior leads II, III, aVF or lateral leads V5, V6

Multiple studies have shown that most commonly missed diagnosis of MI are those caused by LCX occlusion. In patients with a right-dominant coronary anatomy, occlusion of the LCX produces evidence of ST elevation MI (ST elevation, or ST depression V1–V3) on the standard ECG in about 40% of cases. Sensitivity improves almost 30% by obtaining posterior leads V7–V9 [13].

Although the LAD, RCA, and LCX are implicated with equal frequency in non-ST elevation MI, only 15% of diagnosed STEMIs are attributed to LCX occlusion [14]. Because there is no evidence that the LCX is less susceptible to acute coronary syndrome, the lower frequency of circumflex artery related STEMI is more likely due to underdiagnosis of the condition because of the traditional reliance on the standard 12-lead ECG, a test unlikely to show ST elevation in the event of LCX occlusion.

Kulkarni et al. showed that transient occlusion of the left circumflex during balloon angioplasty caused ST elevation in leads V7–V9 in 68% of cases [15]. This was the most common ECG finding in patients with left circumflex occlusion, and of those, 25% had ST-segment elevation in posterior leads alone. In this study, only 63% of LCX occlusions were identified by the standard 12-lead ECG while all of these patients were identified with posterior leads.

Even though a standard 12-lead ECG may show ST-segment elevation inferiorly and the diagnosis of STEMI made in a timely fashion, obtaining posterior leads is important as ST elevation in posterior leads indicates a larger region of infarction and portends a worse prognosis. For example, Matetzky et al. noted an increased incidence in post-MI mitral insufficiency in patients who presented with infarction of the inferolateral wall [16]. Figure 2.6.5 is an example of the utility of posterior leads in diagnosis of posterior MI.

Serial ECG Monitoring

A single ECG only provides a snapshot of the electrical state of the heart at a given time. In patients having stuttering chest pain with symptoms waxing and waning, a single,

normal ECG may provide a false sense of reassurance for a disease process that presents as a continuum. Acute coronary syndromes (ACS) display an array of temporal changes and in order to make an accurate diagnosis, serial ECG sampling may help identify dynamic changes consistent with myocardial ischemia. Coronary artery spasm or intermittent coronary artery occlusion with recanalization may be missed if only one ECG is obtaining to make a diagnosis. An accurate diagnosis can be made by obtaining continuous ST segment monitoring (STM-ECG) or serial ECGs (S-ECG).

STM-ECG

Simple telemetry monitoring lacks the sensitivity of continuous ST segment monitoring to detect ischemia. STM-ECG has been available since the mid-1980s however they are utilized by less than half of critical care units [17]. The purpose of STM-ECG is to alert the provider to ongoing dynamic ischemia. A prior study showed that up to 17% of patients admitted for ACS to telemetry units have transient myocardial ischemia seen on STM-ECG [18]. These patients were 8.5 times more likely to have in-hospital complications. In the absence of prospective randomized clinical trials to determine the optimal approach to monitoring these patients, guidelines recommend inpatient ECG monitoring continuous for up to 24 hours to rule out MI in patients with signs of ischemia on initial ECG along with a risk factor for CAD [19, 20].

Serial ECG Monitoring

If an initial ECG is nondiagnostic, subsequent ECGs may be performed through the admission. A study by Silber et al. showed that up to 20% of patients presenting to the ER with ACS developed thrombolytic criteria on subsequent ECG when the initial presenting ECG was nondiagnostic [21]. Another study by Fesmire et al. looked at 1000 patients admitted to the ER with chest pain. Compared with an initial single standard 12-lead ECG, a 12-lead S-ECG performed every 20 minutes improved sensitivity (68.1% vs 55.4%, $p < 0.001$) and detected injury in an additional 16.2% of patients presenting with chest pain syndrome [22]. The ongoing ASAP Cath trial is comparing S-ECG to Troponin testing in predicting acute coronary syndrome [23]. At the current time, most clinicians obtain an initial ECG with repeat 12-lead ECGs obtained with ongoing symptoms or change in symptoms.

The following cases exemplify the use of serial ECG in diagnosis of acute MI:

(a)

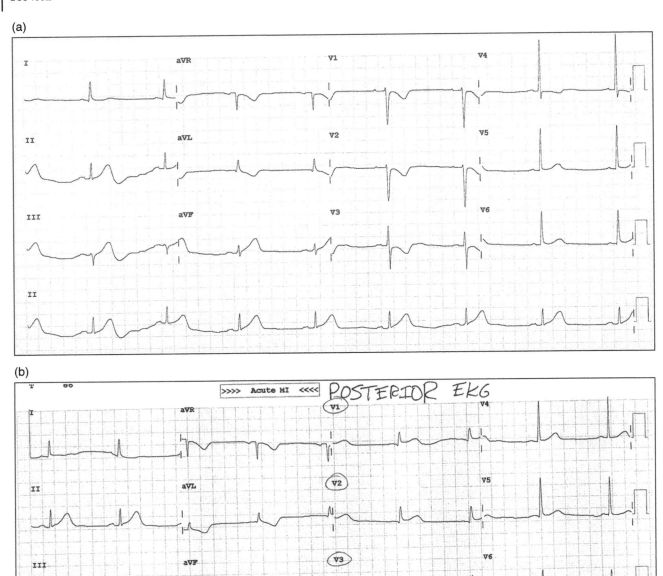

(b)

Figure 2.6.5 (a) Patient A (posterior leads section): Standard 12-lead ECG of an African American male with a history of hypertension and hyperlipidemia presenting with unrelenting chest pain. A small R wave with downsloping ST segments and T-wave inversion is noted in V1–V3, giving the appearance of anterior wall ischemia. Criteria for STEMI are not present. (b) Posterior leads were obtained. Note V1 = V7, V2 = V8, V3 = V9. 1 mm of ST elevation is seen on the posterior leads. The patient was taken emergently to the cardiac catheterization laboratory and found to have a completely occluded nondominant left circumflex artery.

Case 2.6.1

A 48-year-old male called EMS for sudden onset chest pain while exerting. On arrival, an ECG was obtained by EMS that is shown in Figure 2.6.6. The initial ECG showed peaked T waves and the patient was taken to the Emergency Room. Subsequent ECG suggests infarction, given the development of Q waves and ST segment changes in leads V2 and V3. The patient was referred for emergent coronary angiography that showed an occluded proximal LAD. After percutaneous coronary intervention, the ST segment changes resolved.

(a)

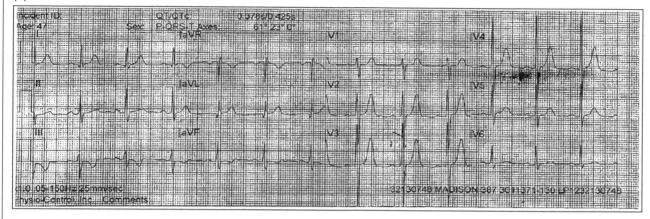

(b)

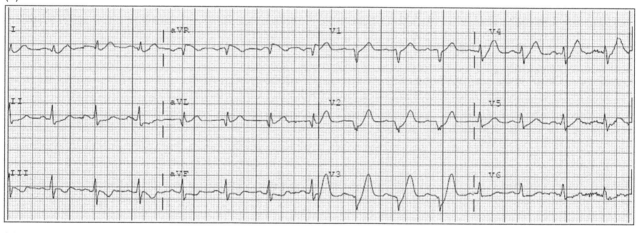

(c)

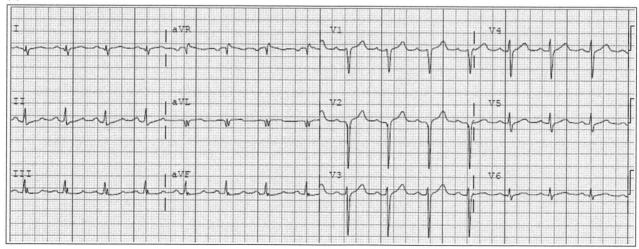

Figure 2.6.6 (a) ECG obtained by EMS showing peaked T waves and nonspecific ST/T wave changes in the anterior leads. (b) An ECG obtained an hour later in the ED upon arrival shows development of Q waves in the anteroseptal leads, ST elevation in aVR and ST depressions in the inferior leads. (c) ECG post-coronary intervention to a lesion in the proximal left anterior descending artery.

Case 2.6.2

A 62-year-old male presented to the emergency room with intermittent substernal chest pressure. An initial ECG on admission was normal. Twenty minutes later, another ECG was obtained shown in Figure 2.6.7 with ST segment elevation in leads V2 and V3 suggesting occlusion of the left anterior descending coronary artery. He was referred for emergent coronary angiography that showed an occluded LAD, and percutaneous coronary intervention was performed.

(a)

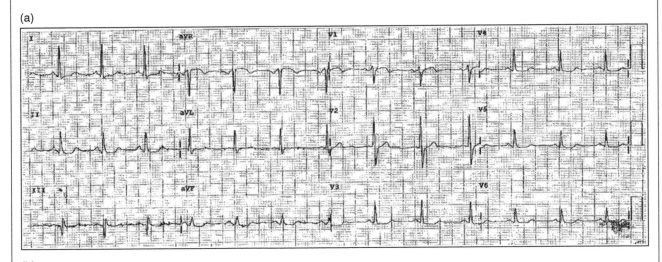

(b)

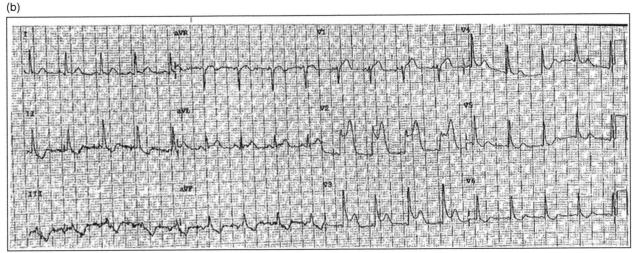

Figure 2.6.7 Serial electrocardiography for acute coronary syndromes: (a) No ST/T wave changes noted on initial ECG on admission to the emergency room. (b) ECG obtained after 21 minutes showed ST-segment elevation in the anteroseptal leads.

References

1 Wartman, W.B. and Hellerstein, H.K. (1948). The incidence of heart disease in 2,000 consecutive autopsies. *Ann. Intern. Med.* 28 (1): 41–65.

2 Haji, S.A. and Movahed, A. (2000). Right ventricular infarction – diagnosis and treatment. *Clin. Cardiol.* 23: 473–482.

3 Cohn, J.N., Guhu, N.H., Broder, M.I., and Limas, C.J. (1974). Right ventricular infarction clinical and hemodynamic features. *Am. J. Cardiol.* 33: 209–214.

4 Dell'Italiea, L.J., Starling, M.R., and O'Rourke, R.A. (1983). Physical examination for exclusion of hemodynamically important right ventricular infarction. *Ann. Intern. Med.* 99: 608–611.

5 Braat, S.H., Brugada, P., de Zwaan, C. et al. (1983 Apr). Value of electrocardiogram in diagnosing right ventricular involvement in patients with an acute inferior wall myocardial infarction. *Br. Heart J.* 49 (4): 368–372.

6 Robalino, B.D., Whitlow, P.L., Underwood, D.A., and Salcedo, E.E. (1989). Electrocardiographic manifestations of right ventricular infarction. *Am. Heart J.* 118: 138–144.

7 Morgera, T., Alberti, E., Silvestri, F. et al. (1984). Right precordial ST and QRS changes in the diagnosis of right ventricular infarction. *Am. Heart J.* 108: 13–18.

8 Khaw, K., Moreyra, A.E., Tannenbaum, A.K. et al. (1999). Improved detection of posterior wall ischemia with the 15-lead electrocardiogram. *Am. Heart J.* 138: 934–940.

9 O'Gara, P.T., Kushner, F.G., Ascheim, D.D. et al. (2013). ACCF/AHA guidelines for the management of ST-elevation myocardial infarction. *JACC* 61 (4): e78–e140.

10 Somers, M.P., Brady, W.J., Bateman, D.C. et al. (2003). Additional electrocardiographic leads in the ED chest pain patient: right ventricular and posterior leads. *Am. J. Emerg. Med.* 21: 563–573.

11 Aqel, R.A., Hage, F.G., Ellipedi, P. et al. (2009). Usefulness of three posterior chest leads for the detection of posterior wall acute myocardial infarction. *Am. J. Cardiol.* 103: 159–164.

12 Wung, S.F. and Drew, B.J. (2001). New electrocardiographic criteria for posterior wall acute myocardial ischemia validated by a percutaneous transluminal coronary angioplasty model of acute myocardial infarction. *Am. J. Cardiol.* 87: 970–974.

13 Schmidt, C., Lehmann, G., Schmieder, S. et al. (2001). Diagnosis of acute myocardial infarction in angiographically documented occluded infarct vessel. *Chest* 120: 1540–1546.

14 Krishnaswamy, A., Lincoff, A.M., and Menon, V. (2009). Magnitude and consequences of missing the acute infarct-related circumflex artery. *Am. Heart J.* 158: 706–712.

15 Kulkarni, A.U., Banka, V.S. et al. (1996). Clinical use of posterior electrocardiographic leads: a prospective electrocardiographic analysis during coronary occlusion. *Am. Heart J.* 131: 736–741.

16 Matetzky, S., Freimark, D., Feinber, M.S. et al. (1999). Acute myocardial infarction with isolated ST-segment elevation in posterior chest leads V7-9: "hidden" ST-segment elevation revealing acute posterior infarction. *JACC* 34: 748–753.

17 Parron, J.A. and Funk, M. (2001). Survey of use of ST-segment monitoring in patients with acute coronary syndrome. *Am. J. Crit. Care* 10: 23–34.

18 Pelter, M.M., Adams, M.G., and Drew, B.J. (2003). Transient myocardial ischemia is an independent predictor of adverse in-hospital outcomes in patients with acute coronary syndromes treated in the telemetry unit. *Heart Lung* 32: 71–78.

19 Drew, B.J., Califf, R.M., Funk, M. et al. (2004). Practice standards of electrocardiographic monitoring in Hosppital settings: an American Heart Association scientific statement from the councils on cardiovascular nursing, clinical cardiology, and cardiovascular disease in the young: endorsed by the International Society of Computerized Electrocardiology and the American Association of Critical-Care Nurses. *Circulation* 110: 2721–2746.

20 Sandau, K.E. and Smith, M. (2009). Continuous ST-segment monitoring: protocol for practice. *Crit. Care Nurse* 29: 39–49.

21 Silber, S.H., Leo, P.J., and Katapadi, M. (1996 Feb). Serial electrocariograms for chest pain patients with initial nondiagnosti electrocardiograms: implications for thrombolytic therapy. *Acad. Emerg. Med.* 3 (2): 147–152.

22 Fesmire, F.M., Percy, R.F., Bardoner, J.B. et al. (1998 Jan). Usefulness of automated serial 12-lead ECG monitoring during the initial emergency department evaluation of patients with chest pain. *Ann. Emerg. Med.* 31 (1): 3–11.

23 American Heart Association.2013. Are Serial Electrocardiograms Additive to the Serial Second-generation Troponin in Predicting Acute Coronary Syndromes in Patients with Undifferentiated Chest Pain (ASAP Cath). https://clinicaltrials.gov/ct2/show/NCT01953276.

7

Electrocardiographic Changes of Ischemia during Stress Testing

Michael J. Lipinski[1] and Victor F. Froelicher[2]

[1] *Cardiovascular Associates of Charlottesville, Charlottesville, VA, USA*
[2] *Division of Cardiovascular Medicine, Stanford University/Palo Alto Veterans Affairs Health Care System, Palo Alto, CA, USA*

Introduction

Cardiac stress testing, whether with exercise or pharmacologic stress, enables clinicians in a controlled setting to recreate ischemia with the cardiovascular system under stress. For patients experiencing exertional angina or chest pain, exercise is the most practical test of cardiac perfusion and function as it most often mimics the physiologic conditions that induce symptoms. The exercise electrocardiogram (ECG) stress test, regardless of whether it incorporates noninvasive imaging modalities, provides information critical in assessing patients with chest pain. The exercise stress test not only shows electrocardiographic changes with exercise but also can provide information regarding maximal or symptom limited exercise capacity, spirometry with oxygen consumption, timing for symptom onset, changes in hemodynamics and blood pressure, changes in the QT interval and/or inducement of arrhythmias. These data can not only provide diagnostic information but also help clinicians determine the prognosis of their patients.

In cardiac stress testing, exercise should be the preferred method of stress and is most typically achieved using established treadmill or bicycle protocols, as described elsewhere [1]. The guidelines specify though that heart rate targets should not be used to end a test or judge its adequacy. Furthermore, estimated METs and not time of exercise should be reported with testing adjusted to the patient so that the test lasts 6–10 minutes. RAMP testing is preferred over rigid stepped protocols.

In patients who are unable to exercise or have specific conditions (i.e. left bundle branch block, LBBB), pharmacologic stress testing may be necessary. Pharmacologic stress testing typically utilizes two very different mechanism, either vasodilation or catecholamine stress. Agents used for vasodilation are adenosine, regadenosine (Lexiscan), or dipyridimole (Persantine) and result in coronary vasodilation, which result in a "steal" phenomena from occluded vessels. This requires radionuclide imaging to identify myocardial perfusion defects during stress that may imply the presence of underlying obstructive coronary artery disease (CAD). In the case of catecholamine stress, dobutamine or arbutamine is infused intravenously using an established protocol until a certain heart rate is achieved. During dobutamine infusion, stress echocardiography can be utilized to assess left ventricular function and identify regional wall motion abnormalities. Alternatively, injection of radionuclide tracer at the time of maximal dobutamine stress can enable radionuclide stress imaging to identify abnormalities in myocardial perfusion. In the case of pharmacologic stress testing, it is important to recognize that a noninvasive imaging modality is required to assess for myocardial ischemia, as pharmacologic stress testing can generate nonspecific ECG changes that may or may not reflect myocardial ischemia.

The ACC/AHA guidelines for the diagnostic use of the standard exercise test have stated that it is appropriate for testing of adult male or female patients (including those with complete right bundle branch block (RBBB) or with less than 1 mm of resting ST depression) with an *intermediate pretest probability* of CAD based on gender, age, and symptoms [2]. Pretest risk assessment is critical to determine whether stress testing is appropriate. Furthermore, interpretation of the ECG in cardiac stress testing can be heavily influenced by the patient history and the stress modality. In this chapter, we will review ECG interpretation in cardiac stress testing with a focus on identification of myocardial ischemia.

Exercise Physiology

Prior to assessment of the ECG in patients undergoing exercise testing, a basic understanding of exercise physiology is

Electrocardiogram in Clinical Medicine, First Edition. Edited by William J. Brady, Michael J. Lipinski, Andrew E. Darby, Michael C. Bond, Nathan P. Charlton, Korin Hudson, and Kelly Williamson.

critical to understanding how changes in blood pressure and heart rate during exercise may also identify patients with myocardial ischemia. In the case of exercise-induced ischemia, the basic physiologic principle is that myocardial oxygen demand outstrips myocardial oxygen supply. The determinants of myocardial oxygen uptake, which is the amount of oxygen consumed by the heart muscle, include intramyocardial wall tension (left ventricular pressure and end-diastolic volume), contractility, and heart rate. It has been shown that myocardial oxygen uptake can be reasonably estimated by the product of heart rate and systolic blood pressure (double product). Exercise-induced angina often occurs at the same myocardial oxygen demand (double product) with a higher double product implying better myocardial perfusion. Thus, double product during exercise testing is an established predictor of myocardial ischemia [3] and prognosis [4, 5]. Exercise-induced ischemia can cause cardiac dysfunction, which results in exercise impairment and an abnormal systolic blood pressure response. Thus, it is important not only to assess the ECG for evidence of myocardial ischemia but to also clinically assess the patient for symptoms and signs of ischemia, such as changes to systolic blood pressure and heart rate during exercise.

The body initially responds to exercise by a coordinated response of the sympathetic and parasympathetic nervous system, leading to an increase in heart rate. The heart rate initially increases by as much as 10–30 bpm through vagal withdrawal, while the following increase in heart rate is thought to be largely driven by increased sympathetic response. The increase in cardiac output with exercise is largely driven by an increase in heart rate rather than change in stroke volume. During exercise, stroke volume increases up to approximately 50–60% of maximal capacity, after which increases in cardiac output are caused by further increases in heart rate. Autonomic physiology during recovery from exercise involves reactivation of the parasympathetic system and deactivation of sympathetic activity.

The decline of heart rate after cessation of exercise is a measure of autonomic function, and a delay in heart rate recovery following exercise is a marker of autonomic dysfunction and/or failure of the cardiovascular system to respond to the normal autonomic responses to exercise. This delay has been shown to be a powerful prognostic marker [6, 7] and may also identify patients with significant CAD [8]. Having the patient perform a cool-down walk after the test can delay or eliminate the appearance of ST-segment depression, while having patients lie down enhances ST-segment abnormalities in recovery [9]. Monitoring should continue for at least five minutes after exercise or until changes stabilize. ST depression occurring only in the recovery period is neither unusual nor necessarily suggestive of a false-positive result. The recovery period, particularly the third minute is critical for ST analy-sis. ST depression at that time has important implications regarding the presence and severity of CAD [10, 11]. In general, ST depression during exercise alone is more sensitive but less specific while depression in recovery is less sensitive but more specific for myocardial ischemia.

The increased demand for myocardial oxygen required by dynamic exercise is the key to the use of exercise testing as a diagnostic tool for CAD. Increased heart rate is particularly important in patients who have obstructive CAD. An increase in heart rate results in a shortening of the diastolic filling period, the time during which coronary blood flow is the greatest. In normal coronary arteries, dilation occurs. In obstructed vessels, however, dilation is limited and flow can be decreased by the shortening of the diastolic filling period. This causes inadequate blood flow and therefore insufficient oxygen supply.

Systolic blood pressure should rise during exercise while diastolic blood pressure usually remains the same or drops. Exertional hypotension has been shown to predict severe angiographic CAD and is associated with a poor prognosis [12]. A drop in systolic blood pressure below pre-exercise values is the most ominous criterion. In patients with prior myocardial infarction (MI), failure of systolic blood pressure to adequately increase is particularly worrisome. This response is the most ominous for adverse events during testing, and that is why manual methods of BP monitoring are important for test safety.

Normal ECG Changes with Exercise

Studies in normal individuals have been performed to assess the impact of exercise on changes in the ECG [13]. These studies demonstrate that the P-wave amplitude increases with exercise while there is typically a decrease in the T-wave amplitude in early exercise. Additionally, there does not appear to be a significant change in the QRS magnitude and rarely a shortening of the QRS complex with exercise. The R-wave amplitude initially increases early in exercise and then begins to decrease in amplitude immediately before maximal exercise [14]. During maximal exercise, there is depression of the J junction, peaking of the T waves, and marked ST-segment upsloping [15], which may be confused with myocardial ischemia by clinicians lacking experience in exercise ECG interpretation.

ECG Changes with Ischemia

Changes in the Q Wave, R Wave, and S Wave

Exercise-induced R-wave and S-wave amplitude changes do not associate with changes in left ventricular volume, ejection fraction, or ischemia. Several studies assessed

R-wave amplitude during exercise and found either little or no correlation with left ventricular volume or ejection fraction [16, 17]. A case of left ventricular ejection fraction is shown in Figure 2.7.1. Initial studies suggested patients with CAD and myocardial ischemia had R-wave amplitude increase, suggesting left ventricular dilation in the setting of ischemia. However, these patients with myocardial ischemia had limited exercise capacity and were unable to

(a)

(b)

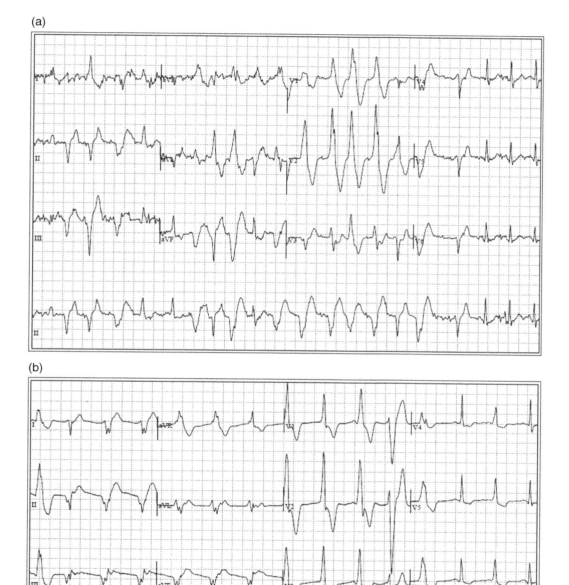

Figure 2.7.1 A 59-year-old male with no cardiac risk factors was referred for worsening dyspnea on exertion and atypical chest pain. During exercise (a), the patient developed frequent and erratic ventricular complexes and ventricular tachycardia and exercise was terminated. The patient developed shortness of breath and the same tight atypical chest pain in the top of his chest. During recovery (b), the ventricular rhythm persisted with different morphologies, as seen in the rhythm strip. An echocardiogram was performed and demonstrated a left ventricular ejection fraction of 20% with global hypokinesis. A subsequent coronary angiogram confirmed the diagnosis of non-ischemic cardiomyopathy, which after careful history was felt to be the result of a viral myocarditis.

achieve the degree of maximal exercise necessary to see the R-wave amplitude decrease seen at maximal exercise in normal individuals [14]. There is an increase in the S-wave in the lateral precordial leads during exercise but this likely results from exercise-induced axis shifts and conduction alterations rather than changes in ventricular contractility. Septal Q-wave amplitude during exercise was studied in normal individuals and in patients with CAD [18]. These data reveal that the septal Q waves were smaller in patients with CAD than in normal subjects, and the loss of Q waves and development of ST-segment depression is highly specific for CAD. The hypothesis is that the loss of the Q wave during exercise in patients with CAD may reflect abnormal activation and loss of septal wall contraction in the setting of myocardial ischemia.

Changes in the ST-Segment

Exercise-induced myocardial ischemia can lead to two possible changes in the ST-segment: elevation or depression.

ST Depression

ST-segment depression during exercise can represent global subendocardial ischemia, and its presence typically occurs in the lateral precordial leads V4–V6. Abnormal exercise-induced ST depression is 1 mm or greater of horizontal or downsloping ST depression measured at the end of the QRS complex/beginning of the ST segment (J junction) and lasting at least 60 ms. Downsloping ST depression is more indicative of ischemia and more serious than horizontal depression. Slow upsloping ST depression is less serious than downsloping or horizontal ST depression but can be a precursor to abnormal ST depression during recovery or at higher workloads. It is also important to assess three or more contiguous beats in the same lead to make sure ST depression is accurately assessed given the possibility of baseline wander or artifact during exercise. If upsloping ST depression is included as a positive test, this will decrease test specificity while increasing sensitivity. In the case of borderline ST segment depression or upsloping ST segment depression, it is important to include the clinical context in the decision of whether to call the test abnormal. A case of borderline ST depression can be seen in Figure 2.7.2. ST depression does not localize coronary artery lesions. ST depression in the inferior leads (II, III, and AVF) is most often caused by the atrial repolarization wave, which begins in the PR segment and can extend to the beginning of the ST-segment.

Exercise-induced ST-depression loses its diagnostic power in patients with LBBB, Wolff-Parkinson-White

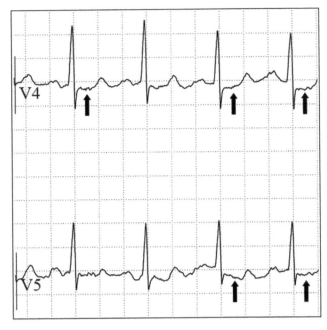

Figure 2.7.2 A 55-year-old male with past medical history of diabetes was referred for exercise stress testing due to worsening dyspnea on exertion. His resting ECG was unremarkable and his ECG at maximal exertion (shown below) only achieved 100 beats per minute at 5 METs. His electrocardiogram had significant baseline wander and showed evidence of borderline ST-segment depression with what appeared to be horizontal ST depression in V4, though not consistent due to wander, and even some downsloping ST depression in V5. The ST depression resolved immediately during recovery. Exercise single photon emission computed tomography (SPECT) imaging suggested a possible inferior defect. The patient was referred for coronary angiography, which did not show any significant obstructive coronary artery disease.

(WPW) syndrome, electronic pacemakers, intraventricular conduction defects (IVCDs) with inverted T waves and in patients with more than 1 mm of resting ST depression. An example of exercise-induced LBBB can be seen in Figure 2.7.3. Digoxin is well known to result not only in baseline ST and T-wave abnormalities but to induce ST depression during exercise in normal subjects [19, 20]. Left ventricular hypertrophy is well known to result in false-positive ST-segment depression and a classic example of this is found in Figure 2.7.4. False-positive ST depression is also seen in patients with valvular heart disease, congenital heart disease, cardiomyopathies, pericardial disease, or RBBB. Patients with RBBB are known to have exercise-induced ST depression in the anterior precordial leads but no ST depression in the inferior and lateral leads [21]. An example exercise-induced RBBB can be found in Figure 2.7.5. In the case of ST-segment changes isolated to the inferior leads are more likely to be false-positive responses unless profound (i.e. more than 1 mm).

(a)

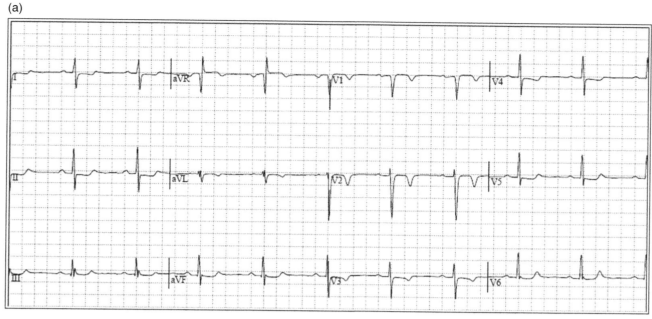

(b)

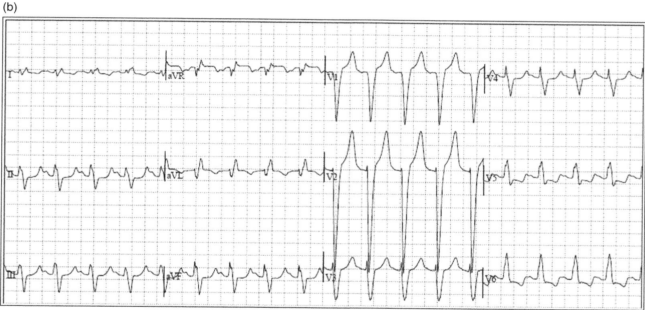

Figure 2.7.3 A 72-year-old man with atypical chest pain was referred for exercise nuclear stress testing given his history of multi-vessel CAD with imaging to identify whether myocardial ischemia was present and to localize the territory or territories if it is present to guide potential revascularization. Resting ECG (a) showed diffuse ST-segment depression and T-wave abnormalities, which are unchanged from previous ECGs. At two minutes exercise, the patient developed LBBB with ST depression (b). Due to septal wall artifacts with nuclear imaging, the patient was converted to a regadenosine stress test, which revealed transient ischemic dilation and findings consistent with multi-vessel coronary disease. This was confirmed by coronary angiography and the patient was referred for coronary artery bypass surgery.

Due to the high false-positive rate of the inferior leads [22], precordial lead V5 alone consistently outperforms the inferior leads or the combination of leads V5 with II. Exercise-induced ST-segment depression isolated to the inferior limb leads has been shown to be a poor marker for CAD [23]. ST depression in precordial lead V5 along with V4 and V6 are reliable markers for CAD in patients with normal resting ECGs without prior MI, and the monitoring of inferior limb leads adds little additional diagnostic information. However, as previously shown, ST-segment

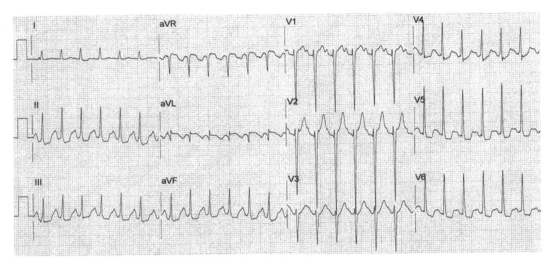

Figure 2.7.4 A 73-year-old male with hypertension was referred for exercise nuclear stress testing for atypical chest pain. His electrocardiogram at maximal exercise is shown below and is significant for left ventricular hypertrophy and ST segment depression in multiple leads. He achieved 10 METS (metabolic equivalents) while exercising nine minutes on the Bruce protocol and nuclear imaging showed no reversible perfusion defects with exercise.

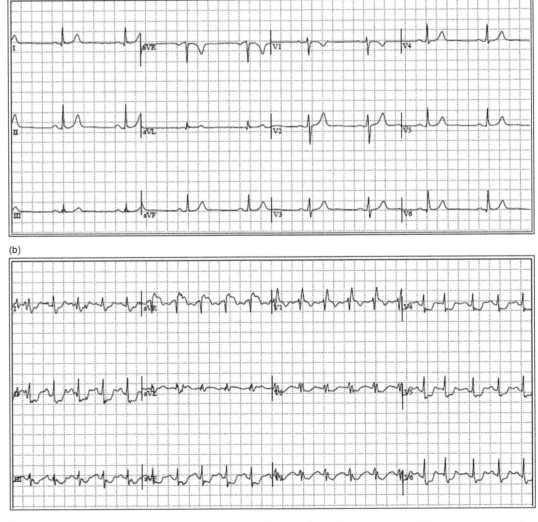

Figure 2.7.5 A 62-year-old male with hypertension, hypercholesterolemia, and atypical symptoms was referred for exercise testing. The patient had a largely unremarkable resting ECG (a) but during exercise developed a RBBB. Toward maximal exercise he developed ST depression in multiple leads (b) and began to have symptoms of chest pain which only improved after five minutes of recovery. He was referred for coronary angiography, which revealed multi-vessel CAD.

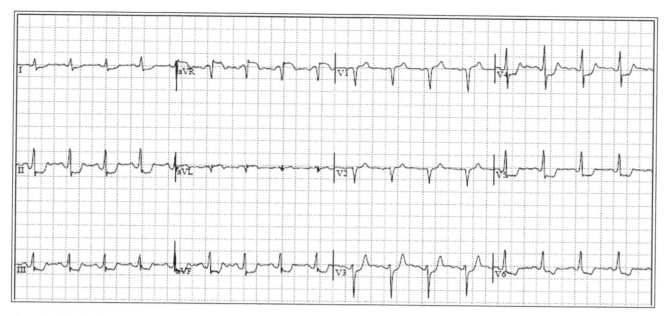

Figure 2.7.6 A 70-year-old male with hypercholesterolemia and diabetes was referred for exercise stress testing due to dyspnea on exertion. He exercised to eight minutes on the Bruce protocol and was limited due to shortness of breath which continued into recovery. His ECG with Max HR of 140 BPM was largely unremarkable at maximal exercise aside from some poor R-wave progression, raising the question of prior anteroseptal myocardial infarction. During recovery, the patient developed significant horizontal and downsloping ST depression shown below starting a two minutes of recovery and reached a maximum at five minutes of recovery (shown below). Coronary angiography demonstrated a severe stenosis of the mid-left anterior descending coronary artery.

elevation in the inferior leads in the absence of prior MI or Q waves should not be ignored.

ST-segment depression limited to the recovery period does not generally represent a "false-positive" response. Inclusion of analysis during this time period increases the diagnostic yield of the exercise test. In Figure 2.7.6, a classic example of ST depression is seen that was limited to recovery. Other criteria, including downsloping ST changes in recovery and prolongation of depression, can improve test performance.

ST Elevation

Severe transmural ischemia, resulting in wall motion abnormalities, causes a shift of the vector in the direction of the wall motion abnormality resulting in ST elevation (STE). The elevation occurs in the leads over lying the ischemia. However, preexisting areas of wall motion abnormality, such as prior MI typically accompanied by Q waves, also cause such a shift resulting in STE without ischemia being present. When the resting ECG shows Q waves of an old MI, ST elevation is caused by ischemia or wall-motion abnormalities or both, whereas accompanying ST depression can be caused by a second area of ischemia or reciprocal changes. Examples of changes to the ST-segment elevation during exercise can be found in Figure 2.7.7. In the case of a normal resting ECG, severe

myocardial ischemia due to either a critical coronary lesion or coronary spasm can lead to STE and is often accompanied by reciprocal ST depression. Such STE is

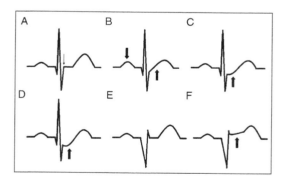

Figure 2.7.7 The effects of exercise on the ST-segment with (a) showing the normal P wave, QRS complex, and T wave at rest. In an individual at maximal exercise (b), the P-wave amplitude is increased (downward arrow), the j point is depressed with an upsloping ST segment (upward arrow), and T-wave amplitude is decreased. The standard criterion for abnormal is 1 mm of horizontal or downsloping ST-segment depression below the PR isoelectric line or 1 mm further depression if there is baseline depression. Horizontal or slow-upsloping of the ST-segment can be seen in (c). Patients with greater than 1.5 mm of slow-upsloping ST-segment depression should usually be considered to have an abnormal test. Downsloping ST-segment depression (d) is also shown. Patients with Q waves on the resting ECG (e) may often develop ST-segment elevation during exercise (f) without being considered abnormal.

(a)

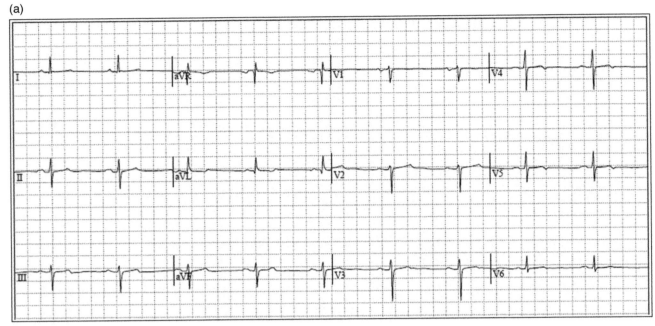

(b)

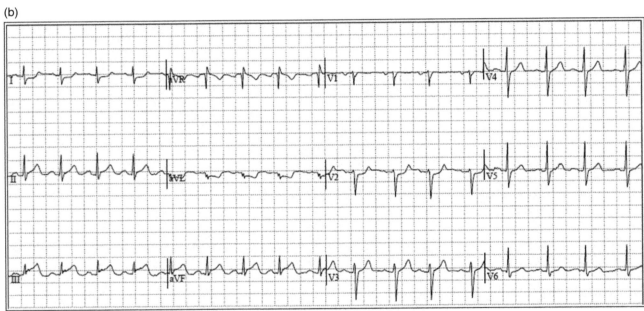

Figure 2.7.8 A 64-year-old male with hypertension, hyperlipidemia, smoking history, and symptoms of typical angina was referred for an exercise nuclear stress testing. Given his pretest probability of disease, initial referral to diagnostic coronary angiography was likely warranted. His resting ECG (a) showed some nonspecific T-wave abnormalities, but the patient developed chest discomfort at 4 minutes of exercise and at minute 5, the physician stopped his exercise when ST-segment elevation was noted in leads II, III, and aVL with reciprocal ST-segment depression in leads I and aVL (b). The patient was taken for urgent cardiac catheterization, which showed a subtotal occlusion of the right coronary artery, which was treated with percutaneous coronary intervention and stenting.

uncommon, very arrhythmogenic, and it localizes. An example of exercise-induced ST-segment elevation can be found in Figure 2.7.8.

Computerized ST-segment measurements should be used cautiously and require physician overreading as choice of isoelectric line and the beginning of the ST segment can lead to erroneous estimation of the degree of ST-segment depression. Filtering and averaging can cause false ST depression because of distortion of the raw data.

Silent Ischemia

Patients with painless ST-segment depression, also known as silent ischemia, usually have milder forms of CAD and a better prognosis and evidence supporting urgent cardiac catheterization in these patients is lacking. The evidence base for silent ischemia being more prevalent in diabetics is not as convincing as one would think given its widespread clinical acceptance. Though many physicians advocate screening for silent ischemia and CAD in diabetics with routine treadmill testing, evidence does not support this practice [24].

Exercise-Induced Arrhythmias

In both patients with CAD and asymptomatic individuals, exercise-induced ventricular arrhythmias have an independent association with death [25]. This risk tends to be a long-term risk (more than six years) rather than the risk associated with ST depression, which carries a higher short-term risk. Examples of ventricular tachycardia at the time of exercise stress testing are shown in Figure 2.7.9. Nonsustained ventricular tachycardia is uncommon during routine clinical treadmill testing and is usually well-tolerated. In patients with a history of syncope, sudden death, physical examination suggesting an enlarged heart, murmurs, ECG showing prolonged QT, preexcitation, Q waves, and heart failure (HF), then exercise-testing–induced ventricular arrhythmias are more worrisome. As an example, when healthy individuals exhibit premature ventricular contractions (PVCs) during testing, there is no need for immediate concern. However, in patients referred for exercise stress testing, frequent PVCs during recovery have been shown to be associated with increased mortality during follow-up while PVCs during exercise were related to heart rate increase with exercise [26, 27]. Exercise-testing–induced supraventricular arrhythmias are relatively rare compared to ventricular arrhythmias and appear to be benign except for their association with the development of atrial fibrillation in the future.

Women

The guidelines are clearly stated regarding testing women: concern about false-positive ST responses can be addressed by careful assessment of pretest probability and selective use of a stress imaging test before proceeding to angiography. The optimal strategy for circumventing false-positive test results for the diagnosis of coronary disease in women requires the use of scores. There is insufficient data to justify routine stress imaging tests as the initial test for women.

Diagnostic Scores

Studies considering non-ECG data consistently demonstrate that the multivariable equations outperform simple ST diagnostic criteria. These equations generally provide a predictive accuracy of 80% (ROC area of 0.80). To obtain the best diagnostic characteristics with the exercise test, clinical and non-ECG test responses should be considered. We have validated simple scores for both men [28] and women [29]. Diagnostic scores should be applied during every exercise test because they are easy to use and significantly improve the prediction of angiographic CAD [30].

Termination of Exercise Testing

The absolute and relative indications for test termination are listed in Table 2.7.1. If none of these endpoints are met, the test should be symptom-limited. An example of a test that was terminated due to ominous ST depression can be found in Figure 2.7.10. Another example of an indication for termination of a test can be found in Figure 2.7.11 with a rare example of regadenosine-induced complete heart block. To ensure the safety of exercise testing, the following list of the most dangerous circumstances in the exercise testing laboratory should be recognized:

- When patients exhibit ST-segment elevation (without baseline diagnostic Q waves), this can be associated with dangerous arrhythmias and infarction. The incidence is approximately 1 in 1000 clinical tests and usually occurs in V2–V3 (LAD involvement) or II/aVF (RCA involvement) rather than V5.
- When a patient with an ischemic cardiomyopathy exhibits severe chest pain because of ischemia (angina pectoris), a cool-down walk is advisable.
- When a patient develops exertional hypotension accompanied by ischemia (angina or ST-segment depression) or when it occurs in a patient with a history of congestive heart failure, cardiomyopathy, or recent MI, safety is a serious issue.
- When a patient with a history of sudden death or collapse during exercise develops premature ventricular contractions that become frequent, a cool-down walk is advisable.

(a)

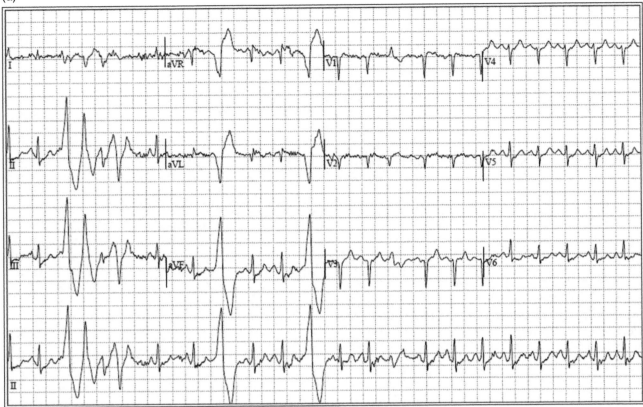

(b)

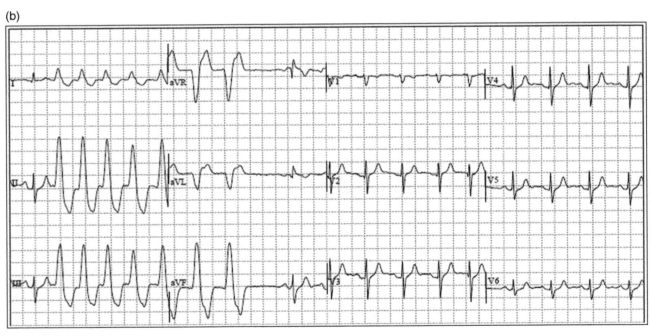

Figure 2.7.9 In the first example (a), a 54-year-old male with hypertension and a significant smoking history was referred for atypical chest pain and feeling lightheaded with exertion. At five minutes of exercise, the patient developed polymorphic ventricular tachycardia characterized by the wide complex tachycardia that changes axis and has variable rate and amplitude (b). It is best seen in the inferior leads and the rhythm strip in lead II. It is important to pay close attention during testing as the ventricular tachycardia could have been missed if one thought it was artifact or "noise". Exercise was terminated and the patient developed frequent premature ventricular complexes and endorsed lightheadedness. Coronary angiography demonstrated a severe stenosis in the proximal left anterior descending artery. In the second example, a 67-year-old male with hypertension developed chest pain during his exercise stress test but did not have significant ST depression. However, at three minutes into recovery (b), the patient experienced an asymptomatic seven beat run of nonsustained ventricular tachycardia. Given the constellation of chest pain and nonsustained ventricular tachycardia despite the negative ST segments, the patient underwent coronary angiography which revealed a severe stenosis in the mid right coronary artery.

Table 2.7.1 Indications for terminating exercise testing.

ABSOLUTE INDICATIONS

Moderate to severe angina

Increasing nervous system symptoms (e.g. ataxia, dizziness, or near-syncope)

Signs of poor perfusion (cyanosis or pallor)

Technical difficulties in monitoring ECG or systolic blood pressure

Subject's desire to stop

Sustained ventricular tachycardia

ST-segment elevation (≥1.0 mm) in leads without diagnostic Q waves (other than V1 or aVR)

RELATIVE INDICATIONS

Drop in systolic blood pressure of ≥10 mmHg from baseline blood pressure despite an increase in workload in the absence of other evidence of ischemia

ST or QRS changes such as excessive ST-segment depression (>2 mm of horizontal or downsloping ST-segment depression) or marked axis shift

Arrhythmias other than sustained ventricular tachycardia, including multifocal PVCs, triplets of PVCs, supraventricular tachycardia, heart block, or bradyarrhythmias

Fatigue, shortness of breath, wheezing, leg cramps, or claudication

Development of bundle branch block or intraventricular conduction delay that cannot be distinguished from ventricular tachycardia

Increasing chest pain

Hypertensive response[a]

---

[a] In the absence of definitive evidence, the committee suggests systolic blood pressure of >250 mmHg and/or a diastolic blood pressure of >115 mmHg.

Source: Modified from Gibbons et al. [2]

Exercise Testing and Acute Coronary Syndromes

The guidelines state that patients who are pain free, have either a normal or nondiagnostic ECG or one that is unchanged from previous tracings, and have a normal set of initial cardiac enzymes are candidates for further evaluation. If the patient is low risk and does not experience any further ischemic discomfort and a follow-up 12-lead ECG and cardiac marker measurements after 6–8 hours of observation are normal, the patient can be considered for an early exercise test to provoke ischemia. This test can be performed before discharge and should be supervised by an experienced physician. In the conservative arm of the Treat Angina with aggrastat and determine Cost of Therapy with an Invasive or Conservative Strategy – Thrombolysis In Myocardial Infarction (TACTICS-TIMI) 18 trial, patients with appropriate medical therapy can safely undergo exercise or pharmacologic stress testing within 48–72 hours of admission as only one death occurred following stress testing in 847 patients with unstable angina or non-ST elevation MI [31]. However, a recent study randomizing patients with acute coronary syndrome and a negative troponin to either stress echocardiography or symptom-limited ECG treadmill testing suggested that the incorporation of the imaging modality resulted in better risk stratification and significant cost benefit. Fewer patients were classified as intermediate risk with stress echocardiography, which would have required further testing [32].

Exercise Testing after Myocardial Infarction

An exercise test prior to discharge is important for giving patients guidelines for exercise at home, reassuring them of their physical status, advising them to resume or increase their activity level, advising them on timing of return to work and determining the risk of complications. Psychologically, it can cause an improvement in the patient's self-confidence by making the patient less anxious about daily physical activities and help them to rehabilitate themselves. The test has been helpful in reassuring spouses of post-MI patients of their physical capabilities. Exercise testing is also an important tool in exercise training as part of comprehensive cardiac rehabilitation, where it can be used to develop and modify the exercise prescription, assist in providing activity counseling, and assess the patient's response at the initiation of, and progress in, the exercise training program. One consistent finding in the review of

(a)

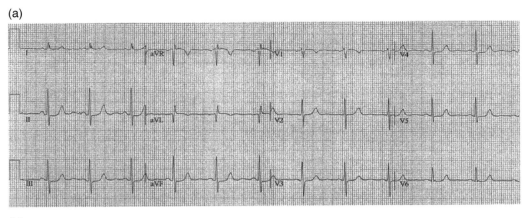

(b)

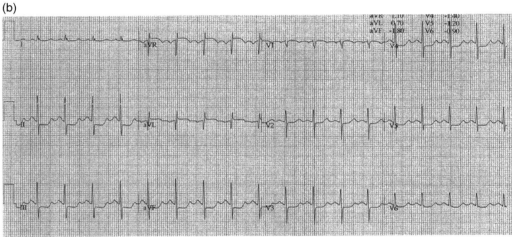

(c)

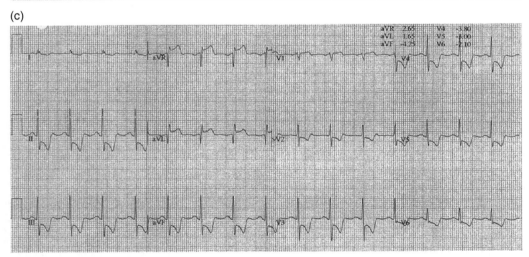

Figure 2.7.10 A 81-year-old female with hypertension was referred for exercise stress testing due to progressive dyspnea on exertion and atypical chest pain. Her resting ECG (a) demonstrated some diffuse minimal ST-segment depression and isolated Q wave with T-wave inversion in aVL. After only two minutes of the Bruce protocol, the test was terminated due to symptoms of significant dyspnea along with ECG evidence concerning for ischemia and potentially left main coronary artery disease (b). There was diffuse ST depression with greater than 2 mm of depression in several leads and ST elevation in leads aVR and aVL. This series of ECGs highlights the importance of the ECG in recovery. The included ECG from recovery (c) is taken at 18 minutes after termination of the test and shows profound ischemia and the patient was carefully monitored until she underwent urgent cardiac catheterization which revealed a 95% stenosis of the distal left main coronary artery along with a 80% stenosis of the proximal right coronary artery. The patient experienced a significant rise in her cardiac troponins as a result of the stress test.

(a)

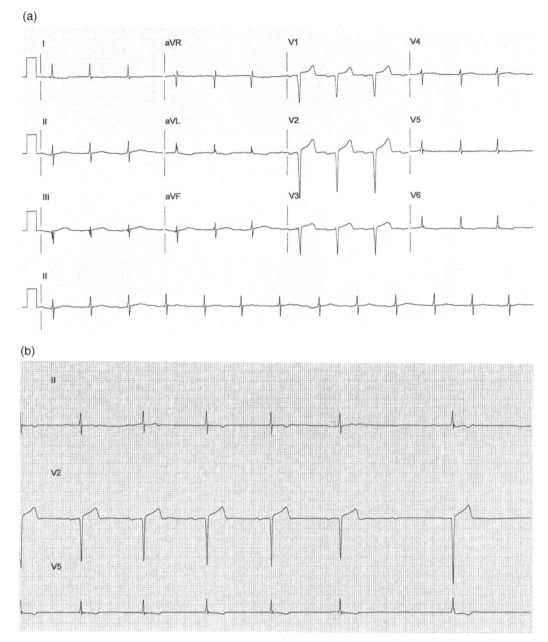

(b)

Figure 2.7.11 A 68-year-old female with coronary artery disease and prior coronary artery bypass surgery was referred for regadenosine nuclear stress testing given atypical chest pain that does not resemble her prior angina. It was hoped angiography could be avoided as her baseline creatinine was elevated at 1.6 mg/dl. Her baseline ECG (a) demonstrated prior anteroseptal myocardial infarction with Q waves in V1–V3 and lateral T-wave abnormalities. Almost immediately following slow injection of the regadenosine (b), the patient developed third-degree atrioventricular block with complete dissociation of the P waves and QRS complexes but maintained a junctional escape rhythm with heart rate of 30 beats per minute. Her blood pressure fell with systolic blood pressure of 65 mmHg and the patient was immediately administered aminophylline to reverse the regadenosine, atropine, and eventually required initiation of dopamine until her blood pressure improved. The patient eventually underwent coronary angiography, which demonstrated severe three-vessel native coronary disease, a patent left internal mammary artery to the distal left anterior descending artery, and occluded vein grafts to the right posterior descending artery and the obtuse marginal artery.

the post-MI exercise test studies that included a follow-up for cardiac end points is that patients who met whatever criteria set forth for exercise testing were at lower risk than patients not tested. From meta-analyses of multiple studies, only an abnormal SBP response or a low exercise capacity were consistently associated with a poor outcome and were more predictive of adverse cardiac events after MI than measures of exercise-induced ischemia [33, 34].

Conclusions

The exercise test complements the medical history and the physical examination, and it remains the second most commonly performed cardiologic procedure next to the routine ECG. ST depression is most important for diagnosing obstructive coronary lesions while exercise capacity is a strong predictor of prognosis. The Duke treadmill score (DTS) should be calculated as part of every test.

The addition of echocardiography or myocardial perfusion imaging does not negate the importance of the ECG or clinical and hemodynamic responses to exercise. The renewed efforts to control costs undoubtedly will support the role of the exercise test. Convincing evidence that treadmill scores enhance the diagnostic and prognostic power of the exercise test certainly has cost-efficacy implications. Thus, a basic understanding of the exercise ECG can not only enhance the clinicians' understanding of ischemic manifestations on the ECG but also help clinicians to risk-stratify patients based on their ECG findings during exercise.

Recommended Reading

Froelicher, V.F. and Myers, J.N. (2006). *Exercise and the Heart*, 5e. Philadelphia, PA: WB Saunders Company.

Froelicher, V.F. and Myers, J.N. (2007). *Manual of Exercise Testing*, 3e. Philadelphia, PA: Mosby Elsevier.

References

1 Froelicher, V.F. and Myers, J.N. (2006). *Exercise and the Heart*, 5e. Philadelphia, PA: WB Saunders Company.

2 Gibbons, R.J., Balady, G.J., Bricker, J.T. et al. (2002). ACC/AHA 2002 guideline update for exercise testing: summary article: a report of the American College of Cardiology/American Heart Association Task Force on Practice Guidelines (Committee to Update the 1997 Exercise Testing Guidelines). *Circulation* 106: 1883–1892.

3 Berman, J.L., Wynne, J., and Cohn, P.F. (1978). A multivariate approach for interpreting treadmill exercise tests in coronary artery disease. *Circulation* 58: 505–512.

4 Villella, M., Villella, A., Barlera, S. et al. (1999). Prognostic significance of double product and inadequate double product response to maximal symptom-limited exercise stress testing after myocardial infarction in 6296 patients treated with thrombolytic agents. GISSI-2 investigators. Grupo Italiano per lo Studio della Sopravvivenza nell-Infarto Miocardico. *Am. Heart J.* 137: 443–452.

5 Sadrzadeh Rafie, A.H., Sungar, G.W., Dewey, F.E. et al. (2008). Prognostic value of double product reserve. *Eur. J. Cardiovasc. Prev. Rehabil.* 15: 541–547.

6 Nishime, E.O., Cole, C.R., Blackstone, E.H. et al. (2000). Heart rate recovery and treadmill exercise score as predictors of mortality in patients referred for exercise ECG. *JAMA* 284: 1392–1398.

7 Shetler, K., Marcus, R., Froelicher, V.F. et al. (2001). Heart rate recovery: validation and methodologic issues. *J. Am. Coll. Cardiol.* 38: 1980–1987.

8 Lipinski, M.J., Vetrovec, G.W., and Froelicher, V.F. (2004). Importance of the first two minutes of heart rate recovery after exercise treadmill testing in predicting mortality and the presence of coronary artery disease in men. *Am. J. Cardiol.* 93: 445–449.

9 Gutman, R.A., Alexander, E.R., Li, Y.B. et al. (1970). Delay of ST depression after maximal exercise by walking for 2 minutes. *Circulation* 42: 229–233.

10 Savage, M.P., Squires, L.S., Hopkins, J.T. et al. (1987). Usefulness of ST-segment depression as a sign of coronary artery disease when confined to the postexercise recovery period. *Am. J. Cardiol.* 60: 1405–1406.

11 Froelicher, V.F., Thompson, A.J., Longo, M.R. Jr. et al. (1976). Value of exercise testing for screening asymptomatic men for latent coronary artery disease. *Prog. Cardiovasc. Dis.* 18: 265–276.

12 Le, V.V., Mitiku, T., Sungar, G. et al. (2008). The blood pressure response to dynamic exercise testing: a systematic review. *Prog. Cardiovasc. Dis.* 51: 135–160.

13 Simoons, M.L. and Hugenholtz, P.G. (1975). Gradual changes of ECG waveform during and after exercise in normal subjects. *Circulation* 52: 570–577.

14 Myers, J., Ahnve, S., Froelicher, V., and Sullivan, M. (1985). Spatial R wave amplitude changes during exercise: relation with left ventricular ischemia and function. *J. Am. Coll. Cardiol.* 6: 603–608.

15 Wolthuis, R.A., Froelicher, V.F., Hopkirk, A. et al. (1979). Normal electrocardiographic waveform characteristics during treadmill exercise testing. *Circulation* 60: 1028–1035.

16 Battler, A., Froelicher, V., Slutsky, R., and Ashburn, W. (1979). Relationship of QRS amplitude changes during exercise to left ventricular function and volumes and the

diagnosis of coronary artery disease. *Circulation* 60: 1004–1013.

17 De Feyter, P.J., de JP, J., Roos, J.P. et al. (1982). Diagnostic incapacity of exercise-induced QRS wave amplitude changes to detect coronary artery disease and left ventricular dysfunction. *Eur. Heart J.* 3: 9–16.

18 Morales-Ballejo, H., Greenberg, P.S., Ellestad, M.H., and Bible, M. (1981). Septal Q wave in exercise testing: angiographic correlation. *Am. J. Cardiol.* 48: 247–251.

19 Sundqvist, K., Atterhog, J.H., and Jogestrand, T. (1986). Effect of digoxin on the electrocardiogram at rest and during exercise in healthy subjects. *Am. J. Cardiol.* 57: 661–665.

20 Sketch, M.H., Mooss, A.N., Butler, M.L. et al. (1981). Digoxin-induced positive exercise tests: their clinical and prognostic significance. *Am. J. Cardiol.* 48: 655–659.

21 Whinnery, J.E., Froelicher, V.F. Jr., Longo, M.R. Jr., and Triebwasser, J.H. (1977). The electrocardiographic response to maximal treadmill exercise of asymptomatic men with right bundle branch block. *Chest* 71: 335–340.

22 Viik, J., Lehtinen, R., Turjanmaa, V. et al. (1998). Correct utilization of exercise electrocardiographic leads in differentiation of men with coronary artery disease from patients with a low likelihood of coronary artery disease using peak exercise ST-segment depression. *Am. J. Cardiol.* 81: 964–969.

23 Miranda, C.P., Liu, J., Kadar, A. et al. (1992). Usefulness of exercise-induced ST-segment depression in the inferior leads during exercise testing as a marker for coronary artery disease. *Am. J. Cardiol.* 69: 303–307.

24 Young, L.H., Wackers, F.J., Chyun, D.A. et al. (2009). Cardiac outcomes after screening for asymptomatic coronary artery disease in patients with type 2 diabetes: the DIAD study: a randomized controlled trial. *JAMA* 301: 1547–1555.

25 Beckerman, J., Wu, T., Jones, S., and Froelicher, V.F. (2005). Exercise test-induced arrhythmias. *Prog. Cardiovasc. Dis.* 47: 285–305.

26 Frolkis, J.P., Pothier, C.E., Blackstone, E.H., and Lauer, M.S. (2003). Frequent ventricular ectopy after exercise as a predictor of death. *N. Engl. J. Med.* 348: 781–790.

27 Dewey, F.E., Kapoor, J.R., Williams, R.S. et al. (2008). Ventricular arrhythmias during clinical treadmill testing and prognosis. *Arch. Intern. Med.* 168: 225–234.

28 Raxwal, V., Shetler, K., Morise, A. et al. (2001). Simple treadmill score to diagnose coronary disease. *Chest* 119: 1933–1940.

29 Morise, A.P., Lauer, M.S., and Froelicher, V.F. (2002). Development and validation of a simple exercise test score for use in women with symptoms of suspected coronary artery disease. *Am. Heart J.* 144: 818–825.

30 Lipinski, M., Do, D., Froelicher, V. et al. (2001). Comparison of exercise test scores and physician estimation in determining disease probability. *Arch. Intern. Med.* 161: 2239–2244.

31 Karha, J., Gibson, C.M., Murphy, S.A. et al. (2004). Safety of stress testing during the evolution of unstable angina pectoris or non-ST-elevation myocardial infarction. *Am. J. Cardiol.* 94: 1537–1539.

32 Jeetley, P., Burden, L., Stoykova, B., and Senior, R. (2007). Clinical and economic impact of stress echocardiography compared with exercise electrocardiography in patients with suspected acute coronary syndrome but negative troponin: a prospective randomized controlled study. *Eur. Heart J.* 28: 204–211.

33 Froelicher, V.F., Perdue, S., Pewen, W., and Risch, M. (1987). Application of meta-analysis using an electronic spread sheet to exercise testing in patients after myocardial infarction. *Am. J. Med.* 83: 1045–1054.

34 Shaw, L.J., Peterson, E.D., Kesler, K. et al. (1996). A metaanalysis of predischarge risk stratification after acute myocardial infarction with stress electrocardiographic, myocardial perfusion, and ventricular function imaging. *Am. J. Cardiol.* 78: 1327–1337.

Section III

The Dysrhythmic ECG

1

Bradycardia

Andrew E. Darby

University of Virginia Health System, Charlottesville, VA, USA

Introduction

There is considerable variation in the resting heart rate among healthy, asymptomatic patients. Evidence suggests the average resting heart rate ranges between 50 and 90 bpm [1]. A patient's baseline heart rate and conduction velocity are determined by the balance between the output of the parasympathetic and sympathetic nervous systems and characteristics of the individual's conduction system. Parasympathetic tone decreases sinus node automaticity and slows atrioventricular (AV) nodal conduction while sympathetic output increases automaticity and enhances conduction. Nocturnal heart rates are generally slower than during waking hours due to increased parasympathetic tone.

Under normal conditions, the primary cardiac pacemaker is the sinoatrial (SA) node located in the right atrium near the junction with the superior vena cava (Figure 3.1.1). It receives blood supply from the SA nodal artery, which most often branches from the right coronary artery (RCA) [2, 3]. The impulse spreads through interatrial pathways to the AV node, which is located in the posteromedial portion of the right atrium, along the interatrial septum adjacent to the coronary sinus and tricuspid annulus. It receives blood supply from the AV nodal artery, which also tends to branch off the right coronary artery. The AV node connects to the His bundle, which travels along the interventricular septum before branching into the right and left bundle branches. The left bundle branch further divides into the left anterior and posterior fascicles. The right bundle branch is supplied by the AV nodal artery and branches of the left anterior descending (LAD) artery. The left anterior fascicle is supplied by branches of the LAD, and the left posterior fascicle receives dual blood supply from the LAD and posterior descending artery (branch of the RCA).

Once depolarization exits, the SA node and spreads through the atria the P wave is generated on the 12-lead electrocardiogram (ECG). P waves during sinus rhythm tend to be upright in the inferior leads II, III, and aVF (due to the superior location of the sinus node) and inverted in lead aVR (because the sinus node is a rightward structure) [3]. When the impulse reaches the sinus node there is a delay represented by the PR interval on the ECG. Delay in the AV node permits complete ventricular filling and protects the ventricles from rapid transmission of impulses as may occur with supraventricular arrhythmias. After exiting the AV node, the impulse travels through the His bundle, then the right and left bundle branches, and, finally, exits through Purkinje fibers to depolarize the ventricles.

Bradycardia may result from decreased automaticity within the sinus node or conduction block in the SA or AV node [4]. Primary (intrinsic) or secondary (extrinsic) abnormalities of the conduction system may produce bradycardia (Table 3.1.1). The SA and AV nodes are innervated by the parasympathetic nervous system, and increased parasympathetic tone may slow SA node automaticity and AV node conduction, thereby resulting in bradycardia. Common causes of vagally mediated bradycardia include painful stimuli, vomiting, endotracheal intubation or airway suctioning, nasal packing, increased intracranial pressure, and malignant hypertension.

Abnormalities of Sinus Node Function

Sinus node dysfunction, or sick sinus syndrome, is a common cause of bradycardia, particularly in older individuals. Clinical features of sinus node dysfunction include sinus bradycardia with chronotropic

Electrocardiogram in Clinical Medicine, First Edition. Edited by William J. Brady, Michael J. Lipinski, Andrew E. Darby, Michael C. Bond, Nathan P. Charlton, Korin Hudson, and Kelly Williamson.

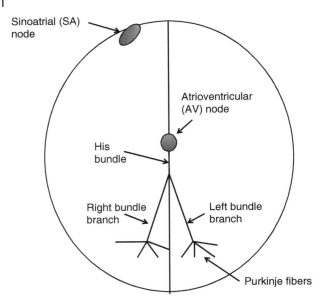

Figure 3.1.1 Anatomy of the cardiac conduction system. The sinoatrial (SA) node functions as the pacemaker for the heart and is located in the superior portion of the right atrium. After the wavefront of depolarization exits the sinus node, it travels through both atria and then meets at the atrioventricular (AV) node. From there, conduction courses through the Bundle of His, then the right and left bundle branches, and, finally, the Purkinje fibers which ramify throughout both ventricles.

Table 3.1.1 Primary and secondary causes of bradycardia.

Primary/Intrinsic	Secondary/Extrinsic
Idiopathic-degenerative changes within structures of the conduction system	Vagal tone
Cardiomyopathy	Medications
Myocarditis	Acute myocardial infarction
Infiltrative diseases	Metabolic (hyperkalemia, acidosis)
Collagen-vascular diseases	Hypothyroidism, hypothermia
Hypertensive heart disease	Infection (endocarditis, Lyme)
Cardiac trauma/surgery	Sepsis

incompetence (i.e. failure to appropriately increase the sinus rate with exertion), sinus pauses or arrest, and paroxysmal atrial tachyarrhythmias (if sinus bradycardia is also present, the patient is considered to have "tachycardia-bradycardia" syndrome (Table 3.1.2 and Figures 3.1.2–3.1.4). Sinus pauses may result from an abrupt decrease in automaticity or failure of the impulse to conduct out of the sinus node (sinus exit block). Sinus pauses <3 seconds are generally not symptomatic or worrisome, but pauses >3 seconds may indicate sinus node pathology and place

Table 3.1.2 Clinical features of sinus node dysfunction.

Sinus bradycardia

Sinus pauses/arrest

Chronotropic incompetence

Paroxysmal atrial tachyarrhythmias

the patient at risk for syncope (Figure 3.1.3) [5–7]. Complete sinus arrest may result in a junctional escape rhythm (generally with a narrow QRS complex and heart rate ranging from 40 to 60 bpm) with either no identifiable P waves on the 12-lead ECG or, alternatively, retrograde P waves closely following each QRS complex (Figure 3.1.5). Nocturnal pauses are common and are not indicative of sinus node pathology.

Abnormalities of Atrioventricular Nodal Conduction

Abnormalities of AV nodal conduction may manifest in several ways: (i) first-degree AV block; (ii) second-degree type I AV block (Mobitz type 1 or Wenckebach); (iii) second-degree type II (Mobitz type 2); or (iv) third-degree (complete heart block) [3]. Another way of categorizing AV nodal conduction block is by location of block (Table 3.1.3): at the AV nodal level or below the level of the AV node at a site in the more distal His-Purkinje system (infra-nodal). Infra-nodal block generally manifests as second-degree type II or complete heart block and is associated with increased morbidity and mortality when compared with type I second-degree AV block, as there is a higher rate of progression to complete heart block and the resultant ventricular escape rhythm tends to be less reliable and slower should complete heart block occur.

First-degree AV block is defined as a PR interval > 200 milliseconds without nonconducted atrial impulses (Figure 3.1.6 a and b). The delay almost always occurs at the level of the AV node. First-degree AV block does not cause bradycardia, although bradycardia may result from concomitant disease of the conduction system such as concurrent sinus node dysfunction. Type I second-degree AV block also typically results from slowing of conduction through the AV node. The pathognomic feature of type I second-degree AV block (i.e. Wenckebach block) is progressive prolongation of the PR interval prior to the nonconducted beat. There is often a pattern of "grouped" beating on the ECG or rhythm strip. Second-degree type II AV block, as opposed to second-degree type I, has no lengthening of the PR interval prior to the nonconducted atrial impulse. The level of block is typically in portions of

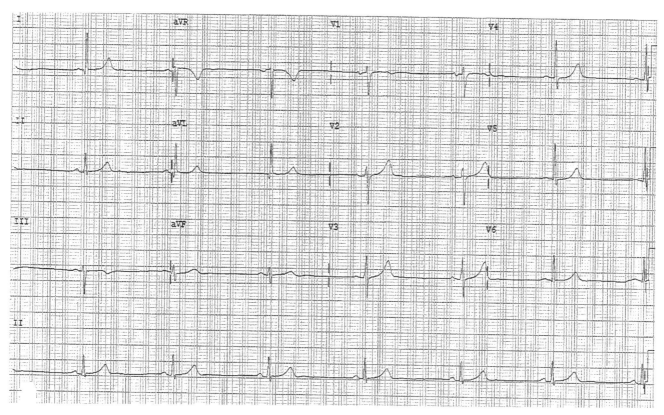

Figure 3.1.2 ECG demonstrating sinus bradycardia. Note the presence of P waves prior to each QRS complex with a normal PR interval. The sinus rate (and, hence, ventricular rate) is approximately 45 beats per minute.

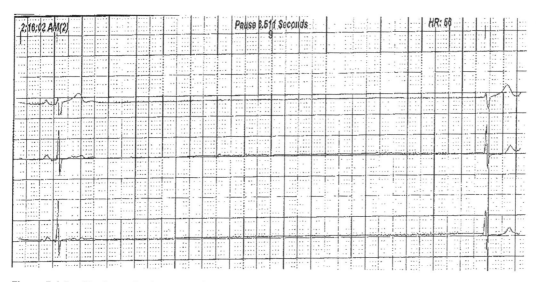

Figure 3.1.3 Rhythm strip demonstrating a sinus pause in a patient with syncope. There is one beat of sinus rhythm after which there is sinus arrest with an approximate 6.5 second pause followed by a junctional escape beat.

the conduction system distal to the AV node, such as the His bundle or Purkinje system. Type II second-degree AV block is more worrisome than Wenckebach block, as there is a higher risk of progression to complete heart block. When atrial to ventricular conduction occurs in a 2 : 1 ratio, Mobitz type II cannot be distinguished from Wenckebach, as there are not enough conducted impulses to assess for PR prolongation (characteristic of Wenckebach conduction). In this scenario, the patient should generally be assumed to have Mobitz type II block so that management

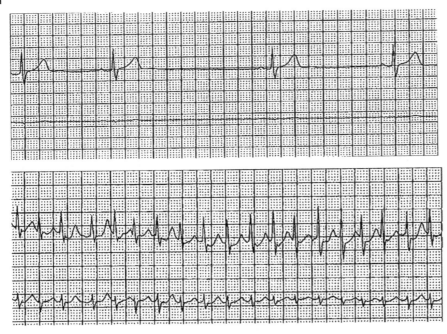

Figure 3.1.4 Rhythm strips from the same patient demonstrating a sinus pause as well as narrow complex tachycardia (likely atrial fibrillation) indicating the patient likely has sinus node dysfunction with tachycardia-bradycardia syndrome.

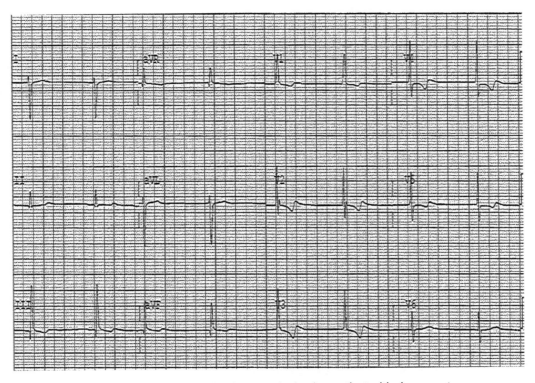

Figure 3.1.5 ECG demonstrating a junctional escape rhythm in a patient with sinus arrest.

is based on the worse of the two possibilities (Figure 3.1.7) [2]. Third-degree AV block occurs in the infra-nodal conduction system and results in atrial and ventricular dissociation (Figure 3.1.8).

Patients with underlying conduction system disease who develop atrial fibrillation (AF) may present with slow ventricular rates (Figure 3.1.9). In this setting, one must distinguish slowly conducted AF from complete AV block with

Table 3.1.3 Clinical features to distinguish conduction abnormalities in the AV node versus infranodal (His-Purkinje) conduction system.

AV nodal block	Infra-nodal block
PR prolongation prior to block	Sudden block without PR prolongation
Escape rate 40–60 bpm	Escape rate < 40 bpm
QRS < 120 milliseconds	QRS > 120 millliseconds
Hemodynamically stable	May be unstable hemodynamically
Increased HR in response to atropine (improvement in conduction with increased sympathetic tone)	Increased block, decreased HR in response to atropine (worsening of AV block with increased sympathetic tone)

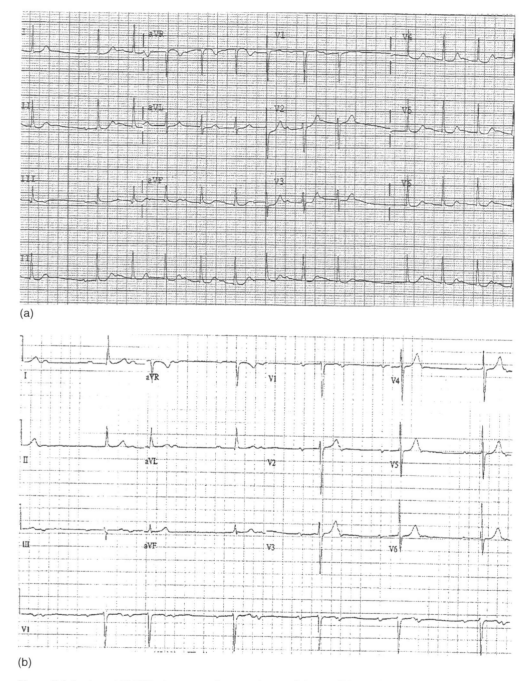

(a)

(b)

Figure 3.1.6 (a and b) ECGs demonstrating type I second degree (Wenckebach) AV block. Note the characteristic lengthening of the PR interval prior to the nonconducted P wave. Type I second degree AV block may produce an irregular rhythm with pauses and, occasionally, bradycardia if there are frequent non-conducted P waves (b). Note b demonstrates predominantly 2 : 1 AV block. In the absence of other clues it would be difficult to determine if the rhythm disturbance is type I vs type II second degree AV block. However, the 2 beats with intact conduction at the beginning of the tracing exhibit clear prolongation of the PR interval prior to the nonconducted P wave revealing type I second degree AV block as the primary cause of bradycardia.

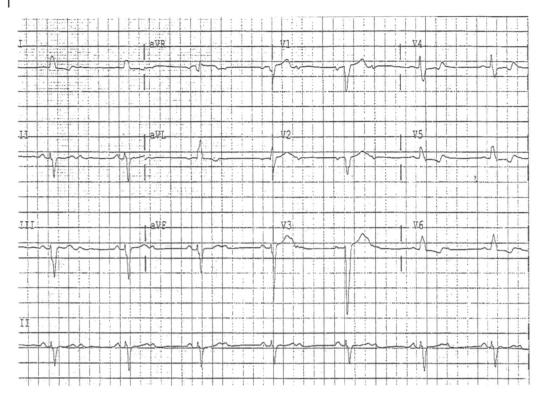

Figure 3.1.7 ECG demonstrating 2 : 1 AV block. Note that every other P wave is conducted to the ventricles. By ECG alone, one cannot distinguish between type I and type II second-degree AV block when there is a pattern of 2 : 1 conduction. Based on the prolonged QRS duration (LBBB pattern), one would assume that the abnormality in the conduction system is below the AV node in the more distal conduction system thereby making type II second degree AV block more likely.

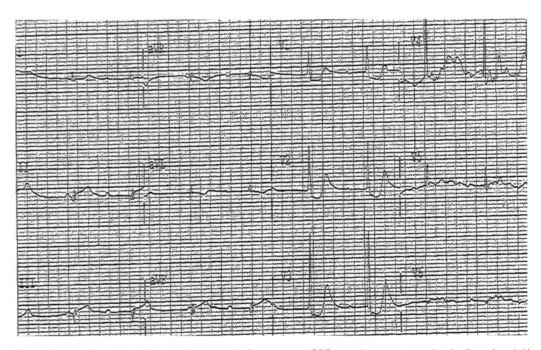

Figure 3.1.8 Complete AV block. Note that the P waves and QRS complexes are completely dissociated. Also of note are the depressed ST segments in the precordial leads, indicative of an acute posterior MI. This patient presented with complete AV block complicating an acute myocardial infarction.

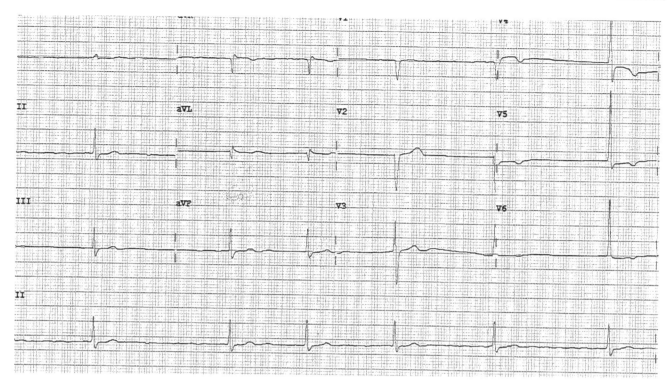

Figure 3.1.9 ECG demonstrating slowly-conducted atrial fibrillation with a mean ventricular rate of approximately 35 beats per minute.

underlying AF. The regularity of the ventricular rhythm is often key, as slowly conducted AF will produce an irregular ventricular rhythm, whereas complete AV block with underlying AF tends to have a regular ventricular rate resulting from the escape rhythm.

Indications for Cardiac Pacing

The American College of Cardiology, American Heart Association, and Heart Rhythm Society recently updated the guidelines for cardiac pacing (Table 3.1.4) [7]. Class I indications for pacing for *sinus node dysfunction* include symptomatic sinus bradycardia, symptomatic sinus pauses, and documented chronotropic incompetence with symptoms. Pacing is indicated for symptomatic bradycardia secondary to third-degree or second-degree type II AV block; ventricular arrhythmias secondary to bradycardia resulting from AV block; asymptomatic bradycardia due to third-degree or second-degree type II AV block with pauses ≥3 seconds or an escape rate < 40 bpm; and patients with AF and bradycardia with pauses ≥5 seconds. Pacing is also indicated for patients with intermittent type II second-degree AV block or third-degree AV block and alternating bundle branch block. Pacing is generally *not* indicated for asymptomatic sinus bradycardia and second-degree AV

Table 3.1.4 Indications for cardiac pacing in sinus node dysfunction and AV block.

Sinus node dysfunction	AV block
Symptomatic bradycardia (including sinus pauses)	Third-degree or second-degree type 2 associated with bradycardia and symptoms
Chronotropic incompetence	Ventricular arrhythmias due to AV block
	Third-degree and type 2 second-degree AV block in asymptomatic patients with pauses ≥3 seconds or escape rate < 40 bpm
	AF and bradycardia with pauses ≥5 seconds

block type I (Wenckebach). In addition, pacing is generally not indicated in situations where bradycardia is secondary to a reversible cause.

Conclusions

Bradycardia is often encountered clinically. When deciding if therapy is indicated, it is critical to determine the relationship between bradycardia and symptoms. It is also important to be able to identify evidence of advanced conduction system pathology on the ECG or rhythm strip. In situations where bradycardia is symptomatic and irreversible, pacemaker therapy is very effective in relieving symptoms.

References

1 Spodick, D.H. (1996). Normal sinus heart rate: appropriate rate thresholds for sinus tachycardia and bradycardia. *South. Med. J.* 89: 666.

2 Brady, W.J. and Harrigan, R.A. (1998). Evaluation and management of bradyarrhythmias in the emergency department. *Emerg. Med. Clin. North Am.* 16: 361.

3 Wagner, G.S. (2001). *Marriott's Practical Electrocardiography*, 10e, 397. Philadelphia: Lippincott Williams & Wilkins.

4 Kaushik, V., Leon, A.R., Forrester, J.S., and Trohman, R.G. (2000). Bradyarrhythmias, temporary and permanent pacing. *Crit. Care Med.* 28: 121.

5 Mangum, J.M. and DiMarco, J.P. (2000). The evaluation and management of bradycardia. *N. Engl. J. Med.* 342: 703.

6 Eraut, D. and Shaw, D.B. (1971). Sinus bradycardia. *Br. Heart J.* 33: 742.

7 Epstein, A.E., DiMarco, J.P., Ellenbogen, K.A. et al. (2013). 2012 ACCF/AHA/HRS Focused Update Incorporated Into the ACCF/AHA/HRS 2008 Guidelines for Device-Based Therapy of Cardiac Rhythm Abnormalities. *J. Am. Coll. Cardiol.* 61 (3): e6.

2

Atrioventricular (AV) Block

Mark Marinescu[1] and Andrew E. Darby[2]

[1] Cardiovascular Medicine, Ohio State University, Columbus, OH, USA
[2] University of Virginia Health System, Charlottesville, VA, USA

Atrioventricular block is defined as delay, or interruption, in the transmission of an impulse from atria to ventricles due to anatomical or functional impairment in the conduction system (Figure 3.2.1) [1–4]. The conduction disturbance may be transient or permanent and can have many causes (Table 3.2.1). AV conduction may be delayed, intermittent, or absent. The PR interval is the electrocardiographic representation of the time required to conduct from atria to ventricles through the AV node. Inspection of the PR interval and determination of the atrioventricular relationship (or lack, thereof) assist in determining the presence and type of AV block. The normal PR interval measures ≤200 milliseconds. Commonly used technology includes first-degree AV block (slowed conduction with fixed prolongation of the PR interval but without loss of AV synchrony); second-degree AV block (intermittent loss of atrioventricular conduction); and third-degree AV block (no AV association with no consistent PR interval).

First-Degree AV Block

First-degree AV block manifests as fixed prolongation of the PR interval (≥200 milliseconds) with intact AV conduction (Figure 3.2.2). In first-degree AV block there is no true block, rather delayed or slowed AV conduction. The conduction delay is most often at the level of the AV node but may also be in the more distal conduction system (i.e. His-Purkinje system). First-degree AV block is a common finding and may be identified in 2–9% of patients depending upon the population studied (more common in older individuals and patients with a history of heart disease) [5–8]. It is generally deemed a benign finding and not associated with an increased mortality risk. First-degree AV block

may result from underlying structural abnormalities of the AV node; increased vagal tone; and AV nodal blocking agents that slow impulse propagation through the AV node. No specific therapy is indicated in the absence of symptoms.

Second-Degree AV Block

Second-degree AV block is defined as an occasional nonconducted P wave that results in a prolonged RR interval on the electrocardiogram (ECG). Second-degree AV block may be subclassified as either Mobitz type I (Wenckebach) in which there is progressive prolongation of the PR interval prior to the nonconducted P wave or Mobitz type II in which there is *no* PR lengthening prior to AV block.

Type I Second-Degree AV Block (Mobitz Type I, or Wenckebach)

Type I second-degree AV block (Wenckebach) results from intermittent failure of an atrial impulse to pass through the AV node and reach the ventricles thereby producing a pause on the electrocardiogram (Figure 3.2.3) [4, 9]. Progressive prolongation of the PR interval is observed prior to AV block. Any pattern of AV block (e.g. 2 : 1, 3 : 1, 4 : 1, etc. or a variable pattern) may be seen, but there is only 1 nonconducted P wave at a time. Also included in the differential diagnosis for a pause on the ECG are sinus pause/exit block as well as premature atrial contractions that occur prior to repolarization of the AV node resulting in loss of AV conduction. The PR interval after the nonconducted beat in type I second-degree AV block is less than the PR interval preceding the nonconducted P wave. The

Sinoatrial (SA)
node

Atrioventricular
(AV) node

His
bundle

Right bundle
branch

Left bundle
branch

Purkinje fibers

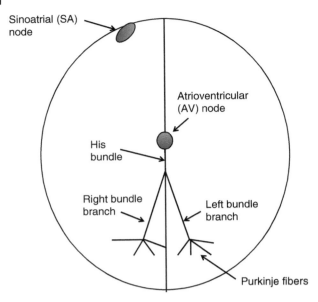

Figure 3.2.1 Anatomy of the cardiac conduction system.

Table 3.2.1 Potential etiologies of impaired atrioventricular conduction.

Physiologic and Pathophysiologic	Iatrogenic
Increased vagal tone	Drugs (AV nodal blocking agents)
Fibrosis of the conduction system	Cardiac surgery
Ischemic heart disease	Catheter ablation
Cardiomyopathy, myocarditis, and infiltrative heart diseases	Transcatheter aortic valve implantation
Congenital heart disease	
Hyperkalemia	
Endocrine and autoimmune conditions	

PR interval at baseline is typically normal but may be prolonged. A hallmark of type I second-degree AV block is the appearance of "grouped" beating on the ECG. Like first-degree AV block, type I second-degree AV block is generally felt to be a benign condition and rarely requires treatment [10, 11].

Type II Second-Degree AV Block (or Mobitz Type II)

Mobitz type II AV block manifests as intermittent failure of an atrial impulse to conduct to the ventricles but, as opposed to Mobitz type I, there is *no* prolongation of the PR interval prior to the nonconducted P wave (Figure 3.2.4) [12–14]. Mobitz type II is often indicative of underlying disease in the His-Purkinje system and typically indicates more advanced conduction disease as opposed to Mobitz type I. Mobitz type II has a higher risk of complete heart

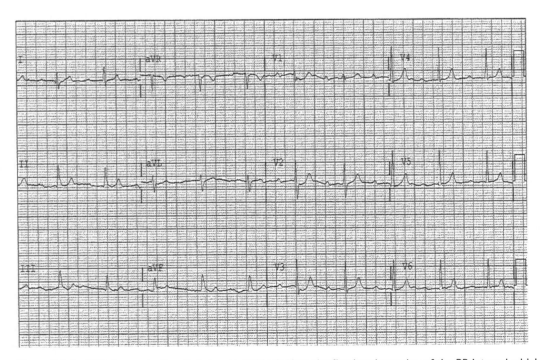

Figure 3.2.2 ECG demonstrating first-degree AV block. Note the fixed prolongation of the PR interval which, in this case, measures approximately 350 milliseconds with no loss of AV conduction.

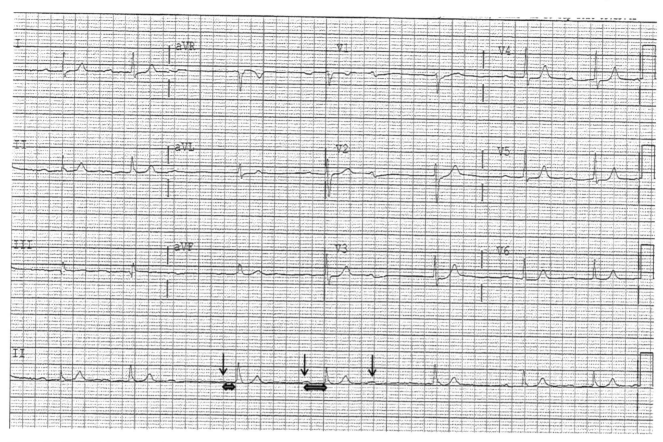

Figure 3.2.3 ECG demonstrating type I second-degree AV block. Note progressive PR interval prolongation prior to the nonconducted P wave (arrows indicate the location of the P waves and blue bars indicate the PR interval).

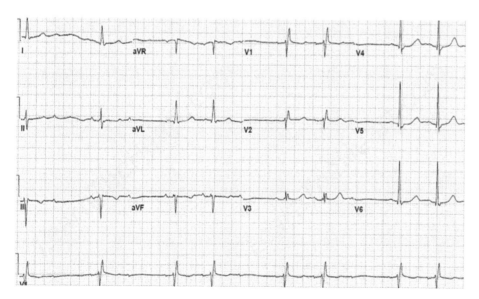

Figure 3.2.4 ECG demonstrating type II second-degree AV block with no appreciable prolongation of the PR interval prior to the nonconducted P waves. There is also evidence of right bundle branch block and probable left anterior fascicular block indicating advanced conduction system disease.

(a)

(b)

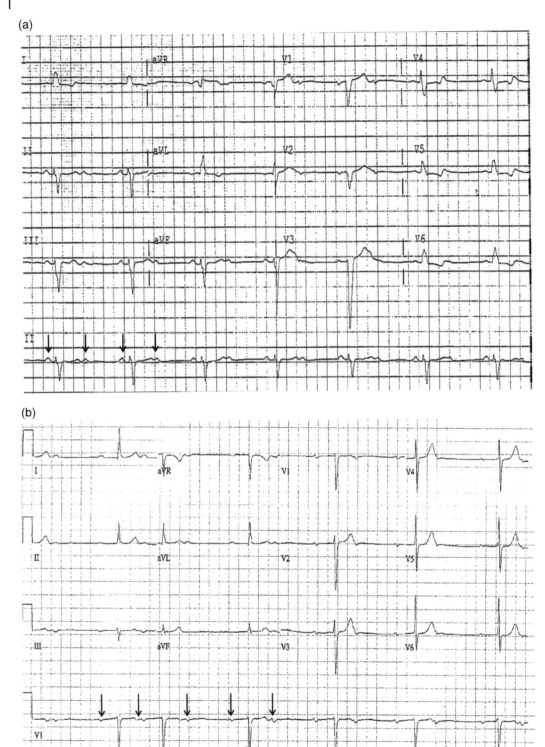

Figure 3.2.5 (a and b) ECGs demonstrating 2 : 1 AV block (arrows indicate P waves). In this setting, it can be difficult to determine if the patient has type I or type II second-degree AV block, as there are not enough conducted P waves to determine if the PR interval prolongs prior to the loss of AV synchrony. The presence of a prolonged QRS duration (LBBB pattern) indicates there is disease in the conduction system beyond the AV node thereby making type II second-degree AV block more likely. (b) Demonstrates an ECG with mostly 2 : 1 AV block although the initial portion of the rhythm strip reveals two consecutive P waves that conduct with prolongation of the PR interval prior to the nonconducted P wave. The remainder of the rhythm strip demonstrates 2 : 1 AV block. Due to evidence of type I second-degree AV block on the early portion of the rhythm strip, type I second-degree AV block with conduction slowing in the AV node is the most likely cause of 2 : 1 AV block in this case.

block than Mobitz type I and is usually an indication for permanent pacing, even in the absence of symptoms.

2 : 1 AV Block

Patients occasionally present with a pattern of 2 : 1 conduction on the electrocardiogram in which every other P wave fails to conduct to the ventricles (Figure 3.2.5). In this situation, it can be difficult to determine if the patient has Mobitz type I or II block (there are not enough conducted P waves to determine if the PR interval prolongs (Mobitz type I) or not (Mobitz type II) prior to AV block). A clue to the presence of Mobitz type II is additional conduction disease on the ECG (e.g. bundle branch and/or fascicular block). A patient presenting with 2 : 1 AV block should generally be assumed to have Mobitz type II block so that management is based on the worse of the two possibilities.

Third-Degree AV Block

Third-degree, or complete, AV block occurs when there is complete failure of the AV node to conduct atrial impulses to the ventricles (Figure 3.2.6) [15]. The ECG in third-degree AV block demonstrates complete AV dissociation with no consistent PR relationship. The ventricular rate is driven by a junctional or ventricular escape rhythm and may have a narrow or wide QRS complex, respectively. Complete AV block may be the result of intrinsic AV nodal disease or disease within the His-Purkinje system (Table 3.2.1). A difficult distinction may occur when trying to differentiate atrial fibrillation with slowed conduction and a bradycardic rate from complete AV block with underlying atrial fibrillation (Figure 3.2.7a and b). The regularity of the ventricular rhythm is a useful clue. Atrial fibrillation with very slow conduction through the AV node will result in an irregular ventricular rhythm, whereas complete AV block with underlying atrial fibrillation will typically have a regular escape rhythm (narrow or wide QRS complexes depending on the origin of the escape rhythm).

Indications for Permanent Pacing

In general, implantation of a permanent cardiac pacemaker is not indicated in situations where AV block is asymptomatic, transient, or reversible. Pacing is indicated for symptomatic third-degree or second-degree type II AV block; ventricular arrhythmias secondary to bradycardia resulting from AV block; asymptomatic bradycardia due to third-degree or second-degree type II AV block with pauses ≥3 seconds or an escape rate < 40 bpm; and patients with

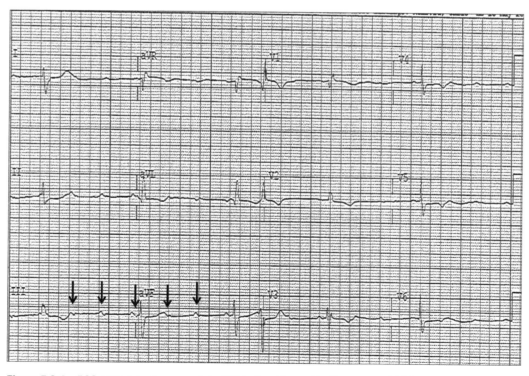

Figure 3.2.6 ECG demonstrating complete AV block evidenced by P waves and QRS complexes occurring at regular but independent intervals (arrows indicate P waves, fourth arrow highlights a P wave near-superimposed on a T wave).

(a)

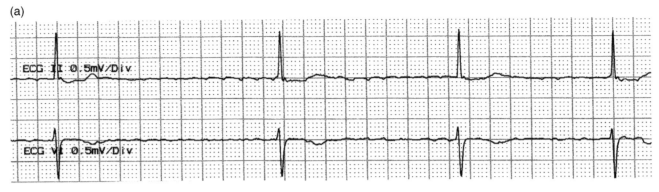

(b)

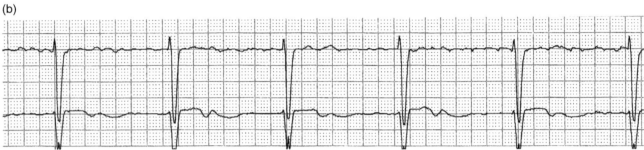

Figure 3.2.7 (a and b) Demonstrate atrial fibrillation with slowed ventricular response and complete AV block with underlying atrial fibrillation, respectively. The primary indicator of AV block in (b) is the *regular* ventricular rhythm (the ventricular response should be irregular with conducted AF).

Table 3.2.2 Indications for cardiac pacing in the setting of impaired atrioventricular conduction.

Third-degree and advanced second-degree (Mobitz type II) AV block associated with symptoms or ventricular arrhythmias presumed due to AV block

Third-degree and advanced second-degree AV block in awake, symptom-free patients in sinus rhythm with documented periods of asystole ≥ 3 seconds or any escape rate < 40 bpm or with an escape rhythm below the AV node

Third-degree and advanced second-degree AV block in awake, symptom-free patients with AF and bradycardia with 1 or more pauses ≥ 5 seconds

Third-degree and advanced second-degree AV block after catheter or surgical ablation of the AV node

Second-degree AV block with associated symptomatic bradycardia regardless of type or site of block

Asymptomatic third-degree AV block with escape rates ≥ 40 bpm if cardiomegaly or LV dysfunction is present

Second- or third-degree AV block during exercise

AF and bradycardia with pauses ≥ 5 seconds (see Table 3.2.2). Pacing is also indicated for patients with intermittent type II second-degree AV block or third-degree AV block and alternating bundle branch block. Pacing is generally *not* indicated for asymptomatic first-degree and second-degree AV block type I (Wenckebach).

Conclusions

Atrioventricular block is encountered commonly in clinical practice. First-degree and type I second-degree AV block may be readily diagnosed by ECG, are typically benign, and rarely require treatment. Permanent cardiac pacing is typically indicated for type II second-degree and complete AV block. Reversible causes for AV block should be sought and corrected prior to considering pacemaker therapy.

References

1 Zoob, M. and Smith, K.S. (1963). The aetiology of complete heart-block. *Br. Med. J.* 2: 1149.

2 Lev, M. (1964). Anatomic basis for atrioventricular block. *Am. J. Med.* 37: 742.

3 Lev, M. (1964). The pathology of complete atrioventricular block. *Prog. Cardiovasc. Dis.* 6: 317.

4 Johnson, R.L., Averill, K.H., and Lamb, L.E. (1960). Electrocardiographic findings in 67,375 asymptomatic

subjects. VII. Atrioventricular block. *Am. J. Cardiol.* 6: 153.

5 Packard, J.M., Graettinger, J.S., and Graybiel, A. (1954). Analysis of the electrocardiograms obtained from 1000 young healthy aviators; ten year follow-up. *Circulation* 10 (3): 384.

6 Erikssen, J. and Otterstad, J.E. (1984). Natural course of a prolonged PR interval and the relation between PR and incidence of coronary heart disease. A 7-year follow-up study of 1832 apparently healthy men aged 40 -59 years. *Clin. Cardiol.* 7 (1): 6.

7 Cheng, S., Keyes, M.J., Larson, M.G. et al. (2009). Long-term outcomes in individuals with prolonged PR interval or first-degree atrioventricular block. *JAMA* 301 (24): 2571.

8 Aro, A.L., Anttonen, O., Kerola, T. et al. (2014 Jan). Prognostic significance of prolonged PR interval in the general population. *Eur. Heart J.* 35 (2): 123.

9 Friedman, H.S., Gomes, J.A., and Haft, J.I. (1975). An analysis of Wenckebach periodicity. *J. Electrocardiol.* 8: 307.

10 Shaw, D.B., Gowers, J.I., Kekwick, C.A. et al. (2004). Mobitz type I atrioventricular block benign in adults? *Heart* 90: 169.

11 Coumbe, A.G., Naksuk, N., Newell, M.C. et al. (2013). Long-term follow-up of older patients with Mobitz type I second degree atrioventricular block. *Heart* 99: 334.

12 Narula, O.S. (1979). Atrioventricular block. In: *Cardiac Arrhythmias: Electrophysiology, Diagnosis, and Management*, 85. Baltimore: Williams & Wilkins.

13 Dhingra, R.C., Denes, P., Wu, D. et al. (1974). The significance of second degree atrioventricular block and bundle branch block. Observations regarding site and type of block. *Circulation* 49: 638.

14 Strasburg, B., Amat-Y-Leon, F., Dhingra, R.C. et al. (1981). Natural history of chronic second-degree atrioventricular nodal block. *Circulation* 63: 1043.

15 Bar, F.W., Den Dulk, K., and Wellens, H.J.J. (1989). Atrioventricular dissociation. In: *Comprehensive Electrocardiology: Theory and Practice in Health and Disease* (eds. M.F. PW and T.D.V. Lawrie), 933. New York: Pergamon Press.

3

The Dysrhythmic ECG

Intraventricular Block

Andrew E. Darby

University of Virginia Health System, Charlottesville, VA, USA

Introduction

Delayed intraventricular conduction is a common abnormality detected on the electrocardiogram (ECG) [1, 2]. Intraventricular conduction delay may manifest as right bundle branch block (RBBB), left bundle branch block (LBBB), nonspecific intraventricular conduction delay (IVCD), left anterior fascicular block (LAFB), or posterior fascicular block (LPFB). These conduction abnormalities may occur in isolation or combination. Right and LBBBs usually reflect intrinsic conduction abnormalities in either the right or left bundle branch system, respectively. Complete bundle branch block leads to prolongation of the QRS interval (≥120 ms); an incomplete bundle branch block results in slight prolongation of the QRS interval between 100 and 120 ms.

Anatomy and Electrophysiology

The bundle of His is the ventricular extension of the AV node. It divides into the left and right bundle branches at the junction of the fibrous and muscular boundaries of the intraventricular septum (Figure 3.3.1). The right bundle branch courses along the right side of the interventricular septum. Near the base of the right anterior papillary muscle, it divides into fascicles that spread to the septal and free walls of the right ventricle. It receives most of its blood supply from septal branches of the left anterior descending artery.

The left bundle branch penetrates the muscular portion of the interventricular septum near the aortic valve annulus and then divides into left anterior and posterior fascicles. The left anterior fascicle courses across the left ventricular outflow tract and terminates in the anterolat-eral portion of the left ventricle. The left posterior fascicle extends inferiorly and posteriorly along the interventricular septum and then divides into Purkinje fibers. The left bundle branch primarily receives blood supply from the left anterior descending artery and its branches.

Right Bundle Branch Block

The prevalence of RBBB increases with age and can occur in an otherwise normal heart. In one prospective study of 855 men followed over 30 years, the prevalence was 0.8% in subjects by age 50 and 11.3% by age 80 [3]. The study found no significant association with ischemic heart disease, myocardial infarction, or cardiovascular death, suggesting that RBBB is usually benign and results from slowly progressive degenerative disease affecting the myocardium and conduction system. Other studies have estimated the prevalence of RBBB to be 0.2–2.3% [4, 5].

RBBB may be caused by a number of conditions. The right bundle branch is vulnerable to trauma during two-thirds of its course as it mostly courses along the subendocardial surface on the right side of the interventricular septum. Conduction through the right bundle branch may be compromised by both structural and functional factors. The most common cause of RBBB is likely idiopathic degenerative disease of the cardiac conduction system. Several structural heart conditions may cause RBBB, such as chronically elevated pulmonary pressures (resulting in increased right ventricular pressure and stretching of the right ventricle, which may compromise conduction in the right bundle branch); a sudden increase in pulmonary pressure (as may occur with a pulmonary embolism); or myocardial ischemia/infarction or inflammation. RBBB may be iatrogenic, as it

Electrocardiogram in Clinical Medicine, First Edition. Edited by William J. Brady, Michael J. Lipinski, Andrew E. Darby, Michael C. Bond, Nathan P. Charlton, Korin Hudson, and Kelly Williamson.

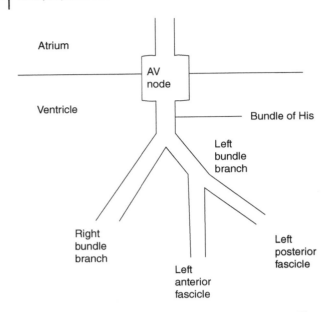

Figure 3.3.1 Anatomy of the normal conduction system. The Bundle of His is the ventricular extension of the AV node. It divides into the right and left bundle branches. The left bundle branch further divides into the left anterior and posterior fascicles.

may occur with catheter insertion into the right side of the heart as well as surgical interventions such as ventricular septal defect repair. RBBB may also be functional occurring as a rate-related bundle branch block (i.e. bundle branch block when the heart rate exceeds some critical value but normal intraventricular conduction with a narrow QRS complex at baseline). Finally, patients may have a "pseudo"-RBBB with conditions such as Brugada syndrome and arrhythmogenic right ventricular cardiomyopathy.

The criteria for diagnosis of RBBB on an electrocardiogram consist of: QRS duration greater than 120 millliseconds in adults; rsR′ pattern in lead V1 (typically the "s" wave goes below the isoelectric baseline and the R′ wave is taller than the initial r wave); and S wave of greater duration than R wave or greater than 40 ms in leads I and V6 (Figures 3.3.2–3.3.3) [6]. RBBB alters the sequence of ventricular repolarization resulting in depression of the ST segments and T wave inversions in the right precordial leads. Because electrical activation of the interventricular septum and left ventricular myocardium are unaffected and the majority of the ventricular muscle mass is in the left ventricle, the QRS axis is generally unaffected by a bundle branch block. Deviation in the QRS axis should raise suspicion for a concomitant fascicular block. Importantly,

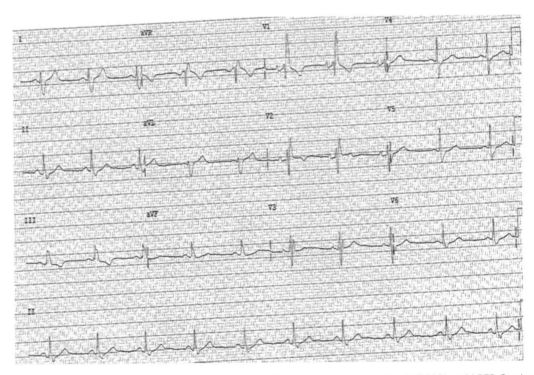

Figure 3.3.2 The ECG demonstrates sinus rhythm with right bundle branch block (RBBB) and LPFB. Pertinent findings with RBBB include QRS duration >120 ms; rsR′ in lead V1 (note the s wave crosses the isoelectric baseline and the R′ wave is taller than the r wave); and the duration of the s wave in V6 is >40 millseconds. Findings indicative of LPFB include right axis deviation, small R waves with deep S waves in aVL, and positive R waves in III and aVF. RBBB does not typically alter the QRS axis, which is a clue to the presence of concomitant fascicular block. The prolonged QRS duration is due to the RBBB and not the fascicular block.

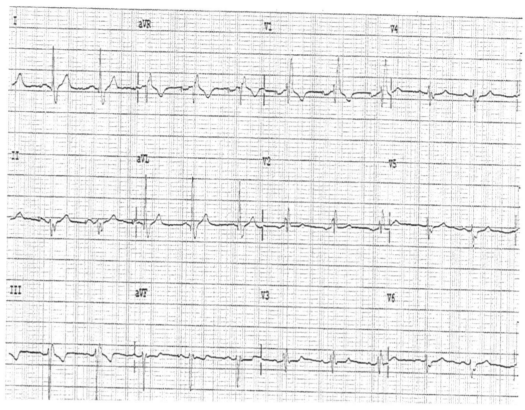

Figure 3.3.3 The ECG demonstrates atrial pacing with capture and right bundle branch block (RBBB) with left anterior fascicular block (LAFB). Findings indicative of RBBB include QRS duration >120 ms; rsR′ in lead V1 (note the s wave crosses the isoelectric baseline and the R′ wave is taller than the r wave); and prominent s wave in V6. The LAFB results in left axis deviation (−52° on this ECG) with a small r wave and deep S wave in lead III and small q wave with prominent R wave in lead I.

RBBB does not interfere with the diagnosis of ST segment elevation myocardial infarction.

The prognosis in patients with RBBB is largely related to the type and severity of concurrent underlying heart disease. RBBB does not have negative prognostic implications in patients without concomitant heart disease [7]. For asymptomatic patients with an isolated RBBB (i.e. no additional cardiac disease), no further diagnostic evaluation or specific therapy is recommended. Pacemaker insertion could be considered for patients with syncope, particularly if other conduction disturbances are present (such as complete heart block or type II second degree AV block).

Left Bundle Branch Block

The prevalence of LBBB increases with age and is relatively infrequent in young, healthy subjects. LBBB occurs in less than 1% of the general population with estimates ranging from 0.2 to 1.1% [5, 8–11]. There is conflicting data regarding the association between LBBB and underlying cardiovascular disease, although there is evidence supporting the association between new onset LBBB and heart disease,

particularly among older individuals. Among more than 5000 people enrolled in the Framingham Heart Study and followed for 18 years, 55 developed LBBB at an average age of 62 years [12]. Patients who developed LBBB had higher rates of hypertension, cardiomegaly, and coronary disease. Over the period of follow-up, only 11% of persons with LBBB remained free of cardiovascular disease compared to 50% in an age-matched control group without LBBB. Because of the association between LBBB and cardiovascular disease, it is reasonable to consider evaluating middle-aged or older persons with LBBB for hypertension, coronary disease, or myopathic conditions.

The electrocardiogram in LBBB (Figures 3.3.4 and 3.3.5) has two major changes compared with a normal ECG: loss of normal early septal forces (absence of R waves in the right precordial leads) and development of large and prolonged QRS complexes in the leftward and lateral leads (I, aVL, V6). Criteria for diagnosis of LBBB have been developed and consist of: QRS duration ≥120 ms in adults; broad, notched, or slurred R waves in leads I, aVL, and V6; absent Q waves in leads I, V5, and V6; and ST and T wave deflections usually opposite in direction to the QRS complex in any given lead [6]. LBBB confounds the electrocardiographic diagnosis of

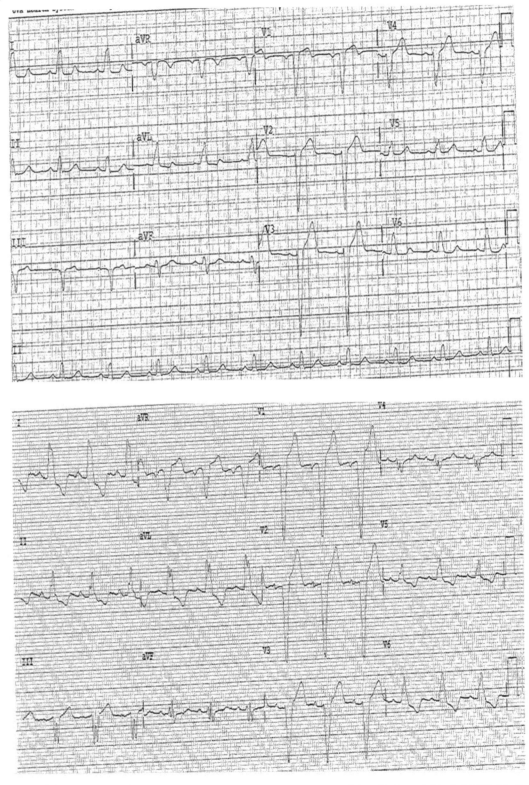

Figures 3.3.4 and 3.3.5 The ECGs demonstrate sinus rhythm with left bundle branch block (LBBB). Findings indicative of LBBB include a prolonged QRS interval (174 ms on this ECG); absence of R waves in leads V1–V3 with prominent, broad R waves in leads I, aVL, and V6.

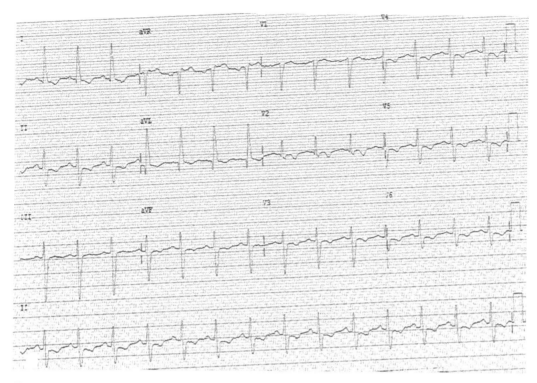

Figure 3.3.6 The ECG demonstrates sinus rhythm with a nonspecific IVCD and probable left ventricular hypertrophy (R wave in lead aVL > 11 mm). Findings indicative of IVCD include prolonged QRS duration (124 ms on this ECG) with features of both RBBB (prominent S wave in lead V6) and LBBB (predominantly negative QRS in V1). Note there was also likely misplacement of lead V2 given the pattern break (negative QRS in V1, positive QRS in V2, negative QRS in V3).

left ventricular hypertrophy and acute ST-segment elevation myocardial infarction. However, depressed ST segments and/or negative T waves in leads with negative QRS complexes should generally be considered abnormal and suggestive of myocardial ischemia. Criteria have been developed to assist with detection of acute myocardial infarction in the setting of LBBB [13].

In general, no specific therapy is required for asymptomatic patients with LBBB. Middle-aged and older individuals should be evaluated for coronary artery disease, hypertension, and underlying cardiomyopathy as mentioned above. Permanent pacemaker insertion would be indicated for patients with LBBB and syncope, particularly if the syncope is felt to be cardiac in etiology. Pacemaker insertion would be indicated if a patient with LBBB also has third-degree or type II second-degree AV block not associated with a reversible condition.

Nonspecific Intraventricular Conduction Delay

A nonspecific IVCD refers to QRS complexes that are wide (>110–120 ms) but without classical left or RBBB morphology (or widened QRS complexes with features of both

RBBB and LBBB). Figure 3.3.6 illustrates a typical example. An IVCD may result from anything that disturbs the passage of electrical impulses through the ventricular portion of the conduction system (e.g. myocardial infarction; age-related degeneration of the conduction system; myocardial infiltration or inflammation).

Fascicular Block

LAFB Is characterized by a left axis deviation in the frontal limb leads, defined as an axis >−45° and up to 90° (Figure 3.3.7). LAFB alone does not prolong the QRS interval. The QRS complex in lead I is upright while the QRS complexes in leads II, III, and aVF are negative (small R wave, deep S wave). There is often a small Q wave and tall R wave in lead aVL. LAFB primarily results from conduction system disease affecting the left anterior fascicle of the left bundle branch, although fibrosis of the peri-fascicular tissue (such as may occur with myocardial infarction) may also cause LAFB.

LPFB occurs when there is conduction delay or block in the left posterior fascicle of the left bundle branch (Figure 3.3.2). LPFB results in right axis deviation in the frontal plane (>+90°). As with LAFB, the QRS interval is

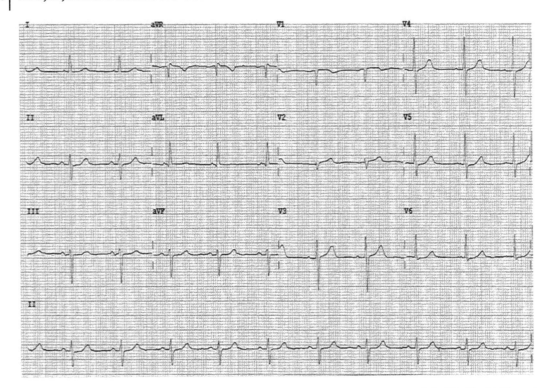

Figure 3.3.7 The ECG demonstrates sinus rhythm with left anterior fascicular block (LAFB). The LAFB results in left axis deviation (−43° on this ECG) with a small r wave and deep S wave in lead III and prominent R wave in lead I.

not prolonged with LPFB. There are small R and deep S waves in leads I and aVL with small q and tall R waves in leads III and aVF. Other conditions which may cause right axis deviation should be excluded such as lateral wall myocardial infarction; right ventricular hypertrophy; dextrocardia; and ventricular pre-excitation.

No specific therapy is recommended for patients with LAFB or LPFB in isolation. Permanent pacemaker insertion may be considered in patients with syncope, presumably cardiac in etiology, in the presence of bifascicular (e.g. RBBB and LAFB) or trifascicular (e.g. RBBB, LPFB, and first-degree AV block) block [14].

References

1 Goldberger, A.L. (2006). A Simplified Approach, 7e. St. Louis: Mosby, Inc.

2 Mirvis, D.M. and Goldberger, A.L. (2011). Electrocardiography. In: Braunwald's Heart Disease: A Textbook of Cardiovascular Medicine, 9e (eds. R.O. Bonow, D.L. Mann, D.P. Zipes and P. Libby), 149. Philadelphia: W.B. Saunders Company.

3 Eriksson, P., Hansson, P.O., Eriksson, H., and Dellborg, M. (1998). Bundle-branch block in a general male population: the study of men born in 1913. *Circulation* 98 (22): 2494.

4 Rotman, M. and Triebwasser, J.H. (1975). A clinical and follow-up study of right and left bundle branch block. *Circulation* 51 (3): 477.

5 Badheka, A.O., Singh, V., Patel, N.J. et al. (2013). Cohen MG. QRS duration on electrocardiography and cardiovascular mortality (from the national health and nutrition examination survey-III). *Am. J. Cardiol.* 112 (5): 671.

6 Surawicz, B., Childers, B., Bj, D. et al., American Heart Association Electrocardiography and Arrhythmias Committee, Council on Clinical Cardiology, American College of Cardiology Foundation, Heart Rhythm Society. (2009). AHA/ACCF/HRS recommendations for the standardization and interpretation of the electrocardiogram: part III: intraventricular conduction disturbances: a scientific statement from the American Heart Association Electrocardiography and Arrhythmias Committee, Council on Clinical Cardiology; the American College of Cardiology Foundation; and the Heart Rhythm Society. *J. Am. Coll. Cardiol.* 53 (11): 976.

7 Miller, W.L., Hodge, D.O., and Hammill, S.C. (2008). Association of uncomplicated electrocardiographic conduction blocks with subsequent cardiac morbidity in a community-based population (Olmstead County, MN). *Am. J. Cardiol.* 101: 102.

8 Siegman-Igra, Y., Yahini, J.H., Goldbourt, U., and Neufeld, H.N. (1978). Intraventricular conduction disturbances: a review of prevalence, etiology, and progression for ten years within a stable population of Israeli adult males. *Am. Heart J.* 96: 669.

9 Ostrander, L.D. Jr., Brandt, R.L., Kjelsberg, M.O., and Epstein, F.H. (1965). Electrocardiographic findings among the adult population of a total natural community, Tecumseh, Michigan. *Circulation* 31: 888.

10 Hiss, R.G. and Lamb, L.E. (1962). Electrocardiographic findings in 122,043 individuals. *Circulation* 25: 947.

11 Zhang, Z.M., Rautaharju, P.M., Soliman, E.Z. et al. (2012). Mortality risk associated with bundle branch blocks and related repolarization abnormalities (from the Women's Health Initiative [WHI]). *Am. J. Cardiol.* 110: 1489.

12 Schneider, J.F., Thomas, H.E. Jr., Kreger, B.E. et al. (1979). Newly acquired left bundle-branch block: the Framingham study. *Ann. Intern. Med.* 90: 303.

13 Sgarbossa, E.B., Pinski, S.L., Barbagelata, A. et al. (1996). Electrocardiographic diagnosis of evolving acute myocardial infarction in the presence of left bundle-branch block. *N. Engl. J. Med.* 334: 481.

14 Epstein, A.E., DiMarco, J.P., Ellenbogen, K.A. et al. (2013). 2012 ACCF/AHA/HRS focused update incorporated into the ACCF/AHA/HRS 2008 guidelines for device-based therapy of cardiac rhythm abnormalities. *J. Am. Coll. Cardiol.* 61 (3): e6.

4

Narrow QRS Complex Tachycardia

Augustus E. Mealor[1] and Andrew E. Darby[2]

[1] University of Tennessee College of Medicine, Erlanger Heart and Lung Institute, Chattanooga, TN, USA
[2] University of Virginia Health System, Charlottesville, VA, USA

Introduction

Narrow complex tachycardias (NCTs) are heart rhythms with a rate greater than 100 beats per minute, QRS duration <120 ms, and are most often supraventricular in origin. NCTs may originate from the sinus node, atrial tissue, the vessels attached to the atria, or the AV node. The mechanism of dysrhythmia may be due to abnormal impulse formation, impulse conduction, or a combination of the two [1]. Abnormal impulse formation occurs when cells other than the sinus node depolarize abnormally rapidly and generate abnormal electrical activity. Known as ectopic beats, these premature impulses may be caused by enhanced automaticity of cells with latent pacemaking ability or by abnormal depolarization of cells caused by increased sympathetic activity, hypothermia, electrolyte imbalances, or drug toxicities. Abnormal impulse conduction, primarily in the form of reentry, is the most common cause of NCT. It occurs when an impulse is conducted between adjacent tissue with different conduction velocities and refractory periods so that a self-sustaining circuit is made in which the impulse is conducted over one portion of the circuit while the other portion of the circuit repolarizes. Reentrant circuits may be very small and localized within a small portion of the atrium or very large and travel between atria and ventricle. Regardless of mechanism, the abnormal electrical activity conducts from atria to ventricles through the His-Purkinje system so that the ventricles depolarize normally creating a narrow QRS complex on the 12-lead electrocardiogram (ECG). (Narrow complex rhythms originating from sites below the AV node have been reported, but these are rare and usually involve a component of the conduction system.)

Nomenclature of NCTs can be confusing and reflects that NCTs can be described alternatively based on their appearance on the 12-lead ECG and the mechanism as determined during a catheter electrophysiology study. The American College of Cardiology and American Heart Association distinguish atrial fibrillation from *supraventricular arrhythmias,* which includes all forms of narrow complex tachycardia other than atrial fibrillation. The term *paroxysmal supraventricular tachycardia* (PSVT) most often refers to a subset of rhythms, namely atrial tachycardia (AT), atrioventricular nodal reentrant tachycardia (AVNRT), and atrioventricular reciprocating tachycardia (AVRT) [2].

The diagnostic evaluation of narrow complex tachycardia can be challenging and in some circumstances requires a formal cardiac electrophysiology study. However, several general principles should be noted. When possible, comparison should be made to prior ECGs, and changes in P-wave axis, P-wave morphology, and QRS morphology should be noted. A high burden of premature atrial beats suggests a predisposition toward atrial fibrillation or an ectopic AT. In patients with Wolff-Parkinson-White syndrome, a delta wave may be apparent on the baseline ECG providing a possible clue to the diagnosis. During narrow complex tachycardia, subtle deflections on the terminal portions of the QRS complexes may represent P waves conducted in a retrograde fashion to the atria as seen with reentrant tachycardias such as AVNRT or AVRT. Changes in rhythm (e.g. onset of tachycardia; change in rate during running tachycardia; or NCT termination) may also be helpful in providing clues to the etiology.

Electrocardiogram in Clinical Medicine, First Edition. Edited by William J. Brady, Michael J. Lipinski, Andrew E. Darby, Michael C. Bond, Nathan P. Charlton, Korin Hudson, and Kelly Williamson.
© 2021 John Wiley & Sons Ltd. Published 2021 by John Wiley & Sons Ltd.

Approach to the ECG Diagnosis of NCT

Various algorithms have been developed to assist in the ECG diagnosis of NCT. We find the following steps most helpful for approaching NCT in a systematic way (Figure 3.4.1):

Step 1: Determine whether the ventricular rhythm is regular or irregular. Sinus tachycardia (ST), AT, AVRT, AVNRT, and junctional tachycardia typically present as *regular* NCTs because the R-R intervals have consistent timing. Atrial fibrillation and multifocal AT have variable R-R intervals. Supraventricular rhythms with extremely rapid rates such as atrial flutter and rapid AT may have regular or irregular R-R intervals depending on whether AV conduction is fixed or variable.

Step 2: Ascertain the presence of P waves. Among the irregular rhythms (i.e. atrial fibrillation; multifocal AT; atrial flutter), atrial fibrillation has no organized atrial activity and, consequently, no consistent P waves on the 12-lead ECG. Multifocal AT presents as an irregular rhythm

with a single P wave preceding each QRS complex although the P waves vary from beat to beat (more than 3 P-wave morphologies is characteristic). Atrial flutter characteristically displays a series of flutter waves (i.e. >1 flutter wave per QRS complex) with a characteristic "sawtooth" appearance. The atrial rate in atrial flutter is classically 300 bpm and often conducts in a 2 : 1 pattern. Consequently, a narrow complex tachycardia with a ventricular rate of 150 bpm should prompt consideration of atrial flutter. Of the regular NCTs, the absence of P waves suggests AVNRT since P waves are retrogradely conducted and often concealed within the QRS.

Step 3: If P waves are present, determine the number of P waves per QRS. The presence of any AV conduction pattern greater than 1 : 1 (i.e. 2 : 1, 3 : 1, etc.) makes AVNRT and AVRT unlikely (completely rules out AVRT). AV conduction patterns of 2 : 1, 3 : 1, or higher are commonly seen in atrial flutter and may occur with rapid ATs. Vagotonic maneuvers or adenosine can have diagnostic value by revealing the underlying rhythm by slowing AV conduction (Figure 3.4.2).

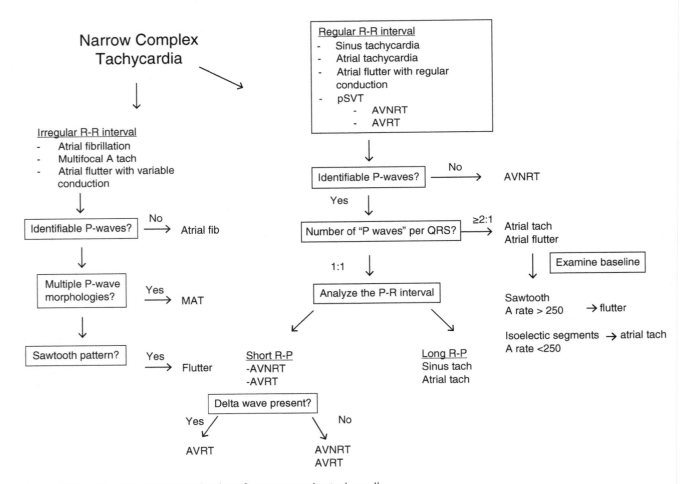

Figure 3.4.1 Algorithm for the evaluation of narrow complex tachycardia.

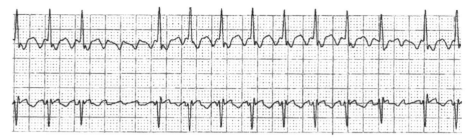

Figure 3.4.2 Rhythm strip demonstrating initiation of a narrow complex tachycardia. The tachy-arrhythmia starts with a premature atrial contraction. During tachycardia there is a retrograde P wave (inverted deflection) immediately following each QRS complex.

Step 4: For NCTs with *1 : 1* AV conduction, analyze the R-P interval. This is done by selecting any two QRS complexes and drawing an arbitrary line half the distance between the two complexes. The RP interval is deemed long if the P wave falls during the latter half of the R-R interval and short if it falls less than half the distance between the two QRS complexes. Long R-P tachycardia, in which atrial depolarization precedes ventricular depolarization, is typical of atrial and ST. A short RP interval suggests the impulse is originating from the AV node (e.g. AVNRT) or an A-V accessory/bypass tract (e.g. AVRT) since atrial depolarization is occurring concomitantly with or slightly after ventricular depolarization (i.e. the P waves are conducted in a retrograde fashion). The differential diagnosis for short RP tachycardia consists primarily of AVNRT and AVRT, and these rhythms can be difficult to distinguish on the 12-lead ECG. The following are clues to the diagnosis: In 95% of cases, patients with a delta wave and short PR interval on the baseline ECG will have AVRT. Epidemiologically, AVNRT has a higher prevalence in the general population and is more likely than AVRT among patients with a regular, narrow complex tachycardia and short RP interval.

anemia, infection, hypovolemia, medication, pain, or emotional stress can be identified. ST should resolve with treatment of the stressor. The sinus rate is typically less than 130 bpm, although higher rates can be achieved in young patients [3]. Very fast rates are rare in ST but more likely to be present in younger patients.

When compared to a baseline ECG in sinus rhythm, the P-wave morphology and axis should be similar. Because the sinus node is located high in the right atrium, the P waves are typically upright in leads I and II. The P-R interval may prolong slightly during tachycardia (decremental conduction is an intrinsic response of the AV node to rapid rates). Onset and offset are typically gradual and coincide with progression and remission of the cause of the ST.

Atrial Tachycardia

- Typically presents as a 1 : 1 tachycardia with a long RP interval.
- P wave morphology is different than sinus P wave.
- Atrial rate is typically 150–250 bpm.

The Regular Narrow Complex Tachycardias

Sinus Tachycardia

- P-wave morphology and axis are identical to sinus P wave.
- Maximum rate 220 – age.
- Slow onset and termination "ramp up and cool down."
- Often an underlying cause is present.

The most common form of narrow complex tachycardia, physiological ST, is a normal response to stress (Figure 3.4.3). Usually, an underlying cause such as

ATs include dysrhythmias arising from atrial myocardium or atrial conduction fibers between the sinus and AV nodes (Figure 3.4.4a and b). It is important to note that the categories of atrial dysrhythmia – AT, multifocal AT, atrial flutter, and atrial fibrillation – exist along a spectrum. There is often overlap between diagnostic categories, and patients will sometimes convert from one form of atrial dysrhythmia to another.

AT may be caused by a variety of mechanisms. The most common form, paroxysmal atrial tachycardia (PAT) is caused either by abnormal depolarization by an irritable focus or by a reentrant circuit. Digitalis toxicity is a classic trigger of abnormally early depolarization. Digitalis simultaneously exerts sympathetic effects on atrial myocytes, predisposing it to depolarization, and parasympathetic effects on the AV node, causing slowed conduction [4]. The result is

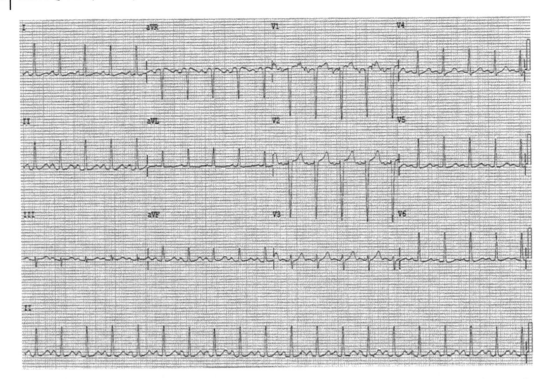

Figure 3.4.3 ECG demonstrating sinus tachycardia with a ventricular rate of ~ 120 bpm. Note the deep S wave in lead V2, which may also be indicative of left ventricular hypertrophy.

an atrial tachyarrhythmia with AV block. Indeed, PAT is often referred to as ectopic AT with block. AT may also result from continuous depolarization of the atrial by a reentrant circuit. As discussed below, atrial flutter is a specific form of reentrant AT that traverses the cavotricuspid isthmus.

PAT is typically brief, self-limited, and is often rapid. Incessant AT is a distinct classification of AT that is present for more than 50% of the day. The mechanism is often increased automaticity, whereby an atrial pacemaker depolarizes at an increased rate, exceeding the sinus node. The danger of prolonged tachycardia is the risk of developing tachycardia-induced cardiomyopathy and heart failure.

Focal AT may have a variable atrial rate of 110–250 bpm. Incessant AT typically occurs at the lower end of this spectrum. Occasionally, there may be a warm-up period of a few seconds in which the rate ramps up. Although AT most often conducts in a 1 : 1 AV pattern (i.e. 1 P: QRS complex), higher rates may exceed the conduction capacity of the AV node resulting in 2 : 1 conduction. An important ECG clue for differentiating focal AT from ST is the P-wave morphology (both may present as a long RP tachycardia as mentioned above). The P-wave morphology is frequently different than the sinus P wave and is dependent on the location of the initial impulse within the atria. Because the ectopic source is typically lower that the sinus node, the PR interval may be shorter than in sinus rhythm, and if the focus is low in the atrium the P wave

will be negative in the inferior leads. Focal AT may occasionally be mistaken for atrial flutter. Clues for distinguishing them on the ECG include the presence or absence of an isoelectric baseline between the atrial deflections (i.e. a return to baseline between atrial deflections) and the atrial rate. In focal AT with AV conduction pattern >2 : 1, there is an isoelectric interval between P waves, whereas atrial flutter produces a "sawtooth" pattern with continuous undulation of the baseline (no isoelectric interval between atrial deflections). The atrial rate in focal AT is generally 150–250 bpm, while that of atrial flutter often exceeds 250 bpm.

AT is often sensitive to adenosine. Vagal maneuvers rarely have any effect on the atrial rate, although transient AV block may be induced, allowing the P waves to be identified. Treatment includes search for an underlying cause (similar to ST) and AV nodal blocking agents to slow the ventricular rate.

Atrial Flutter

- May produce regular or irregular RR intervals.
- Continuous atrial deflections ("sawtooth" waves) are often seen
- Atrial rate approaches 300 bpm.
- 2:1 AV conduction produces a ventricular rate of 150 bpm.

(a)

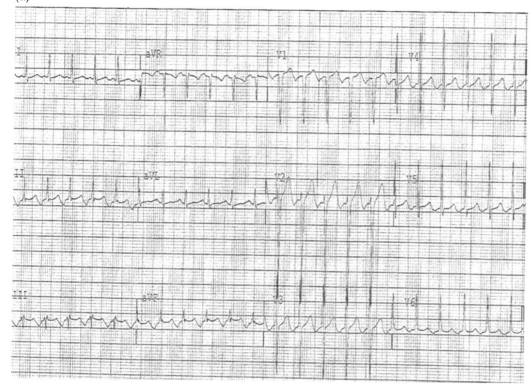

(b)

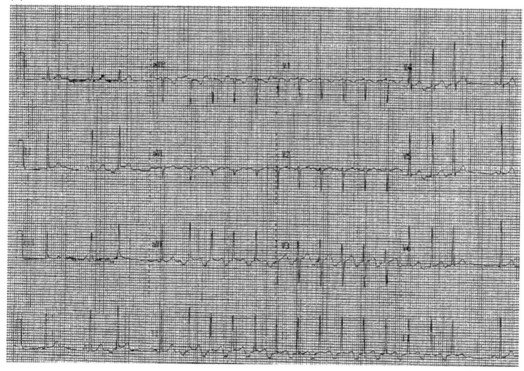

Figure 3.4.4 (a and b) ECG demonstrating an atrial tachycardia: note the rhythm is regular with a single P wave per QRS complex. There is a long RP interval and inverted P waves in leads II, III, and aVF indicating the rhythm is of nonsinus origin (likely from a site in the low right atrium). In ECG 4b, one sees a short run of tachycardia with a clear change in P-wave axis from "positive" at the beginning of the rhythm strip (first two beats are of sinus origin) to negative on beat 5. During the run of tachycardia one notes similar findings as seen in (a) – regular tachycardia; single P wave per QRS; long RP interval; and change in P-wave axis with tachycardia.

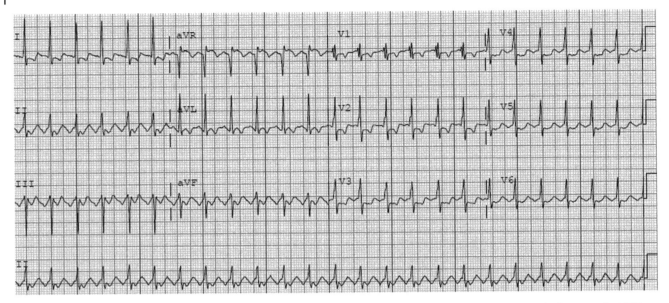

Figure 3.4.5 ECG demonstrating atrial flutter in which there is 2 : 1 AV conduction, resulting in a mean ventricular rate of ~ 150 bpm. The "sawtooth" flutter waves are most clearly visible in the inferior leads (II, III, aVF).

Classic atrial flutter is a re-entrant tachycardia that processes through the atrial tissue in a broad circuit (Figure 3.4.5). In typical atrial flutter part of the circuit passes through the cavotricuspid isthmus, a tract of tissue between the tricuspid valve annulus and inferior vena cava. The atrial rate is approximately 300 bpm, corresponding to an interval of 200 ms or one large box on the ECG. The orientation of the reentrant cycle within the atrium and its characteristic rate result in the pathognomic "sawtooth" pattern recognizable on the ECG, with the "teeth" pointed down in inferior leads II, III, aVF and upwards in V1. The AV node cannot accommodate rates this high in normal circumstances so a proportion of the flutter waves are not conducted. At lower conduction rates, e.g. 3 : 1 and 4 : 1 conduction, with rates of approximately 100 bpm and 75 bpm, respectively, the flutter waves are usually appreciable. At 2 : 1 conduction, the flutter waves are often buried within the QRS complex and T wave and may be difficult to discern. Transient slowing of AV conduction with vagal maneuvers or adenosine can reveal flutter waves that would otherwise be buried within the QRS and T wave. Any regular narrow complex tachycardia with a rate of about 150 bpm should prompt a careful search for flutter waves. In some circumstances, atrial flutter has variable AV conduction producing an irregular NCT.

Treatment of atrial flutter consists of anticoagulation for stroke prevention and AV nodal blocking agents to slow the ventricular response. Consideration should also be given to restoration of sinus rhythm with cardioversion or catheter ablation.

Paroxysmal Supraventricular Tachycardia

This subset of supraventricular arrhythmias is an umbrella term typically encompassing AVNRT and AVRT. They are characterized by recurrent episodes of rapid, regular tachycardia with abrupt onset and termination. Ventricular rates are often unusually rapid, typically 180–220 bpm. Patients may be asymptomatic or they may present with palpitations, chest comfort, dizziness, or more rarely, syncope. Patients with SVT often present at young age, and women have a twofold higher incidence than men.

Atrioventricular Nodal Reciprocating Tachycardia (AVNRT)

- Regular narrow complex tachycardia.
- Abrupt onset and offset.
- P waves may be hidden within QRS complexes or occur just after the QRS producing a short RP interval.
- Often responds to vagal maneuvers or adenosine.

AVNRT is the most common form of paroxysmal SVT, causing up to 50% of all regular narrow complex tachycardias [5]. The rhythm is predicated on the existence of unique AV nodal conducting properties termed "dual AV nodal physiology" in which there are two atrial inputs into the AV node – fast fibers, which conduct quickly but repolarize more slowly, and slower fibers, which conduct

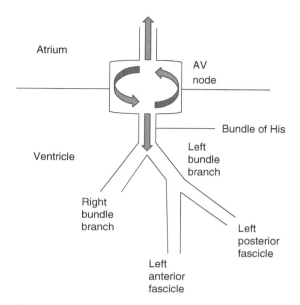

Atrium

AV node

Ventricle

Bundle of His

Left bundle branch

Right bundle branch

Left posterior fascicle

Left anterior fascicle

Figure 3.4.6 Diagram illustrating the mechanism of AV nodal reentrant tachycardia (AVNRT). A reentrant circuit revolves around the AV node resulting in near simultaneous depolarization of the atria and ventricles.

slower but repolarize faster. This creates the potential for reentry between these two sets of fibers around the AV node which is the mechanism of AVNRT (Figure 3.4.6). It is thought that 10–35% of the general population has dual AV nodal physiology but only a very small percentage ever develop SVT [5]. Patients with AVNRT are typically young, although they may present at any age.

In most cases, AVNRT occurs when a premature atrial or ventricular beat reaches the AV node after the slow fibers have repolarized but the fast fibers remain refractory. In this scenario, the impulse uses the slow fibers to conduct into the AV node. If the fast fibers have repolarized and are capable of retrograde conduction, depolarization will conduct retrograde to the atria over the fast fibers. At this point, the impulse may "reenter" the AV node through the slow fibers if they have now repolarized. In this manner, a circuit of reentry is created between the fast and slow inputs into the AV node thereby generating AVNRT.

During AVNRT, the circuit is small and centered around the AV node. Each revolution of the tachycardia circuit around the AV node generates simultaneous atrial and ventricle depolarization. Consequently, the P waves may be hidden within the QRS complexes. The absence of P waves in a rapid, regular tachycardia is fairly specific for AVNRT. In scenarios where the P wave is visible, it tends to occur on the terminal portion of the QRS complex producing a short RP tachycardia (Figure 3.4.7a and b). It occasionally takes careful inspection to identify the P wave and comparison with an ECG in sinus rhythm can

be helpful. Slight differences on the terminal portion of the QRS complex in tachycardia may be secondary to retrograde P waves. It can be particularly helpful to examine the inferior leads where the retrograde P wave may appear as a negative deflection at the end of the QRS (often mistaken for an s wave or V1 where the P wave may produce a terminal upward deflection resembling an r' wave [3, 5]. The presence of a pseudo-S wave in II, III, aVF and/or pseudo-r' in V1 is characteristic for AVNRT.

On the 12-lead ECG, AVNRT is characterized by a narrow complex rhythm with regular RR intervals and ventricular rate of 140–220 bpm. Onset and termination are abrupt. Classically, an atrial premature complex immediately precedes onset of tachycardia. As described in the preceding paragraph, the P wave may not be visible because it is obscured by the QRS or apparent as a slight deflection noted at the terminal portion of the QRS complex.

Vagal maneuvers are sometimes effective at terminating AVNRT and should be attempted initially. Adenosine is the drug of choice and will often terminate AVNRT. For recurrent episodes, the preferred treatment is electrophysiology study and catheter ablation.

Atrioventricular Reciprocating Tachycardia (AVRT)

- An accessory AV connection (bypass tract) participates in the tachycardia.
- Typically abrupt onset and offset.
- AVRT typically has regular RR intervals but may produce a narrow or wide QRS complex tachycardia.
- Like AVNRT, it tends to produce a short RP interval in tachycardia.
- Ventricular "pre-excitation" (short PR interval and delta waves) on the baseline 12-lead ECG suggests AVRT as the tachycardia mechanism.
- Typically terminates with adenosine or vagal maneuvers.

In the normal heart, the fibrous skeleton of the mitral and tricuspid valves electrically isolate the atria from the ventricles so that the AV node and His bundle are the sole pathway for atrioventricular conduction. In approximately 0.1–0.3% of the general population, a small muscular band forms an accessory pathway connecting atrium to ventricle potentially producing an alternate route for conduction [6–8].

Accessory pathways may conduct in variable directions with some only capable of conducting from atrium to ventricle, others conduct solely from ventricle to atrium, while some are capable of conducting in either direction. If an accessory pathway is capable of conducting from atrium to ventricle, AV conduction will occur over both the accessory

(a)

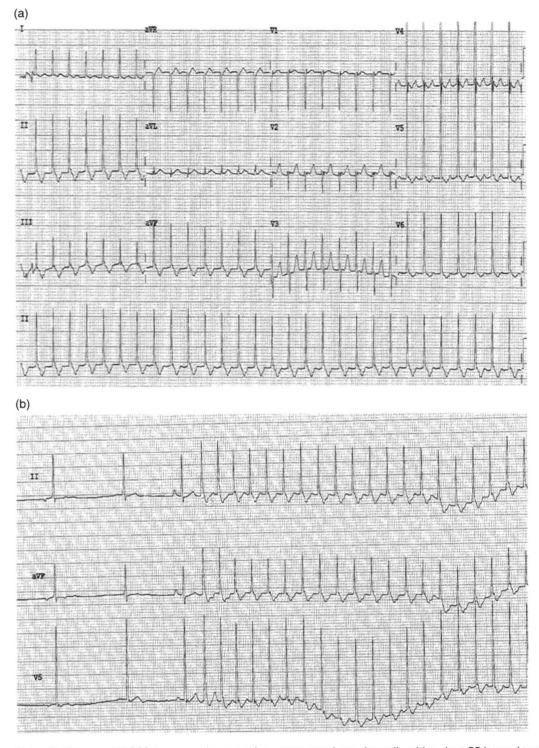

(b)

Figure 3.4.7 (a and b) ECG demonstrating a regular, narrow complex tachycardia with a short RP interval typical of AV nodal reentrant tachycardia (AVNRT). The rhythm strip in (b) reveals the onset of tachycardia, which is initiated by a premature atrial contraction.

pathway and the AV node. In most cases, the accessory pathway conducts more rapidly than the AV node and depolarizes a portion of the ventricle by the time rapid ventricular depolarization occurs via the His-Purkinje system.

The early activation of the ventricle by an accessory pathway is termed *preexcitation* and is manifested on the 12-lead ECG by a shortened PR interval followed by a slurred onset of the QRS complexes (delta wave) giving the

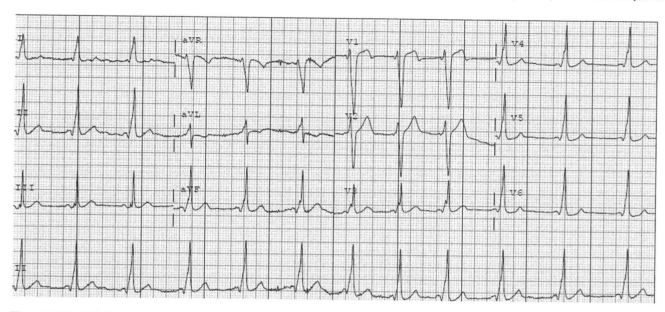

Figure 3.4.8 ECG demonstrating ventricular pre-excitation: note the patient is in sinus rhythm with a short PR interval and delta waves apparent in all leads, particularly the inferior and lateral precordial leads.

appearance of a slightly widened QRS complex (Figure 3.4.8). Accessory pathways capable of only conducting from ventricle to atrium will not produce a short PR interval or delta wave on the 12-lead ECG because the ventricles are not "pre-excited." Such accessory pathways are termed *concealed* as the presence of an accessory pathway is not apparent in sinus rhythm.

AVRT occurs when depolarization alternately transverses atrium and ventricle in a circuit that involves both the AV node and an accessory pathway (Figure 3.4.9). AVRT is also referred to as *circus movement AV tachycardia,* and depending on the direction of the circuit, AVNRT may be *orthodromic* or *antidromic* from the Greek words for "straight course" and "opposite course," respectively. Orthodromic AVRT occurs when depolarization proceeds antegrade down the AV node, resulting in normal ventricular depolarization and a narrow QRS, and retrograde ventricle-to-atrium (VA) conduction over the accessory pathway. The circuit of antidromic AVRT proceeds in the opposite direction and results in a wide complex tachycardia as ventricular depolarization occurs over the accessory pathway with the normal conduction system facilitating retrograde VA conduction. Concealed accessory pathways may participate in AVRT but will only produce narrow QRS complex tachycardia because the accessory pathway is only used for retrograde conduction from ventricle to atrium. Accessory pathways capable of conducting in either direction may produce AVRT with a narrow or wide QRS complex depending on the direction of conduction.

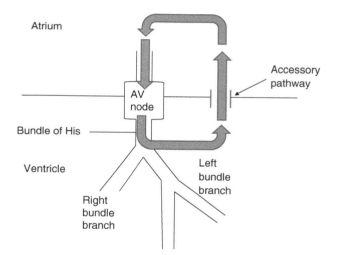

Figure 3.4.9 Diagram of the activation pattern in atrioventricular reciprocating tachycardia (AVRT). With this pattern of conduction (AV conduction over the normal conduction system and retrograde VA conduction by the accessory pathway), the tachycardia will have a narrow QRS complex tachycardia. The opposite pattern of conduction (antegrade over the bypass tract and retrograde over the AV node) will produce a wide complex tachycardia because the ventricles are activated over an accessory pathway rather than the normal conduction system.

On the 12-lead ECG, orthodromic AVRT is a regular, narrow-complex tachycardia with a short RP interval (if P waves are identifiable) (Figure 3.4.10). The ventricular rate may be quite rapid and can range from 150 to >230 bpm. Because the wave of depolarization reciprocates between

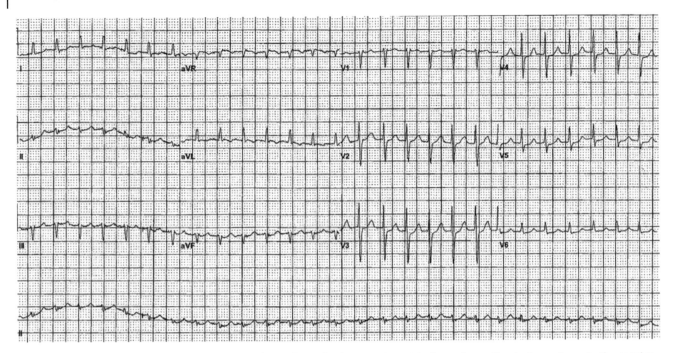

Figure 3.4.10 ECG demonstrating a narrow complex tachycardia due to atrioventricular reciprocating tachycardia: note the regular rhythm, narrow QRS complexes, and ST depressions in the inferolateral leads (not uncommon with supraventricular tachycardia). P waves are difficult to discern but appear to be in the ST segment just prior to the T waves in some leads.

atrium and ventricle the P waves and QRS complexes will not be superimposed as is often the case in AVNRT. A short PR interval and delta waves on the baseline 12-lead ECG suggest AVRT as the tachycardia mechanism.

In the acute setting, vagal maneuvers may terminate the rhythm by inducing AV block. Adenosine is effective at terminating AVRT but should be used with caution and expert guidance. In addition to blocking AV nodal conduction, adenosine can trigger atrial fibrillation. Atrial fibrillation with preexcitation is a potentially lethal arrhythmia as AV conduction over the accessory pathway is not rate-limited. This effect is exacerbated by suppressed AV nodal conduction. Patients with ventricular preexcitation and documented tachycardia should be referred to a cardiologist to discuss catheter ablation of the accessory pathway.

The Irregular Narrow Complex Tachycardias

In comparison to the regular NCTs, the irregular NCTs are more easily distinguishable on the ECG. Atrial fibrillation has no organized atrial activity and, consequently, no P waves; multifocal AT is characterized by multiple P wave morphologies; and atrial flutter produces a "sawtooth" appearance. Atrial flutter has already been discussed in

detail but is mentioned here because, with variable AV conduction, the RR interval appears irregular.

Atrial Fibrillation

- Irregularly, irregular rhythm.
- No consistently identifiable P waves on the 12-lead ECG.

Atrial fibrillation is the most common sustained arrhythmia encountered in adults. It accounts for 30% of hospitalizations for dysrhythmia and effects up to 8% of patients over the age of 80 [9]. The prevalence is expected to increase with advancements in the survival of patients with ischemic heart disease and congestive heart failure [9].

Conditions that increase atrial volume and pressure such as valvular heart disease, hypertension, and congestive heart failure lead to increased atrial stretching and fibrosis and account for the most important risk factors for atrial fibrillation. Atrial fibrillation may also be induced by states that lead to increased myocardial excitability such as sepsis, hyperthyroidism, and decompensated heart failure.

Electrocardiographically, AF is characterized by the absence of regular atrial activity (Figure 3.4.11). Atrial depolarizations are of low and variable amplitude and duration and irregular intervals, *resulting in the irregular baseline often seen on ECG.*

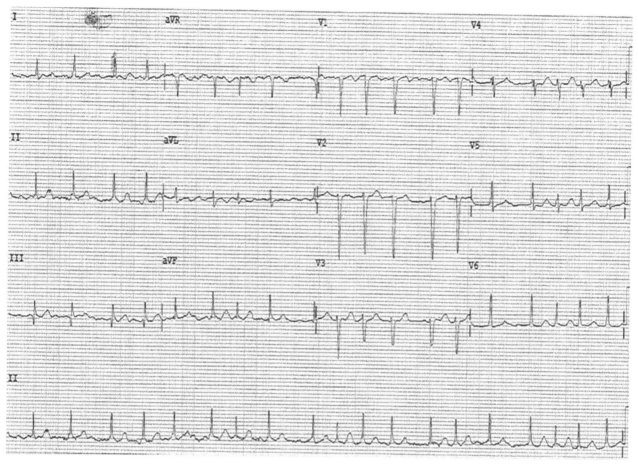

Figure 3.4.11 ECG demonstrating atrial fibrillation: note the irregular ventricular rhythm without organized atrial activity (no consistent P waves).

The ventricular rhythm is classically "irregularly irregular" with beat-to-beat variation in the RR intervals. However, at very fast rates, ventricular conduction may appear regular to the naked eye, and in these circumstances atrial fibrillation may be confused with SVT or atrial flutter with 2 : 1 conduction. Comparison of RR intervals with calipers will usually reveal beat-to-beat variation.

Therapy for atrial fibrillation begins with anticoagulation for stroke prevention and AV nodal blocking agents to slow the ventricular rate. Consideration should also be given to restoration of sinus rhythm and the utility of long-term maintenance of sinus rhythm with either antiarrhythmic drug therapy or catheter ablation.

Multifocal Atrial Tachycardia

- Irregularly, irregular RR intervals.
- Variable P-wave morphologies (>3).
- Often associated with critical illness and/or pulmonary disease.

Also known as chaotic AT, multifocal AT is an irregular NCT characterized by at least three different P-wave morphologies in the same lead. The rhythm is completely irregular with varying PR, RP, and RR intervals (Figure 3.4.12) [3, 5]. The atrial rate usually does not exceed

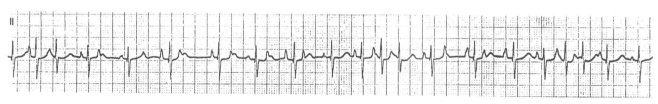

Figure 3.4.12 ECG demonstrating multifocal atrial tachycardia: note the irregular ventricular rhythm but, in contradistinction to atrial fibrillation, P waves are present (1 P wave per QRS complex) with variable P wave morphologies across the ECG.

140 bpm but may be higher [3, 5]. The arrhythmia is more common in elderly and severely ill patients and is classically associated with pulmonary disease. It is often preceded by sinus rhythm with frequent APCs and may precipitate atrial fibrillation or atrial flutter.

References

1 Lilly, L.S. *Pathophysiology of Heart Disease*, 3e. Lipincott Williams and Wilkins.

2 Page, R.L., Joglar, J.A., Caldwell, M.A. et al. (2016). 2015 ACC/AHA/HRS guideline for the management of adult patients with supraventricular tachycardia. *J. Am. Coll. Cardiol.* 67 (13): e27–e115.

3 Kahn, M.G. *Rapid ECG Interpretation*, 3e. Humana Press.

4 Wagner, G.S. *Marriott's Practical Electrocardiography*, 10e. Lipincott Williams and Wilkins.

5 Surawicz, B. and Knilans, T. *Chou's Electrocardiography in Clinical Practice*, 6e. Saunders Elsevier.

6 Rosner, M.H., Brady, W.J. Jr., Kefer, M.P., and Martin, M.L. (1999). Electrocardiography in the patient with the Wolff–Parkinson–White syndrome: diagnostic and initial therapeutic issues. *Am. J. Emerg. Med.* 17 (7): 705–714.

https://doi.org/10.1016/S0735-6757(99)90167-5. PMID 10597097.

7 Sorbo, M.D., Buja, G.F., Miorelli, M. et al. (1995). The prevalence of the Wolff–Parkinson–White syndrome in a population of 116,542 young males. *Giornale Italiano di Cardiologia (in Italian)* 25 (6): 681–687. PMID 7649416.

8 Munger, T.M., Packer, D.L., Hammill, S.C. et al. (1993). A population study of the natural history of Wolff–Parkinson–White syndrome in Olmsted County, Minnesota, 1953–1989. *Circulation* 87 (3): 866–873. https://doi.org/10.1161/01.CIR.87.3.866. PMID 8443907.

9 Fuster, V., Rydén, L.E., Cannom, D.S. et al. (2011). 2011 ACCF/AHA/HRS focused updates incorporated into the ACC/AHA/ESC 2006 guidelines for the management of patients with atrial fibrillation. *JACC* 57: e101–e198.

5

Wide QRS Complex Tachycardia

Andrew E. Darby

University of Virginia Health System, Charlottesville, VA, USA

Tachycardias may be broadly categorized based on the width of the QRS complex on the surface 12-lead electrocardiogram (ECG). Narrow QRS complex tachycardias have a QRS duration <120 milliseconds and are most often supraventricular in origin. Wide QRS complex tachycardias (WCTs) have a QRS duration >120 milliseconds. The prolonged QRS duration seen in WCT reflects abnormally slow ventricular activation, which may result from ventricular activation outside the normal conduction system (e.g. ventricular tachycardia); abnormalities within the intraventricular conduction system (e.g. supraventricular tachycardia (SVT) with preexisting or rate-related bundle branch block); or ventricular activation over an accessory pathway (i.e. preexcited tachycardias).

Diagnosing a wide complex tachycardia by ECG can be challenging due to the multiple potential etiologies, and the diagnostic algorithms are imperfect (see Figure 3.5.1). There a number of clues, however, which can help differentiate ventricular tachycardia (VT) from the various supraventricular rhythms that may present with a WCT. Differentiating VT from SVT is important, as urgent therapy may be required for VT.

The differential diagnosis for wide QRS complex tachycardia is listed in Table 3.5.1. Several important clinical pearls are worth noting. Ventricular tachycardia accounts for up to 80% of WCT in unselected populations and more than 90% of cases in patients with prior myocardial infarction [1–3]. Thus, if a definitive diagnosis of WCT cannot be made with certainty, an unknown rhythm should be presumed to be VT in the absence of contrary evidence. Making the assumption of VT protects against providing inappropriate and potentially dangerous therapies (e.g. adenosine in the setting of a preexcited tachycardia), and treatment of SVT as if it were VT (e.g. iv amiodarone or external cardioversion) is safe and often effective in restoring sinus rhythm. Hemodynamic instability should not be regarded as suggestive of SVT.

Ventricular Tachycardia

Ventricular tachycardia is the most common type of WCT (Figures 3.5.2–3.5.4). VT originates within the ventricular myocardium outside the normal conduction system and, as a result, leads to abnormal ventricular activation, thereby producing a wide QRS complex on the surface ECG. VT is the most common cause of WCT accounting for 80–90% of cases [1–3]. VT may either be monomorphic (uniform or stable QRS morphology during an episode) or polymorphic (continuously varying QRS morphologies during an episode) [4, 5]. "Nonsustained" VT is defined as an episode lasting less than 30 seconds, whereas "sustained" VT lasts longer than 30 seconds [3]. Evidence of AV dissociation greatly facilitates the diagnosis of ventricular tachycardia and rules out a supraventricular rhythm as the cause of WCT.

Supraventricular Tachycardia

Supraventricular tachycardia may produce a wide QRS complex rhythm if there is a rate-related bundle branch block (i.e., aberrancy) or preexisting bundle branch block. Consequently, the baseline 12-lead electrocardiogram can be very helpful for comparison. SVT with aberrancy occurs when supraventricular impulses are delayed or blocked in the bundle branches or distal Purkinje fibers resulting in delayed ventricular activation and a widened QRS complex [6]. Aberrant conduction is the most common reason for a widened QRS complex during SVT, but aberrantly conducted SVT is less common than VT (21% of cases in one series) [7].

Electrocardiogram in Clinical Medicine, First Edition. Edited by William J. Brady, Michael J. Lipinski, Andrew E. Darby, Michael C. Bond, Nathan P. Charlton, Korin Hudson, and Kelly Williamson.

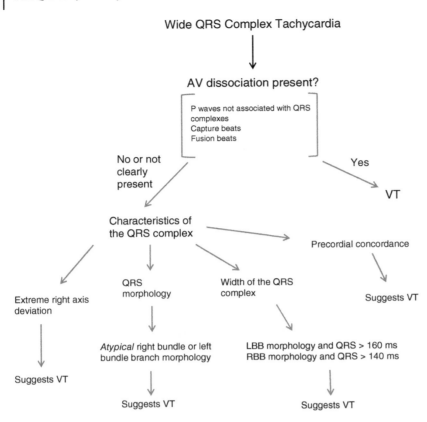

Figure 3.5.1 Algorithm for approaching an ECG or rhythm strip with wide QRS complex tachycardia.

Table 3.5.1 Differential diagnosis of wide QRS complex tachycardia.

Ventricular tachycardia

Supraventricular tachycardia with preexisting bundle branch block

Supraventricular tachycardia with rate-related bundle branch block (aberrancy)

Preexcited tachycardia

Ventricular paced rhythm

Preexcited Tachycardia

In preexcited rhythms, an accessory pathway is present and conduction from atrium to ventricle can occur over the normal conduction system as well as the accessory pathway. Accessory pathways are abnormal extranodal muscle fibers connecting atrium to ventricle across either the mitral valve annulus or tricuspid valve annulus. In the absence of an accessory pathway, atrial to ventricular conduction occurs as depolarization passes through the AV node and His bundle, through the bundle branches, and out the Purkinje fibers which ramify out from the apices of the ventricles. Consequently, the ventricular tissue adjacent to the mitral and tricuspid valve annuli is the latest to depolarize during ventricular activation. *Preexcitation* refers to the premature

activation of a portion of one of the ventricles at the site of accessory pathway insertion. Consequently, the ventricular myocardium in this area is depolarized earlier than would occur through the normal conduction system. Accessory pathways may conduct from atrium to ventricle (so-called "manifest" accessory pathways as they are apparent on the baseline 12-lead by producing a short PR interval and delta waves) or only from ventricle to atrium (so called "concealed" accessory pathways as there are no delta waves at baseline). Patients with accessory pathways may develop a variety of arrhythmias, including atrial fibrillation and paroxysmal SVT (more specifically, atrioventricular reciprocating tachycardia, or AVRT) [3]. Atrioventricular reciprocating tachycardia may occur in an orthodromic or antidromic fashion [4, 8]. In orthodromic AVRT, ventricular activation occurs over the normal conduction system, with the accessory pathway facilitating conduction from ventricle to atrium. This pattern of activation produces a narrow complex tachycardia due to the activation of the ventricles over the normal conduction system. In antidromic AVRT, conduction from atrium to ventricle occurs over the accessory pathway and the normal conduction system is used for retrograde conduction from ventricle to atrium. Antidromic AVRT produces a wide complex tachycardia as the ventricles are preexcited by activation over the accessory pathway. Orthodromic AVRT is more common than antidromic

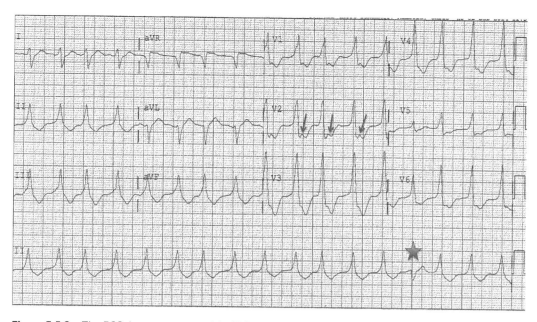

Figure 3.5.2 The ECG demonstrates a wide QRS complex tachycardia with right bundle branch block morphology (upright QRS complex in lead V1). The patient presented with ventricular tachycardia at a rate of ~105 bpm. The patient was taking amiodarone, which slowed the VT rate. It is important to note that VT may occasionally present with a slow rate, and rate by itself cannot distinguish VT from SVT. The monophasic R wave in V1 (atypical RBBB morphology) and positive precordial concordance indicate that the rhythm is VT. There appear to be retrograde P waves after each QRS complex (arrows) and a fusion beat (star).

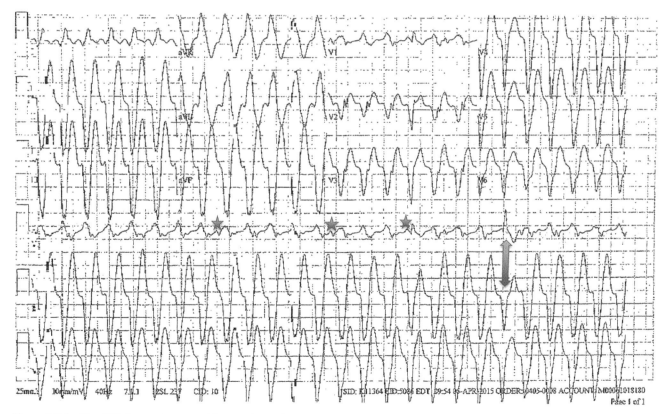

Figure 3.5.3 The ECG demonstrates a wide complex tachycardia with right bundle branch block morphology, rate ~160 bpm. The rhythm was ventricular tachycardia, and the primary clues to the diagnosis are the atypical bundle branch block morphology, fusion beat (double arrow), and P waves independent of QRS complexes (indicated by stars). The fusion beat and P waves occurring independent of QRS complexes are both signs of AV dissociation and indicate the rhythm is of ventricular origin, as it is occurring independent of atrial activity. The patient had experienced a prior inferior myocardial infarction, increasing the probability that the wide complex rhythm is VT.

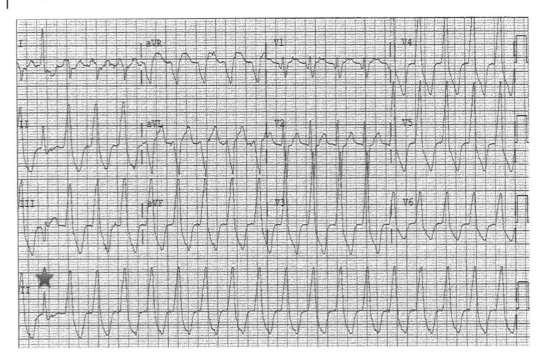

Figure 3.5.4 ECG demonstrating a wide QRS complex tachycardia with a ventricular rate of ~110 bpm. The star indicates a capture beat, which reveals evidence of AV dissociation and thereby confirms ventricular tachycardia as the diagnosis.

tachycardia, which occurs in only about 10% of individuals with accessory pathways [9]. Atrial fibrillation in a patient with a manifest accessory pathway may result in preexcited atrial fibrillation. This condition may be quite dangerous, as it can result in extremely rapid ventricular rates and potentially degenerate into ventricular fibrillation [8]. Preexcited atrial fibrillation presents as an *irregular* wide complex tachycardia on ECG (Figure 3.5.5). Additional characteristic findings include delta waves at the onset of the QRS complexes and QRS complexes, which vary in width throughout the ECG recording. The variation in QRS width is due to changing mechanisms of ventricular depolarization: some QRS complexes result purely from activation through the normal conduction system; some are created solely by depolarization over the accessory pathway when the AV node is refractory; and some QRS complexes result from fusion of depolarization over the normal conduction system and accessory pathway. This rhythm may be relatively easily distinguished from atrial fibrillation occurring in the presence of preexisting bundle branch block as the latter has a more consistent QRS morphology and typical bundle branch block QRS morphology (Figure 3.5.6). AV nodal blocking agents should *not* be administered to patients suspected of having preexcited atrial fibrillation, as doing so may result in acceleration of the ventricular rate thereby producing hemodynamic instability.

Ventricular Paced Rhythm

Ventricular pacing may result in a wide complex rhythm by creating a pattern of ventricular depolarization different than occurs through the normal conduction system. Most ventricular pacemakers pace the right ventricular apex, which creates a wide QRS complex with a left bundle branch morphology (broad R wave in lead I and often broad R waves in leads aVL and V6 with a negative QRS complex in lead V1). If a patient has a pacemaker with leads in the right atrium and right ventricle and develops a supraventricular arrhythmia, the pacemaker may "track" the atrial rhythm and pace the ventricles rapidly in response, thereby producing a wide QRS complex tachycardia (Figure 3.5.7). Pacemaker spikes or artifact may be seen prior to each QRS when this is the cause of wide QRS complex tachycardia. Device interrogation may then reveal the underlying mechanism of tachycardia if not readily apparent from the 12-lead electrocardiogram.

Other Causes of Wide Complex Tachycardia

Certain medications and electrolyte abnormalities may result in wide QRS complex tachycardia. Medications that block cardiac sodium channels (e.g. class I anti-arrhythmic drugs; citalopram; tricyclic antidepressants; venlafaxine)

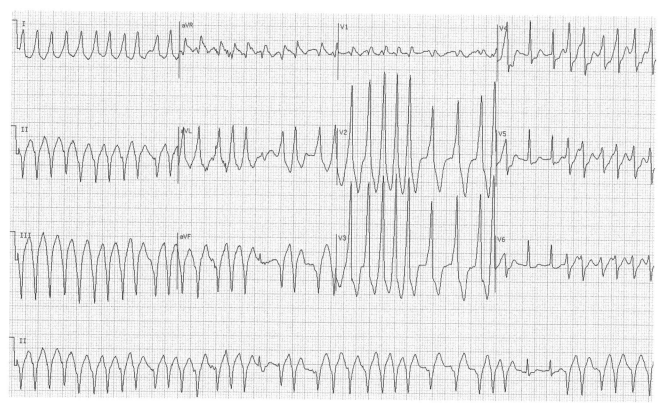

Figure 3.5.5 The ECG demonstrates an irregular wide complex rhythm with a rate, at times, approaching 300 bpm. The patient has an accessory pathway, and the rhythm is preexcited atrial fibrillation. Clues to the diagnosis include an irregularly, irregular rhythm with delta waves best seen in leads V2 through V4. Note the QRS complexes vary in width from beat to beat, which results from changing ventricular activation. The ventricles may be depolarized solely by the accessory pathway when the AV node is refractory (widest QRS complexes); solely by the normal conduction system when the accessory pathway is refractory (narrow QRS complexes); and by fusion of depolarization over the accessory pathway and normal conduction system (intermediate QRS complexes).

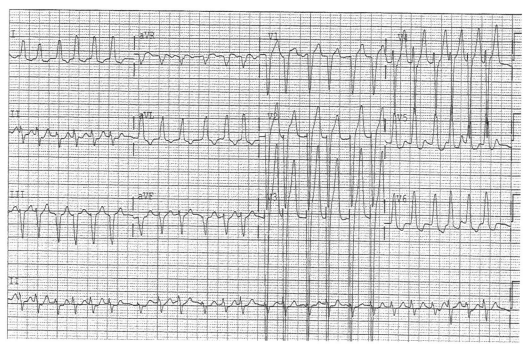

Figure 3.5.6 Atrial fibrillation occurring in a patient with preexisting LBBB.

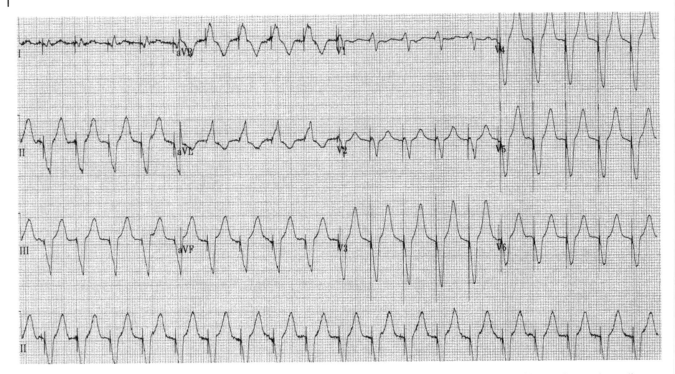

Figure 3.5.7 The ECG is from a patient presenting with a regular, wide QRS complex tachycardia, HR ~120 bpm. Pacemaker spikes are consistently present before each QRS complex indicating this is a paced rhythm. Device interrogation confirmed an underlying atrial tachycardia which was being tracked by the patient's pacemaker.

may widen the QRS complex by slowing ventricular depolarization. If a patient develops a supraventricular arrhythmia in this setting, the ECG may demonstrate a wide QRS complex tachycardia. Severe hyperkalemia may also result in a WCT. Characteristic ECG findings of hyperkalemia include peaked T waves, PR prolongation, diminished P-wave amplitude, widening of the QRS complex, and, if uncorrected, may eventually result in sine-wave formation and then ventricular fibrillation and asystole [10].

Diagnosis of Wide QRS Complex Tachycardia by Electrocardiogram

Numerous algorithms and ECG criteria have been developed to assist in the identification of WCT on the ECG, but none has proven definitive. The diagnostic criteria proposed by Brugada and colleagues is among the most widely used [11]. The algorithm suggests evaluating the ECG for: (i) absence of an RS complex in all precordial leads; (ii) an RS interval > 100 milliseconds in any one precordial lead; (iii) AV dissociation; (iv) various QRS morphologies in leads V1–V2 and V6. The presence of any one of the four criteria was considered diagnostic of VT while the absence of all four criteria ruled out VT in 98% of cases. Attempts to validate the Brugada criteria have demonstrated significant interobserver variability, and using the Brugada algorithm may

misdiagnose VT as SVT in 9–21% of cases [12, 13]. Although there is no perfect algorithm to rule VT in or out by the ECG, there are a number of clues that are suggestive of VT.

AV Dissociation

The presence of AV dissociation is virtually pathognomonic of VT [14, 15]. Evidence of AV dissociation include: (i) P waves independent of QRS complexes with the ventricular rate exceeding the atrial rate; (ii) fusion beats; (iii) capture beats. P waves independent of QRS complexes may be difficult to identify on a single 12-lead ECG but may be more readily identifiable on a longer recording such as a rhythm strip. Occasionally ventricular tachycardia may produce retrograde P waves resulting in a 1 : 1 tachycardia. One pitfall is to avoid mistaking retrograde P waves for sinus P waves and misdiagnosing VT as sinus tachycardia with bundle branch block.

Capture and fusion beats are additional evidence of AV dissociation and, when present, suggest VT as the diagnosis. Capture beats arise when a sinus P wave activates the entire ventricle through the normal conduction system in the midst of tachycardia. A capture beat appears as a narrow complex beat with morphology identical or very similar to the native QRS complex. A fusion beat is a QRS complex that occurs when the ventricles have two sources of activation – a P wave that has activated the ventricles through the normal conduction system merging with the next VT complex. Fusion beats appear as a QRS complex of intermediate width.

Characteristics of QRS Complexes

There are several features of QRS complexes during wide complex tachycardia that suggest VT as the diagnosis. The width of the QRS complex may be suggestive of VT for it has been proposed that the wider the QRS complex, the more likely the rhythm is to be ventricular in origin. Some authors have suggested that a QRS duration >140 milliseconds with right bundle branch morphology and a QRS duration >160 milliseconds with left bundle branch pattern are indicative of VT [11, 12]. However, approximately 20% of patients with VT have a QRS duration <140 milliseconds [16].

The QRS axis may also provide a clue as to the etiology of wide QRS complex tachycardia. Extreme right axis deviation (−90° to ±180°) favors VT over SVT [2]. Identification of concordance in the precordial leads can be helpful. Concordance refers to the polarity of the QRS complexes in the precordial leads. When the QRS complexes are all negative (negative precordial concordance) or all positive (positive precordial concordance), a diagnosis of VT is supported.

Inspecting the QRS morphologies in leads V1 and V6 can also be very helpful in the diagnosis of wide complex tachycardia. Ventricular tachycardia results in either a left bundle branch morphology (negative QRS complex in V1, broad R wave in V6) or right bundle branch morphology (predominantly positive QRS complex in V1). The site of origin within the ventricles dictates the pattern, as VT from the right ventricle tends to produce left bundle branch morphology while VT from the left ventricle often results in right bundle branch morphology. In differentiating VT from SVT with bundle branch block, it is helpful to inspect the QRS complexes in leads V1 and V6. SVT with bundle branch block produces QRS complexes with morphology identical to those present in typical bundle branch block. With a wide complex tachycardia of right bundle branch block (RBBB) morphology due to SVT, the QRS complex in V1 will have an rsR' pattern in which the s wave crosses the isoelectric baseline and the R' wave is taller than the r wave, and there is a deep S wave in V6 (in other words, the QRS complexes appears consistent with typical RBBB). VT with right bundle branch morphology produces an upright QRS complex in lead V1 similar to RBBB, but the QRS complex often has a qR pattern or monophasic R wave without the classic features of typical RBBB [3, 11]. Conversely, SVT with left bundle branch block (LBBB) produces a negative QRS complex in lead V1 with broad R waves in leads I, aVL, and V6. VT with left bundle branch morphology produces a wide QRS complex tachycardia with a negative QRS complex in lead V1, but the QRS complexes do not have all the classic features of typical LBBB [17]. Essentially, the QRS complexes in SVT with bundle branch block tend to have all the features typical of either right or left bundle branch block. However, the QRS complexes in VT often appear *similar* to right or left bundle branch block, but the QRS complexes have atypical features and do not meet classic criteria for either bundle branch block.

Conclusions

The diagnosis of wide complex tachycardia by ECG can be challenging due to the multiple potential etiologies, and the diagnostic algorithms are imperfect. When uncertain, wide complex tachycardia should be considered ventricular tachycardia until proven otherwise. Evidence of AV dissociation is particularly helpful to distinguish ventricular tachycardia from other mechanisms of wide QRS complex tachycardia. Preexcited atrial fibrillation is another important rhythm to recognize as administration of AV nodal blocking agents in this setting may be potentially harmful.

References

1 Stewart, R.B., Bardy, G.H., and Greene, H.L. (1986). Wide complex tachycardia: misdiagnosis and outcome after emergent therapy. *Ann. Intern. Med.* 104: 766.

2 Akhtar, M., Shenasa, M., Jazayeri, M. et al. (1988). Wide QRS complex tachycardia. Reappraisal of a common clinical problem. *Ann. Intern. Med.* 109: 905.

3 Gupta, A.K. and Thakur, R.K. (2001). Wide QRS complex tachycardias. *Med. Clin. North. Am.* 85: 245.

4 Ray, I. (2004). Wide complex tachycardia: recognition and management in the emergency room. *J. Assoc. Phys. India* 52: 882.

5 Wellens, H. (2001). Ventricular tachycardia: diagnosis of broad QRS complex tachycardia. *Heart* 86: 579.

6 Akhtar, M. (1983). Electrophysiological bases for wide QRS complex tachycardia. *Pacing Clin. Electrophysiol.* 6: 81.

7 Miller, J.M., Hsia, H.H., Rothman, S.A., and Buxton, A.E. (2000). Ventricular tachycardia versus supraventricular tachycardia with aberration: electrocardiographic distinctions. In: *Cardiac Electrophysiology From Cell to Bedside* (eds. D.P. Zipes and J. Jalife), 696. Philadelphia: W.B. Saunders.

8 Atiga, W. and Calkins, H. (2002). Catheter ablation of supraventricular tachycardia. In: *Management of Cardiac Arrhythmias* (ed. L. Ganz), 56. Totowa, New Jersey: Human Press.

9 Hollowell, H., Mattu, A., Perron, A. et al. (2005). Wide-complex tachycardia: beyond the traditional differential diagnosis of ventricular tachycardia vs supraventricular tachycardia with aberrant conduction. *Am. J. Emerg. Med.* 23: 876.

10 Gennari, F. (2002). Disorders of potassium homeostasis: hypokalemia and hyperkalemia. *Crit. Care Clin.* 18: 273.

11 Brugada, P., Brugada, J., Mont, L. et al. (1991). A new approach to the differential diagnosis of a regular tachycardia with a wide QRS complex. *Circulation* 83 (5): 1649.

12 Herbert, M.E., Votey, S.R., Morgan, M.T. et al. (1996). Failure to agree on the electrocardiographic diagnosis of ventricular tachycardia. *Ann. Emerg. Med.* 27: 35.

13 Isenhour, J., Craig, S., Gibbs, M. et al. (2000). Wide-complex tachycardia: continued evaluation of diagnostic criteria. *Acad. Emerg. Med.* 7 (7): 769.

14 Steinman, R.T., Herrara, C., Schluger, C.D., and Lehmann, M.H. (1989). Wide QRS tachycardia in the conscious adult: ventricular tachycardia is the most frequent cause. *JAMA* 261: 1013.

15 Wellens, H., Bar, F.W., and Lie, K.I. (1978). The value of the electrocardiogram in the differential diagnosis of a tachycardia with widened QRS complex. *Am. J. Med.* 64: 27.

16 Wellens, H.H.J. and Brugada, P. (1987). Diagnosis of ventricular tachycardia from the 12-lead electrocardiogram. *Cardiol. Clin.* 5: 511.

17 Kindwall, E., Brown, J., and Josephson, M.E. (1988). Electrocardiographic criteria for ventricular tachycardia in wide complex left bundle branch block morphology tachycardias. *Am. J. Cardiol.* 61: 1279.

6

Non-Sinus Rhythms with Normal Rates

Will Dresen[1] and Andrew E. Darby[2]

[1] Cardiovascular Medicine, University of Virginia Health System, Charlottesville, VA, USA
[2] University of Virginia Health System, Charlottesville, VA, USA

Introduction

A variety of nonsinus rhythms with normal heart rates may be encountered clinically and are important to recognize. These rhythms may present with narrow or wide QRS complexes on the 12-lead electrocardiogram (ECG). They tend to be well-tolerated hemodynamically and typically do not require emergency treatment.

Ectopic Atrial Rhythm

An ectopic atrial rhythm occurs when the dominant pacemaker is an ectopic (nonsinus) focus in either the right or left atrium [1]. Ectopic atrial rhythms may result from failure of the sinus node (e.g. sinus arrest or sinus exit block) and the development of an atrial escape rhythm or acceleration of an ectopic atrial focus to a rate exceeding that of the sinus node. The heart rate is generally 40–60 bpm but may be faster, depending on sympathetic tone. The site of origin of the ectopic focus dictates the morphology, axis, and duration of the P wave on the 12-lead ECG (Figure 3.6.1) [2, 3]. The QRS complexes will resemble those seen in sinus rhythm since ventricular activation is over the normal conduction system. In the absence of symptoms or prolonged pauses from sinus node dysfunction, there is no indication for specific therapy for ectopic atrial rhythms.

Wandering Atrial Pacemaker

A wandering atrial pacemaker is present when there are three or more ectopic foci acting as dominant pacemakers without a single, consistent (i.e. dominant) P wave identifiable (Figure 3.6.2). Due to the presence of multiple foci, the

P-wave morphology and axis vary on the ECG or rhythm strip. The ventricular rate is <100 beats per minute. If the rate exceeds 100 beats per minute, the rhythm is referred to as multifocal atrial tachycardia. Wandering atrial pacemaker results in an irregular ventricular rhythm and could be confused for atrial fibrillation. It could also be mistaken for sinus rhythm with frequent premature atrial contractions although, in this situation, a dominant sinus P wave can often still be identified.

Accelerated Junctional Rhythm

Accelerated junctional rhythm results from acceleration of impulse generation within the atrioventricular junction, which then assumes the role of the dominant cardiac pacemaker if it exceeds the rate of the sinus node [4]. P waves may not be visible on the ECG if occurring simultaneous with the QRS complexes or may be visible just after the QRS complexes (i.e. retrograde). Junctional escape rhythms typically have a rate of 40–60 bpm. When the junctional rhythm exceeds 100 beats per minute it is referred to as junctional tachycardia. If there is retrograde block of the junctional impulse to the atrium, the sinus node will not be suppressed by the retrograde depolarizations and sinus P waves may be seen occurring independently of the QRS complexes (Figure 3.6.3). The QRS complexes typically resemble those in sinus rhythm (i.e. narrow with duration <120 ms) since ventricular activation is over the normal conduction system.

Occasionally another form of junctional rhythm, referred to as isorhythmic dissociation, may be encountered clinically. It is most often seen in young, athletically conditioned individuals whose sinus rates are slow. In isorhythmic dissociation, the junctional rate may, at times,

Electrocardiogram in Clinical Medicine, First Edition. Edited by William J. Brady, Michael J. Lipinski, Andrew E. Darby, Michael C. Bond, Nathan P. Charlton, Korin Hudson, and Kelly Williamson.

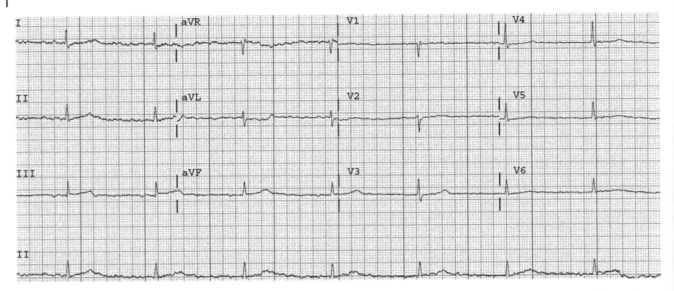

Figure 3.6.1 Electrocardiogram demonstrating an example of an ectopic atrial rhythm. Note that the P wave is inverted (superior axis) in the inferior leads suggesting a site of origin in the lower portion of the atrium (sinus P waves have an inferior axis (i.e. are upright) in the inferior leads).

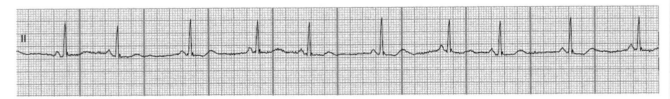

Figure 3.6.2 Rhythm strip demonstrating a wandering atrial pacemaker. Note the irregular rhythm with P waves of varying morphologies.

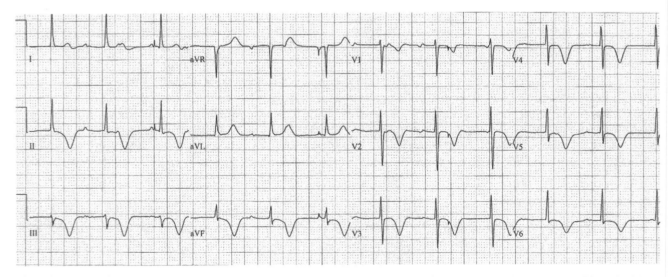

Figure 3.6.3 ECG demonstrating junctional rhythm with complete heart block: note the ventricular rate is normal (~70 bpm) with a junctional rhythm and no clear relationship between the QRS complexes and P waves. There are also widespread T-wave inversions concerning for possible ischemia.

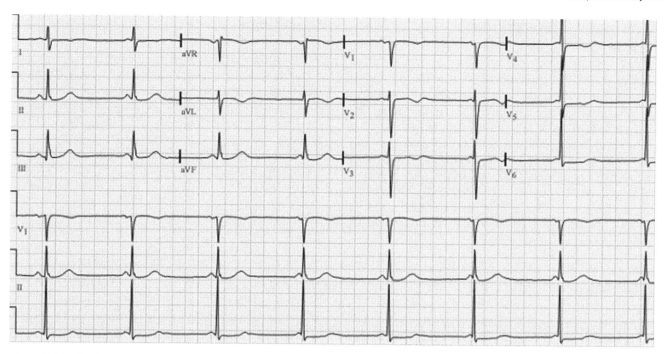

Figure 3.6.4 ECG demonstrating isorhythmic dissociation: Note the regular QRS intervals and narrow QRS complexes with gradual "blending" of the P wave into the QRS complexes when the junctional rate slightly exceeds that of the sinus node.

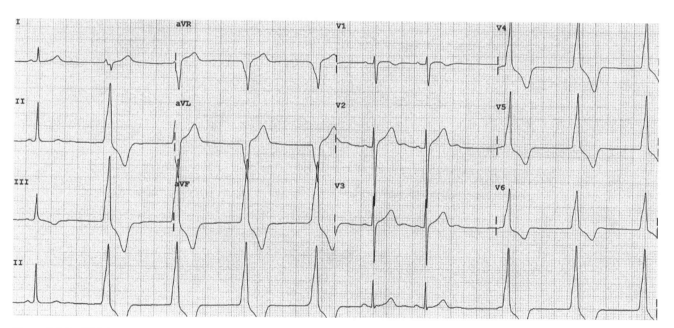

Figure 3.6.5 ECG demonstrating runs of accelerated idioventricular rhythm: Note the patient has sinus rhythm with two episodes of accelerated idioventricular rhythm in which the QRS complexes clearly are wider than sinus, and a P wave merges with a ventricular beat (fusion) on the first beat of the second run (eighth beat on the rhythm strip).

exceed the rate of the sinus node (Figure 3.6.4). Consequently, the rhythm may alternate between sinus and junctional, and the patient may appear to have AV dissociation when the junctional rate exceeds that of the sinus node. Patients are typically asymptomatic with this rhythm. Increasing sympathetic tone, such as through exercise, should increase the rate of the sinus node and restore sinus rhythm with normal atrial to ventricular conduction.

Accelerated Idioventricular Rhythm (AIVR)

An accelerated idioventricular rhythm (AIVR) is a rhythm of ventricular origin typically occurring with a rate of 60–100 bpm (Figure 3.6.5). It often results from an accelerated ventricular focus generating an impulse faster than the sinus node and therefore assumes control as the dominant cardiac pacemaker. Atrioventricular (AV) dissociation may or may not be seen. AIVR may be a marker of spontaneous or induced reperfusion in the peri-myocardial infarction setting (seen in up to 50% of acute infarcts) [5, 6]. AIVR typically does not require acute therapy as the patient is often hemodynamically stable.

Conclusions

Ectopic atrial rhythms, wandering atrial pacemaker, junctional rhythm, isorhythmic dissociation, and AIVR represent nonsinus rhythms, which are important to recognize. It is important to distinguish junctional rhythm and isorhythmic dissociation from complete heart block. These rhythms are rarely symptomatic and generally do not require treatment. AIVR may accompany reperfusion in the setting of myocardial infarction, and a recent ischemic event should be considered when this rhythm is identified.

References

1 Josephson, M.E. (2002). Clinical Cardiac Electrophysiology, Techniques and Interpretations, 3e, 155. Philadelphia: Lippincott, Williams, and Wilkins.

2 Hoffman, B.F. (1970). The P wave and PR interval. Effects of the site of origin of atrial depolarization. *Circulation* 42: 653.

3 Waldo, A.L. (1975). P waves during ectopic atrial rhythms in man. A study utilizing atrial pacing with fixed electrodes. *Circulation* 52: 426.

4 Scherlag, B.J., Lazzara, R., and Helfant, R.H. (1973). Differentiation of "A-V junctional rhythms.". *Circulation* 48: 304.

5 Gorgels, A.P., Vos, M.A., Letsch, I.S. et al. (1988). Usefulness of the accelerated idioventricular rhythm as a marker for myocardial necrosis and reperfusion during thrombolytic therapy in acute myocardial infarction. *Am. J. Cardiol.* 61: 231.

6 Rothfeld, E.L., Zucker, I.R., Parsonnet, V., and Alinsonorin, C.A. (1968). Idioventricular rhythm in acute myocardial infarction. *Circulation* 37: 203.

7

Rhythms of Cardiac Arrest

Erich Kiehl[1] and Andrew E. Darby[2]

[1] *Cardiovascular Medicine, Cleveland Clinic Foundation, Cleveland, OH, USA*
[2] *University of Virginia Health System, Charlottesville, VA, USA*

Introduction

Sudden cardiac arrest (SCA) is the abrupt onset of physiologic malfunction such that sufficient blood flow (cardiac output) cannot be supplied to the body's organs in order to sustain life. SCA is a common cause of sudden death with over 300 000 events per year in the United States making it the leading cause of both cardiovascular and overall mortality [1]. Among EMS-treated out-of-hospital cardiac arrest (OHCA), 23% have an initial rhythm of ventricular fibrillation (VF) or ventricular tachycardia (VT). Survival to hospital discharge following EMS-treated OHCA approaches 10% compared with an approximate 30% survival rate among bystander-witnessed OHCA in which the initial rhythm is treatable with a defibrillator (VT or VF). Furthermore, these statistics do not take into account post-arrest morbidity. Mild to severe permanent neurologic dysfunction is common, even in survivors receiving post-arrest therapeutic hypothermia, the current standard of care.

The cardiac electrical activity at the time of SCA can be subdivided into "shockable" and "nonshockable" rhythms (Table 3.7.1). Shockable rhythms are those that may be terminated with electrical cardioversion or defibrillation and include VF, ventricular tachycardia VT, and supra-ventricular tachycardias (SVT). Non-shockable rhythms can be further subdivided into pulseless electrical activity (PEA) or asystole. PEA includes variants of sinus rhythm (bradycardia to tachycardia), nonsinus bradycardias (junctional or ventricular), and atrioventricular blocks (all without a palpable pulse) whereas asystole is defined as the complete absence of organized electrical activity. Although not foolproof, when determining the underlying disease process leading to SCA, shockable rhythms are more likely to be cardiovascular in etiology whereas nonshockable rhythms

are more likely to be noncardiovascular (Table 3.7.2). Four rhythms may produce pulseless cardiac arrest: VF; rapid VT; PEA; and asystole. Survival from these rhythms depends on prompt recognition and initiation of appropriate basic life support (BLS) and advanced cardiac life support (ACLS) techniques. During SCA, basic cardiopulmonary resuscitation (CPR) and early defibrillation (when appropriate) are of utmost importance.

Ventricular Fibrillation

VF is the most common arrhythmia in cardiac arrest patients. There is no organized ventricular activity on the electrocardiogram (ECG). Instead, the ECG demonstrates irregular, disorganized, and chaotic ventricular activity (Figure 3.7.1). If the rhythm continues, it may degenerate further into asystole. The most common cause of VF is myocardial ischemia. Other potential causes of VF include myocardial scar secondary to a prior heart attack, myocarditis, electrolyte abnormalities (particularly potassium disorders), hypoxemia, and hypothermia. Treatment include prompt initiation of ACLS techniques including prompt defibrillation [2].

Ventricular Tachycardia

VT originates within the ventricular myocardium outside the normal conduction system and, as a result, leads to abnormal ventricular activation thereby producing a wide QRS complex on the surface ECG (Figure 3.7.2). VT is the most common cause of wide complex tachycardia accounting for 80–90% of cases [3]. VT may either be monomorphic (uniform or stable QRS morphology during an episode) or polymorphic (continuously varying QRS morphologies

Electrocardiogram in Clinical Medicine, First Edition. Edited by William J. Brady, Michael J. Lipinski, Andrew E. Darby, Michael C. Bond, Nathan P. Charlton, Korin Hudson, and Kelly Williamson.
© 2021 John Wiley & Sons Ltd. Published 2021 by John Wiley & Sons Ltd.

Table 3.7.1 Rhythms associated with cardiac arrest.

"Shockable" rhythms	"Nonshockable" rhythms
Ventricular fibrillation	Pulseless electrical activity
Ventricular tachycardia	Asystole
Hemodynamically intolerable atrial fibrillation	

Table 3.7.2 Treatable conditions associated with cardiac arrest.

Condition	Predisposing factors
Acidosis	Renal failure, diarrhea, sepsis, drug overdose
Anemia	Gastrointestinal bleeding, trauma
Cardiac tamponade	Recent cardiac procedure, malignancy, pericarditis, post-MI
Disorders of potassium	Renal failure, hemolysis, rhabdomyolysis, trauma
Hypothermia	Exposure, drug overdose
Hypovolemia	Significant burns, gastrointestinal losses, hemorrhage
Hypoxemia	Pulmonary disease, airway obstruction, hypoventilation
Myocardial infarction	
Pulmonary embolism	Recent surgery or period of immobilization
Tension pneumothorax	Recent chest procedure, trauma

during an episode; Figure 3.7.3). "Nonsustained" VT is defined as an episode lasting less than 30 seconds, whereas "sustained" VT lasts longer than 30 seconds.

The etiologies of VT differ, depending on whether the patient presents with monomorphic or polymorphic VT. Etiologies of monomorphic VT include acute or prior myocardial infarction, myocarditis, prior cardiac surgery (particularly repair of congenital heart disease involving the ventricles, such as ventricular septal defect), and certain genetic arrhythmia syndromes such as arrhythmogenic ventricular cardiomyopathy. Polymorphic VT is often associated with acute myocardial ischemia, electrolyte abnormalities, and prolonged QT interval (either genetic or drug-induced). Ventricular tachycardia may also be precipitated by significant medical illness in a patient with prior myocardial infarction who has the underlying substrate for development of VT. As with VF, initial treatment for the SCA patient with VT should include basic ACLS and cardioversion. Amiodarone is the most common pharmacologic agent to prevent recurrent VT [2, 3].

Torsade de Pointes

Torsade de pointes (TdP) is a specific type of ventricular arrhythmia that can lead to sudden cardiac death. TdP is a polymorphic ventricular tachycardia exhibiting distinct characteristics on the electrocardiogram, specifically a "twisting" of the QRS complex around the isoelectric baseline (Figure 3.7.4). It is typically polymorphic VT occurring in the setting of a prolonged QT interval. Predisposing factors include congenital or acquired prolongation of the QT interval; electrolyte abnormalities (hypokalemia; hypomagnesemia; hypocalcemia); severe bradycardia; and myocardial ischemia. Treatment is directed toward withdrawal of the offending agent (if the patient is taking a QT prolonging medication such as a fluoroquinolone antibiotic or haloperidol); infusion of magnesium sulfate; and temporary pacing to increase the heart rate and secondarily shorten the QT interval if profound bradycardia is the culprit [4].

Preexcited Atrial Fibrillation

Atrial fibrillation (AF) rarely precipitates hemodynamic instability, although patients with advanced structural heart disease (particularly severe aortic or mitral stenosis) may become hemodynamically unstable in the setting of AF with rapid ventricular response. In addition, patients with atrial

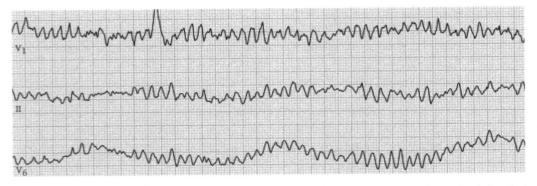

Figure 3.7.1 Rhythm strip demonstrating ventricular fibrillation: Note the absence of organized electrical activity (i.e. no appreciable QRS complexes).

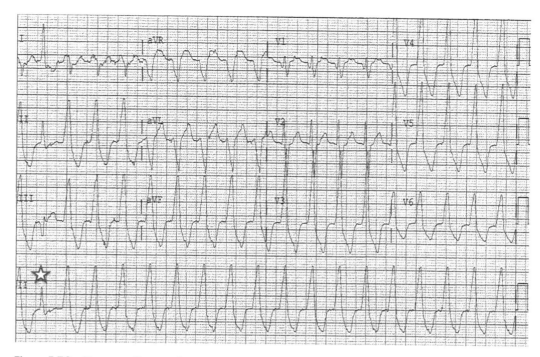

Figure 3.7.2 Electrocardiogram demonstrating a wide complex tachycardia with left bundle branch block morphology due to sustained monomorphic VT: the star denotes a capture beat indicative of AV dissociation.

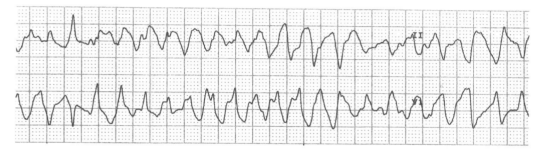

Figure 3.7.3 Rhythm strip demonstrating polymorphic ventricular tachycardia in which the ventricular rhythm is irregular without organized QRS complexes.

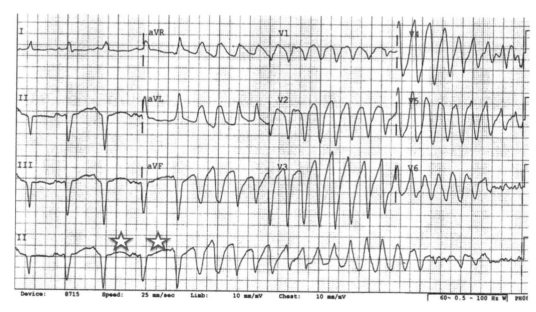

Figure 3.7.4 ECG demonstrating torsade de pointes (TdP) with the characteristic "twisting" of the QRS complexes around the isoelectric baseline. Note the prolonged QT interval prior to the onset of TdP.

(a)

(b)

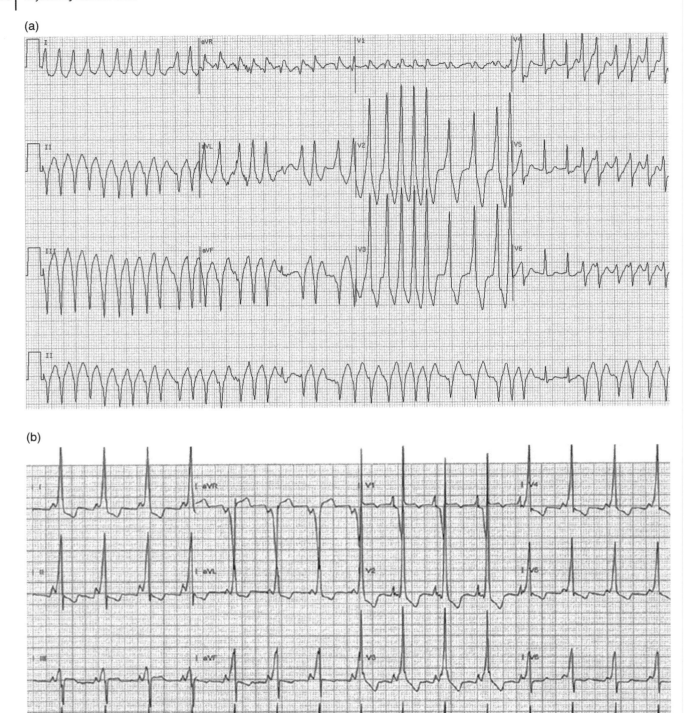

Figure 3.7.5 (a) The electrocardiogram demonstrates preexcited atrial fibrillation. Note the irregular rhythm due to underlying AF, delta waves most readily apparent in the precordial leads and lead I, and beat-to-beat variation in QRS width and degree of pre-excitation. (b) The 12-lead electrocardiogram demonstrates sinus rhythm with ventricular preexcitation (very short PR interval with delta waves at the onset of the QRS complexes).

fibrillation occurring in a patient with an accessory pathway capable of anterograde conduction may potentially result in extremely rapid ventricular rates and hemodynamic instability. Accessory pathways may be manifest (anterograde conduction with ventricular preexcitation at baseline) or concealed (only retrograde conduction, so not visible on the baseline 12-lead ECG as there are no delta waves). Manifest accessory pathways are present in 0.1–0.3% of the population [5]. Patients with manifest accessory pathways may develop atrioventricular reciprocating tachycardia (AVRT) or preexcited atrial fibrillation. Rapid anterograde accessory pathway conduction during atrial fibrillation can result in sudden cardiac death with a 10-year risk of 0.15–0.24% [6, 7]. It is critical that preexcited atrial fibrillation be recognized promptly so that appropriate therapy be administered (Figure 3.7.5). The ECG typically demonstrates an irregular rhythm due to the underlying AF; delta waves due to ventricular preexcitation; and beat-to-beat variability in the degree of ventricular preexcitation (QRS width). The changes in QRS width are due to variable degrees of fusion of anterograde conduction over the AV node and accessory pathway. At times, the AV node may be refractory and unable to conduct resulting in increased conduction over the accessory pathway and greater preexcitation (wider QRS, more evident delta wave). At other times, anterograde conduction may be over both the AV node and accessory pathway resulting in a narrower QRS with perhaps less evident delta wave. Importantly, AV nodal-blocking agents are contraindicated in patients at risk of rapid conduction down the accessory pathway during AF. Administration of such medications may slow AV nodal conduction but result in more rapid conduction down the accessory pathway leading to potential hemodynamic instability. Appropriate therapy may be either synchronized cardioversion or intravenous ibutilide or procainamide. Both ibutilide and procainamide may decrease the ventricular rate by slowing conduction over the accessory pathway and may potentially chemically convert AF to sinus rhythm [5].

Pulseless Electrical Activity

PEA, also occasionally known as electromechanical dissociation, refers to a cardiac arrest situation in which electrical activity is present on telemetry or a 12-lead electrocardiogram, but there is no palpable pulse. Most practitioners are familiar with the etiologies of PEA arrest at the 6 Hs and 6 Ts: **h**ypovolemia; **h**ypoxia; **h**ydrogen ions (acidosis); **h**yperkalemia or **h**ypokalemia; **h**ypoglycemia; **h**ypothermia; **t**ablets or **t**oxins (drug overdose); cardiac **t**amponade; **t**ension pneumothorax; **t**hrombosis (myocardial infarction or pulmonary embolism); **t**achycardia; **t**rauma (hypovolemia from blood loss) [8]. The electrocardiogram may occasionally provide clues to the etiology, particularly in the setting of myocardial ischemia, electrolyte abnormalities, drug toxicity or overdose, pulmonary embolism, and cardiac tamponade. Myocardial ischemia triggering PEA may potentially occur with an ST-elevation myocardial infarction (STEMI, Figure 3.7.6). A massive ischemic event may result in PEA arrest through several

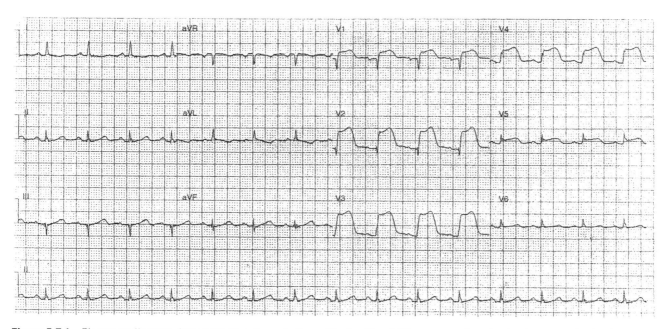

Figure 3.7.6 Electrocardiogram demonstrating sinus rhythm with significant ST segment elevation in the precordial leads indicating acute myocardial infarction.

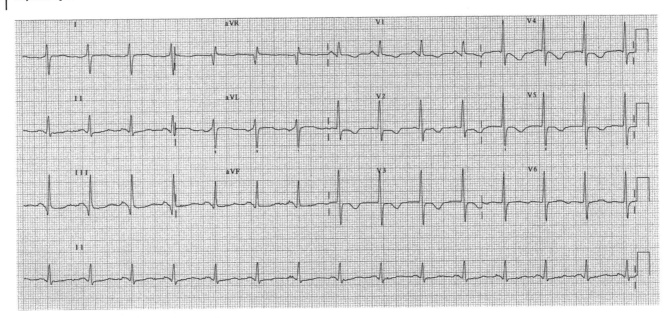

Figure 3.7.7 Electrocardiogram in a patient presenting with acute pulmonary embolism: note the prominent R waves in leads V1–V3 with accompanying T-wave inversions indicating acute right heart strain as well as the S wave in lead I and Q wave in lead III.

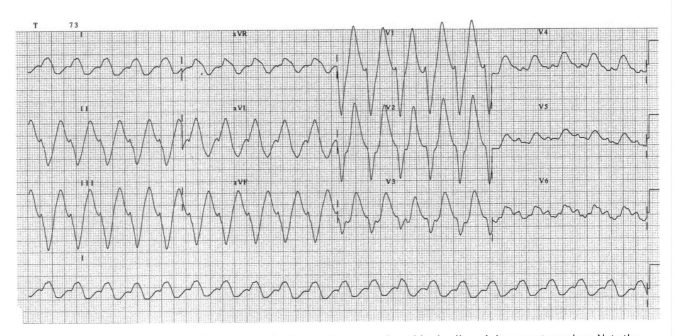

Figure 3.7.8 This 12-lead electrocardiogram was taken in a patient presenting with tricyclic anti-depressant overdose: Note the significant prolongation of the QRS complexes (may potentially be misdiagnosed as hyperkalemia).

mechanisms, including pump failure, secondary ventricular tachycardia or VF, or myocardial rupture as a late complication of STEMI.

A hemodynamically significant pulmonary embolism may also result in PEA arrest if not promptly treated. Various changes may be seen on the 12-lead electrocardiogram in a patient presenting with acute pulmonary

embolism, although none are sensitive or specific enough to rule the diagnosis in or out [9]. The 12-lead electrocardiogram in a patient presenting with acute pulmonary embolism most often demonstrates sinus tachycardia. The ECG may also show signs of right heart strain with incomplete or complete right bundle branch block; inverted T waves in leads V1–V4; and right axis deviation. The "classic"

ECG signs of a large S wave in lead I, Q wave in lead III, and an inverted T wave in lead III (S1Q3T3) occurs in 12–50% of patients with the diagnosis but also occur in 12% of patients without pulmonary emboli (Figure 3.7.7) [10].

Drug toxicity or overdose may also produce PEA arrest along with certain ECG changes. Class III anti-arrhythmic agents block K^+ channels and, in cases of overdose or reduced clearance, excessive QT prolongation may result. Tricyclic anti-depressant agents have Na + channel blocking properties and, in cases of toxicity or overdose, may produce both bradycardia and QRS widening (prolongation of the QRS complexes results from slowing of depolarization and impulse propagation). Excessive QRS prolongation may predispose patients to ventricular dysrhythmias (Figure 3.7.8).

Conclusions

The 12-lead electrocardiogram or rhythm strip in a patient presenting with cardiac arrest may provide clues to the diagnosis or underlying etiology. Prompt initiation of ACLS protocols are imperative, and "shockable" rhythms should be treated with prompt cardioversion or defibrillation.

References

1 Mozaffarian, D., Benjamin, E.J., Go, A.S. et al. (2015). Heart disease and stroke statistics – 2015 update: a report from the American Heart Association. *Circulation*: e1–e294.

2 Neumar, R.W., Shuster, M., Callaway, C.W. et al. (3 November 2015). Part 1: executive summary: 2015 American Heart Association guidelines update for cardiopulmonary resuscitation and emergency cardiovascular care. *Circulation* 132 (18 Suppl 2): S315–S367.

3 John, R.M., Tedrow, U.B., Koplan, B.A. et al. (October 2012). Ventricular arrhythmias and sudden cardiac death. *Lancet* 380 (9852): 1520–1529.

4 Napolitano, C., Priori, S.G., and Schwartz, P.J. (1994). Torsade de pointes. Mechanisms and management. *Drugs* 47 (1): 51–65.

5 Page, R.L., Joglar, J.A., Caldwell, M.A. et al. (2015). 2015 ACC/AHA/HRS guideline for the management of adult patients with supraventricular tachycardia. *Circulation* 132: 1–131.

6 Brembilla-Perrot, B., Moulin-Zinsch, A., Sellal, J.M. et al. (2013). Impact of transesophageal electrophysiologic study to elucidate the mechanism of arrhythmia on children with supraventricular tachycardia and no preexcitation. *Pediatr. Cardiol.* 34: 1695–1702.

7 Villain, E., Bonnet, D., Acar, P. et al. (1998). Recommendations for the treatment of recurrent supraventricular tachycardia in infants. *Arch. Pediatr.* 157: 101–106.

8 American Heart Association Guidelines for Cardiopulmonary Resuscitation and Emergency Cardiovascular Care (November 2010). Part 8: adult advanced cardiovascular life support. *Circulation* 122 (18 Suppl): S729–S767.

9 Brown, G. and Hogg, K. (October 2005). Best evidence topic report. Diagnostic utility of electrocardiogram for diagnosing pulmonary embolism. *Emerg. Med. J.: EMJ.* 22 (10): 729–730.

10 Rodger, M., Makropoulos, D., Turek, M. et al. (October 2000). Diagnostic value of the electrocardiogram in suspected pulmonary embolism. *Am. J. Cardiol.* 86 (7): 807–809, A10.

8

Premature Atrial and Ventricular Complexes

Adrián I. Löffler[1] and Andrew E. Darby[2]

[1] Cardiovascular Medicine, University of Virginia Health System, Charlottesville, VA, USA
[2] University of Virginia Health System, Charlottesville, VA, USA

Premature atrial and ventricular complexes are disturbances of the cardiac rhythm in which ectopic impulses arise from a muscle fiber or group of fibers within the atria or ventricles producing irregularity in the heart rhythm. Ectopic impulses from the atria are correspondingly termed premature atrial contractions (PACs) while ectopic impulses from the ventricles are referred to as premature ventricular contractions, or complexes (PVCs). Atrial and ventricular ectopy may or may not be associated with symptoms (palpitations, most commonly) and may occur in the presence or absence of structural heart disease.

Premature Atrial Contractions

PACs are the most common arrhythmia seen during ECG monitoring [1, 2]. Although the exact cause of PACs is unclear, they are a premature activation of the atria from ectopic electrical impulses that trigger the atria before depolarization from the sinus node. PACs can occur in any decade of life, but the incidence increases with age and presence of structural heart disease. PACs by themselves are not considered an abnormal finding. Patients are often asymptomatic but can experience palpitations or a fluttering sensation in the chest [3]. Occasionally, PACs can initiate supraventricular arrhythmias, particularly atrial fibrillation. Table 3.8.1 displays some of the underlying conditions associated with PACs [4, 5].

ECG Findings of PACs

On an electrocardiogram, PACs manifest as premature beats (i.e. occurring earlier than the next expected sinus beat), typically with a P wave different than that occurring in sinus rhythm (Figure 3.8.1). If the ectopic focus is near the sinus node, however, the P-wave may appear similar to the sinus P wave. Typically, the atrial impulse propagates normally through the atrioventricular node resulting in a narrow QRS complex. In addition to generating a P wave sooner than would be expected from the baseline sinus rate, the following ECG findings may be seen with PACs:

1) A normal or short PR interval with a normal QRS complex.
2) A prolonged PR interval with a normal QRS complex.
3) A conducted but aberrant QRS complex.
4) A nonconducted PAC, resulting in no QRS complex.

Treatment

Atrial ectopy may require no treatment other than reassurance when asymptomatic. If associated with symptoms, behavior modification (decreasing alcohol, caffeine, smoking, and stress) should be tried first. For highly symptomatic patients who have persistent symptoms despite lifestyle modifications, beta blockers or calcium-channel blockers may be tried and have modest efficacy. Antiarrhythmic agents may eliminate PACs but often have undesirable side effects or risks that preclude their routine use. Catheter ablation to eliminate the repetitive focus is another option if drug-refractory.

Multifocal Atrial Tachycardia (MAT)

An extreme form of atrial ectopy is multifocal atrial tachycardia in which multiple ectopic foci are depolarizing rapidly and at irregular intervals. MAT is characterized by a heart rate greater than 100 beats per minute with at least three

Electrocardiogram in Clinical Medicine, First Edition. Edited by William J. Brady, Michael J. Lipinski, Andrew E. Darby, Michael C. Bond, Nathan P. Charlton, Korin Hudson, and Kelly Williamson.

Table 3.8.1 Potential etiologies for premature atrial contractions.

Cardiac	Noncardiac	Behavior/Other
Acute myocardial infarction	Acute and chronic pulmonary disease	Smoking
Coronary artery disease	Chronic renal failure	Caffeine
Valvular heart disease	Neurologic disorders	Alcohol
Cardiomyopathy		Theophylline
		Thyroid disease

Premature Atrial Contractions

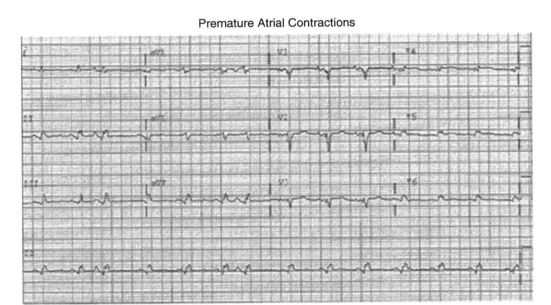

Figure 3.8.1 The ECG demonstrates sinus rhythm with anterior Q waves and poor R-wave progression, suggesting a prior anterior myocardial infarction. Note the third and seventh beats are premature atrial contractions. These beats may be distinguished from sinus beats by the earlier timing and P-wave morphology different from sinus with identical QRS complexes.

different P-wave morphologies on the electrocardiogram. Because the ectopic foci are generated by multiple foci throughout the atria, the resulting P waves have variable morphologies often with variable PR intervals. It can mimic atrial fibrillation given its irregular rhythm as shown in Figure 3.8.2. It may be differentiated from atrial fibrillation electrocardiographically as atrial fibrillation does not produce organized atrial activity, or P waves, whereas MAT displays clear P waves prior to each QRS although the P wave morphology varies. This arrhythmia occurs most often in patients with chronic lung disease, particularly in patients presenting with an acute exacerbation of their chronic lung condition. It is also associated with hypoxia, pulmonary embolism, hypokalemia, or stimulants.

Treatment of MAT consists of correcting the underlying condition (hypoxia, electrolyte abnormality) and discontinuation of medications thought to exacerbate the arrhythmia. It generally resolves as the patient's underlying condition

improves; however, the most efficacious drugs are metoprolol and IV magnesium [6].

Pulmonary Vein Tachycardia

Premature atrial depolarizations may occasionally trigger atrial fibrillation. It has been shown that atrial ectopic beats originating from the pulmonary veins are common triggers of atrial fibrillation [6]. These foci can be targeted for catheter ablation as part of the treatment for atrial fibrillation. P waves generated by ectopic foci from the pulmonary veins are characteristically positive in V1 and throughout the other precordial leads owing to the posterior location of the pulmonary veins where they connect to the left atrium [7].

The P-wave morphology and axis in the limb leads may be helpful in determining the site of origin, which can be useful if catheter ablation is considered. Because the left-sided pulmonary veins are lateral structures and farther from the

Multifocal Atrial Tachycardia

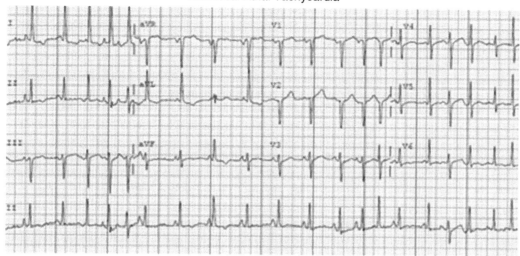

Figure 3.8.2 This ECG is from a patient with severe sepsis due to pneumonia and acute respiratory failure. Multifocal atrial tachycardia (MAT) characteristically presents as a narrow complex tachycardia with an irregularly, irregular rhythm and multiple (>3) P-wave morphologies. This rhythm can be distinguished from atrial fibrillation for MAT has organized atrial activity with a P wave visible before each QRS complex, whereas there is no organized atrial activity (i.e. P waves) in AF.

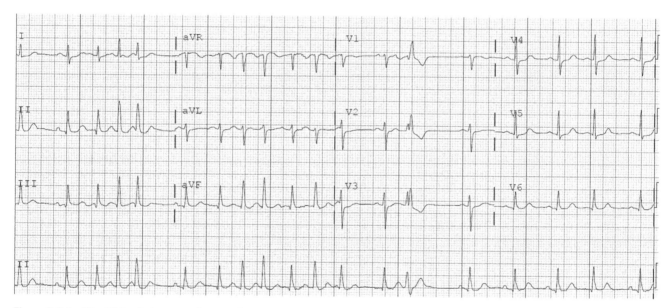

Figure 3.8.3 The 12-lead electrocardiogram from a patient with atrial fibrillation displays sinus rhythm with a burst of PACs originating from one of the pulmonary veins. Atrial fibrillation originating from the pulmonary veins often behaves in this manner with repetitive, paroxysmal bursts of irregular tachycardia.

midline, total atrial activation time is longer compared with impulses from the right-sided veins, resulting in a longer P-wave duration and characteristic notching in the inferior leads. The lateral limb leads are also useful given the anatomical relationship of the veins. Ectopic impulses from the right-pulmonary veins are typically positive in limb lead I, whereas ectopy from the left pulmonary veins tends to be associated with isoelectric or negative P-waves. The inferior limb leads help to discriminate between the upper and lower pulmonary veins. Foci from the superior pulmonary veins tend to have a more inferiorly directed (or positive) P-wave compared with impulses from the inferior pulmonary veins [4]. Figure 3.8.3 is an example of pulmonary vein tachycardia. Characteristic features of this entity include frequent, repetitive bursts of narrow complex tachycardia in a patient with a history of atrial fibrillation.

Premature Ventricular Contractions

Ventricular ectopy or premature ventricular contractions (PVCs) result from abnormal electrical discharges from Purkinje fibers in the ventricles rather than the sinoatrial node. These electrical discharges produce a premature heartbeat and irregularity in the heart rhythm. PVCs are ubiquitous, usually benign, and may or may not be associated with underlying structural heart disease. Ventricular bigeminy occurs when a PVC follows each normal QRS complex, as shown in Figures 3.8.4 and 3.8.5. Three or more consecutive PVCs would be considered nonsustained ventricular tachycardia.

Symptoms

PVCs are often asymptomatic but can cause palpitations, a pounding sensation in the neck, dizziness, or, rarely, presyncope or syncope [3]. Patients with infrequent PVCs and no or minimal symptoms may not warrant any additional investigation, whereas patients with a high burden of PVCs and/or concerning symptoms (i.e. syncope) should be evaluated for underlying structural heart disease (Table 3.8.2).

Differential Diagnosis

Evaluation

A high burden of ventricular ectopy (generally >15–20% of all beats on 24-hour Holter monitoring) has been associated

with the potential development of left ventricular dysfunction (PVC-induced cardiomyopathy) [8]. Patients with a high burden of ventricular ectopy and/or symptoms should undergo assessment of the PVC frequency by cardiac monitoring such as by continuous 24-hour Holter monitoring. Echocardiography is useful to assess for valvular pathology, regional wall motion abnormalities, cardiomyopathies, or other myocardial abnormalities, which may cause or be a result of frequent ventricular ectopy. PVC-induced cardiomyopathy is a diagnosis of exclusion, but typical features on TTE include: deceased left ventricular ejection fraction, increased left ventricular systolic and diastolic dimensions, wall motion abnormalities (often global instead of regional), and mitral regurgitation (due to mitral annular dilation) [8]. Thyroid disease and electrolyte abnormalities should also be excluded, as they are potentially reversible causes of ventricular ectopy.

PVC Origin

PVCs most often occur in the absence of underlying structural heart disease and are termed *idiopathic* if no identifiable cause can be determined. Approximately two-thirds of idiopathic PVCs originate from the ventricular outflow tracts, mainly the right ventricular outflow tract near the pulmonic valve. PVCs originating from the outflow tracts are often monomorphic and not associated with underlying heart disease [5]. They have a typical appearance on the 12-lead ECG as the PVCs display a left bundle branch block

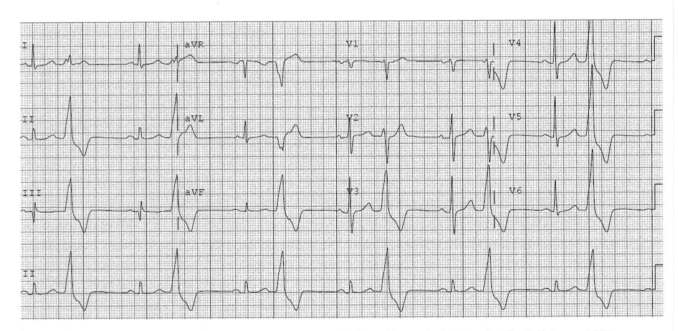

Figure 3.8.4 The 12-lead electrocardiogram demonstrates sinus rhythm with ventricular bigeminy. The PVCs have a LBBB morphology (given that they are predominantly negative in lead V1 and positive in V6) with an inferiorly directed axis (positive in leads II, III, and aVF) suggestive of origin in the ventricular outflow tracts.

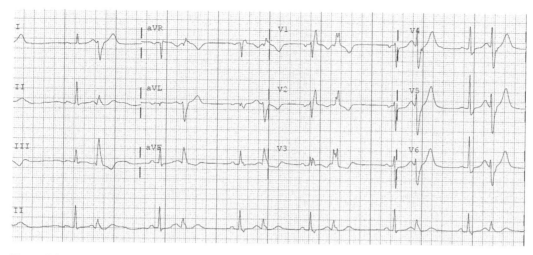

Figure 3.8.5 The electrocardiogram demonstrates sinus rhythm with ventricular bigeminy. The sinus QRS displays a RBBB, and the PVCs also have a right bundle branch block pattern given that they are positive in lead V1 and predominantly negative in lead V6 suggestive of origin from the left ventricle.

Table 3.8.2 Possible causes of premature ventricular contractions [1, 2].

Cardiac	Pulmonary	Endocrinopathies	Behavior/Other
Heart failure	COPD	Thyroid abnormalities	Nicotine
Acute myocardial infarction	Sleep apnea	Adrenal abnormalities	Caffeine
Hypertension with left ventricular hypertrophy	Pulmonary Hypertension	Gonadal abnormalities	Alcohol
Hypertrophic cardiomyopathy	Other Pulmonary diseases		Sympathomimetic agents (e.g., beta-agonists, antihistamines)
Congenital heart disease			Illicit drugs (e.g., cocaine, amphetamines)
Idiopathic ventricular tachycardia			

(LBBB) morphology (negative QRS in lead V1, positive QRS in lead V6) and upright QRS complexes in the inferior leads (Figure 3.8.4).

Understanding the anatomy of lead placement can help identify PVC origin. The inferior leads (i.e. leads II, III, aVF) are most useful because all outflow tract arrhythmias show positive deflections (i.e. upright QRS complexes) in these leads. This results from the superior location of the ventricular outflow tracts. Premature depolarizations from these areas produce a wavefront that spreads from superior to inferior through the heart. Leads aVR and aVL are both superior leads; thus, the vast majority of outflow tract arrhythmias show simultaneous negative (QS complex) deflections in these two leads. Lead V1 is a right-sided and anterior lead; thus, RVOT PVCs are all negative in this lead with a LBBB morphology [9]. PVCs that display a positive QRS in lead V1 (right bundle branch block (RBBB) morphology) originate from the left ventricle, with depolarization spreading from

left to right across the heart (the wavefront travels toward lead V1 resulting in a predominantly positive QRS complex) as seen in Figure 3.8.5.

PVCs may also arise from ventricular locations other than the musculature surrounding the aortic and pulmonic valves in the ventricular outflow tracts. Less common sites of origin include the ventricular free walls, around the mitral or tricuspid valves, interventricular septum, and papillary muscles. PVCs from these areas tend to be monomorphic and occur as single complexes, although nonsustained ventricular tachycardia may also occur. Frequent ventricular ectopy from *non*-outflow tract sites of origin should prompt evaluation for underlying structural heart disease.

Treatment

As mentioned above, PVCs are frequently seen in clinical practice, typically benign, and often do not require treatment.

The patient should be evaluated for the presence of underlying structural heart disease, and if absent, the prognosis is very favorable. If behavioral etiologies are identified (Table 3.8.2), lifestyle modifications should be the first intervention. If symptomatic, beta blockers and calcium channel blockers are generally safe and may be effective. Antiarrhythmic agents can be considered but often have a higher side-effect profile. Catheter ablation is another option for highly symptomatic patients who have failed medical therapy [10, 11].

References

1 Brodsky, M., Wu, D., Denes, P. et al. (1977). Arrhythmias documented by 24 hour continuous electrocardiographic monitoring in 50 male medical students without apparent heart disease. *Am. J. Cardiol.* 39 (3): 390.

2 Folarin, V.A., Fitzsimmons, P.J., and Kruyer, W.B. (2001). Holter monitor findings in asymptomatic male military aviators without structural heart disease. *Aviat. Space Environ. Med.* 72 (9): 836.

3 Zimetbaum, P. and Josephson, M.E. (1998). Evaluation of patients with palpitations. *N. Engl. J. Med.* 338 (19): 1369.

4 Macfarlane, P.W., SpringerLink. (2011). Comprehensive Electrocardiology, 2e. New York; London: Springer.

5 Longo, D.L., Harrison, T.R., Kasper, D.L. et al. (2012). Harrison's Principles of Internal Medicine, 18e. New York: McGraw.

6 McCord, J. and Borzak, S. (1998). Multifocal atrial tachycardia. *Chest* 113 (1): 203–209.

7 Haïssaguerre, M., Jaïs, P., Shah, D.C. et al. (1998 Sep 3). Spontaneous initiation of atrial fibrillation by ectopic beats originating in the pulmonary veins. *N. Engl. J. Med.* 339 (10): 659–666.

8 Lee, G.K., Klarich, K.W., Grogan, M., and Cha, Y.M. (2012 Feb). Premature ventricular contraction-induced cardiomyopathy: a treatable condition. *Circ. Arrhythm. Electrophysiol.* 5 (1): 229–236.

9 Asirvatham, S.J. (2009 Aug). Correlative anatomy for the invasive electrophysiologist: outflow tract and supravalvar arrhythmia. *J. Cardiovasc. Electrophysiol.* 20 (8): 955–968.

10 Ng, G.A. (2006. Nov). Treating patients with ventricular ectopic beats. *Heart* 92 (11): 1707–1712. Review.

11 Bala, R. and Marchlinski, F.E. (2007). Electrocardiographic recognition and ablation of outflow tract ventricular tachycardia. *Heart Rhythm.* 4: 366.

9

Nontraditional Rhythm Disorders

Dysrhythmias Related to Metabolic and Toxicologic Conditions

Andrew E. Darby

University of Virginia Health System, Charlottesville, VA, USA

Introduction

A variety of metabolic and toxicologic conditions may affect the electrical properties of the heart thereby producing heart rhythm disturbances. Depending on the underlying metabolic or toxicologic condition, the patient may present with either a tachyarrhythmia or bradyarrhythmia. Certain QRS complex and ST segment abnormalities may also occur with various metabolic and toxic conditions and are important to recognize.

Hyperkalemia

Hyperkalemia may result in a variety of changes on the 12-lead electrocardiogram (ECG). The classic finding, and often one of the first changes, is tall peaked T waves [1]. Classically, "peaked T waves" has been defined as T waves exceeding 6 mm in height in the limb leads and 10 mm in the precordial leads. Peaking of the T waves typically develops with serum potassium concentrations of 5.5–6.5 mEq/l [2–4]. Serum potassium concentrations in this range may also produce shortening of the QT interval and possibly reversible left anterior or posterior fascicular block. If the serum potassium concentration continues to rise into the range of 6.5–7.5 mEq/l, additional changes may be observed, including first degree AV block, flattening of the P waves, and ST segment depression with widening of the QRS complexes (Figure 3.9.1). Further increase in the serum potassium concentration exceeding 7.5 mEq/l may result in disappearance of the P waves, left or right bundle branch block, or markedly widened and diffuse intraventricular conduction delay resembling a "sine wave" pattern, ST-segment elevation in the right precordial leads resembling a Brugada pattern, and potentially life-threatening arrhythmias, including VT, VF, or asystole [5]. Although the aforementioned ECG changes have been associated with the serum potassium ranges as mentioned above, it is important to note that the progression and severity of ECG changes do not correlate perfectly with serum potassium concentration.

Hypokalemia

A variety of arrhythmias may be seen in patients presenting with hypokalemia. These include premature atrial and ventricular beats, sinus bradycardia, and paroxysmal atrial or junctional tachycardia [6]. Hypokalemia may also produce characteristic ECG changes, including ST-segment depression, decreased T-wave amplitude, and an increase in the amplitude of the U waves, which occur at the end of the T wave (Figure 3.9.2) [7, 8]. U waves are often best seen in the lateral precordial leads (i.e. V4–V6). Hypokalemia may also prolong the QT interval (in contrast to hyperkalemia, which may shorten the QT interval). The QRS duration may increase with severe hypokalemia, and the ST segments may become markedly depressed along with inversion of the T waves.

Hypercalcemia

Hypercalcemia may result in shortening of the QT interval, primarily due to a decrease in the ST-segment duration (Figure 3.9.3) [9]. In addition to hypercalcemia, the differential diagnosis for QT interval shortening includes hyperkalemia, digitalis, and beta-blocker effect. Hypercalcemia typically produces little, if any, effect on the P wave, QRS complex, or T wave. PR-segment prolongation may rarely occur.

Electrocardiogram in Clinical Medicine, First Edition. Edited by William J. Brady, Michael J. Lipinski, Andrew E. Darby, Michael C. Bond, Nathan P. Charlton, Korin Hudson, and Kelly Williamson.

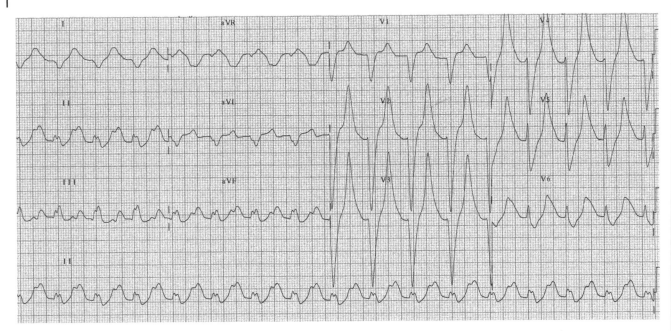

Figure 3.9.1 12-lead electrocardiogram demonstrating features of hyperkalemia: Note the "peaked" T waves in the precordial leads; widening of the QRS complexes; diffuse ST abnormalities. The P waves are difficult to visualize but are typically flattened with hyperkalemia.

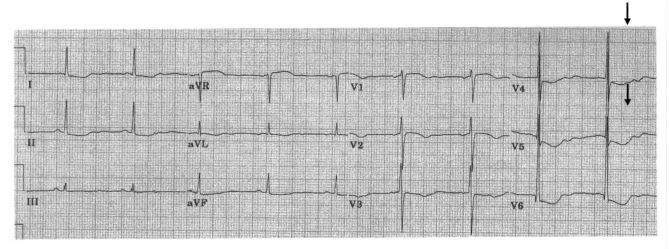

Figure 3.9.2 12-lead electrocardiogram demonstrating features of hypokalemia: Note the ST segment depression; relatively short QT interval; and U waves (arrows).

Hypocalcemia

The primary ECG manifestation of hypocalcemia is QT-interval prolongation. The QT interval prolongs as a result of lengthening of the ST segment. Occasionally, flattening or inversion of the T waves may be seen.

Antiarrhythmic Drug Toxicity

With the rising prevalence of atrial fibrillation, patients taking antiarrhythmic drugs will be increasingly encountered in clinical practice [10–13]. It is therefore worth having familiarity with the commonly used antiarrhythmic drugs, their mechanism of action, and potential toxicities (Figure 3.9.4a–c). The most frequently used class I antiarrhythmic drugs are flecainide and propafenone. Their primary antiarrhythmic effects are achieved by blocking sodium channels, thereby slowing conduction and increasing cardiac tissue refractoriness. By slowing myocardial conduction, sodium channel toxicity may manifest as widening of the QRS complexes on the ECG (Figure 3.9.5). Flecainide and propafenone exhibit "*use dependent*" sodium channel blockade in which the drugs are more tightly bound to the sodium channels at *faster*

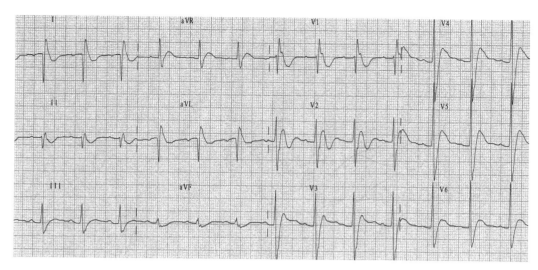

Figure 3.9.3 12-lead electrocardiogram demonstrating features of hypercalcemia including ST segment abnormalities and QT interval shortening.

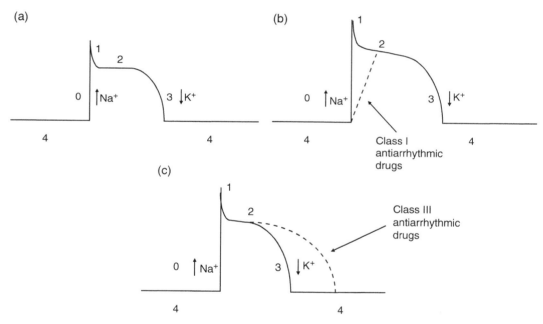

Figure 3.9.4 (a) The cardiac myocyte action potential: Phase 0 corresponds with the resting phase of the cardiac action potential. In phase 1, the cardiac myocytes depolarize, which is driven by influx of sodium ions. Phase 2 consists of transient repolarization (driven by efflux of potassium), and phase 3 is the plateau phase which is calcium-dependent. During phase 4 the myocytes repolarize secondary to efflux of potassium, which delivers them back to the resting membrane potential. (b) Mechanism of action of class I antiarrhythmic drugs: the class I antiarrhythmic agents block sodium channels, blunting phase 1 of the cardiac action potential and thereby slowing depolarization. The primary electrocardiographic manifestation of sodium channel-blocker toxicity is widening of the QRS complexes secondary to conduction slowing. (c) Mechanism of action of class III antiarrhythmic drugs: the class III antiarrhythmic agents block potassium channels, thereby prolonging phase 4 (repolarization) of the cardiac action potential. The primary electrocardiographic manifestation of potassium channel-blocker toxicity is QT prolongation secondary to slowing of repolarization.

heart rates. Consequently, patients taking these drugs who then develop atrial fibrillation or atrial flutter with rapid ventricular response may present with a wide QRS complex tachycardia as a result of increased sodium channel blockade achieved at faster heart rates (may be mistaken for ventricular tachycardia). In addition, the class I antiarrhythmic drugs may convert atrial fibrillation into atrial flutter and, by slowing atrial conduction, result in atrial flutter which may be conducted in a 1 : 1 pattern with rapid ventricular rates.

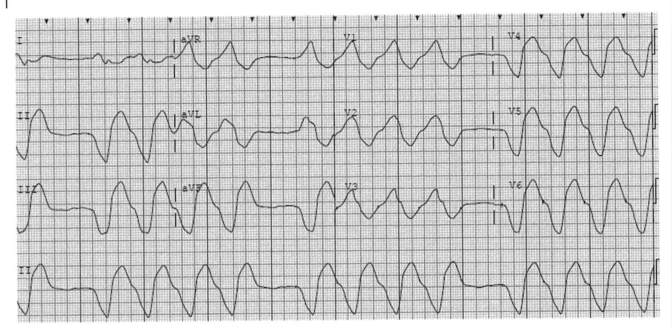

Figure 3.9.5 12-lead ECG demonstrating features of class I anti-arrhythmic dug toxicity: the patient was taking flecainide for suppression of atrial fibrillation and also had a dual chamber pacemaker. Development of renal failure resulted in reduced clearance of flecainide and sodium-channel blocker toxicity, manifesting as QRS widening and intermittent failure of the pacemaker to capture.

The class III antiarrhythmic agents include sotalol, dofetilide, dronedarone, and amiodarone, and they primarily exert their antiarrhythmic effects through blockade of cardiac potassium channels. Blocking potassium channels prolongs repolarization and the cardiac action potential, resulting in increased tissue refractoriness. Potassium channel blockade may result in QT prolongation in situations of drug toxicity (e.g. excessive dosage; reduced clearance). Sotalol and dofetilide also exhibit *"reverse* use dependence," meaning their potassium channel blocking effects are exaggerated at *slower* heart rates (i.e. increased risk for QT prolongation at slower heart rates). Potassium channel toxicity may produce excessive QT prolongation, placing the patient at risk for torsade de pointes (Figure 3.9.6).

Digoxin, although not considered an antiarrhythmic drug, is occasionally used to control the ventricular response to atrial fibrillation. In nontoxic situations, the ECG often has characteristic findings in patients taking digoxin. Specifically, the ST segments may have downsloping depression with a "sagging" appearance. The QT interval may be slightly shortened, and the T waves may be flat, biphasic, or inverted. A variety of dysrhythmias may be encountered with digoxin toxicity [14–16]. The classic rhythms associated with digoxin toxicity are secondary to increased automaticity and decreased atrioventricular (AV) conduction and include paroxysmal atrial tachycardia

with 2 : 1 AV block, accelerated junctional rhythm, and bidirectional ventricular tachycardia. Sinus bradycardia and premature ventricular contractions are common, and first-, second-, or third-degree AV block may also occur. In acute digoxin toxicity, hyperkalemia may be observed and correlates with prognosis [17]. Patients presenting with digoxin toxicity and serum potassium level > 5.5 mg/dl have a worse prognosis than those with serum potassium < 5.5 mg/dl. If patients present with hypokalemia, potassium repletion may help to improve arrhythmias related to digoxin toxicity. Acute, severe toxicity may be treated by administration of antibodies against digoxin (i.e. digoxin immune Fab).

Tricyclic Antidepressant Toxicity

Tricyclic antidepressants (e.g. amitriptyline, nortriptyline) are used in the treatment of clinical depression, attention deficit hyperactivity disorder, and chronic pain. They are primarily referred to as serotonin-norepinephrine reuptake inhibitors because their pharmacologic activities consist of blocking serotonin and norepinephrine transporters. Most tricyclic antidepressants (TCAs) are also potent inhibitors of sodium and calcium channels and therefore act as sodium channel blockers and calcium channel blockers, respectively [18]. Potent

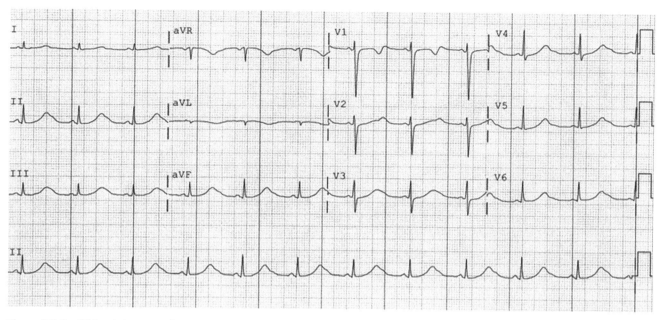

Figure 3.9.6 12-lead electrocardiogram demonstrating QT prolongation in a patient taking a class III anti-arrhythmic agent.

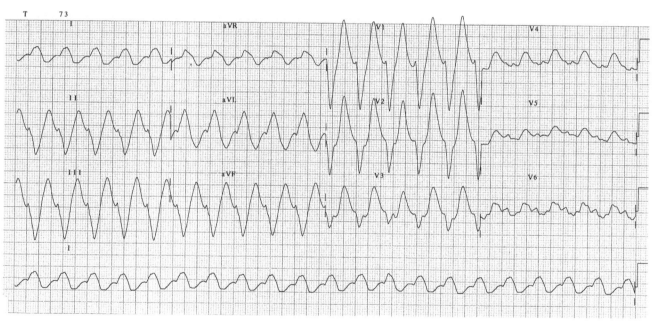

Figure 3.9.7 12-lead electrocardiogram in a patient with tricyclic antidepressant overdose. Note: the excessive QRS prolongation (resulting from sodium channel blockade/toxicity), which may be mistaken for ventricular tachycardia or hyperkalemia.

sodium channel inhibition is primarily responsible for the high mortality rate with TCAs. TCA overdose may result in prolongation of the QRS, QT, and PR intervals and may lead to ventricular tachycardia or ventricular fibrillation (Figure 3.9.7) [19]. The risk of ventricular arrhythmias complicating TCA overdose increases with QRS prolongation over 160 msec.

Conclusions

Metabolic and toxicologic conditions may have a variety of effects on the cardiac conduction system and heart rhythm. Most affect the QRS and QT intervals and may place patients at risk for both atrial and ventricular arrhythmias. The ECG may not only assist with diagnosis but also affect prognosis.

References

1 Montague, B.T., Ouellette, J.R., and Buller, G.K. (2008). Retrospective review of the frequency of ECG changes in hyperkalemia. *Clin. J. Am. Soc. Nephrol.* 3: 324.

2 Surawicz, B., Chlebus, H., and Mazzoleni, A. (1967). Hemodynamic and electrocardiographic effects of hyperpotassemia. Differences in response to slow and rapid increases in concentration of plasma K. *Am. Heart J.* 73: 647.

3 Somers, M.P., Brady, W.J., Perron, A.D., and Mattu, A. (2002). The prominent T wave: electrocardiographic differential diagnosis. *Am. J. Emerg. Med.* 20: 243.

4 Mattu, A., Brady, W.J., and Robinson, D.A. (2000). Electrocardiographic manifestations of hyperkalemia. *Am. J. Emerg. Med.* 18: 721.

5 Littmann, L., Monroe, M.H., Taylor, L. 3rd, and Brearley, W.D. Jr. (2007). The hyperkalemic Brugada sign. *J. Electrocardiol.* 40 (1): 53.

6 Rose, B.D. and Post, T.W. (2001). Hypokalemia. In: *Clinical Physiology of Acid-Base and Electrolyte Disorders*, 5e (eds. B.D. Rose and T.W. Post), 836. New York: McGraw-Hill.

7 Yelamanchi, V.P., Molnar, J., Ranade, V., and Somberg, J.C. (2001). Influence of electrolyte abnormalities on interlead variability of ventricular repolarization times in 12-lead electrocardiography. *Am. J. Ther.* 8 (2): 117.

8 Nia, A.M., Gassanov, N., Ortega, M., and Er, F. (2011). Drunk potassium channels. *Europace* 13 (9): 1352.

9 Edelson, G.W. and Kleerekoper, M. (1995). Hypercalcemic crisis. *Med. Clin. North Am.* 79: 79.

10 Naccarelli, G., Varker, H., Lin, J., and Schulman, K.L. (2009). Increasing prevalence of atrial fibrillation and flutter in the United States. *Am. J. Cardiol.* 104 (11): 1534.

11 Al-Khatib, S.M., LaPointe, N.M.A., Curtis, L.H. et al. (2003). Outpatient prescribing of antiarrhythmic drugs from 1995 to 2000. *Am. J. Cardiol.* 91 (1): 91.

12 Kowey, P.R. (1998). Pharmacological effects of antiarrhythmic drugs. Review and update. *Arch. Intern. Med.* 158 (4): 325.

13 Zimetbaum, P. (2012). Antiarrhythmic drug therapy for atrial fibrillation. *Circulation* 125: 381.

14 Thacker, D. and Sharma, J. (2007). Digoxin toxicity. *Clin. Pediatr. (Phila)* 46 (3): 276.

15 Yang, E.H., Shah, S., and Criley, J.M. (2012). Digitalis toxicity: a fading but crucial complication to recognize. *Am. J. Med.* 125 (4): 337.

16 Kelly, R.A. and Smith, T.W. (1992). Recognition and management of digitalis toxicity. *Am. J. Cardiol.* 69 (18): 108G.

17 Bismuth, C., Gaultier, M., Conso, F., and Efthymiou, M.L. (1973). Hyperkalemia in acute digitalis poisoning: prognostic significance and therapeutic implications. *Clin. Toxicol.* 6 (2): 153.

18 Pancrazio, J.J., Kamatchi, G.L., Roscoe, A.K., and Lynch, C. (1998). Inhibition of neuronal Na+ channels by antidepressant drugs. *J. Pharmacol. Exp. Ther.* 284 (1): 208–214.

19 Harrigan, R.A. and Brady, W.J. (1999). ECG abnormalities in tricyclic antidepressant ingestion. *Am. J. Emerg. Med.* 17 (4): 387–393.

10

Dysrhythmia-Related Syndromes

Michele Murphy[1] and Andrew E. Darby[2]

[1] Cardiovascular Medicine, University of Virginia Health System, Charlottesville, VA, USA
[2] University of Virginia Health System, Charlottesville, VA, USA

Introduction

A number of electrical and structural cardiac conditions have characteristic electrocardiographic findings, and the ability to recognize key ECG features associated with these conditions can facilitate diagnosis and proper treatment. Such conditions include primary electrical abnormalities such as Wolff-Parkinson-White syndrome, long QT syndrome, and Brugada syndrome and primary structural abnormalities such as hypertrophic cardiomyopathy (HCM) and arrhythmogenic right ventricular cardiomyopathy (i.e. arrhythmogenic right ventricular cardiomyopathy (ARVC)) in which arrhythmias are a prominent feature.

Dysrhythmia-Related Syndromes – Primary Electrical Abnormalities

Several primary cardiac electrical abnormalities, most of which are genetic or heritable conditions, have characteristic findings on the electrocardiogram (ECG). Important conditions to recognize are Wolff-Parkinson-White syndrome, long QT syndrome, and Brugada syndrome.

Wolff-Parkinson-White Syndrome

In the normal heart, the fibrous skeleton of the mitral and tricuspid valves electrically isolates the atria from the ventricles so that the AV node and His bundle are the sole pathway for atrioventricular (AV) conduction. In approximately 0.1–0.3% of the general population, a small muscular band forms an accessory pathway connecting atrium to ventricle potentially producing an alternate route for conduction [1, 2].

Accessory pathways may conduct in variable directions with some only capable of conducting from atrium to ventricle, others conducting solely from ventricle to atrium, and still others capable of conducting in either direction. If an accessory pathway is capable of conducting from atrium to ventricle, AV conduction in sinus rhythm will occur over both the accessory pathway and the AV node. In most cases, the accessory pathway conducts more rapidly than the AV node and depolarizes a portion of the ventricle (at the site of accessory pathway insertion) earlier than would occur solely via the normal conduction system. The early activation of the ventricle by an accessory pathway is termed *pre-excitation* and is manifest on the 12-lead ECG by a shortened PR interval followed by a slurred onset of the QRS complexes (delta wave), giving the appearance of a slightly widened QRS complex (Figure 3.10.1). Ventricular pre-excitation as well as the occurrence of arrhythmias associated with an accessory pathway (e.g. atrioventricular reciprocating tachycardia (AVRT) or "preexcited" atrial fibrillation) fulfill the criteria necessary to diagnose Wolff-Parkinson-White syndrome.

Accessory pathways capable of only conducting from ventricle to atrium will not produce a short PR interval or delta wave on the baseline 12-lead ECG because the ventricles are not "preexcited." Such accessory pathways are termed *concealed* as the presence of an accessory pathway is not apparent in sinus rhythm. Patients with concealed accessory pathways are not diagnosed with Wolff-Parkinson-White syndrome, as they do not have manifest ventricular preexcitation on the 12-lead ECG.

Electrocardiogram in Clinical Medicine, First Edition. Edited by William J. Brady, Michael J. Lipinski, Andrew E. Darby, Michael C. Bond, Nathan P. Charlton, Korin Hudson, and Kelly Williamson.

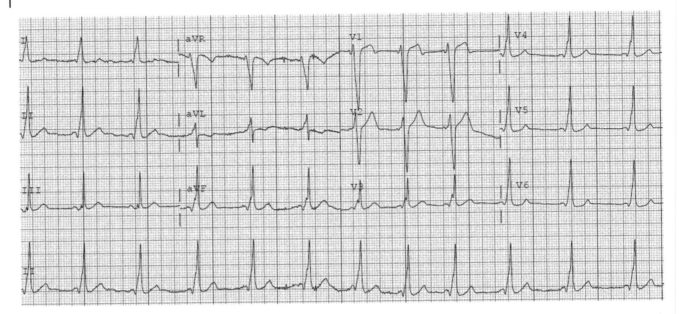

Figure 3.10.1 12-lead electrocardiogram demonstrating sinus rhythm with ventricular preexcitation: note the short PR interval and delta waves most apparent in the inferior leads (II, III, aVF) and lateral precordial leads (V4–V6).

In addition to ventricular preexcitation (i.e., short PR interval and delta wave) on the baseline 12-lead ECG, patients with Wolff-Parkinson-White syndrome may have several associated arrhythmias. AVRT occurs when depolarization alternately transverses the atrium and ventricle in a circuit that involves both the AV node and an accessory pathway. AVRT is also referred to as *circus movement AV tachycardia,* and depending on the direction of the circuit, AVRT may be *orthodromic* or *antidromic* from the Greek words for "straight course" and "opposite course," respectively. Orthodromic AVRT occurs when depolarization proceeds to the ventricle over the AV node, resulting in normal ventricular depolarization and a narrow QRS, with retrograde ventricle-to-atrium (VA) conduction over the accessory pathway (Figure 3.10.2). Antidromic AVRT proceeds in the opposite direction and results in a wide complex tachycardia as ventricular depolarization occurs over the accessory pathway with the normal conduction system facilitating retrograde VA conduction (Figure 3.10.3). Concealed accessory pathways may participate in AVRT but will only produce narrow QRS complex tachycardia because the accessory pathway is only used for retrograde conduction from ventricle to atrium. Accessory pathways capable of conducting in either direction may produce AVRT with a narrow or wide QRS complex, depending on the direction of conduction. In addition to AVRT, in which the RR intervals in tachycardia are regular, patients with Wolff-Parkinson-White syndrome may also

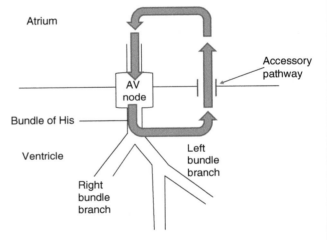

Figure 3.10.2 Diagram of the activation pattern in orthodromic atrioventricular reciprocating tachycardia (AVRT). With this pattern of conduction (AV conduction over the normal conduction system and retrograde VA conduction by the accessory pathway), the tachycardia will have a narrow QRS complex tachycardia. The opposite pattern of conduction (antegrade over the bypass tract and retrograde over the AV node) will produce a wide complex tachycardia because the ventricles are activated over an accessory pathway rather than the normal conduction system.

have preexcited atrial fibrillation. In this rhythm, the RR intervals are irregularly irregular, and the QRS complexes vary in width due to changing patterns of ventricular activation (Figure 3.10.4). Delta waves are apparent at the onset of most QRS complexes.

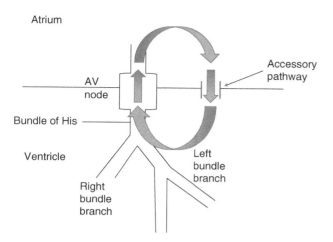

Figure 3.10.3 Diagram of the activation pattern in antidromic atrioventricular reciprocating tachycardia (AVRT). With this pattern of conduction (AV conduction over an accessory pathway and VA conduction by the normal conduction system), the tachycardia will have a wide QRS complex.

Recognition of ventricular preexcitation, particularly preexcited atrial fibrillation, is important to ensure proper therapy is administered [3]. AVRT often responds acutely to AV nodal blocking agents. Adenosine, which transiently halts AV nodal conduction, can be both diagnostic and therapeutic, as it will terminate AVRT. AV nodal blocking agents are *contraindicated* in patients with preexcited atrial fibrillation. Treatment options for this rhythm include synchronized electrical cardioversion or intravenous medication such as procainamide (preferred drug) or ibutilide.

Long QT Syndrome

Long QT syndrome is a relatively rare inherited heart condition in which cardiac repolarization is prolonged, thereby increasing the risk of torsade de pointes. The condition is so named because the QT interval is prolonged (i.e. >440 ms) on the baseline electrocardiogram [4]. Some individuals with long QT syndrome may have a normal QT interval at times with an abnormally prolonged QT interval occurring only after the administration of certain medications or with exercise. The prevalence of long QT syndrome is higher than previously thought, occurring in up to 1 in 2500 individuals [5]. The diagnosis hinges on the presence of a prolonged QT interval on the ECG (Figure 3.10.5) and exclusion of other reasons for a prolonged QT interval (e.g. myocardial ischemia; electrolyte abnormalities; bradycardia; thyroid abnormalities). Genetic testing may be confirmatory, as a number of the genetic mutations responsible for the common forms of long QT syndrome have been identified.

Patients with long QT syndrome should avoid agents that may prolong the QT interval and increase the risk of ventricular arrhythmias. The characteristic rhythm associated with long QT syndrome is torsade de pointes,

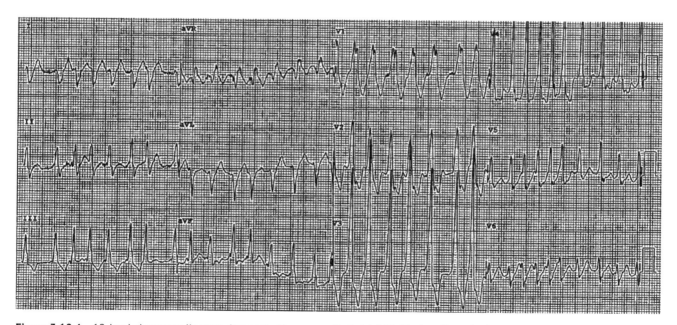

Figure 3.10.4 12-lead electrocardiogram demonstrating preexcited atrial fibrillation: Note the irregular rhythm (from the underlying AF), delta waves at the onset of the QRS complexes, and variability in QRS width related to varying degrees of ventricular preexcitation.

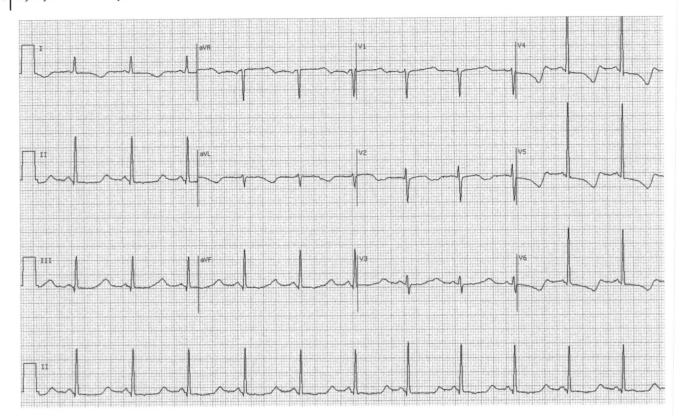

Figure 3.10.5 12-lead electrocardiogram demonstrating sinus rhythm with marked QT prolongation along with ST depression/repolarization abnormalities in the lateral leads. The QT interval measures approximately 600 ms with a QTc of nearly 660 msec.

polymorphic VT with characteristic alternating axis with waxing and waning QRS amplitude (Figure 3.10.6). Patients with a corrected QT interval > 500 ms are generally at high risk for ventricular arrhythmias and/or sudden cardiac death [6]. The characteristic symptoms associated with this rhythm are syncope and/or palpitations. In the acute setting, patients with repetitive episodes of torsade de pointes are best treated with intravenous magnesium and isoproterenol or temporary cardiac pacing to increase the heart rate and consequently shorten the QT interval. Patients with long QT syndrome types 1 and 2 (potassium channel defects confirmed by genetic testing) often respond well to beta-blocker therapy for prophylaxis against torsade de pointes [7].

Brugada Syndrome

Brugada syndrome is an inherited cardiac electrical condition predisposing patients to ventricular fibrillation and sudden cardiac death. There are no precise data on the epidemiology of Brugada syndrome, but its prevalence is much higher in Southeast Asian countries. A

variety of genetic abnormalities have been associated with Brugada syndrome, including a specific sodium channel defect. Symptoms associated with Brugada syndrome include palpitations, syncope, nocturnal agonal respiration (as a result of ventricular arrhythmias during sleep), and ventricular fibrillation or aborted sudden cardiac death. Brugada syndrome should be considered in a patient presenting with cardiac arrest/ventricular fibrillation in the absence of obvious underlying cause. ECG clues include baseline ST-segment elevation in at least one right precordial lead (V1 and V2) [7]. The ST segments in these leads may have either coved or saddleback elevation with an incomplete right bundle branch block (RBBB) appearance (Figure 3.10.7). Occasionally, the ECG may be normal when patients are in their baseline state of health, but the ECG changes (and symptoms) may develop with febrile illness. The ECG differential diagnosis includes a number of conditions producing ST-segment elevation in right precordial leads, including atypical right bundle branch block, left ventricular hypertrophy, early repolarization, acute pericarditis, and acute myocardial infarction.

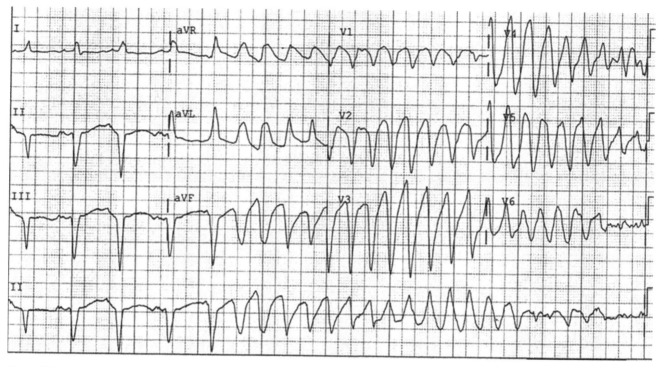

Figure 3.10.6 12-lead electrocardiogram demonstrating the onset of torsade de pointes in a patient with a prolonged QT interval: note the characteristic variability in QRS amplitude and apparent "twisting" of the QRS complexes around the isoelectric baseline.

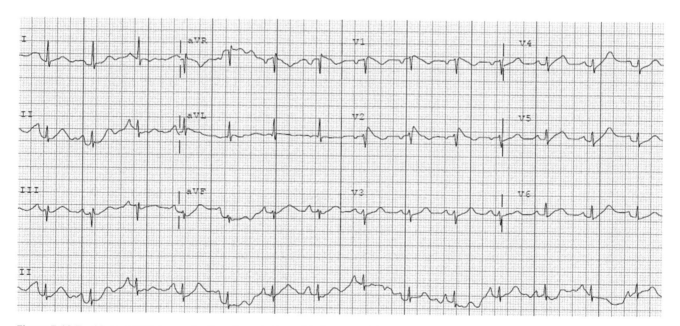

Figure 3.10.7 12-lead ECG demonstrating sinus rhythm with features of Brugada syndrome, notably downsloping ST depression in leads V1 and V2 in the absence of other causes of ST elevation in these leads (ischemia, ventricular hypertrophy, pericarditis).

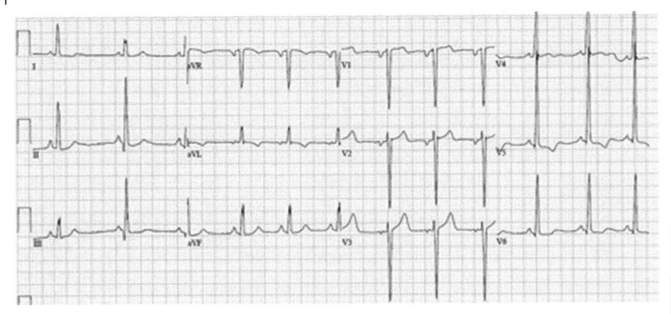

Figure 3.10.8 12-lead ECG demonstrating features of hypertrophic cardiomyopathy: the rhythm is sinus with evidence of LVH (note the deep S waves in leads V2, V3, and the tall R waves in lead V5 with ST depression in the lateral leads).

Dysrhythmia-Related Syndromes – Primary Cardiac Structural Conditions

Hypertrophic Cardiomyopathy

HCM is a primary disease of the ventricular myocardium in which a portion of the myocardium is abnormally thickened or hypertrophied (usually the basal portion of the interventricular septum) [8, 9]. Both atrial and ventricular arrhythmias may occur in patients with HCM. It is also a leading cause of sudden cardiac death, particularly among young athletes. The typical ECG in a patient with hypertrophic cardiomyopathy demonstrates increased QRS voltage consistent with left ventricular hypertrophy and localized or widespread repolarization changes (ST segment depression ± T-wave inversions). Other findings include prominent abnormal Q waves in the inferior and lateral leads (reflecting depolarization of hypertrophied tissue in the interventricular septum), P-wave abnormalities reflecting atrial enlargement, and left-axis deviation (Figure 3.10.8). The apical variant of HCM, in which hypertrophy is restricted to the apical portion of the left ventricle, may present with deeply inverted T waves in the mid-precordial leads (V2–V4) and may be misdiagnosed as myocardial ischemia.

PRKAG-2 Mutation

The *PRKAG2* gene encodes part of AMP-activated protein kinaase, an enzyme responsible for regulating adenosine triphosphate (ATP) metabolism in muscle cells. ATP is the primary energy source of muscle cells, and mutation in *PRKAG2* leads to abnormal energy regulation as well as abnormalities in ion channels involved in the heart's electrical system. *PRKAG2* mutation results in a unique genetic syndrome of familial hypertrophic cardiomyopathy, ventricular preexcitation, and progressive conduction system disease. As a result, the 12-lead ECG of patients with this syndrome is quite unique, with features of both ventricular hypertrophy and preexcitation (Figure 3.10.9). Patients with this genetic syndrome may have complete degeneration of the normal conduction system such that accessory pathway(s) may be the only route for atrioventricular conduction.

Arrhythmogenic Right Ventricular Cardiomyopathy

ARVC is a cardiomyopathy characterized by replacement of the normal ventricular myocardium with fibro-fatty infiltrates [10, 11]. It more often affects the right ventricle but can affect the left ventricle as well. The prevalence of ARVC in the general adult population is approximately 1 in 2000 to 1 in 5000. It is an important cause of sudden death in young adults due to the development of ventricular arrhythmias. The sensitivity of the ECG alone for the presence of ARVC is suboptimal, as 40–50% of patients have a normal ECG at presentation [12]. ECG abnormalities observed in ARVC include QRS prolongation in leads V1–V6 (due to delayed right ventricular activation); incomplete or complete RBBB; epsilon wave (sharp deflection at the end of the QRS complex most often seen in lead V1); and inversion of T waves in the right precordial leads (V1–V3) (Figure 3.10.10) [13].

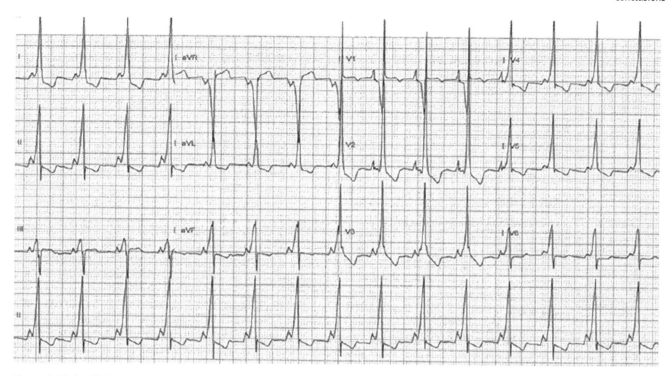

Figure 3.10.9 12-lead electrocardiogram from a patient with PRKAG2 mutation demonstrating ventricular preexcitation and ventricular hypertrophy.

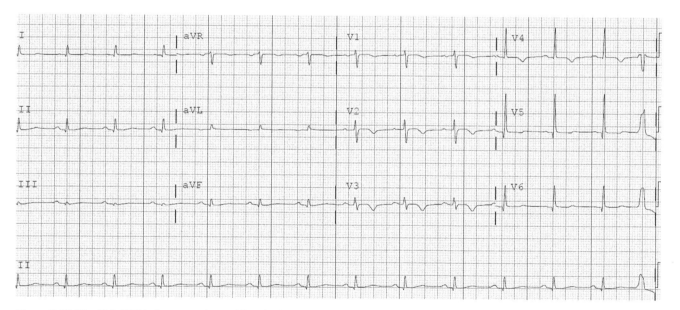

Figure 3.10.10 This ECG is from a patient with arrhythmogenic right ventricular cardiomyopathy (ARVC) and demonstrates typical anterior T-wave inversions. Other common findings include incomplete or complete RBBB and epsilon waves (sharp upward deflections at the end of the QRS complexes in leads V1, V2).

Conclusions

A number of primary electrical and structural cardiac conditions may present with arrhythmias as their chief manifestation. Clues to their presence may be evident on the baseline ECG, and recognition of these ECG features is important to ensure proper diagnosis and treatment.

References

1 Rosner, M.H., Brady, W.J. Jr., Kefer, M.P., and Martin, M.L. (1999). Electrocardiography in the patient with Wolff-Parkinson-White syndrome: diagnostic and initial therapeutic issues. *Am. J. Emerg. Med.* 17 (7): 705.

2 Munger, T.M., Packer, D.L., Hammill, S.C. et al. (1993). A population study of the natural history of Wolff-Parkinson-White syndrome in Olmsted County, Minnesota, 1953 – 1989. *Circulation* 87 (3): 866.

3 Fengler, B.T., Brady, W.J., and Plautz, C.U. (2007). Atrial fibrillation in the Wolff-Parkinson-White syndrome: ECG recognition and treatment in the ED. *Am. J. Emerg. Med.* 25 (5): 576.

4 Morita, H., Wu, J., and Zipes, D.P. (2008). The QT sydromes: long and short. *Lancet* 372: 750.

5 Schwartz, P.J., Stramba-Badiale, M., Crotti, L. et al. (2009). Prevalence of the congenital long-QT syndrome. *Circulation* 120 (18): 1761.

6 Ellinor, P.T., Milan, D.J., and MacRae, C.A. (2003). Risk stratification in the long-QT syndrome. *N. Engl. J. Med.* 349 (9): 908.

7 Priori, S.G., Wilde, A.A., Horie, M. et al. (2013). HRS/EHRA/APHRS expert consensus statement on the diagnosis and management of patients with inherited primary arrhythmia syndromes. *Heart Rhythm.* 10 (12): 1932.

8 Nishimura, R.A. and Holmes, D.R. Jr. (2004). Hypertrophic obstructive cardiomyopathy. *N. Engl. J. Med.* 350: 1320.

9 Maron, B.J. (2002). Hypertrophic cardiomyopathy: a systematic review. *JAMA* 287 (10): 1308.

10 Gemayel, C., Pelliccia, A., and Thompson, P.D. (2001). Arrhythmogenic right ventricular cardiomyopathy. *J. Am. Coll. Cardiol.* 38 (7): 1773.

11 Sen-Chowdhry, S., Lowe, M.D., Sporton, S.C., and McKenna, W.J. (2004). Arrhythmogenic right ventricular cardiomyopathy: clinical presentation, diagnosis, and management. *Am. J. Med.* 117 (9): 685.

12 Nava, A., Bauce, B., Basso, C. et al. (2000). Clinical profile and long-term follow-up of 37 families with arrhythmogenic right ventricular cardiomyopathy. *J. Am. Coll. Cardiol.* 36 (7): 2226.

13 Marcus, F.I., McKenna, W.J., Sherrill, D. et al. (2010). Diagnosis of arrhythmogenic right ventricular cardiomyopathy/dysplasia: proposed modification of the task force criteria. *Circulation* 121 (13): 1533.

Section IV

The ECG in Cardinal Presentations and Scenarios

1

The Patient with Cardiac Arrest

Michael Cirone[1,2], Mitchell Lorenz[3], and Karis Tekwani[1,2]

[1] *Advocate Christ Medical Center Emergency Medicine Residency, Chicago, IL, USA*
[2] *Department of Emergency Medicine, University of Illinois at Chicago, Chicago, IL, USA*
[3] *Advocate Good Samitarian Hospital, Downer's Grove, IL, USA*

Introduction

The patient arriving at the emergency department (ED) in cardiac arrest requires expert electrocardiography interpretation to accurately identify the presenting rhythm and to determine the underlying pathology that may have contributed to the arrest. This chapter will focus on review, identification, and management of ventricular fibrillation (VF), pulseless ventricular tachycardia (VT), asystole, and pulseless electrical activity (PEA) and will briefly review reperfusion rhythms.

Ventricular Fibrillation

VF is a life-threatening arrhythmia that must be immediately recognized and treated appropriately. As it is a rhythm that is only encountered in cardiac arrest, it should never be diagnosed on a formal 12-lead electrocardiogram (ECG).

Classic ECG findings include an erratic ECG with a wandering baseline and deflections without discernible waves (Figure 4.1.1). The rate of fibrillation is typically 350–450 beats per minute (bpm), although it can reach 500 bpm. It should be immediately treated with defibrillation per advanced life-support guidelines.

VF may be caused by untreated VT or other abnormal tachydysrhythmias and is most likely to occur in patients with preexisting cardiac disease. Other causes include drug toxicity, electrolyte abnormalities, or heart strain as caused by massive pulmonary embolism (PE), cardiac tamponade, or commotio cordis alli [1]. It is characterized at the myocardial level by numerous small foci of ectopic ventricular pacemakers firing nearly simultaneously. The end result is many small patches of myocardium becoming depolarized at random times, leading to fibrillation of the ventricle without any true contraction [2]. As cardiac output drops, the coronary arteries do not receive adequate flow and ischemic damage quickly follows, decreasing the chances of return on spontaneous circulation (ROSC).

As the duration of VF lengthens and myocardial death occurs, the deflections may become smaller (Figure 4.1.1). VF can thus be subdivided into coarse, intermediate, fine, and very fine fibrillation (Figure 4.1.1). While these rhythms may appear slightly different on the monitor, they are both treated with immediate defibrillation. Per advanced life-support guidelines, if the initial defibrillation is not successful, epinephrine and amiodarone should be administered while undergoing a second round of CPR until the next pulse check when defibrillation may be attempted again.

VF and VT occur in only about 26% of out of hospital cardiac arrests yet make up the vast majority of survivors [3]. For this reason, it is imperative that these rhythms be rapidly identified and treated.

Pulseless Ventricular Tachycardia

Ventricular tachycardia is another life-threatening rhythm that must be rapidly identified and treated. The spectrum of presentation is broad: some patients complain only of palpitations while others present in cardiac arrest. Electrocardiographically, VT is defined as three or more wide complex ventricular beats in succession; sustained VT occurs when these wide complex beats persist for more than 30 s. The rate is typically between 120 and 200 bpm. There are many types of VT, the most common of which is monomorphic VT (Figure 4.1.2a). In monomorphic VT, the

Electrocardiogram in Clinical Medicine, First Edition. Edited by William J. Brady, Michael J. Lipinski, Andrew E. Darby, Michael C. Bond, Nathan P. Charlton, Korin Hudson, and Kelly Williamson.

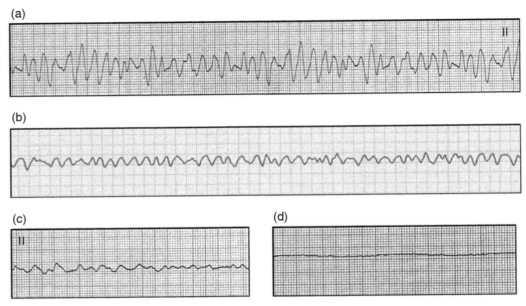

Figure 4.1.1 Ventricular fibrillation, separated by waveform types: (a) Coarse; (b) Intermediate; (c) Fine; (d) Very fine.

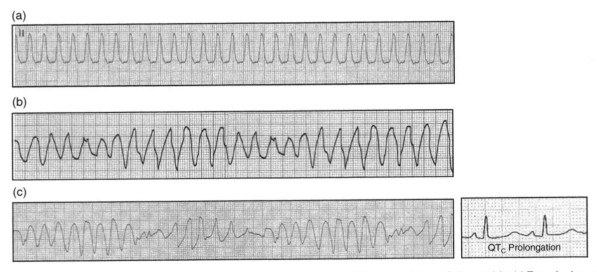

Figure 4.1.2 Ventricular tachycardia, separated by waveform types: (a) Monomorphic; (b) Polymorphic; (c) Torsade des pointes.

rhythm will look almost perfectly regular but may have some slight variation from beat to beat [4]. No matter the type, cardiac arrest secondary to VT requires emergent defibrillation in order to return to a perfusing rhythm.

VT most commonly presents in patients who have sustained previous ischemic damage to the heart or who are experiencing acute myocardial infarction or ischemia. Tissue damage leads to changes in myocardial conduction and development of dangerous reentrant pathways. Additional inciting events include hypoxia, toxic exposures, and electrolyte abnormalities. Normally

overdrive-suppressed by the sinoatrial node, irritated ventricular myocytes increase their inherent automaticity leading to VT. The fast rate and poor output of VT create a perfect storm of increased oxygen demand with decreased supply to the cardiac myocytes. It is important to identify and treat the cause of VT rapidly, as it may quickly degenerate to VF.

Polymorphic VT (Figure 4.1.2b) is a result of multiple irritated ventricular foci and is characterized by varying QRS morphology from beat to beat along a single ECG lead. A specific subtype of polymorphic VT, torsades de pointes (Figure 4.1.2c), can develop as a result of delayed repolarization and prolongation of the QT interval. Torsades is characterized by the classic "twisting ribbon" appearance of the ECG. If it occurs in a patient with a pulse, pharmacologic measures may be taken; however, the pulseless patient should be immediately defibrillated.

Asystole

Asystole is defined as the complete absence of cardiac electrical activity (Figure 4.1.3). As with VF, this rhythm should never be detected on ECG as it is not compatible with life. When a cardiac arrest patient presents with asystole, treatment should follow ACLS protocol with special attention to the reversible causes of cardiac arrest.

Asystole has a grave prognosis, as the complete absence of cardiac electrical activity is indicative of severe myocardial injury. Most cardiac myocytes have some inherent automaticity function, yet in asystole none are functioning well enough to continue to generate a rhythm. It is important when you encounter asystole to check your monitor and pads and to ensure proper connection and mode. Defibrillators have multiple modes and settings, and it is imperative not to miss a treatable arrhythmia due to equipment failure.

One unusual circumstance in which an emergency provider may encounter asystole is following a lightning strike. The significant electrical current conducted through the myocardium acts as a defibrillation-like force and can temporarily halt normal cardiac automaticity. Asystole is the most common presenting rhythm in these patients; however, ischemia soon sets in and VF may develop. For this reason, lightning-strike victims should be treated in an order opposite of typical disaster triage, and cardiac arrest patients should be resuscitated first, as asystole secondary to lightning is likely reversible and high-quality CPR in the interim can preserve neurologic function in these critically ill patients.

Pulseless Electrical Activity

PEA is a cardiac arrest rhythm (Figure 4.1.4) defined as the presence of an organized electrical rhythm without a pulse (Figure 4.1.4). Patients with PEA account for roughly 30% of cardiac arrest victims, yet their survival rate is significantly lower than patients with shockable rhythms [4]. It is hypothesized that this poor survival rate may be due to the diverse pathophysiology that contributes to a PEA arrest.

Before considering emergent interventions, it is essential that medical providers differentiate PEA from cases where a pulse is not palpable yet there is evidence of end-organ perfusion. For example, patients with profound vasoconstriction due to hypothermia can appear to be in PEA due to an absent palpable pulse. A quick assessment of the patient's blood pressure or mental status may help to estimate their true cardiac output.

Once PEA is identified, providers should implement standard advanced life support protocol and attempt to identify the cause of the arrest. Studies have shown that cause-specific interventions to treat PEA are more effective than general advanced life support guidelines alone[11]. As a result, advanced life support guidelines explicitly stress the importance of identifying and treating the cause of PEA arrests as quickly as possible [5].

Classically, medical providers are taught to recall their "H's and T's" when considering potentially reversible causes of PEA arrests (Figure 4.1.5).

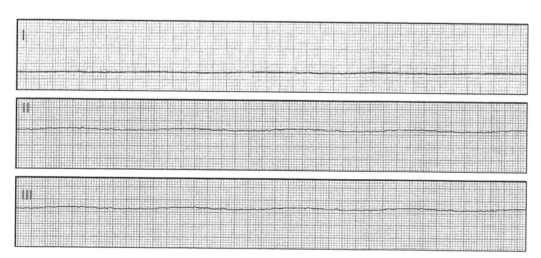

Figure 4.1.3 Asystole. No electrical activity detected on 10 s rhythm strip.

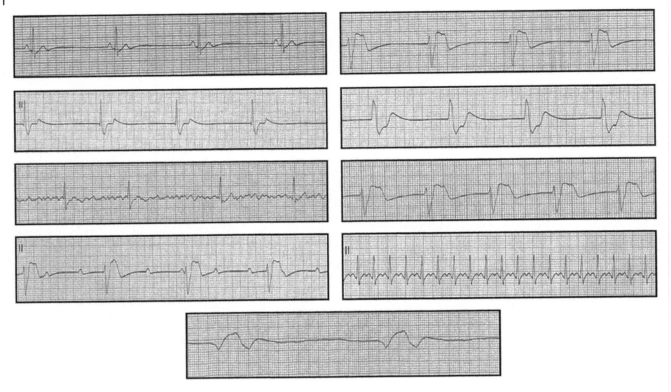

Figure 4.1.4   Various rhythms encountered in the PEA presentation.

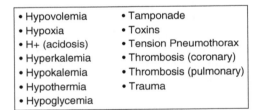

- Hypovolemia
- Hypoxia
- H+ (acidosis)
- Hyperkalemia
- Hypokalemia
- Hypothermia
- Hypoglycemia
- Tamponade
- Toxins
- Tension Pneumothorax
- Thrombosis (coronary)
- Thrombosis (pulmonary)
- Trauma

Figure 4.1.5   Common causes of PEA.

Conclusion

In conclusion, cardiac arrest patients are the most critical patients to which physicians provide care. Rapid and accurate interpretation of the ECG and/or rhythms strip can help the provider determine the cause for cardiac arrest and ultimately guide management and treatment.

References

1 Tintinalli, J. (2011). *Emergency Medicine: A Comprehensive Study Guide*, 8e, 2011. New York: McGraw-Hill.

2 Dubin, D. (2009). *Rapid Interpretation of ECGs*, 6e. Tampa: Cover Publishing Company.

3 Weisfeldt, M.L., Everson-Stewart, S., Sitlani, C. et al. (2011). Ventricular tachyarrhythmias after cardiac arrest in public versus at home. *N Engl J Med*. 364 (4): 313–321.

4 Engdahl, J., Bang, A., Lindqvist, J., and Herlitz, J. (2001). Factors affecting short- and long-term prognosis among 1,069 patients with out-of-hospital cardiac arrest and pulseless electrical activity. *Resuscitation*. 51 (1): 17–25.

5 Neumar, R.W., Otto, C.W., Link, M.S. et al. (2010). Part 8: adult advanced cardiovascular life support: 2010 American Heart Association guidelines for cardiopulmonary resuscitation and emergency cardiovascular care. *Circulation*. 122 (18 Suppl 3): S729–S767.

2

The Patient with Chest Pain

Paul Basel[1], Lane Thaut[1], and Nathan Olson[2]

[1] *Emergency Medicine Physician, United States Air Force*
[2] *Section of Emergency Medicine, University of Chicago, Chicago, IL, USA*

Introduction

Chest pain is one of the most common symptoms, prompting patients to seek medical care. Due to the density of anatomic structures in the thorax, pathology ranges from benign musculoskeletal strain to life-threatening emergencies such as ST segment myocardial infarction.

The ECG thereby becomes an invaluable clinical tool in the evaluation of the etiology of this complaint. The ECG findings associated with acute coronary syndrome (ACS), pericarditis and myocarditis, and Takotsubo cardiomyopathy will be discussed in this chapter.

Acute Coronary Syndrome

Myocardial ischemia is a common and life-threatening etiology of chest pain; approximately 15% of patients with chest pain presenting to the emergency department will ultimately be diagnosed with ACS [1]. The spectrum of ACS is broad and describes the constellation of signs and symptoms associated with injury to myocardial tissue due to ischemia caused by narrowed or occluded coronary vessels. Pathology ranges from ST segment elevation myocardial infarction (STEMI), non-ST segment elevation myocardial infarction (NSTEMI), and unstable angina (UA). Obtaining an ECG in a rapid fashion is essential in the diagnosis of ACS, as ischemic tissue causes findings such as ST-segment elevation (STE) or depression as well as T-wave changes. In addition, the ECG in ACS is dynamic; as myocardial ischemia progresses, the ECG findings can evolve. Serial ECGs are therefore imperative if ACS is suspected; comparison with an old ECG can also be invaluable when available.

The ECG findings associated with ACS are representative of the underlying ischemia. STE is caused by transmural ischemia that is most often the result of complete occlusion of the culprit vessel [2]. Early diagnosis is critical, as these patients require emergent revascularization via percutaneous coronary intervention (PCI), coronary artery bypass grafting, or, in rare instances, thrombolysis [3]. ST depression and T-wave changes are typically due to subendocardial ischemia that does not extend through the full thickness of the myocardium [4]. These lesions are often at least initially amenable to medical therapy: anti-platelet and anti-coagulation agents to prevent thrombus extension, combined with nitrates and beta blockers to decrease myocardial oxygen demand, as well as consideration of prompt cardiac catheterization to define the underlying anatomy. It is important to note that ECG changes alone do not diagnose acute myocardial infarction (AMI). The Third Universal Definition of myocardial infarction establishes two criteria that indicate myocardial injury: a significant rise and fall of cardiac biomarkers (ideally troponin), as well as evidence of acute myocardial ischemia seen by any one of the following: clinical symptoms consistent with cardiac ischemia, new Q waves, new ST changes, new left bundle branch block (LBBB) and finally, imaging showing angiographic coronary blockage or wall motion abnormalities [5].

The diagnosis of ST segment elevation MI is accompanied by specific ECG findings. Current AHA guidelines require ST elevation at the J point, the junction between the end of the QRS and the beginning of the ST segment, in at least two contiguous leads (Figure 4.2.1). Furthermore, the STE must be at least 2 mm in men and 1.5 mm in women at V2–V3 or 1 mm in all other leads in the absence of left ventricular hypertrophy and LBBB [3]. While new LBBB was previously considered a STEMI equivalent, the finding has recently been removed as a criterion as it was a poor predictor of AMI [6].

Electrocardiogram in Clinical Medicine, First Edition. Edited by William J. Brady, Michael J. Lipinski, Andrew E. Darby, Michael C. Bond, Nathan P. Charlton, Korin Hudson, and Kelly Williamson.
© 2021 John Wiley & Sons Ltd. Published 2021 by John Wiley & Sons Ltd.

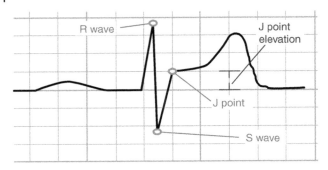

Figure 4.2.1 The J point is the junction between the end of the QRS and the beginning of the ST segment.

Table 4.2.1 Localization of cardiac ischemia based on ECG findings.

Location	ECG changes	Coronary vessel
Anterior	STE: V2–4	LAD
Lateral	STE: I, aVL, V5, V6 Reciprocal STD: inferior leads	Circumflex
Inferior	STE: II, III, aVF Reciprocal STD: aVL	RCA
Posterior	STD: V1-V3	Usually RCA

ST elevation can have different morphological appearances on ECG, which can aid the clinician in determining whether the changes are truly related to ischemia. Convex STE is very concerning for ischemia (Figure 4.2.2); a study by Brady et al. found a 97% specificity for nonconcave ST elevation (convex or horizontal) indicating ischemia. However, this morphology was only 82% sensitive [7]. Conversely, concave elevation is less specific for AMI.

An understanding of coronary anatomy and ECG lead placement allows a clinician to localize the likely culprit lesion based on the pattern of STE (Table 4.2.1).

Leads II, III, and aVF are typically referred to as the "inferior" leads, reflecting the territory supplied by the right coronary artery (RCA) or less frequently the left circumflex artery (LCX). RCA occlusion typically leads to greater STE in lead III as compared to lead II [8]. This distinction can be important as occlusion of the RCA can lead to right ventricular (RV) ischemia. As a result, all patients with inferior STEMI patterns should have a right sided ECG performed to evaluate for RV ischemia or infarction (Figure 4.2.3). Elevation of 0.5 mm, or 1 mm in males less than 30 years old, in V3R or V4R is diagnostic of RV infarction [3].

Patients experiencing RV ischemia or infarction are often hypotensive, due to lack of preload from a poorly functioning RV, and bradycardic, due to vagal stimulation or AV nodal ischemia. Noting these changes on ECG is important as patients with RV infarcts should not be given nitrates and often need intravenous fluids and other measures to maintain preload.

STE in the precordial leads, V1–V4, is referred to as an anterior STEMI and indicates a left anterior descending (LAD) artery lesion. The number of leads affected with STE depends upon the location of the lesion within the LAD. STE isolated to V1 and V2 is referred to as a "septal" infarct; proximal occlusion of the LAD prior to the first septal perforator can lead to STE in aVR as discussed later in the chapter. Isolated lateral STEMIs (elevation in I, aVL or V5, V6) are rare, but result from occlusion of distal branches of either LAD or LCX.

The posterior wall of the heart, supplied by derivatives of the RCA or LCX, is not directly evaluated on a standard 12-lead ECG. However, findings of ST depression or upright, broad-based R waves in V1 and V2 should prompt the clinician to obtain a posterior ECG to assess for STE. Only 0.5 mm of STE is required in the posterior leads to make a diagnosis of STEMI (Figures 4.2.4 and 4.2.5).

In addition to STE, the ECG in STEMI may also demonstrate ST depression, which is typically downsloping or horizontal in nature (Figure 4.2.6) [8]. The ECG may also demonstrate reciprocal ST depression in the leads opposite of those with STE, a finding that can be useful in confirming the diagnosis of AMI.

While lack of reciprocal changes does not rule out STEMI, it should trigger the clinician to consider alternate etiologies of the symptoms, including pericarditis, left ventricular aneurysm, and early repolarization. The mnemonic PAILS (Posterior, Anterior, Inferior, Lateral, Septal) is applied to indicate where expected reciprocal changes

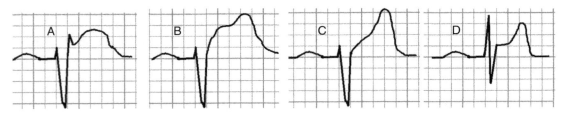

Figure 4.2.2 A and B are convex ST elevations, high risk for STEMI; C and D are concave, less specific for STEMI.

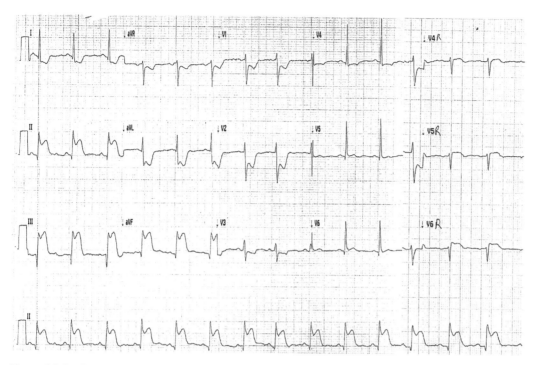

Figure 4.2.3 Classic inferior and right-sided STEMI due to RCA occlusion. STE in III > II, > 0.5 mm STE in VR4–VR6. Reciprocal changes seen in I, aVL, V1–V3.

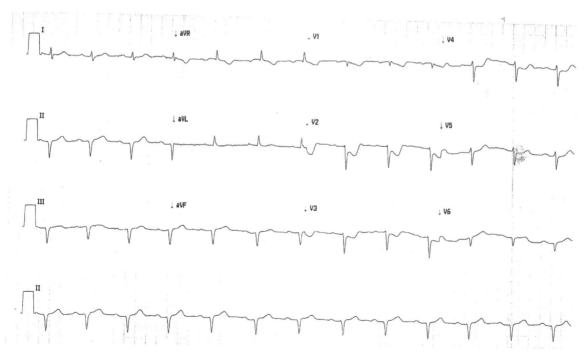

Figure 4.2.4 Isolated STD in V2–V4. No other STEMI criteria. The astute care provider knows to order a posterior ECG to evaluate for posterior STEMI.

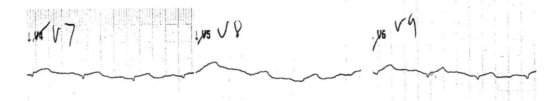

Figure 4.2.5 While voltage is quite low in the posterior leads, 0.5 mm of STE is present. Cath confirmed distal LCX occlusion.

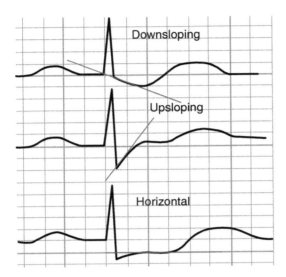

Figure 4.2.6 Types of ST depression. Horizontal and downsloping are more concerning for ischemia.

Table 4.2.2 Definition of pathologic Q waves.

Pathologic Q waves
• Any Q-wave in leads V2–V3 ≥ 0.02 s or QS complex in leads V2 and V3
• Q-wave ≥ 0.03 s and > 0.1 mV deep or QS complex in any 2 contiguous leads excepting V1–3
• R-wave ≥ 0.04 s in V1–V2 and R/S ≥ 1 with a concordant positive T-wave in the absence of a conduction defect (reflecting posterior Q waves)

occur. For example, in posterior STEMI, one would expect to find anterior reciprocal changes; in inferior STEMI, lateral reciprocal changes may be found.

Prior to the development of ST elevation, well-described T-wave changes may occur. Hyperacute T waves are an enlargement of the T waves that can be present in the early stages of STEMI [9]. Additional T-wave findings include asymmetry and broad base to the T wave [10]. While these ECG changes are typically transient as ST elevation soon evolves, when present they can lead to earlier diagnosis of STEMI resulting in earlier intervention and potentially better outcomes.

Prolonged myocardial ischemia will ultimately lead to tissue infarction and electrically silent myocardium. This evolution is represented on ECG by decreased amplitude of R waves and the development of pathologic Q waves (Table 4.2.2).

It should be noted the reciprocal of a Q wave is an R wave; in the setting of a posterior MI, upright R waves develop in V1 and V2. Ultimately, as the infarction completes, the ST segment returns to baseline though inverted T waves may persist for weeks to months (Figure 4.2.7) [11].

If a patient develops a left ventricular aneurysm following an AMI then the STE can persist for weeks.

There are a few special situations in STEMI that warrant discussion, including LBBB, Wellens syndrome, De Winter's T waves, and STE in lead aVR. In LBBB, depolarization starts in the RV and spreads through the LV creating a wide, slurred QRS and dramatic repolarization abnormalities, which preclude the standard assessment for STE; ventricular paced rhythms with RV leads have a very similar depolarization pattern. In 1996, Sgarbossa and colleagues created a three-item scoring system to allow for the diagnosis of AMI in the presence of LBB (Table 4.2.3).

A score of three more provided 90% specificity for AMI, therefore this value was chosen as the cutoff for diagnosis of AMI [13, 14].

While these criteria provide high specificity for AMI in LBBB, the sensitivity in the validation cohort of the study was exceedingly low. Therefore, these criteria are valuable to rule in AMI in the setting of LBBB, but less effective at ruling out the diagnosis. These criteria were also evaluated in ventricular paced rhythms with similar results [15]. In an attempt to improve sensitivity, in 2012 Smith et al. derived a modified Sgarbossa criteria, retaining the first two criteria from the initial study but replacing the third criteria that evaluates the proportional discordance elevation (or depression). A ratio is then formed from the sizes of the R or S wave (whichever is more prominent) to the measurement of discordant ST elevation or depression, called the ST/S ratio. Values <0.25 were considered positive. In this set of criteria, the scoring system was discarded and only one positive was required to diagnose STEMI [15].

Normal Myocardium   Ischemic Myocardium   Infarcted Myocardium

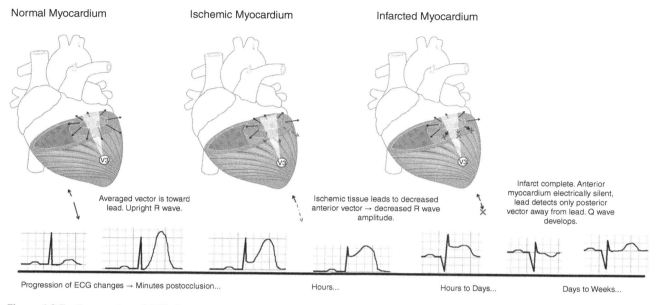

Figure 4.2.7   Progression of ECG changes from a normal myocardium to postinfarcted tissue.

Table 4.2.3   Original Sgarbossa criteria.

Criterion*	Points
ST-segment elevation ≥1 mm and concordant with QRS complex	5
ST-segment depression ≥1 mm in leads V1-V3	3
ST-segment elevation ≥5 mm and discordant with QRS complex	2

*Requires a score of 3 or greater 36% sensitive and 96% specific for AMI [12].

In the derivation group, the researchers reported a much-improved sensitivity of 91% with preserved specificity at 90% (Table 4.2.4).

Wellens syndrome is a well-described phenomenon of ischemia originating in the proximal LAD followed by spontaneous reperfusion. Patients are typically asymptomatic at the time of presentation but report a history of recent chest pain. This phenomenon was described in 1982 after determining that the majority of patients presenting with this ECG pattern who did not undergo coronary revascularization developed extensive anterior myocardial infarction within a few weeks of admission [18].

Criteria for Wellens syndrome include the following:

- Biphasic (Wellens A) or deeply inverted T waves (Wellens B) in leads V2 and V3, and occasionally in leads V1, V4–6
- No or minimal elevation of cardiac enzymes
- No or minimal ST-segment elevation (<1 mm)
- No loss of precordial R-wave progression
- No pathological precordial Q wave
- Recent chest pain

Serial ECGs should be performed in all patients with Wellens syndrome. If patients experience return of pain, a repeat ECG must be performed as these patients are high risk for repeat artery occlusion and STEMI. In addition, these patients should not undergo stress testing, given the severe underlying stenosis and the risk of provocation of STEMI and cardiac arrest [19] (Figures 4.2.8 and 4.2.9).

Another manifestation of ischemia and concern for evolving STEMI is De Winter's T waves, which are significant ST depressions with peaked T waves in the precordial leads and are indicative of acute LAD occlusion. ECG diagnostic criteria include tall, prominent, symmetric T-waves in the precordial leads, upsloping ST segment depression >1 mm at the J-point, absence of ST elevation in the precordial leads, and STE (0.5 mm–1 mm) in aVR. This pattern of upsloping T wave occurs in approximately 2% of patients with a LAD occlusion and requires immediate reperfusion therapy (Figure 4.2.10) [17].

Lead aVR is unique on the standard 12-lead ECG. It is isolated with the positive pole directed to the right superior part of the heart and is often neglected when interpreting ECGs [20]. However, in the setting of clinical ACS, lead aVR can provide valuable diagnostic and prognostic information. While current AHA guidelines do not recognize isolated STE in lead aVR as a STEMI, there is recognition of an association between elevation in this lead and severe left main coronary artery disease (LMCA) [3]. The ECG in this disease process typically reveals STE in lead aVR and

Table 4.2.4 The Modified Sgarbossa criteria and ST/S ratio.

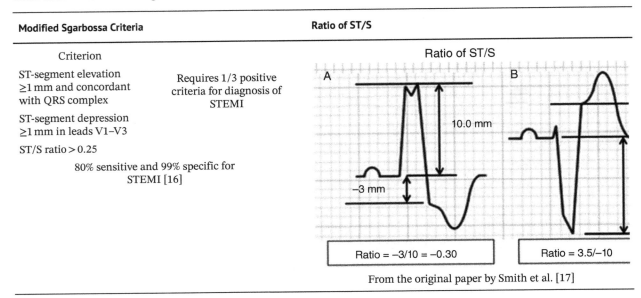

Modified Sgarbossa Criteria		Ratio of ST/S
Criterion		Ratio of ST/S
ST-segment elevation ≥1 mm and concordant with QRS complex	Requires 1/3 positive criteria for diagnosis of STEMI	
ST-segment depression ≥1 mm in leads V1–V3		
ST/S ratio > 0.25		
	80% sensitive and 99% specific for STEMI [16]	Ratio = −3/10 = −0.30 Ratio = 3.5/−10
		From the original paper by Smith et al. [17]

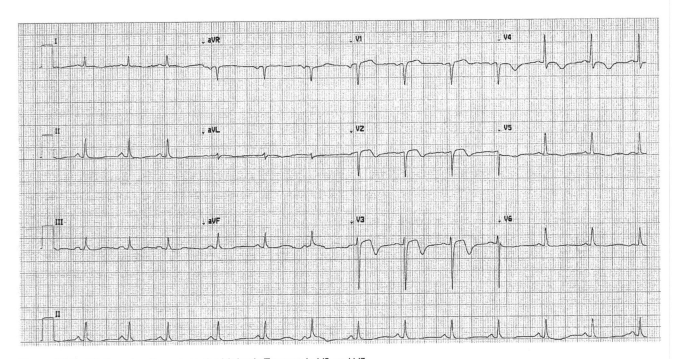

Figure 4.2.8 Wellens A pattern, note the biphasic T waves in V2 and V3.

diffuse ST depressions in other leads. A 2005 study evaluated 310 patients with NSTEMIs and showed STE of aVR (≥0.5 mm) was significantly associated with LMCA or three-vessel disease with an odds ratio of 19.7 [16]. In 2011, researchers demonstrated aVR elevation ≥1 mm strongly predicted severe LMCA or three-vessel disease with 80% sensitivity and 93% specificity [20]. Patients in these stud-

ies with aVR elevation were also significantly more likely to need urgent CABG compared to those without [16, 21].

Elevation in aVR has also been shown to have prognostic value in AMI. A 2003 evaluation of 775 patients with NSTEMIs showed patients with aVR STE (≥0.5 mm) had significantly higher rates of in-hospital mortality and new-onset heart failure [22]. Szymanski et al. also demonstrated

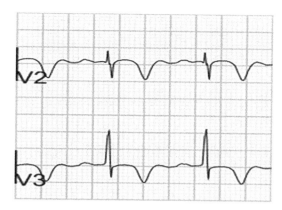

Figure 4.2.9 Type B Wellens T waves in V2 and V3. Image reproduced with permission from http://lifeinthefastlane.com.

that the degree of STE in aVR is associated with increased rates of mortality [23].

Pericarditis

Pericarditis, or inflammation of the pericardium due to a variety of causes, typically presents with chest pain that is described as sharp or stabbing in the precordial or retrosternal area [24]. Typically, the pain is aggravated by movement and a supine position, but relieved when leaning forward [25]. Classically, the ECG in pericarditis evolves as the disease progresses, though can remain normal in up to

60% of patients [26]. In those with ECG abnormalities, initially diffuse ST-segment elevation is present with PR depression in leads I, II, III, and aVF, defined as Stage I pericarditis. The ST elevation decreases in Stage II pericarditis, becoming more isoelectric as the T waves flatten. In stage III, diffuse T-wave inversion occurs [27]. An important distinction between the ST elevation in pericarditis compared to AMI is that there should not be ST depression except in aVR and V1 in pericarditis (Figure 4.2.11).

If the pericarditis is associated with a pericardial effusion, then there will be decreased overall voltage of the QRS complex [28].

Myocarditis is inflammation of the heart muscle that may accompany pericarditis. The disease often presents with systemic illness symptoms, including fever, muscle aches, and chills [24]. The ECG in myocarditis is nonspecific and may range from normal, sinus tachycardia all the way to significant abnormalities, including regional STE and Q waves similar to AMI (Figure 4.2.12). Atrial and ventricular ectopic beats, as well as complex ventricular arrhythmias, may manifest as further electrocardiographic signs of myocarditis [12, 27, 29].

Takotsubo cardiomyopathy was first described in Japan in 1990 [30]. Also known as broken heart syndrome, stress-induced cardiomyopathy, or apical ballooning, it is an acute and reversible dysfunction of the left ventricle following catecholamine surge [31]. Patients most often present with chest pain following a psychological or physical stressor [32]. The ECG in Takotsubo cardiomyopathy

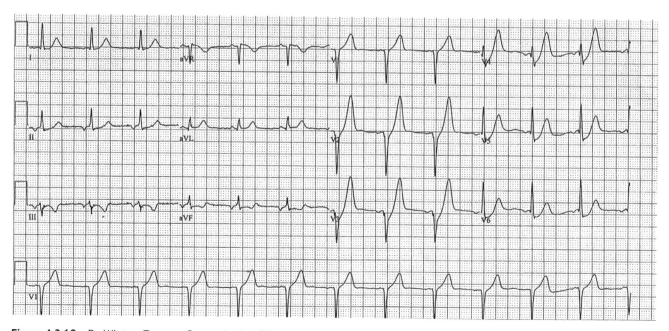

Figure 4.2.10 De Winters T waves. See upsloping ST depression in anterior leads. Image reproduced with permission from http://lifeinthefastlane.com.

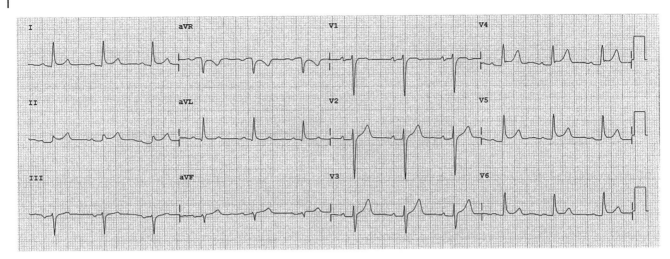

Figure 4.2.11 Stage I Pericarditis: diffuse STE. Image reproduced with permission from http://lifeinthefastlane.com.

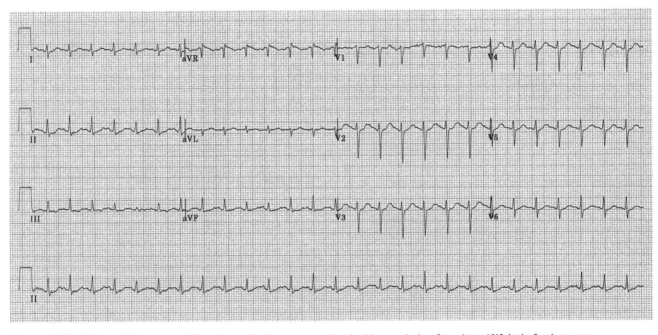

Figure 4.2.12 Myocarditis: nonspecific tachycardia. Image reproduced with permission from http://lifeinthefastlane.com.

demonstrates sinus rhythm in the vast majority of patients, though an elevated heart rate is common. STE occurs in approximately 44% of patients, most often in the anterior leads though some patients will present with solitary ST elevation in an isolated limb lead [31]. Additional findings include ST-depression, T-wave inversion, and prolongation of the QT interval (Figure 4.2.13) [32].

Aortic dissection is an uncommon but deadly disease. The mortality is 10–60% depending on the type (A or B) and underlying comorbidities [33]. Patients classically present with sharp ripping chest pain that radiates into the mid-back. Other symptoms include syncope, abdominal

pain, and, if the carotid arteries are involved, neurologic changes or strokelike symptoms [1]. The ECG is generally nonspecific for aortic dissections and can be normal in about 20–30% of patients [1]. Other ECG changes can include nonspecific ST changes (40–60%), ACS-like changes such as ST depressions and T-wave inversions, and even a STEMI pattern [34]. Any ACS like changes on the ECG that accompany aortic dissection indicate a worse prognosis and likely coronary artery involvement in the dissection [34].

Spontaneous coronary artery dissection is an uncommon but increasingly recognized nonatherosclerotic cause of

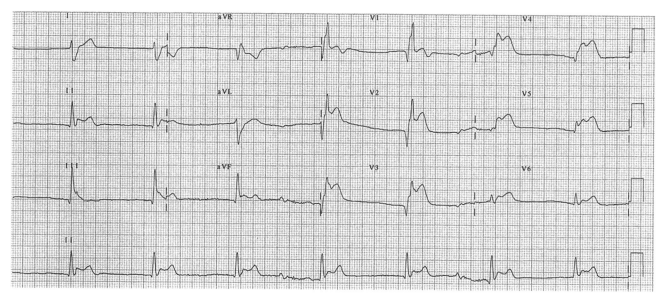

Figure 4.2.13 Takotsubo myocarditis. ST elevations in the anterior and inferior leads. Image reproduced with permission from http://lifeinthefastlane.com.

ACS, now thought to occur in about 4% of all patients presenting with ACS [35]. Patients at higher risk include females 30–50 years old, pregnant patients, cocaine users, smokers, or patients with collagen disease such as Marfan syndrome [36]. Clinically, coronary dissection has a wide range of presentations, from UA to sudden cardiac death, and the ECG can range from nonspecific ST changes to a STEMI [35]. Chest pain has been and will continue to be one of the most commonly encounter problems in the clinical setting.

The ECG is an essential tool in helping to determine if in fact the chest pain involves the heart. It is one of the fastest and most easily reproduced tests available and can change to disposition and management of a patient immediately. As such, it is essential to become familiar with the ECG changes found in various pathologies related to chest pain presented in this chapter.

References

1 Tintinalli, J.E., Stapczynski, J.S., Ma, O.J. et al. (2016). *Tintinalli's Emergency Medicine: A Comprehensive Study Guide*. New York: McGraw-Hill Education.

2 Amsterdam, E.A., Wenger, N.K., Brindis, R.G. et al. (2014). *AHA/ACC Guideline for the Management of Patients with Non-St-Elevation Acute Coronary Syndromes*, vol. 130. American College of Cardiology/American Heart Association Task Force on Practice Guidelines.

3 O'Gara, P.T., Kushner, F.G., Ascheim, D.D. et al. (2013). ACCF/AHA guideline for the management of ST-elevation myocardial infarction: a report of the American College of Cardiology Foundation/American Heart Association Task Force on Practice Guidelines. *J. Am. Coll. Cardiol.* 61 (4): 2013.

4 Li, D., Li, C.Y., Yong, A.C., and Kilpatrick, D. (1998). Source of electrocardiographic ST changes in subendocardial ischemia. *Circ. Res.* 82 (9): 957–970.

5 Thygesen, K., Alpert, J.S., Jaffe, A.S. et al. (2012). Third universal definition of myocardial infarction. *Circulation* 126 (16): 2020–2035.

6 Chang, A.M., Shofer, F.S., Tabas, J.A. et al. (2009). Lack of association between left bundle-branch block and acute myocardial infarction in symptomatic ED patients. *Am. J. Emerg. Med.* 27 (8): 916–921.

7 Brady, W.J., Syverud, S.A., Beagle, C. et al. (2001). Electrocardiographic ST-segment elevation: the diagnosis of acute myocardial infarction by morphologic analysis of the ST segment. *Acad. Emerg. Med.* 8 (10): 961–967.

8 Thygesen, K., Alpert, J.S., White, H.D. et al. (2007). Universal definition of myocardial infarction: Kristian Thygesen, Joseph S. Alpert, and Harvey D. White on behalf of the Joint ESC/ACCF/AHA/WHF Task Force for the Redefinition of Myocardial Infarction. *Eur. Heart J.* 28 (20): 2525–2538.

9 Wagner, G.S., Macfarlane, P., Wellens, H. et al. (2009). AHA/ACCF/HRS recommendations for the standardization and interpretation of the electrocardiogram. Part VI: acute ischemia/infarction a scientific statement from the American Heart Association electrocardiography and arrhythmias committee, Council on Clinical Cardiology; the American College of Cardiology Foundation; and the Heart Rhythm Society. *J. Am. Coll. Cardiol.* 53 (11): 1003–1011.

10 Dressler, W. and Hugo, R. (1947). High T waves in the earliest stage of myocardial infarction. *Am. Heart J.* 34 (5): 627–645.

11 Nable, J.V. and Brady, W. (2009). The evolution of electrocardiographic changes in ST-segment elevation myocardial infarction. *Am. J. Emerg. Med.* 27 (6): 734–746.

12 Friedrich, M.G., Strohm, O., Schulz-Menger, J. et al. (1998). Contrast media-enhanced magnetic resonance imaging visualizes myocardial changes in the course of viral myocarditis. *Circulation* 97 (18): 1802–1809.

13 Sgarbossa, E.B., Pinski, S.L., Barbagelata, A. et al. (1996). Electrocardiographic diagnosis of evolving acute myocardial infarction in the presence of left bundle-branch block. GUSTO-1 (global utilization of streptokinase and tissue plasminogen activator for occluded coronary arteries) investigators. *N. Engl. J. Med.* 334 (8): 481–487.

14 Sgarbossa, E.B., Pinski, S.L., Gates, K.B., and Wagner, G.S. (1996). Early electrocardiographic diagnosis of acute myocardial infarction in the presence of ventricular paced rhythm. *Am. J. Cardiol.* 77 (5): 423–424.

15 Smith, S.W., Dodd, K.W., Henry, T.D. et al. (2012). Diagnosis of ST-elevation myocardial infarction in the presence of left bundle branch block with the ST-elevation to S-wave ratio in a modified Sgarbossa rule. *Ann. Emerg. Med.* 60 (6): 766–776.

16 Kosuge, M., Kimura, K., Ishikawa, T. et al. (2005). Predictors of left main or three-vessel disease in patients who have acute coronary syndromes with non-ST-segment elevation. *Am. J. Cardiol.* 95 (11): 1366–1369.

17 Verouden, N.J., Koch, K.T., Peters, R.J. et al. (2009). Persistent precordial "hyperacute" T-waves signify proximal left anterior descending artery occlusion. *Heart* 95: 1701–1706.

18 Tandy, T.K., Bottomy, D.P., and Lewis, J.G. (1999). Wellens' syndrome. *Ann. Emerg. Med.* 33 (3): 347–351.

19 Zwaan, C.D., Bär, F.W., and Wellens, H.J. (1982). Characteristic electrocardiographic pattern indicating a critical stenosis high in left anterior descending coronary artery in patients admitted because of impending myocardial infarction. *Am. Heart J.* 103 (4): 730–736.

20 Pahlm, U.S., Pahlm, O., and Wagner, G.S. (1996). The standard 11-lead ECG. Neglect of lead aVR in the classical limb lead display. *J. Electrocardiol.* 29 (Suppl): 270–274.

21 Kosuge, M., Ebina, T., Hibi, K. et al. (2011). An early and simple predictor of severe left main and/or three-vessel disease in patients with nonst-segment elevation acute coronary syndrome. *Am. J. Cardiol.* 107 (4): 495–500.

22 Barrabés, J.A., Figueras, J., Moure, C. et al. (2003). Prognostic value of lead aVR in patients with a first non-ST-segment elevation acute myocardial infarction. *Circulation* 108 (7): 814–819.

23 Szymański, F.M., Grabowski, M., Filipiak, K.J. et al. (2008). Admission ST-segment elevation in lead aVR as the factor improving complex risk stratification in acute coronary syndromes. *Am. J. Emerg. Med.* 26 (4): 408–412.

24 Niemann, J.T. (2016). Cardiomyopathies and pericardial disease. In: *Tintinalli's Emergency Medicine: A Comprehensive Study Guide*, 8e (eds. J.E. Tintinalli, J.S. Stapczynski, O.J. Ma, et al.). New York, NY: McGraw-Hill Education.

25 Lange, R.A. and Hillis, L.D. (2004). Acute Pericarditis. *N. Engl. J. Med.* 351 (21): 2195–2202.

26 Imazio, M., Brucato, A., Cemin, R. et al. (2013). A randomized trial of colchicine for acute pericarditis. *N. Engl. J. Med.* 369 (16): 1522–1528.

27 Wang, K., Asinger, R.W., and Marriott, H.J. (2003). ST-segment elevation in conditions other than acute myocardial infarction. *N. Engl. J. Med.* 349 (22): 2128–2135.

28 Punja, M., Mark, D.G., McCoy, J.V. et al. (2010). Electrocardiographic manifestations of cardiac infectious-inflammatory disorders. *Am. J. Emerg. Med.* 28 (3): 364–377.

29 Sarda, L., Colin, P., Boccara, F. et al. (2001). Myocarditis in patients with clinical presentation of myocardial infarction and normal coronary angiograms. *J. Am. Coll. Cardiol.* 37 (3): 786–792.

30 Sato, H., Tateishi, H., Dote, K. et al. (1990). Tako-tsubo-like left ventricular dysfunction due to multivessel coronary spasm. In: *Clinical Aspect of Myocardial Injury: From Ischemia to Heart Failure*, 56–64. Tokyo: Kagakuhyoronsha Publishing Co.

31 Tsuchihashi, K., Ueshima, K., Uchida, T. et al. (2001). Transient left ventricular apical ballooning without coronary artery stenosis: a novel heart syndrome mimicking acute myocardial infarction. *J. Am. Coll. Cardiol.* 38 (1): 11–18.

32 Templin, C., Ghadri, J.R., Diekmann, J. et al. (2015). Clinical features and outcomes of Takotsubo (stress) cardiomyopathy. *N. Engl. J. Med.* 373 (10): 929–938.

33 Hagan, P., Nienaber, C.A., Isselbacher, E.M. et al. (2000). The international registry of acute aortic dissection (IRAD): new insights into an old disease. *JAMA* 283: 897.

34 Biagini, E., Lofiego, C., Ferlito, M. et al. (2007). Frequency, determinants, and clinical relevance of acute coronary syndrome-like electrocardiographic findings in patient with acute aortic syndrome. *Am. J. Cardiol.* 100: 1013.

35 Sultan, A. and Kreutz, R.P. (2015). Variations in clinical presentation, risk factors, treatment, and prognosis of spontaneous coronary artery dissection. *J. Invasive Cardiol.* 27 (8): 363–369.

36 Winchester, D.E. and Pepine, C.J. (n.d.). Nonobstructive atherosclerotic and nonatherosclerotic coronary heart disease. In: *Hurst's the Heart*, 14e, vol. 1), Chapter 35 (eds. V. Fuster, R.A. Harrington, J. Narula and Z.J. Eapen). McGraw-Hill Education.

3

The Patient with Dyspnea

Adriana Segura Olson[1], Anders Messersmith[2], and Matthew Robinson[3]

[1] *Emergency Physician, University of Chicago, Chicago, IL, USA*
[2] *Emergency Physician, Envision Physician Services*
[3] *Emergency Physician, Woodhull Hospital, Brooklyn, NY, USA*

Introduction

Many patients present for the evaluation of dyspnea, and the ECG is an important diagnostic tool for clinicians evaluating these patients. The ECG can be useful not only in ruling out certain diagnoses, but also in directing clinicians toward alternate pathologies. There are a variety of conditions that present with dyspnea including pulmonary embolism (PE), cor pulmonale, cardiomyopathy, heart failure, pneumothorax, pneumonia, obstructive lung disease, anaphylaxis, and metabolic disorders. While the ECG findings associated with these conditions are not always sensitive or specific for a particular pathology, they can be helpful for clinicians in directing further workup and management of the patient with dyspnea.

Pulmonary Embolism

PE is a potentially life-threatening cause of dyspnea. Definitive diagnosis typically relies upon pulmonary CT angiography or ventilation/perfusion scan; however, these tests require significant time and expose patients to considerable ionizing radiation. ECG findings in PE are somewhat variable, and more specific findings are found more commonly in those with heavy clot burden and worse prognosis than those with less severe disease [1–4]. According to the PIOPED group, the most common ECG abnormality was nonspecific ST- and T-wave changes in 49% of patients; tachycardia was only identified in 30% of patients and 18% of patients will have a normal ECG [1, 5, 6]. The traditionally described S1-Q3-T3 pattern is neither sensitive nor specific for PE, found in only 11–28% of patients in various trials [1].

Pathophysiologically, emboli that occlude any portion of the pulmonary vasculature increase the pulmonary vascular resistance (PVR) by reducing the total capillary territory, forcing cardiac output to shunt to the remaining pulmonary vasculature. If the PVR is sufficiently increased, the right ventricle (RV) must either pump at higher pressures or at higher rates to maintain total cardiac output. Thus, for hemodynamically significant PE, ECG findings may represent pressure overload of the RV, distortion of the RV anatomy due to dilatation, or tachycardia [7]. Any conditions that cause pressure or volume overload of the RV are also likely to cause overload of the right atrium (RA) as well. Changes associated with hemodynamically significant PE can primarily be characterized by those consistent with RVH, RV dilatation/strain, RA enlargement, and tachycardia.

Right Ventricular Hypertrophy

RVH develops as the RV attempts to compensate for increased afterload. Normally, the balance of electrical forces between the right and left ventricles strongly favors the left ventricle, thus yielding large R waves in lateral/leftward leads, and large S waves in rightward leads. However, when the RV hypertrophies, the right ventricular bulk increases, and with this increasing bulk, the QRS balance may become neutral or even rightward [7, 8]. Usually, the left ventricle finishes depolarization after the RV due to thickness differences. However, if the RV becomes thicker than the LV, the end of depolarization may have a right ventricular predominance. These hypertrophic changes are seen as tall R waves or rSR′ patterns in V1–V2, and deep S waves in I, aVL, V5–V6, as well as right axis deviation in the frontal leads (R wave in III and aVF, S wave in I and aVL).

Electrocardiogram in Clinical Medicine, First Edition. Edited by William J. Brady, Michael J. Lipinski, Andrew E. Darby, Michael C. Bond, Nathan P. Charlton, Korin Hudson, and Kelly Williamson.

Right Ventricular Strain

Frequently, severe RVH or acute increases to right ventricular overload will lead to right ventricular strain. On the ECG, these are represented by ST depressions and T-wave inversions over the rightward leads V1 and V2. ST depressions are hypothesized to be related to an "injury current" from less injured epicardial tissue toward more injured subendocardial tissue during electrical diastole, which registers as an increased T–P voltage, and ST segment on the baseline [8]. However, due to convention that the ECG baseline is the T–P interval, the affected ECG will demonstrate ST depression from the T–P "baseline." Regarding T-wave inversion, the normal epicardial to endocardial repolarization reverses, reverting to the same endo- to epicardial direction of the initial depolarization wave. As repolarization is transit of positive charge out of the cell, as opposed to an inward flux as in depolarization, the repolarization wave carries opposite polarity to the depolarization wave if traveling in the same direction.

Right Atrial Enlargement

RA enlargement can be characterized by hypertrophy in the chronic setting (chronic or multiple PE) or by dilatation in the acute setting (acute massive PE). Anatomically, the SA node exists within the RA and it thereby depolarizes in the early part of the P wave, while the left atrium represents the terminal portion of the P wave, after conduction across the interatrial septum through the Bachmann's bundle [8]. Because of the posterior, basal, and rightward position of the sinoatrial node, depolarization across the RA proceeds in an anterior, apical, and leftward fashion. Thus, the usual findings of RA enlargement demonstrate accentuation of early P-wave voltage contributions, visible as an early "peaked" P wave in I, II. In anteriorly facing leads such as V1 and V2, this is seen as positive early P-wave deflection. In left atrial enlargement, lengthening of the P wave, "double hump" P wave in lead II, and late negative p-wave deflection in V1 will develop (Figure 4.3.1) [7].

Right Bundle Branch Block (RBBB)

RBBB may also develop in response to the pressure overload and subsequent dilatation of the RV resulting from PE. With RBBB, impulses to the RV are delayed. Thus, unopposed left ventricular forces will predominate early in the ECG, and delayed right ventricular forces may appear late in the QRS complex [8]. This leads to a similar pattern as RVH as discussed above. However, there is not usually QRS axis deviation in the frontal leads, as depolarization proceeds normally through the leftward fascicles (Figure 4.3.2). Other conditions that lead to pressure or volume overload of the ventricle or direct insults to the conduction system (in particular the right bundle branch) will also lead to the RBBB pattern.

The final ECG change that commonly exists with PE is tachycardia. As mentioned previously, this is to some extent due to a compensatory mechanism to maintain cardiac output in the face of suddenly increased PVR. Additionally, elements such as pain and anxiety may contribute to tachycardia in this patient population.

Cor Pulmonale

Cor pulmonale refers to a chronic cardiac condition resulting from underlying pulmonary diseases. Any disease that causes an increase in PVR will in turn force the RV to pump either faster or more forcefully to maintain cardiac output. If the rise in PVR happens slowly, the RV has time to hypertrophy to generate higher driving pressures. In the case of acute increases in PVR, the RV may be unable to cope with the required driving pressure, and will dilate. After this point, tachycardia is required to maintain cardiac output.

Conditions that lead to increased PVR stem from a number of mechanisms: pulmonic stenosis, primary arterial stiffening (connective tissue disorders, atherosclerosis), pulmonary edema/ARDS (occupying of normally compliant airspace with much more resistant fluid), emphysema (hyperinflation of airspace leading to narrowing/lengthening of pulmonary capillaries), any conditions that lead to chronic hypoxia through a maladaptive global hypoxic pulmonary vasoconstrictive response (sleep apnea, chronic obstructive pulmonary disease [COPD], high altitude conditions, and intrinsic lung disease that increases A-a gradients), and chronic thromboembolic lung disease (due to multiple stepwise increases in PVR from emboli).

The ECG changes of cor pulmonale reflect the increased pressure load on the right heart. Changes typical of right atrial enlargement and right ventricular hypertrophy are common (Figure 4.3.3). These changes are discussed more thoroughly in the PE section. Briefly, changes of Cor Pulmonale include prominent RSR' pattern with unusually positive early p-wave in V1; peaked P wave in I, II; R wave predominance in early precordial leads; and right axis deviation [7, 8].

Cardiomyopathy

This section discusses dilated and restrictive cardiomyopathies only. Hypertrophic and obstructive cardiomyopathy is covered in section 4, chapter 4, page 234.

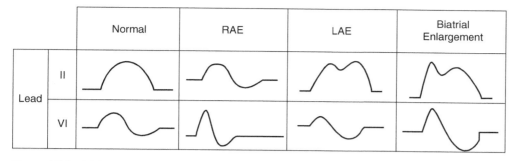

Figure 4.3.1   ECG P-wave changes associated with atrial enlargement.

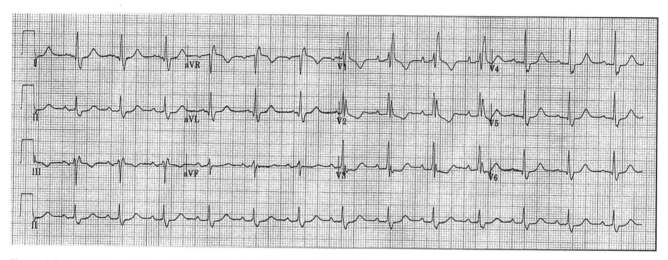

Figure 4.3.2   Right bundle branch block. Note the RSR' pattern in V1–V2, wide S-wave in 1, aVL, V5–V6. Also note the relatively normal frontal plane QRS axis. *Source:* Image reproduced with permission from http://lifeinthefastlane.com.

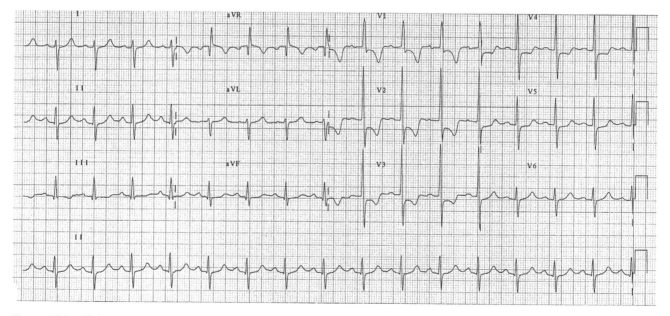

Figure 4.3.3   Right ventricular hypertrophy with RV strain. Note the right axis deviation, prominent R wave in V1–V2, deep S wave in 1, aVL, V5–V6. Additionally, ST depression and T-wave inversion of V1–V2 are seen. *Source:* Image reproduced with permission from http://lifeinthefastlane.com.

In dilated cardiomyopathy (DCM), the myocardium is unable to pump against the increased afterload leading to dilation of the ventricular cavity. Unlike in hypertrophic cardiomyopathy, the ventricle either does not have enough time to develop compensatory hypertrophy, or is incapable of doing so secondary to injury, toxin, or fibrosis. Dilation of the ventricle causes subsequent anatomic changes, often leading to valvular insufficiency, which then results in atrial enlargement. DCM can be separated into two categories: ischemic and nonischemic.

Ischemic DCM develops after completion of a large-territory infarction, most commonly involving the left anterior descending (LAD) artery. As the injury heals, the territory previously supplied by the now infarcted vessels remodels to predominantly fibrotic tissue instead of the previously contractile and electrically conductive myocardium. In LAD disease, this is represented by qS waves in V1–4 on the ECG [7]. Nonischemic DCM results from global insults to the heart, such as toxins, metabolic derangements, deposition of inappropriate tissue, inflammation, infection, or congenital muscular disease. Examples include diabetes, alcoholism, amyloidosis, Chagas disease, Lyme disease, tuberculosis, chemotherapy (especially doxorubicin), and congenital muscular disease such as muscular dystrophy. Other conditions that lead to increased demand on the heart may also lead to DCM, with, or without antecedent LVH. These include hyperthyroidism, anemia, stimulant usage, and pregnancy. Electrocardiographically, replacement of myocardium with fibrotic tissue leads to depolarization vectors away from the distribution of the injury, the resulting imbalance demonstrated as qS-waves in the direction of the injury, or, in globally infiltrative diseases, such as amyloidosis and sarcoidosis, the diffuse replacement of myocardium tissue with electrically inert tissue leads to decreased QRS voltages [7].

Strain patterns develop when myocardium stretches: slowed depolarization conduction through the myocardium yields a prolonged QRS, which can resemble bundle branch block. Repolarization is affected as well, leading to endo-to-epicardial repolarization (the opposite of the normal case) and ion leakage, which yields T-wave inversion and discordant ST-segment changes in leads over the stretched tissue [7]. When the LAD territory is involved, these changes develop in the left ventricle and delayed depolarization yields changes similar to LVH or LBBB: QRS widening and strongly negative S waves in leads over the anterior/right precordium (V1–V3) which develop into strongly positive R waves over the posterior/left precordium (V4–V6, I, AVL). Deranged repolarization leads to

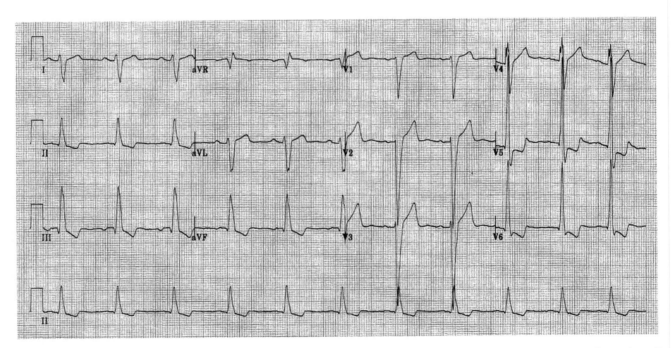

Figure 4.3.4 ECG of a patient with ischemic cardiomyopathy. Note the LVH changes (deep early precordial S waves leading to large R waves in V4–V6), "pseudoinfarct" qS changes in V1–V2, discordant ST elevation in V1–V2 and strain-like ST depression in V5–V6. Of note, this patient likely had biventricular hypertrophy given right axis deviation in the setting of LVH and inferior strain patterning (II, III, AVF downsloping ST depressions). *Source:* Image reproduced with permission from http://lifeinthefastlane.com.

discordant ST depression and T-waves, seen as ST elevation and upright T waves in V1–V3, and ST depression and T-wave inversion in V4–V6, I, AVL (Figure 4.3.4).

The vascular anatomy of the His bundle has dual supply from the AV nodal artery and septal branches of the LAD artery. Thus, LAD infarction may lead to ischemia of the bundle branches, and uni-, bi-, or tri-fasicular block patterns can develop. Similarly, nonischemic cardiomyopathies may cause electrical blockade if the disease process affects the conduction system. If the AV node is affected, the ECG can reveal first- or second-degree blockade instead of fasicular block [8].

Conditions that lead to mechanical failure of a ventricle will often result in dilation/enlargement of the associated atrium. Please see the section on PE for a more detailed discussion of the ECG findings associated with atrial enlargement.

Congestive Heart Failure

Congestive heart failure is a clinical condition wherein one or both ventricles become incapable of maintaining cardiac output, leading to vascular congestion and eventually interstitial edema in tissues that drain into the involved chamber of the heart. There are two schema for development of heart failure: inability to sufficiently pump blood forward due to muscular failure, or systolic heart failure, and inability for the ventricle to sufficiently relax after systole leading to impaired stroke volume, or diastolic heart failure. In systolic heart failure, a variety of insults cause death or injury of myocytes, leading to impaired pumping function. This, in turn, leads to congestion of the associated ventricle. A compensatory hypertrophy may develop, or if the ventricle is unable to compensate for the decreased pumping efficacy, then it will dilate. As the ventricle becomes incapable of generating sufficient stroke volume, blood flow will back up, leading to associated atrial enlargement. In diastolic heart failure, disease of the myocardium leads to impaired relaxation and ultimately decreased stroke volume.

With this pathophysiology in mind, changes of the ECG in heart failure represent hypertrophy and strain patterns with associated atrial enlargement. RVH and atrial enlargement is discussed in further detail in the section on PE. LVH is discussed in the section on hypertrophic cardiomyopathy.

In severe congestive heart failure, patients become increasingly more prone to ventricular arrhythmias, due to increased stretch leading to decreased native conduction and distortion of anatomy leading to pathways for ventricular tachycardia. It is for this reason that patients with severe congestive heart failure are evaluated for implantable cardioverter defibrillator device placement.

Pneumothorax

Pneumothorax, or an abnormal collection of air in the pleural space, is often accompanied by shortness of breath. Historically, this condition was diagnosed by chest radiograph, though more modern techniques, such as computed tomography and ultrasonography, have demonstrated higher sensitivity for detecting pneumothorax. As symptoms of a pneumothorax include dyspnea and chest pain, ECGs are commonly obtained on these patients during their evaluation.

The specific ECG changes seen with pneumothorax develop from three mechanisms: deviation of the heart/ mediastinum due to pressure effects, increased freedom of movement of the heart when surrounded by air instead of lung, and insulation of the heart from the chest wall due to interposed air. Tachycardia may also develop, which may be due to pain in the mild case, or obstructive shock in the case of tension pneumothorax.

Pneumothorax may cause rotation and translation of the heart. Left-sided spontaneous pneumothorax results in rightward rotation of the heart [9], leading to early R-wave progression and right-axis deviation. Right-sided pneumothorax has not demonstrated a strong association with axis deviation [10].

The absence of substantial tissue surrounding the heart, as occurs in left-sided pneumothorax, leads to an increased freedom of movement of the heart. As the heart points in a different direction beat-to-beat, the QRS axis will subsequently follow. Usually this pattern is rhythmic in nature, leading to voltage alternans on the ECG [9].

Finally, the presence of air interposed between the heart and the chest wall attenuates the observed voltages at the skin surface. Right-sided pneumothoraces, thus, do not generally cause significant voltage attenuation, as these do not generally yield air between any of the standard 12 leads [10]. Left-sided pneumothorax shows diminished QRS voltage over lateral and precordial leads (V1–V6, I, AVL), but this may disappear if the patient is placed in the upright or left lateral decubitus position as the heart again makes contact with the chest wall [9].

An additional finding of unknown etiology in left-sided pneumothorax is deep precordial T-wave inversion that resolves upon successful treatment of the pneumothorax [9]. It is important to note that while left-sided pneumothorax causes delayed R-wave progression, T-wave inversion, and decreased QRS voltage, it does not generally disturb the ST segment, which may be useful in differentiating this pathology from acute MI [9].

ASTHMA/COPD

Asthma and COPD are inflammatory diseases of the lungs that cause reversible airflow obstruction and bronchospasm. In the acute exacerbation, many patients will have known diagnosis of obstructive lung disease, but in an undifferentiated patient with dyspnea, ECG changes due to mechanical forces and long-term effects of hypoxic pulmonary vasoconstriction can be an important diagnostic clue. The mechanical and pathophysiological changes are manifested primarily by changes to the P wave and axis, with many similar changes described in the previous section on Cor Pulmonale. Changes to the QRS axis and amplitude along with atrial arrhythmias are also common in COPD and asthma [11–13].

P-Wave Changes

The effects of chronic hypoxia on the pulmonary vasculature leads to pulmonary hypertension that results in right ventricular and right atrial enlargement. The chronic effect of pulmonary hypertension in the late stages of the disease is discussed in the previous section on cor pulmonale, though there are additional more subtle findings earlier in the disease process.

One of the most common ECG findings is a vertical P wave axis (rightward of +80°). In the normal heart, the P wave is upright in lead I with an axis between −50° and +60°, but in obstructive lung disease the P wave shifts inferiorly and away from the left arm. P waves also become peaked in lead II, III, and aVF and when the height of the P waves is >2.5 mm, the pattern is called "P pulmonale" [14]. Late in the disease course, the QRS axis also becomes vertically directed and can lead to a flat P wave and QRS in lead I, called "isoelectric lead I sign." This finding is highly correlative of underlying COPD (Figure 4.3.5) [15].

QRS Changes

The QRS duration is typically shorter in COPD/asthma patients than in other disease processes [16]. The mechanical changes in asthma and COPD occur due to overaeration of the lungs secondary to bronchoconstriction and outflow obstruction. Overaeration of the lungs displaces the diaphragm inferiorly, and subsequently elongates and vertically orients the heart. Due to the attachment of the heart to the great vessels, the heart rotates in the transverse plane with the RV moving anteriorly and the left ventricle moving posteriorly. These mechanical changes change the mean QRS axis of the ECG to >=90° in the frontal plane. A nearly pathognomonic finding for COPD in the absence of acute ischemia or pericardial effusion is low voltage QRS amplitude in limb leads <=5 mm [14]. This change is due to the over-aerated lungs dampening the electrical activity of the heart [11, 12, 14]. $S_1 S_2 S_3$ syndrome is characterized by negative S wave deflections in limb leads I, II, and III

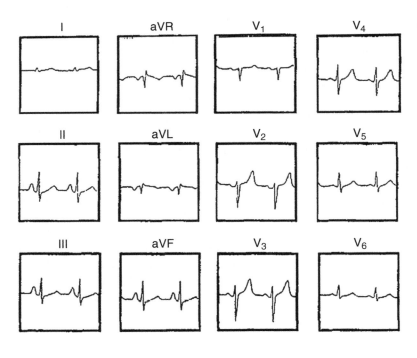

Figure 4.3.5 ECG of a 44-year-old man with precocious emphysema illustrating "lead I sign." Note the isoelectric P wave and the low amplitude of both the QRS complex and T wave. *Source:* Image reproduced with permission from Rodman et al. [15].

(the magnitude of the S wave is near or greater than the R wave) and often has an R′ in lead V_1 and a normal QRS duration (Figure 4.3.6).

Another diagnostic pattern characteristic of COPD is the presence of a prominent R wave in V1, which suggests pulmonary hypertension. However, patients with COPD do not often meet criteria for right ventricular hypertrophy and instead have persistent S waves across the precordium and delayed precordial transition known as *poor R-wave progression*. This pattern is characterized by low amplitude of the R wave in the right-sided leads. V2 is <=1.5 mm, and V3 <=3 mm.

These ECG changes are generally late findings in obstructive airway diseases, and prior authors have demonstrated that having two or more of these findings may correlate with severity of the underlying disease [11, 14].

Arrhythmias

In obstructive lung disease arrhythmias are usually transient, and most often occur with an acute exacerbation of the disease, respiratory failure, or infection. The most common arrhythmia is sinus tachycardia, followed by multifocal atrial tachycardia, in which there are multiple morphologies of the P waves with ectopic uniform atrial tachycardia, atrial flutter and atrial fibrillation (Figure 4.3.7). Most patients with COPD and an arrhythmia have evidence of right ventricular hypertrophy [15].

Anaphylaxis/Kounis Syndrome

Kounis syndrome is a hypersensitivity coronary artery disorder which is induced by drugs, food, environmental factors, or an unknown triggers. There are three types of Kounis syndrome: type I vasospastic allergic angina, type II allergic myocardial infarction, and type III stent thrombosis with occluding thrombus and infiltrating mast cells and eosinophils [17].

The most commonly affected age group for Kounis syndrome is 40–70 years old, and risk factors include history of previous allergy, hypertension, smoking, diabetes, and hyperlipidemia. The most frequently identified causes were antibiotics (27.4%) and insect bites (23.4%) [17]. The pathophysiology involves coronary artery vasospasm or plaque rupture during an allergic reaction and mast cell degranulation with release of inflammatory mediators. The inflammatory mediators released during an allergic reaction including histamine can induce vasospasm in the coronary arteries, activates platelets and decreases oxygen delivery to the myocardium [17].

ECG changes in Kounis syndrome are the same as described in acute myocardial ischemia. Typically the ECG shows acute ST-T changes including elevation of >2 mm in two or more contiguous leads, reciprocal ST depression in the opposite leads. Echocardiogram may demonstrate

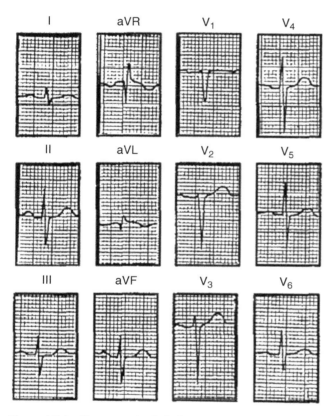

Figure 4.3.6 Illustrates the $S_1 S_2 S_3$ pattern, which is due to right atrial enlargement. *Source:* Figure reproduced with permission from Rodman et al. [15].

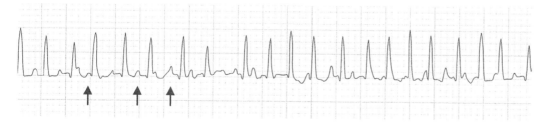

Figure 4.3.7 Multifocal atrial tachycardia. Note the different morphologies of the P waves represented by the arrows. *Source:* Image obtained with permission from http://lifeinthefastlane.com.

regional wall motion abnormalities and cardiac catheterization may reveal coronary vasospasm or stenosis [18, 19].

Metabolic

ECG changes in metabolic acidosis and renal failure are driven by abnormal serum electrolyte concentrations resulting in changes in the transmembrane potential of the cardiac cells. Metabolic acidosis and alkalosis are usually associated with changes in the concentration of both potassium and calcium, often in the setting of renal failure. It is

therefore difficult to distinguish ECG changes due specifically to pH rather than the electrolyte abnormalities commonly associated with them.

Hyperkalemia

It is important to note that changes on an ECG for electrolyte abnormalities exist on a continuum. While ECG changes are often described at happening at a certain concentration of the extracellular potassium level, any of the changes described can occur with varying potassium levels (Figures 4.3.8–4.3.11) [20].

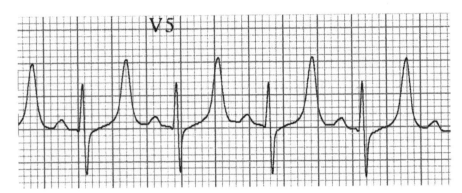

Figure 4.3.8 Potassium level >= 5.5; Peaked T waves. *Source:* Image reproduced with permission from http://lifeinthefastlane.com.

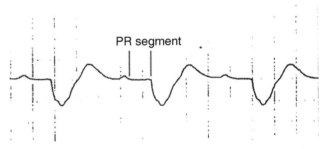

Figure 4.3.9 Potassium level >= 6.5; P wave widens, flattens, and eventually disappears. PR segment lengthens. *Source:* Image reproduced with permission from http://lifeinthefastlane.com.

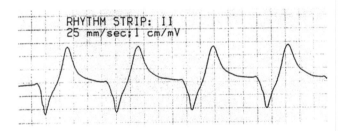

Figure 4.3.11 Potassium level >= 9.0; Ventricular fibrillation, pulseless electrical activity, sine wave. *Source:* Image reproduced with permission from http://lifeinthefastlane.com.

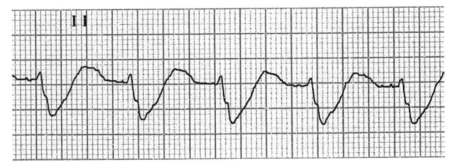

Figure 4.3.10 Potassium level >= 7.0; Prolonged QRS similar to LBBB or RBBB, AV conduction block. *Source:* Image reproduced with permission from http://lifeinthefastlane.com.

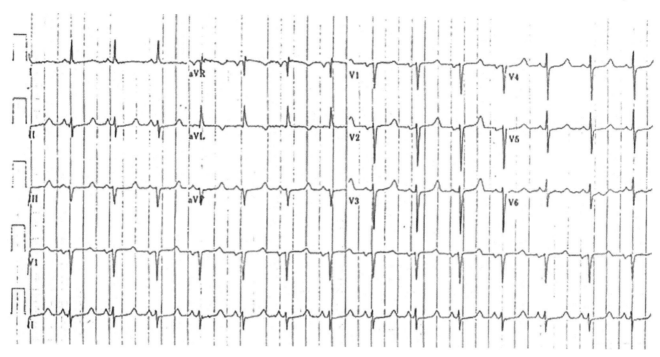

Figure 4.3.12 Showing prolonged QT interval in a patient with hypocalcemia. *Source:* Image reproduced with permission from http:// lifeinthefastlane.com.

Hypermagnesemia

While hypermagnesemia does not reliably produce any specific ECG pattern in humans, infusions of magnesium have been shown to lengthen sinus not recovery time and AV conduction time, and QRS duration in ventricular pacing [21, 22].

Hypocalcemia

In renal failure, hypocalcemia is caused by concomitant hyperphosphatemia binding excess calcium, and causing a decrease in the serum calcium level. Hypocalcemia is associated with ST segment and QTc interval prolongation, though the T wave remains unchanged (Figure 4.3.12) [23].

Summary

Patients presenting for evaluation of dyspnea may have associated ECG findings that can aid the clinician in determining the etiology and appropriate management for the underlying condition.

References

1 Panos, R.J., Barish, R.A., Whye, D.W., and Groleau, G. (1988 Aug 31). The electrocardiographic manifestations of pulmonary embolism. *J. Emerg. Med.* 6 (4): 301–307.

2 Shopp, J.D., Stewart, L.K., Emmett, T.W., and Kline, J.A. (2015 Oct 1). Findings from 12-lead electrocardiography that predict circulatory shock from pulmonary embolism: systematic review and meta-analysis. *Acad. Emerg. Med.* 22 (10): 1127–1137.

3 Ferrari, E., Imbert, A., Chevalier, T. et al. (1997 Mar 31). The ECG in pulmonary embolism: predictive value of negative T waves in precordial leads-80 case reports. *Chest* 111 (3): 537–543.

4 Geibel, A., Zehender, M., Kasper, W. et al. (2005 May 1). Prognostic value of the ECG on admission in patients with acute major pulmonary embolism. *Eur. Respir. J.* 25 (5): 843–848.

5 Stein, P.D., Terrin, M.L., Hales, C.A. et al. (1991 Sep 30). Clinical, laboratory, roentgenographic, and electrocardiographic findings in patients with acute pulmonary embolism and no pre-existing cardiac or pulmonary disease. *Chest* 100 (3): 598–603.

6 Stein, P.D., Saltzman, H.A., and Weg, J.G. (1991 Dec 15). Clinical characteristics of patients with acute pulmonary embolism. *Am. J. Cardiol.* 68 (17): 1723–1724.

7 Wagner, G.S. and Strauss, D.G. (2013 Oct 24). *Marriott's Practical Electrocardiography*. Philadelphia: Lippincott, Williams, and Wilkins.

8 Lipman, B.S., Dunn, M., and Massie, E. (1984 May 1). *Clinical Scalar Electrocardiography*. Maryland Heights, MO: Mosby.

9 Walston, A.B., Brewer, D.L., Kitchens, C.S., and Krook, J.E. (1974 Mar 1). The electrocardiographic manifestations of spontaneous left pneumothorax. *Ann. Intern. Med.* 80 (3): 375–379.

10 Alikhan, M. and Biddison, J.H. (1998 Jul). Electrocardiographic changes with right-sided pneumothorax. *South. Med. J.* 91 (7): 677–680.

11 Burch, G.E. and DePasquale, N.P. (1963). The electrocardiographic diagnosis of pulmonary heart disease. *Am. J. Cardiol.* 11: 622.

12 Schmock, C.L., Pomerantz, B., Mitchell, R.S. et al. (1971). The electrocardiogram in emphysema with and without chronic airway obstruction. *Chest* 60: 328.

13 Chou, T.C. (1996). *Electrocardiography in Clinical Practice. Adult and Pediatric*, 281–295. Philadelphia: Saunders.

14 Selvester, R.H. and Rubin, H.B. (1965). New criteria for the electrocardiographic diagnosis of emphysema and cor pulmonale. *Am. Heart J.* 69: 437.

15 Rodman, D.M., Lowenstein, S.R., and Rodman, T. (1990). The electrocardiogram in chronic obstructive pulmonary disease. *J. Emerg. Med.* 8: 607–615.

16 Zambrano, S.S., Moussavi, M.S., and Spodick, D.H. (1974). QRS duration in chronic obstructive lung disease. *J. Electrocardiol.* 7: 35.

17 Abdelghany, M., Rogin, S., Siddharth, S., and Hani, K. (2017). Kounis Kounis syndrome: a review article on epidemiology, diagnostic findings, management and complications of allergic acute coronary syndrome. *Int. J. Cardiol.* 232 (2): 1–4.

18 Kularatne, K., Kannangare, T., Jayasena, A. et al. (2014). Fatal acute pulmonary oedema and acute renal failure following multiple wasp/hornet(Vespa affinis) stings in Sri Lanka:two case reports. *J. Med. Case Rep.* 8: 188.

19 Kogias, J.S., Sideris, S.K., and Anifadia, S.K. (2007). Kounis syndrome associated with hypersensitivity to hymenoptera stings. *Int. J. Cardiol.* 114 (2): 252–255.

20 Ettinger, P.O., Regan, T.J., and Oldewurtel, H.A. (1974). Hyperkalemia, cardiac conduction and the electrocardiogram: a review. *Am. Heart J.* 88: 360.

21 Surawicz, B. (1989). Is hypomagnesemia or magnesium deficiency arrhythmogenic? *J. Am. Coll. Cardiol.* 14: 1093.

22 DiCarlo, L.A., Morady, F., de Buitleir, M. et al. (1986). Effects of magnesium sulfate on cardiac conduction and refractoriness in humans. *J. Am. Coll. Cardiol.* 7: 1356.

23 Surawicz, B., Lepeschkin, E., and Herrlich, H.C. (1961). Low and high magnesium concentrations at various calcium levels: effect on the monophasic action potential, electrocardiogram, and contractility of isolated rabbit hearts. *Circ. Res.* 9: 811.

4

The Patient with Palpitations/Syncope

Natasha Wheaton[1], Emma Nash[2], and Jeffrey Brown[3]

[1] University of California-Los Angeles, Los Angeles, CA, USA
[2] Department of Anesthesiology, University of Nebraska, Omaha, Nebraska
[3] Unity Point Health, Rock Island, IL, USA

Palpitations are a common presenting symptom to the emergency department accounting for more than 684 000 visits per year [1]. Patients often describe these symptoms as a racing heart, a "flip-flopping or rising feeling," or a pounding sensation in the chest or neck. Many of these symptoms will ultimately be diagnosed as secondary to a benign cause, with up to 20% in an outpatient case series attributed to anxiety or panic disorder [2]. However, there are several life-threatening causes of palpitations that must be considered, including acute arrhythmias. In addition, there are subtle findings on resting ECG that may predispose patients to the development of a malignant arrhythmia. As many patients are asymptomatic at the time of their medical evaluation, it is important to be able to recognize these more subtle findings that indicate Brugada syndrome, Wolf-Parkinson-White syndrome (WPW), prolonged QTc syndrome, hypertrophic cardiomyopathy (HCM), and arrhythmogenic right ventricular dysplasia. Clinicians must maintain a high index of suspicion and screen every resting ECG for these five syndromes in order to identify the at-risk patients. With an overall combined estimated prevalence of 35/1000 for these disorders [3–7], over the course of an average 30-year career, clinicians will encounter more 2000 patients with these syndromes [8].

Supraventricular Tachycardia

Supraventricular tachycardia (SVT) arises from a point that is electro-physiologically above the ventricles. As such, these tachydysrhythmias typically produce a narrow complex QRS as the impulse travels through the bundle of His and subsequently into the ventricles. Here we will focus on AV nodal reentry tachycardia (AVNRT), the most common

of the SVT rhythms and also the arrhythmia most likely to occur in individuals with structurally normal hearts (Figure 4.4.1) [9].

AVNRT presents with a regular tachycardia that is typically 140–280 bmp with a narrow QRS complex. P waves are often absent, or when present are produced via retrograde conduction with the electrical signal traveling backward through the AV node, thereby leading to inversion in leads II, III, and aVF on the ECG (leads where P waves are typically upright). Additionally, the location of the P wave with respect to the QRS complex may provide additional information as to the dominant nodal electrical pathway, which ultimately allows further distinction between the types of AVNRT. Other ECG findings seen less frequently in SVT include diffuse ST segment depression and QRS alternans (Figure 4.4.2).

In summary, SVT is most readily identified on ECG by noting (i) narrow QRS complex; (ii) regular tachycardia; (iii) absent or retrograde P waves (inverted in the inferior leads); and with or without (iv) diffuse ST depression; and (v) QRS alternans.

Atrial Fibrillation

Atrial fibrillation is one of the most commonly encountered sustained arrhythmias, which is increasing in both incidence and prevalence as the population ages [10]. A patient experiencing symptomatic atrial fibrillation may report palpitations, syncope, dypsnea, or chest pain as the atria are no longer functioning to maintain a regular rhythm. Instead, the heart rate is irregular and may have aberrant beats produced either by the atria (as in atrial fibrillation with rapid ventricular response) or through an

Electrocardiogram in Clinical Medicine, First Edition. Edited by William J. Brady, Michael J. Lipinski, Andrew E. Darby, Michael C. Bond, Nathan P. Charlton, Korin Hudson, and Kelly Williamson.
© 2021 John Wiley & Sons Ltd. Published 2021 by John Wiley & Sons Ltd.

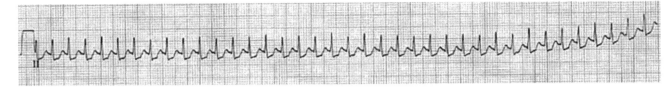

Figure 4.4.1 A typical example of Slow-Fast AVNRT. Note the rate of approximately 200 bpm, the narrow QRS complex, and diffuse ST depression. *Source:* Image reproduced with permission from http://lifeinthefastlane.com.

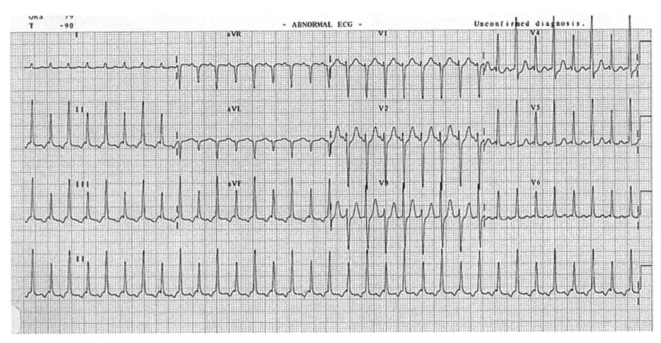

Figure 4.4.2 SVT with QRS Alternans. Note the ST depression in the lateral leads, retrograde P waves before the QRS complex (leads II, III, and aVF). *Source:* Image reproduced with permission from http://lifeinthefastlane.com.

accessory pathway (as in Wolf-Parkinson-White or Ashman's aberrancy) (Figure 4.4.3).

The hallmark of atrial fibrillation as seen on ECG is a lack of discrete P waves resulting from the disorganized nature of the atrial electrical activity. The QRS complex will remain narrow, though there may be several QRS morphologies found in the same 12-lead ECG. Additionally, the rhythm will be irregularly irregular, as the atria are no longer effectively setting the ventricular rate. Finally, there may be low amplitude fibrillations, typically seen in V1, though these are not always present.

In summary, the key findings to identify atrial fibrillation on an ECG are (i) absence of discrete P waves; (ii) irregularly irregular rhythm; (iii) narrow QRS complexes; and possibly (iv) low amplitude fibrillatory waves in V1; and (v) multiple morphologies of the QRS complex. The ventricular response can either be fast, normal, or slow, depending on how many of the atrial fibrillatory impulses are conducted through the AV node (Figure 4.4.4).

Multifocal Atrial Tachycardia

Multifocal atrial tachycardia (MAT) is an ECG finding most commonly seen in patients with severe underlying lung disease and is a poor prognostic indicator (Figure 4.4.5) [11]. Cor pulmonale leads to right atrial dilation that ultimately results in increased atrial automaticity and MAT. Though the exact mechanism remains unclear, increased atrial automaticity induces ectopic foci of electrical activity and atrial activation, resulting in one of the key ECG findings: multiple (at least three) distinct P-wave morphologies. Other key features include tachycardia (>100 bpm) and an irregularly irregular rhythm. The ECG may also reveal evidence of right heart strain in the setting of cor pulmonale, which is discussed more in detail in the previous chapter, but including right axis deviation (the QRS complex is primarily negative in lead I and positive in lead aVF) and right ventricular hypertrophy (dominant R wave in V1 and dominant S wave in V6).

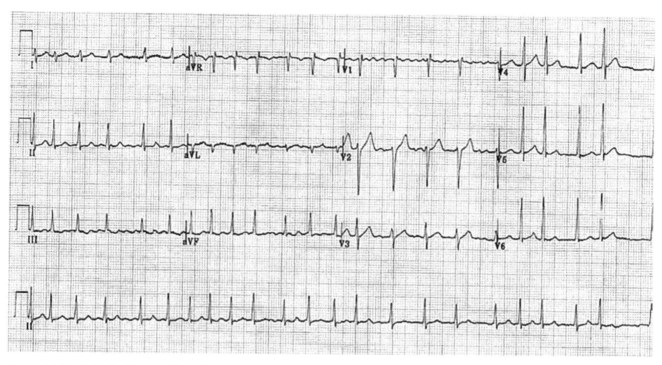

Figure 4.4.3 Atrial fibrillation with rapid ventricular response. Note the narrow complex irregular tachycardia with a rate of approximately 135 bpm. P waves are absent in all leads, though there are fine fibrillations in V1. *Source:* Image reproduced with permission from http://lifeinthefastlane.com.

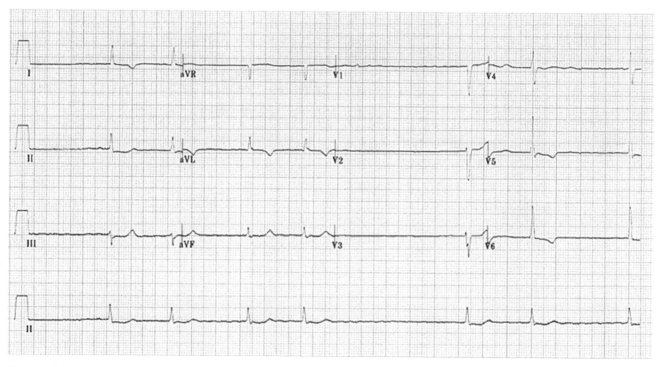

Figure 4.4.4 Atrial fibrillation with slow ventricular response, which may be seen in patients on AV nodal-blocking pharmacologic agents (including digoxin), hypothermia, patients with a dysfunctional AV node and less commonly in certain poisonings (i.e. "mad honey poisoning") [12]. *Source:* Image reproduced with permission from http://lifeinthefastlane.com.

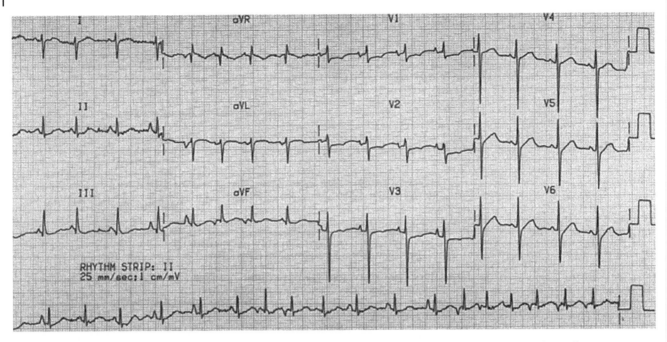

Figure 4.4.5 Multifocal atrial tachycardia. Note the varying P-wave morphologies in lead II as well as the tachycardic rate (approximately 115 bpm) and irregularly irregular rhythm. *Source:* Image reproduced with permission from http://lifeinthefastlane.com.

In summary, the key findings of MAT are (i) tachycardia; (ii) at least three distinct P wave morphologies; and (iii) an irregularly irregular rhythm.

Conduction Blocks

A conduction block describes an electrical impulse that is properly initiated by the atria but fails to produce a regular, sustained ventricular rhythm. As this chapter focuses on ECG findings in patients presenting with palpitations or syncope, we will focus primarily on second- and third-degree heart blocks, as these are more likely to be symptomatic.

Second-degree heart blocks are defined by intermittently transmitted atrial impulses and are further distinguished as Mobitz I and Mobitz II heart blocks. In Mobitz I heart block (Figure 4.4.6) the AV node fails to conduct impulses to the ventricles in a specific pattern: the PR interval gradually increases until there is failed conduction entirely, represented by the absence of a resultant QRS complex. This "dropped beat" typically occurs in a pattern, such as 3 : 2, where for every three P waves there are only two QRS complexes. The primary features on ECG are a gradually increasing PR interval and the ultimate absence of a QRS complex despite a P wave being present.

The Mobitz I pattern may be secondary to both reversible and nonreversible causes, which affect the conduction of atrial impulses through the AV node, including medications, vagal tone, inflammation, or a myocardial infarction (particularly inferior MI) [13].

The second type of second-degree heart block known as Mobitz II, in which there are intermittent P waves with failed ventricular conduction, though the PR interval remains constant and the dropped beats do not follow a regular pattern (Figure 4.4.7). The ECG findings of Mobitz II will show a regular and consistent PR interval when the QRS is present, intermittent absence of the QRS complex, and a regular, sustained rate at which the P waves are produced. The QRS complex is typically narrow as the block often occurs below the AV node. However, if the block occurs distal to the bundle of His, then the QRS complex will be wide [14].

Patients determined to have a Mobitz II rhythm on ECG are at high risk for progression to complete heart block and sudden cardiac death, thereby warranting admission to cardiology for further evaluation and pacemaker placement.

In third-degree heart block, also described as complete heart block, there is complete discordance between the atrial and ventricular rhythms (Figure 4.4.8). None of the impulses originating from the atria are conducted in a normal fashion to the ventricles, thereby creating a high risk for sudden cardiac death. On ECG, there is a regular atrial rhythm and a regular ventricular rhythm which is completely independent of the atrial rhythm. Any patient found to be in complete heart block warrants immediate cardiology consultation and admission [15].

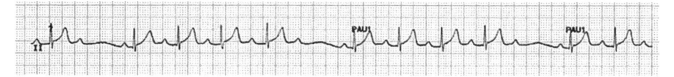

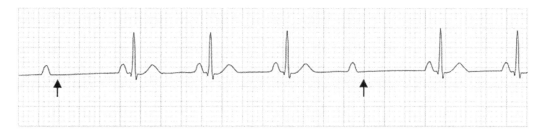

Figure 4.4.6 Second-degree AV block, Mobitz I (Wenckebach Phenomenon). Note the 5:4 pattern, in which there are five P waves with only four QRS complexes. *Source:* Image reproduced with permission from http://lifeinthefastlane.com.

Figure 4.4.7 Second-degree AV block, Mobitz II. Note the sustained P wave rate, consistent PR intervals, and intermittently dropped QRS complexes. *Source:* Image reproduced with permission from http://lifeinthefastlane.com.

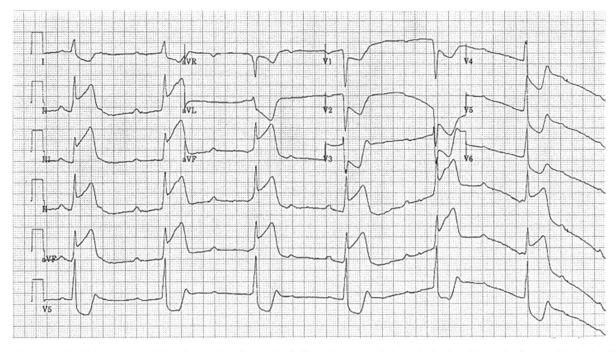

Figure 4.4.8 Third-degree AV block, complete heart block. Note that the atrial rate (calculated from the P waves) is in the 1980s, while the ventricular rate is approximately 40 with no clear pattern between the atrial and ventricular rhythms. In this patient, the third-degree block is resulting from the acute inferior myocardial infarction. *Source:* Image reproduced with permission from http://lifeinthefastlane.com.

The Big 5: Identifying Predisposing Risk for Malignant Arrhythmia on Resting ECG

At this point, we will transition to the more subtle ECG findings that may predispose a patient to the development of a malignant arrhythmia. Any patient presenting with palpitations or syncope should have their ECG scrutinized for these potentially fatal five diagnoses: Brugada syndrome, HCM, WPW, prolonged QTc, and arrhythmogenic right ventricular dysplasia.

Brugada Syndrome

Brugada syndrome is an autosomal dominant genetic disorder that can result in sudden cardiac death from ventricular tachycardia or ventricular fibrillation. In a retrospective study of 104 symptomatic patients presenting with Brugada syndrome, 73% were in ventricular fibrillation and 27% presented with syncope [16]. Brugada syndrome was originally described as a sinus rhythm with right bundle branch block (RBBB), normal QT interval, and ST elevation in V1–V3 in those presenting with sudden ventricular arrhythmia or cardiac arrest [17]. Further study discovered the pattern is actually a pseudo-RBBB, as the S wave is not widened as in a standard RBBB. Of note, the ST elevation creates a dome shape if combined with a T-wave inversion (Figure 4.4.9) or a saddleback-shaped with an upright or positive T wave.

Brugada syndrome is far more common in males than females, is more common in those of Asian descent, and typically presents in the fourth or fifth decade of life. A symptomatic presentation can be incited by illicit drug use, certain medications, electrolyte abnormalities, ischemia, and fever. Any symptomatic patient with a Brugada pattern on resting ECG should be admitted for further workup by electrophysiology and evaluation for placement of an implantable cardioverter-defibrillator.

Hypertrophic Cardiomyopathy

HCM is the leading cause of sudden cardiac death in people under the age of 35 and should be considered in the young patient with exertional syncope, chest pain, or palpitations [18]. Similar to Brugada syndome, HCM has a genetic predisposition and can incite malignant arrhythmias, though while Brugada syndrome is purely an electrical abnormality, the arrhythmias in HCM result from underlying structural abnormalities. While the ECG in patients with HCM may be normal in approximately 6% of patients [18], the typical findings, including narrow and deep ("dagger-like") Q waves in the lateral and inferior leads (Figure 4.4.10). Other common findings include signs of an enlarged left atrium indicated by a biphasic P wave, inverted T waves in inferior and lateral leads, and evidence of left ventricular hypertrophy (Figure 4.4.11). Patients with ECG concerning for HCM need an echocardiogram to further characterize their heart structure and should refrain from any physical activity until that time.

Wolf-Parkinson-White Syndrome

WPW is a preexcitation syndrome caused by an accessory electrical pathway that is present at birth (Figure 4.4.12). Although isolated cases had previously been reported, WPW was termed after the 1930 publication describing 11 cases of tachycardia associated with a bundle branch block and short PR interval. The electrophysiology of this syndrome is quite complicated, but in short, the accessory pathway allows the creation of an electrical circuit that bypasses the AV node, decreasing the time between atrial

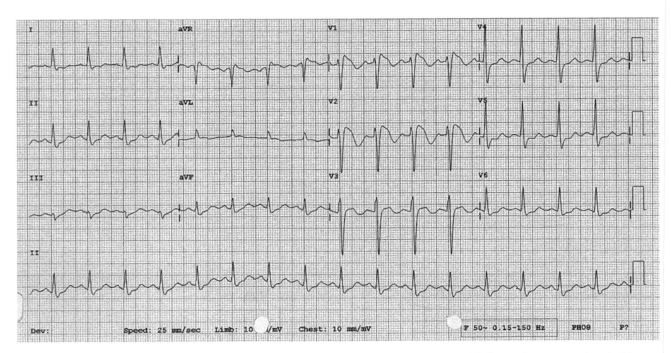

Figure 4.4.9 Brugada pattern on resting ECG. Note the dome-shaped ST segments in V1 and V2. *Source:* Image reproduced with permission from http://lifeinthefastlane.com.

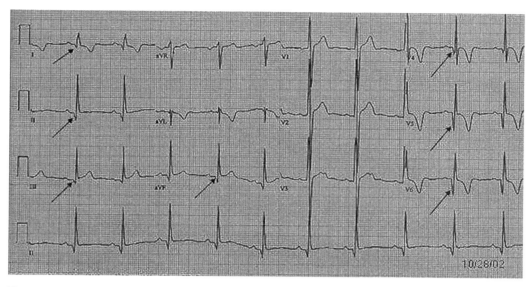

Figure 4.4.10 HCM. Note the narrow and deep Q waves in the inferior and lateral leads. *Source:* Image reproduced with permission from http://lifeinthefastlane.com.

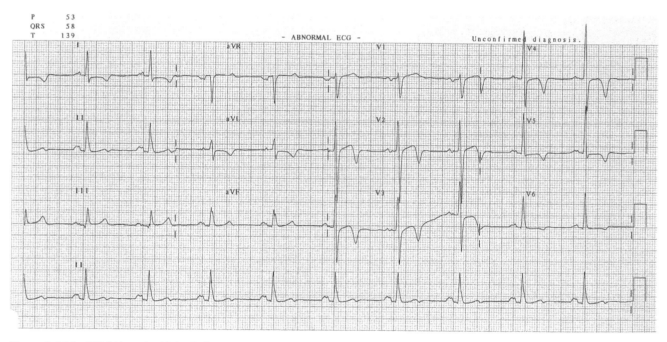

Figure 4.4.11 HCM. Note the biphasic P wave, inverted T waves in the lateral leads, and LVH. *Source:* Image reproduced with permission from http://lifeinthefastlane.com.

and ventricular depolarization, and thereby shortening the PR interval. The premature excitation of the ventricles is seen on the ECG as a "delta wave," a slurred upstroke to the QRS complex, which makes the QRS complex appear widened [19]. However, not every beat on the ECG demonstrates the delta wave, as some beats may be conducted in the traditional manner [20].

WPW predisposes patients to development of arrhythmias as the electrical conduction bypasses the AV node via the accessory pathway, thereby transmitting all atrial signals to the ventricles. SVT is the most commonly encountered arrhythmia, but patients may also experience malignant atrial fibrillation with a wide complex QRS (Figure 4.4.13). These patients should not be given AV

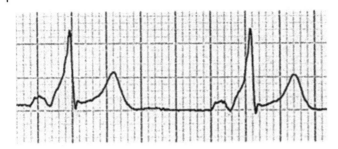

Figure 4.4.12 WPW. Note the shortened PR interval and the delta wave. *Source:* Image reproduced with permission from http://lifeinthefastlane.com.

nodal blocking agents such as diltiazem or beta blockers, as this may trigger ventricular fibrillation.

Long QT Syndrome

The QT interval is measured from the start of the QRS complex to the completion of the T wave and captures both the depolarization and repolarization of the ventricles. While there is some overlap between normal variants and a pathologic long QT interval [21], the typically accepted cutoff is 450 ms for men and 470 ms [22]. Long QT syndrome can be congenital or acquired; the acquired version may result from medications, structural or electrical heart disease, and electrolyte abnormalities including hypokalemia, hypomagnesemia and hypocalcemia. If a provider identifies a long QT interval in a patient with a concerning history, this finding should prompt telemetry admission for further evaluation. In addition, providers must avoid administering medications that are known to prolong the QT interval in patients at risk for long QT syndrome, including those prone to electrolyte abnormalities and those on psychotropic medications; please see Table 7.4.5 in chapter 7 of this section for a list of medications that prolong the QT interval [23]. In these patient populations, it is prudent to order a screening ECG before the administration of medications that could further prolong the QT interval.

Patients with a prolonged QT interval are at risk for developing polymorphic ventricular tachycardia, otherwise known as torsades de pointes (TdP), which occurs when the T wave of the preceding beat encroaches on the subsequent QRS complex, known as the "R on T" phenomena (Figure 4.4.14). In TdP, the resultant QRS complexes vary in amplitude, axis, and duration and appear to "twist" around the isoelectric line resulting from the multiple ventricular foci of electrical activation. TdP with heart rates >220 bpm are particularly prone to degeneration into ventricular fibrillation.

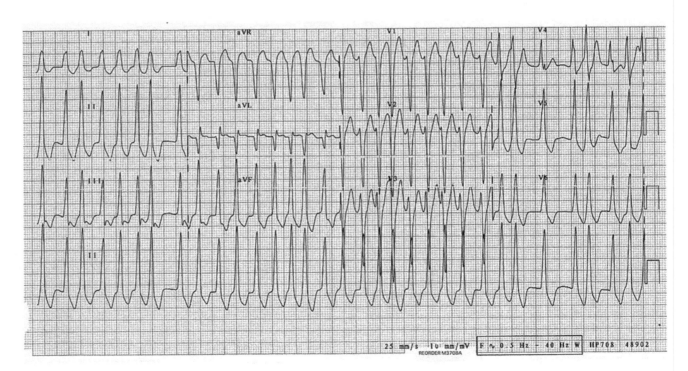

Figure 4.4.13 Wide complex atrial fibrillation in a patient with underlying WPW. *Source:* Image reproduced with permission from http://lifeinthefastlane.com.

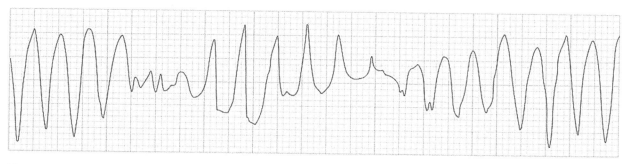

Figure 4.4.14 Torsades de pointes. Note the QRS complexes that vary in morphology and "twist" around the isoelectric line. *Source:* Image reproduced with permission from http://lifeinthefastlane.com.

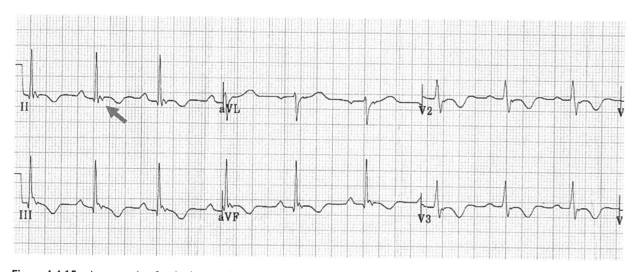

Figure 4.4.15 An example of arrhythmogenic right ventricular dysplasia. Note the deep T-wave inversions in the precordial leads shown (V2, V3), as well as the small epsilon wave just after the QRS complex indicated by the red arrow. *Source:* Reproduced with permission from http://Lifeinthefastlane.com.

Arrhythmogenic Right Ventricular Dysplasia

Arrhythmogenic right ventricular cardiomyopathy, also known as arrhythmogenic right ventricular dysplasia, is a genetically determined disorder characterized by the replacement of right-sided myocardium with fibro-fatty tissue, which ultimately disrupts normal electrical conduction leading to heart failure, arrhythmia and death [24]. Symptoms, ranging from palpitations, lightheadedness, syncope, and sudden death, typically present during strenuous activity; this condition is the second leading cause of sudden cardiac death in people under 35 [25]. This diagnosis can be particularly challenging as the resting ECG is often normal and diagnosis relies on imaging studies, tissue biopsy, and family history [26]. If present, ECG abnormalities include inverted T waves in the precordial leads, conduction abnormalities including *epsilon waves* (a small "blip" between the end of the QRS and the T wave), or isolated QRS widening in V2. If the patient presents with an arrhythmia, it is classically a ventricular tachycardia with a left bundle branch block (LBBB).

As evidenced in Figure 4.4.15, the characteristic epsilon wave of ARVD can be incredible subtle, further reinforcing the need to examine the ECG in every patient presenting with palpitations or syncope for findings that can predispose to a malignant arrhythmia.

References

1 Probst, M.A., Mower, W.R., Kanzaria, H.K. et al. (2014 May 15). Analysis of emergency department visits for palpitations. *Am. J. Cardiol.* 113 (10): 1685–1690.

2 Barsky, A.J. (2001). Palpitations, arrhythmias and awareness of cardiac activity. *Ann. Intern. Med.* 134 (9 pt 2): 932–937.

3 Lu, C.W., Wu, M.H., Chen, H.C. et al. (2014 Jul 1). Epidemiological profile of Wolf-Parkinson-White syndrome in a general population younger than 50 years of age in the era of radiofrequency catheter ablation. *Int. J. Cardiol.* 174 (3): 530–534. https://doi.org/10.1016/j.ijcard.2014.04.134. Epub 2014 Apr 21. (WPW).

4 Semsarian, C., Ingles, J., Maron, M.S., and Maron, B.J. (2015 Mar 31). New perspective on the prevalence of hypertrophic cardiomyopathy. *J. Am. Coll. Cardiol.* 65 (12): 1249–1254. https://doi.org/10.1016/j.jacc.2015.01.019. (HCM).

5 Viskin, S. (2009 May). The QT interval: too long, too short or just right. *Heart Rhythm.* 6 (5): 711–715. Epub 2009 Mar 3. (prolonged QTc).

6 Romero, J., Mejia-Lopez, E., Manrique, C., and Lucariello, R. (2013). Arrhythmogenic right ventricular cardiomyopathy (ARVC/D): a systematic literature review. *Clin. Med. Insights. Cardiol.* 7: 97–114.

7 Brugada. UptoDate. http://www.uptodate.com (accessed May 15, 2017).

8 Collins, M. (August 2009). *Staffing an ED Appropriately and Efficiently*. ACEP News.

9 Fox, D.J., Tischenko, A., Krahn, A.D. et al. (2008 Dec). Supraventricular tachycardia: diagnosis and management. *Mayo Clin. Proc.* 83 (12): 1400–1411. PMID: 19046562.

10 Medi, C., Hankey, G.J., and Freedman, S.B. (2007 Feb 19). Atrial fibrillation. *Med. J. Aust.* 186 (4): 197–202. PMID: 17309423.

11 McCord, J. and Borzak, S. (1998 Jan). Multifocal atrial tachycardia. *Chest* 13 (1): 203–209.

12 Osken, A., Yaylaci, S. et al. (2012 Jul-Sep). Slow ventricular response atrial fibrillation related to mad honey poisoning. *J. Cardiovasc. Dis. Res.* 3 (3): 245–247.

13 Sauers, W.H. Second degree atrioventricular block: Mobitz type I (Wenckebach block). 2019. UptoDate. https://www.uptodate.com/home/about-us.

14 Sauers, W.H.Second degree atrioventricular block: Mobitz type II. 2019. UptoDate. https://www.uptodate.com/contents/second-degree-atrioventricular-block-mobitz-type-ii.

15 Paulk, E.A. et al. Complete heart block in acute myocardial infarction. *Am. J. Cardiol.* 17 (5): 695–706.

16 Littmann, L., Monroe, M.H., Kerns, W.P. 2nd et al. (2003 May). Brugada syndrome and "Brugada sign": clinical spectrum with a guide for the clinician. *Am. Heart J.* 145 (5): 768–778.

17 Brugada, P. and Brugada, J. (1992 Nov 15). Right bundle branch block, persistent ST segment elevation and sudden cardiac death: a distinct clinical and electrocardiographic syndrome. A multicenter report. *J. Am. Coll. Cardiol.* 20 (6): 1391–1396.

18 McLeod, C.J., Ackerman, M.J., Nishimura, R.A. et al. (2009-07-14). Outcome of patients with hypertrophic cardiomyopathy and a normal electrocardiogram. *J. Am. Coll. Cardiol.* 54 (3): 229–233.

19 Wolff, L., Parkinson, J., and White, P.D. (2006). Bundle-branch block with short P-R interval in healthy young people prone to paroxysmal tachycardia. *Ann. Noninvasive Electrocardiol.* 11: 340–353.

20 Kiger, M., McCanta, A., Tong, S. et al. (2016). Intermittent versus persistent Wolf-Parkinson-White syndrome in children: electrophysiologic properties and clinical outcomes. *Pacing Clin. Electrophysiol.* 39 (1): 14–20.

21 Al-Khatib, S.M., Allen LaPointe, N.M., Kramer, J.M., and Califf, R.M. (2003). What clinicians should know about the QT interval. *JAMA* 289 (16): 2120–2127.

22 Viskin, S. (2009-05-01). The QT interval: too long, too short or just right. *Heart Rhythm.* 6 (5): 711–715.

23 Hafermann, M., Namdar, R., and Page, S.G.e.R. (2011). Effect of intravenous ondansetron on QT interval prolongation in patients with cardiovascular disease and additional risk factors for torsades: a prospective, observational study. *Drug Healthc. Patient Saf.* 3: 53–58.

24 Sen-Chowdhry, S., Lowe, M.D., Sporton, S.C., and McKenna, W.J. (2004). Arrhythmogenic right ventricular cardiomyopathy: clinical presentation, diagnosis, and management. *Am. J. Med.* 117 (9): 685–695.

25 Anderson, E. (2006 April 15). Arrhythmogenic right ventricular dysplasia. *Am. Fam. Physician* 73 (8): 1391–1398.

26 Marcus, F.I., McKenna, W.J., Sherrill, D. et al. (2010). Diagnosis of arrythmogenic right ventricular cardiomyopathy/dysplasia: proposed modification of the task force criteria. *Circulation* 121: 1533.

5

The Patient with Preoperative Evaluation

Sarah Chuzi, Jane Wilcox, and Lisa B. Van Wagner

Northwestern University Feinberg School of Medicine, Chicago, IL, USA

Introduction

Electrocardiography is commonly performed as part of a patient's preoperative risk assessment. The prognostic significance of the preoperative electrocardiogram (ECG), however, is unclear. In certain populations of patients, including those with known coronary artery disease (CAD), arrhythmia, peripheral arterial disease (PAD), cerebrovascular disease, structural heart disease, or in patients who are undergoing high-risk surgical procedures, the preoperative ECG may provide useful baseline and prognostic information [1, 2]. In contrast, studies suggest that routine preoperative ECG is of limited value in predicting postoperative complications after low or intermediate risk noncardiac surgery in patients without significant cardiac disease [3–5]. This chapter will review the indications to obtain a preoperative ECG and the significance of the various ECG abnormalities that physicians are most likely to encounter during the routine preoperative evaluation of the asymptomatic patient prior to noncardiac surgery.

Indications

While a number of task forces have published recommendations on the indications for preoperative ECG, the updated American College of Cardiology (ACC)/American Heart Association (AHA) and European Society of Cardiology (ESC)/European Society of Anesthesiology (ESA) guidelines from 2014 are the most widely utilized [6, 7]. A suggested algorithm for determining which patients should undergo preoperative electrocardiography is depicted in Figure 4.5.1. In addition, symptoms of heart disease, such as chest pain, dyspnea, and palpitations, should prompt physicians to perform an ECG regardless of the cardiac risk of upcoming procedure. For asymptomatic patients, the decision to perform an ECG should be based on the level of surgical risk inherent to the procedure [6] (Table 4.5.1) and on the presence or absence of cardiac risk factors. It should be noted that current guidelines and recommendations are based primarily on expert opinion and low-level evidence, and therefore the decision to order an ECG should also be individualized.

Common ECG Abnormalities

Left Ventricular Hypertrophy

Left ventricular hypertrophy (LVH) is a common electrocardiographic finding in patients with and without known cardiac disease. While a number of criteria for LVH have been proposed, general ECG findings of LVH include increased QRS voltage, increased QRS duration, left axis deviation, repolarization (ST-T) changes, and left atrial enlargement or abnormality (Figure 4.5.2) [8]. In particular, ST-T changes, or repolarization abnormalities that were previously known as "strain" pattern, are indicative of greater left ventricular mass and are more common in patients with LVH and concomitant CAD [9]. The characteristic strain pattern is a slight ST segment depression followed by a broadly inverted T wave, which is usually best seen in leads with tall R-waves (Figure 4.5.3). The presence of ST-T wave abnormalities in LVH is a poor prognostic sign that is associated with increased risk of cardiovascular death, myocardial infarction, and stroke compared with patients without strain [10].

LVH is a common finding among adults, particularly those with hypertension, and is associated with increased incidence of heart failure, reduced ejection fraction, sudden cardiac death, and ventricular arrhythmias [11–13].

Electrocardiogram in Clinical Medicine, First Edition. Edited by William J. Brady, Michael J. Lipinski, Andrew E. Darby, Michael C. Bond, Nathan P. Charlton, Korin Hudson, and Kelly Williamson.

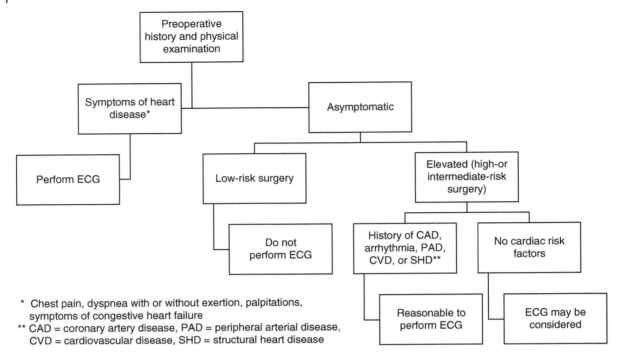

Figure 4.5.1 Indications for preoperative ECG based on the 2014 ACC/AHA and ESC/ESA guidelines.

Table 4.5.1 Cardiac risk stratification for noncardiac surgical procedures.

Surgical risk	Definition	Examples
Elevated (high- or intermediate-risk)	Reported risk of cardiac death or MI is ≥1%	Major vascular surgery Peripheral artery surgery Orthopedic surgery Intraperitoneal surgery Intrathoracic surgery Carotid endarterectomy
Low-risk	Reported risk of cardiac death or MI is <1%	Plastic surgery Cataract surgery Endoscopic surgery Superficial procedures

Importantly, the degree of cardiovascular risk conferred by the increased left ventricular mass is independent of the degree of blood pressure elevation [13], and physicians should be mindful of this when evaluating patients who are either normotensive in clinic or whose LVH seems out of proportion to their hypertension.

Many studies have identified LVH as a strong independent predictor of postoperative myocardial ischemia and adverse events. The most compelling data for this association is from studies conducted in high-risk patients, including those who have CAD or who are at high risk for developing CAD [14], or who are undergoing major vascular surgery [15]. It should be noted, however, that

several other studies have failed to demonstrate an association between LVH and poor outcomes [4, 16, 17]; however, these studies were either smaller in size or limited to younger, healthier patients undergoing lower risk procedures.

Note that many patients with severe LVH develop QRS widening and ST-T changes that resemble a left bundle branch block (LBBB). Physicians should look for the broad notched or slurred R wave in leads I, aVL, V5, and V6 that is characteristic of LBBB to help distinguish this and LVH with QRS widening [8].

Conduction Abnormalities

Atrioventricular (AV) Conduction Delays

Low-grade conduction abnormalities – first-degree and second-degree type I (Wenckebach) AV block – are not uncommon among asymptomatic individuals [18, 19]. In contrast, high-grade cardiac conduction abnormalities, such as second-degree type II or complete atrioventricular block, may increase operative risk and need for temporary or permanent transvenous pacing in the perioperative period [20]. Thus, patients presenting with these arrhythmias during the preoperative evaluation should be promptly referred to a cardiologist or the emergency room, especially if they have associated symptoms of lightheadedness. In contrast, the surgical risk conferred by the less significant conduction disturbances is less clear as few studies have addressed this question. This section

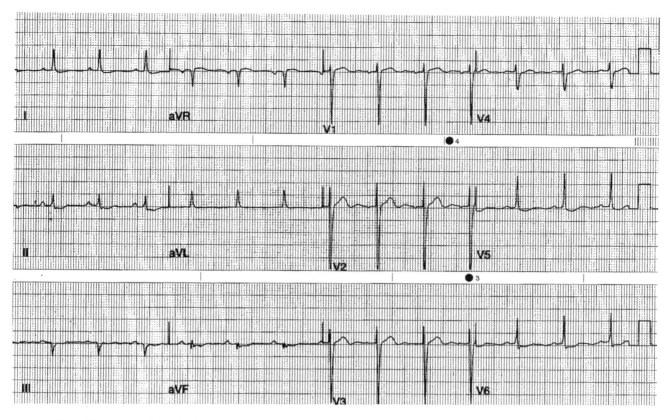

Figure 4.5.2   ECG showing LVH with increased voltages, without strain pattern present.

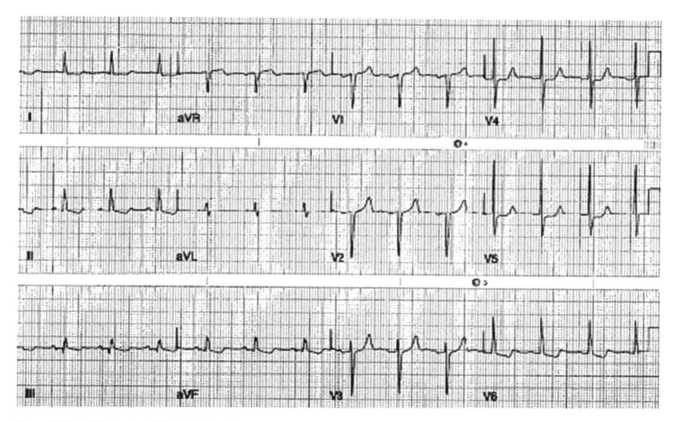

Figure 4.5.3   ECG showing LVH with LV strain pattern.

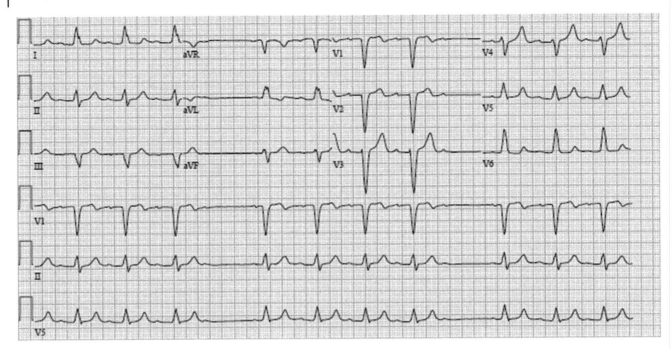

Figure 4.5.4 LBBB with characteristic-wide QRS, wide QS complex in V1, and wide R wave in V6. ST segments are opposite the main vector of the QRS complex.

will focus on the identification and clinical significance of these two rhythms.

First-degree AV block is characterized by PR interval prolongation, with a uniformly prolonged PR interval greater than 200 ms. There is no evidence that first-degree AV block predicts postoperative cardiac complications among individuals undergoing noncardiac surgery [4]. Even in patients who have chronic bifascicular block or complete LBBB (see Figure 4.5.4), an additional first degree AV block does not increase the incidence of severe bradyarrhythmias or the need for pacemaker postoperatively [21]. When detected during the preoperative evaluation, no specific therapy or further evaluation is required. If the patient is taking medications that increase vagal tone and decrease conduction through the AV node, such as beta blockers, the dose of medication may be decreased or stopped if the drug is not essential [22].

In second-degree type I AV block, the AV node becomes increasingly refractory with each stimulus from the atria, ultimately resulting in a "dropped QRS" whereby the atrial stimulus is not conducted at all [8]. The characteristic ECG signature of Wenckebach is progressive lengthening of the QRS from beat to beat until a QRS complex is dropped, thereby producing a pattern of *grouped beating* (Figure 4.5.5).

Physicians should be cautious, however, not to mistake second-degree AV block for the group beating seen with atrial premature beats. In the former, nonconducted P waves come "on time" while in the latter the p waves come "early" (Figure 4.5.6).

As in first-degree block, second-degree AV block type I portends a benign prognosis and in most cases will not necessitate further evaluation when encountered during the pre-operative evaluation. Recall, however, that symptomatic AV block of any kind is an indication for permanent pacing [23]. A thorough history and review of systems should be undertaken when these rhythms are encountered.

Ventricular Conduction Abnormalities – Bundle Branch Blocks

Left and right bundle branch blocks (RBBB) are the result of conduction delays in the left- and right-sided intraventricular conduction systems, respectively. They cause characteristic changes in the QRS complex and ST-T wave (Figures 4.5.4 and 4.5.7). Diagnostic criteria for both LBBB and RBBB require that the QRS duration be greater than 120 ms. More modest prolongation of the QRS (100–119 ms) is referred to as an incomplete bundle. In both LBBB and RBBB, there is appropriate discordance between the ST segments and T waves and the main vector of the QRS complex (in LBBB) or the terminal mean spatial QRS vector (in RBBB). When T-wave inversions are discordant, meaning they cannot be explained solely on the basis of the bundle branch block, a primary abnormality such as ischemia should be suspected.

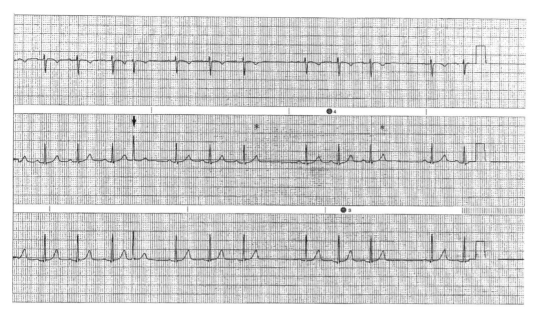

Figure 4.5.5 Second-degree type I AV block with characteristic grouped beating.

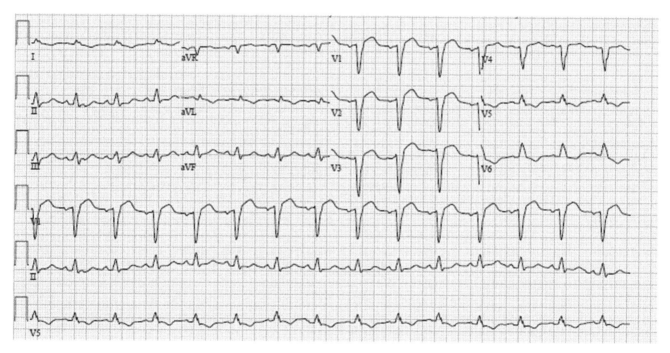

Figure 4.5.6 Sinus rhythm with one conducted atrial premature beat (ê) and nonconducted atrial premature beats (shown with *) leading to a grouped beating pattern.

LBBB, which occurs in fewer than 1% of the overall population but in more than one third of patients with heart failure, has been associated with an increased risk of morbidity and mortality from infarction, heart failure, and arrhythmias in nonsurgical patients, as well as an increased risk of sudden death (relative risk = 2.7) [24]. Among patients with CAD, LBBB correlates with more extensive disease and increased mortality compared to those without a block [25]. In contrast, RBBB is a more common finding in the general population. This condition occasionally occurs in healthy patients, but more often is seen in those with organic heart disease. It often portends a more benign prognosis than LBBB. In patients without underlying cardiac disease, RBBB is generally

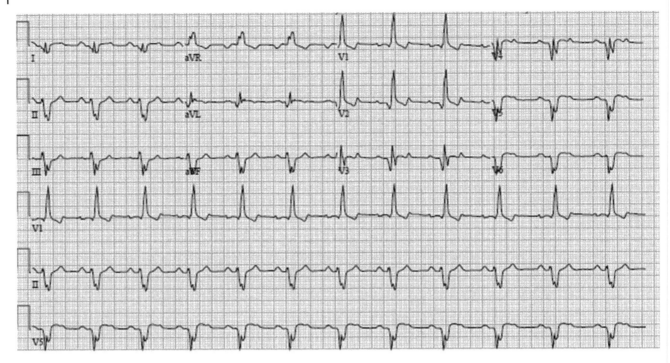

Figure 4.5.7 RBBB with characteristic wide QRS, wide rSR' complex in V1, and qRS complex in V6. ST segments are opposite the terminal deflection of the QRS complex.

not associated with an increased risk of morbidity or mortality [24], however patients with RBBB may have increased right ventricular (RV) size and reduced RV function [26].

The preoperative significance of bundle branch blocks is uncertain. In one study of all patients undergoing noncardiac surgery who were seen at a preoperative testing center, LBBB was associated with an increased risk for death postoperatively compared with controls (OR 6.0, 95% CI 1.2–100) and with RBBB (OR 8.7, 95% CI 1.2–100), however none of the patients in this study died from cardiovascular complications [27]. Another large study looking at a similar population found that the identification of preoperative RBBB and LBBB was associated with postoperative myocardial infarction and death, but did not improve prediction of poor outcomes beyond risk factors (history of ischemic heart disease and high risk surgery) noted on patient interview [28]. Other studies have found no association between preexisting bundle branch blocks and postoperative mortality, need for pacemaker, or adverse cardiac events [3–5, 29]. Clearly the data on this subject is conflicting. Importantly, physicians should be aware that the presence of a BBB, especially LBBB, is often a sign of underlying cardiac disease, and therefore should direct referral to specialist care and further diagnostic testing based on risk factors and symptomatology.

Nonspecific ST-T Changes

Nonspecific ST-T changes commonly occur on ECGs. The types of abnormalities are varied but usually refer to a slight ST-segment depression or T wave inversion or flattening in the absence of a convincing clinical history or symptoms. These changes can be diffuse or may be isolated to contiguous leads, such as the inferior, lateral, or anterior leads. These subtle repolarization abnormalities are often benign, especially in low risk patients, or represent conditions such as ischemia, drug effects, hyperventilation, or electrolyte abnormalities. Interestingly, despite being termed *nonspecific,* these abnormalities have been associated with significant increases in age-adjusted risk of CAD, cardiovascular disease, and total mortality over long-term follow up in middle-aged men and women without known heart disease [30]. Despite this potential increased long-term risk, nonspecific ST-T wave abnormalities on preoperative ECG are not associated with increased morbidity or mortality postoperatively [31], including among older patients [4] and those with known CAD [32].

Pathologic Q Waves

A Q wave is any negative deflection that precedes the R wave in the QRS complex, but physicians should be familiar

Table 4.5.2 Criteria for pathologic Q waves.

Limb leads		Precordial leads	
Lead	Criteria for abnormal	Lead	Criteria for abnormal
I	≥0.03 sec	V1	Any Q
II	≥0.03 sec	V2	Any Q
III	None	V3	Any Q
aVR	None	V4	≥0.02 sec
aVL	≥0.03 sec	V5	≥0.03 sec
aVF	≥0.03 sec	V6	≥0.03 sec

with the commonly accepted criteria for *pathologic* Q waves [33] (Table 4.5.2). Importantly, the presence of a pathologic Q wave does not indicate any specific electrophysiologic mechanism; rather, Q waves can be related to a number of factors that lead to sufficient loss of regional electrical force. This includes but is not limited to physiologic or positional factors (as in the normal variant "septal" Q waves), acute processes such as myocardial ischemia or myocarditis, infiltrative processes that lead to replacement of myocardial tissue with electrically silent tissue (e.g. amyloid or fibrosis), ventricular hypertrophy or enlargement, or conduction abnormalities such as LBBB or Wolf-Parkinson-White (WPW). As such, the clinical history in a patient with pathologic Q waves on ECG is extremely important.

The significance of preoperative Q waves on ECG is controversial and inconsistent across studies, though it may be relevant for patients undergoing major noncardiac surgery. In an analysis of 4315 patients undergoing elective major noncardiac procedures, pathologic Q waves on ECG were associated with a 2.4-fold increased risk for perioperative events [31]. However, it is unclear if this increased risk could have been identified based on history of cardiac ischemia alone. Other studies in the literature have identified similar associations between preoperative Q waves and postoperative cardiac events [5], but this association has not been demonstrated consistently across studies [1, 4, 15, 32]. It is undetermined whether Q waves portend additional risk for patients without known CAD.

QT/QTc Prolongation

The QT interval, which is measured from the beginning of the QRS complex to the end of the T wave, represents ventricular repolarization. The QT should be measured in the ECG lead that shows the longest intervals [8]. Because the QT interval varies with different heart rates, the rate-corrected QT or QTc is used to standardize and compare QT values over time at different heart rates. The finding of a prolonged QT/QTc interval as determined by computer interpretation should always be rechecked manually. There are multiple formulas used to estimate QTc, but the Bazett formula ($QTc = QT/\sqrt{RR}$) is most commonly and widely used due to its simplicity [34].

Studies have shown that a prolonged QTc interval not only places patients at risk for potentially lethal ventricular arrhythmias, but also predicts peri- and postoperative cardiovascular events and therefore this ECG characteristic should be examined closely prior to surgery [35]. The degree of QTc prolongation that confers higher risk is not consistent across studies, but it does appear that the higher the value the greater risk the patient is at for cardiac events. Mean QTc of >440 ms has been shown to be an independent predictor of postoperative major cardiovascular events [2, 36]. Further, Biteker et al. determined that every 10 ms increase in QTc was related to a 13% increase for perioperative events [36]. Other studies have shown that QTc >500 is significantly related to adverse events [37]. If a lengthened QT/QTc is discovered on a preoperative ECG, a thorough review of the patient's medications should be performed to look for offending agents, electrolytes should be checked, and referral to cardiology or alerting of the surgeon should be done.

Conclusion

In summary, the indications for preoperative ECG, the prognostic significance of abnormal findings in asymptomatic patients on such ECG, and the recommended subsequent evaluation of these findings are all uncertain. It is our opinion that a detailed history must be taken, including probing for any subtle symptoms of cardiovascular disease. Experts agree that patients with symptoms of cardiac disease should undergo ECG, and that obtaining ECG in patients with significant cardiac disease who are undergoing high- or intermediate-risk surgery is reasonable to improve risk stratification. However, further studies are needed so that stronger recommendations about the indications for preoperative ECG can be made. Once the preoperative ECG has been obtained, physicians must determine whether an abnormal finding is significant enough to alter the surgical risk/benefit ratio. Table 4.5.3 summarizes the ECG abnormalities discussed in this chapter. Importantly, decisions regarding further workup of abnormal ECG findings should be individualized to each patient.

Table 4.5.3 Summary of preoperative ECG findings and their prognostic significance.

ECG abnormality	Summary of findings
LVH	• Strong predictor of postoperative myocardial ischemia and adverse events in high-risk patients in many studies. • Significance in healthier patients undergoing lower-risk procedures is unclear.
AV conduction delays	• First- and second-degree AVB are unlikely to portend worse prognosis. • High-grade AVB should be referred to cardiology
Bundle branch blocks	• Data are conflicting on prognostic significance. May not improve prediction outcomes beyond risk factor assessment. • LBBB should be interpreted as sign of underlying cardiac disease. Refer to specialist as indicated.
Nonspecific ST-T changes	• Not associated with increased postoperative morbidity or mortality.
Pathologic Q waves	• Associated with 2.4-fold increased risk for perioperative events in one large study. • Other studies have been inconsistent.
Prolonged QT interval	• Increases risk for perioperative adverse events.

References

1 Jeger, R.V., Probst, C., Arsenic, R. et al. Long-term prognostic value of the preoperative 12-lead electrocardiogram before major noncardiac surgery in coronary artery disease. *American Heart Journal* 151 (2): 508–513.

2 Payne, C.J., Payne, A.R., Gibson, S.C. et al. (2011). Is there still a role for preoperative 12-lead electrocardiography? *World Journal of Surgery* 35 (12): 2611–2616.

3 Schein, O.D., Katz, J., Bass, E.B. et al. (2000). The value of routine preoperative medical testing before cataract surgery. *New England Journal of Medicine* 342 (3): 168–175.

4 Liu, L.L., Dzankic, S., and Leung, J.M. (2002). Preoperative electrocardiogram abnormalities do not predict postoperative cardiac complications in geriatric surgical patients. *Journal of the American Geriatrics Society* 50 (7): 1186–1191.

5 Noordzij, P.G., Boersma, E., Bax, J.J. et al. (2006). Prognostic value of routine preoperative electrocardiography in patients undergoing noncardiac surgery. *The American Journal of Cardiology* 97 (7): 1103–1106.

6 Fleisher, L.A., Fleischmann, K.E., Auerbach, A.D. et al. (2014). 2014 ACC/AHA guideline on perioperative cardiovascular evaluation and management of patients undergoing noncardiac surgery. A report of the American College of Cardiology/American Heart Association task force on practice guidelines. *Journal of the American Heart Association* 64 (22): e77–e137.

7 Kristensen, S.D., Knuuti, J., Saraste, A. et al. (2014). 2014 ESC/ESA guidelines on noncardiac surgery: cardiovascular assessment and management. The joint task force on noncardiac surgery: cardiovascular assessment and management of the European Society of Cardiology (ESC) and the European Society of Anaesthesiology (ESA). *European Heart Journal* 35 (35): 2383–2431.

8 Goldberger, A.L.G., Goldberger, Z.D., and Shvilkin, A. (2013). *Goldberger's Clinical Electrocardiography*, 8e. Elsevier, Inc.

9 Okin, P.M., Devereux, R.B., Nieminen, M.S. et al. (2001). Relationship of the electrocardiographic strain pattern to left ventricular structure and function in hypertensive patients: the LIFE study. *Journal of the American College of Cardiology* 38 (2): 514–520.

10 Bang, C.N., Devereux, R.B., and Okin, P.M. (2014). Regression of electrocardiographic left ventricular hypertrophy or strain is associated with lower incidence of cardiovascular morbidity and mortality in hypertensive patients independent of blood pressure reduction – a LIFE review. *Journal of Electrocardiology* 47 (5): 630–635.

11 Levy, D., Garrison, R.J., Savage, D.D. et al. (1990). Prognostic implications of echocardiographically determined left ventricular mass in the Framingham heart study. *New England Journal of Medicine* 322 (22): 1561–1566.

12 Verdecchia, P., Carini, G., Circo, A. et al. (2001). Left ventricular mass and cardiovascular morbidity in essential hypertension: the MAVI study. *Journal of the American College of Cardiology* 38 (7): 1829–1835.

13 Koren, M.J., Devereux, R.B., Casale, P.N. et al. (1991). Relation of left ventricular mass and geometry to

morbidity and mortality in uncomplicated essential hypertension. *Annals of Internal Medicine* 114 (5): 345–352.

14 Hollenberg, M., Mangano, D.T., Browner, W.S. et al. (1992). Predictors of postoperative myocardial ischemia in patients undergoing noncardiac surgery. *JAMA* 268 (2): 205–209.

15 Landesberg, G., Einav, S., Christopherson, R. et al. (1997). Perioperative ischemia and cardiac complications in major vascular surgery: importance of the preoperative twelve-lead electrocardiogram. *Journal of Vascular Surgery* 26 (4): 570–578.

16 Lette, J., Waters, D., Bernier, H. et al. (1992). Preoperative and long-term cardiac risk assessment. Predictive value of 23 clinical descriptors, 7 multivariate scoring systems, and quantitative dipyridamole imaging in 360 patients. *Annals of Surgery* 216 (2): 192–204.

17 Gold, B.S., Young, M.L., Kinman, J.L. et al. (1992). The utility of preoperative electrocardiograms in the ambulatory surgical patient. *Archives of Internal Medicine* 152 (2): 301–305.

18 Aro, A.L., Anttonen, O., Kerola, T. et al. (2014). Prognostic significance of prolonged PR interval in the general population. *European Heart Journal* 35 (2): 123–129.

19 Johnson, R.L., Averill, K.H., and Lamb, L.E. (1960). Electrocardiographic findings in 67,375 asymptomatic subjects. *The American Journal of Cardiology* 6 (1): 153–177.

20 Epstein, A.E., DiMarco, J.P., Ellenbogen, K.A. et al. (2008). ACC/AHA/HRS 2008 guidelines for device-based therapy of cardiac rhythm abnormalities. A report of the American College of Cardiology/American Heart Association task force on practice guidelines (writing committee to revise the ACC/AHA/NASPE 2002 guideline update for implantation of cardiac pacemakers and antiarrhythmia devices): developed in collaboration with the American Association for Thoracic Surgery and Society of Thoracic Surgeons. *Journal of the American College of Cardiology* 117 (21): e350–e408.

21 Gauss, M.D.A., Hubner, M.D.C., Radermacher, M.D.P. et al. (1998). Perioperative risk of bradyarrhythmias in patients with asymptomatic chronic bifascicular block or left bundle branch block does an additional first-degree atrioventricular block make any difference? *Anesthesiology* 88 (3): 679–687.

22 Olshansky, B.C. (2012). *Arrhythmia Essentials*. Jones & Bartlett Learning, LLC.

23 Tracy, C.M., Epstein, A.E., Darbar, D. et al. (2012). 2012 ACCF/AHA/HRS focused update of the 2008 guidelines for device-based therapy of cardiac rhythm abnormalities. A report of the American College of Cardiology Foundation/American Heart Association task force on practice guidelines. *Journal of the American College of Cardiology* 60 (14): 1297–1313.

24 Aro, A.L., Anttonen, O., Tikkanen, J.T. et al. (2011). Intraventricular conduction delay in a standard 12-lead electrocardiogram as a predictor of mortality in the general population clinical perspective. *Circulation. Arrhythmia and Electrophysiology* 4 (5): 704–710.

25 Freedman, R.A., Alderman, E.L., Thomas Sheffield, L. et al. (1987). Bundle branch block in patients with chronic coronary artery disease: angiographic correlates and prognostic significance. *Journal of the American College of Cardiology* 10 (1): 73–80.

26 Kim, J.H., Noseworthy, P.A., McCarty, D. et al. (2011). Significance of electrocardiographic right bundle branch block in trained athletes. *The American Journal of Cardiology* 107 (7): 1083–1089.

27 Dorman, T., Breslow, M.J., Pronovost, P.J. et al. (2000). Bundle-branch block as a risk factor in noncardiac surgery. *Archives of Internal Medicine* 160 (8): 1149–1152.

28 van Klei, W.A., Bryson, G.L., Yang, H. et al. (2007). The value of routine preoperative electrocardiography in predicting myocardial infarction after noncardiac surgery. *Annals of Surgery* 246 (2): 165–170.

29 Pastore, J.O., Yurchak, P.M., Janis, K.M. et al. (1978). The risk of advanced heart block in surgical patients with right bundle branch block and left axis deviation. *Circulation* 57 (4): 677–680.

30 Greenland, P., Xie, X., Liu, K. et al. (2003). Impact of minor electrocardiographic ST-segment and/or T-wave abnormalities on cardiovascular mortality during long-term follow-up. *The American Journal of Cardiology* 91 (9): 1068–1074.

31 Lee, T.H., Marcantonio, E.R., Mangione, C.M. et al. (1999). Derivation and prospective validation of a simple index for prediction of cardiac risk of major noncardiac surgery. *Circulation* 100 (10): 1043–1049.

32 Mangano, D.T., Browner, W.S., Hollenberg, M. et al. (1990). Association of perioperative myocardial ischemia with cardiac morbidity and mortality in men undergoing noncardiac surgery, the study of perioperative ischemia research group. *New England Journal of Medicine* 323 (26): 1781–1788.

33 Wagner, G.S., Freye, C.J., Palmeri, S.T. et al. (1982). Evaluation of a QRS scoring system for estimating myocardial infarct size. I. Specificity and observer agreement. *Circulation* 65 (2): 342–347.

34 Bazett, H.C. (1997). An analysis of the time-relations of electrocardiograms. *Annals of Noninvasive Electrocardiology* 2 (2): 177–194.

35 Moss, A.J. (2003). Long QT syndrome. *JAMA* 289 (16): 2041–2044.

36 Biteker, M., Duman, D., and Tekkeşin, A.İ. (2012). Predictive value of preoperative electrocardiography for perioperative cardiovascular outcomes in patients undergoing noncardiac, nonvascular surgery. *Clinical Cardiology* 35 (8): 494–499.

37 Thomas, W., Michael, W., Thomas, N. et al. (2014). Pathologic Q waves and prolonged QTc time in preoperative ECG are predictive for perioperative cardiovascular events. *World Journal of Cardiovascular Diseases*: 498–509.

6

The Patient in Shock

Meagan R. Hunt and Nicholas D. Hartman

Department of Emergency Medicine, Wake Forest School of Medicine, Winston-Salem, NC, USA

Introduction

Patients present for care in a physiologic state of shock for a multitude of reasons and the electrocardiogram (ECG) serves as a key clinical tool to aid in determination of the etiology. Shock is defined by a condition of poor perfusion to the vital organs, often demonstrating hypotension upon initial presentation. Other indicators of shock include end organ dysfunction, as manifested by altered mental status, respiratory distress, chest pain, or diaphoresis. The ECG is most helpful in identifying a cardiogenic cause for the circulatory collapse that accompanies shock, whether indicating a possible underlying cardiomyopathy or identifying an unstable cardiac arrhythmia. The ECG also provides useful information about other sources of shock, including electrolyte derangements, pulmonary embolism, or cardiac tamponade.

Shock has traditionally been classified into four major categories: cardiogenic, obstructive, distributive, and hypovolemic. Each of these categories includes multiple more specific etiologies. For example, distributive shock includes sepsis, neurogenic shock, anaphylaxis, and various toxicologic and endocrine based shock states. Examples of ECG findings that are associated with each category of shock will be discussed in this chapter.

Cardiogenic Shock

Cardiomyopathy

Sources of cardiogenic shock can be divided into two primary categories: cardiomyopathies and arrhythmias. Ischemic cardiomyopathy is one of the most common causes of cardiogenic shock. As ischemia progresses, the cardiac myocytes become unable to generate sufficient force to maintain adequate perfusion pressures. ECG changes associated with ischemic cardiomyopathy overlap with those detected in acute coronary syndromes as discussed in chapter 2 in this section. In patients suffering from cardiogenic shock from an acute myocardial infarction, certain ECG changes can indicate the potential for an increased benefit from emergency vascularization; in a prospective study of patients in cardiogenic shock, emergency re-vascularization improved outcomes for patients with prolonged QRS duration or inferior MI with precordial ST depression [1].

Exacerbations of heart failure may also result in cardiogenic shock; as heart failure is exacerbated by ischemia, there may be the aforementioned signs of acute coronary syndrome on the ECG. The presence of ST depression has been found to be associated with an increased risk of 30 days mortality among patients presenting with acute heart failure [2]. In addition to morphological ECG changes, heart failure exacerbations leading to cardiogenic shock may be associated with a number of rhythm disturbances, including atrioventricular block, atrial fibrillation or flutter, or ventricular arrhythmias. Identification of the rhythm is critical for guiding the appropriate heart failure therapy, which is discussed in more detail later in the chapter [3]. It is also important to identify these arrhythmias, as they are associated with increased in-hospital and long-term mortality, likely due to their association with more advanced heart disease [4]. ECG findings most closely associated with major structural heart disease or major left ventricular systolic dysfunction include widened QRS (greater than 0.120 seconds) and anterior pathological Q waves [5]. Q waves are an initially negative (or downward) deflection of the QRS complex; pathologic Q waves represent altered ventricular conduction, often due to previous myocardial injury or ventricular enlargement.

Electrocardiogram in Clinical Medicine, First Edition. Edited by William J. Brady, Michael J. Lipinski, Andrew E. Darby, Michael C. Bond, Nathan P. Charlton, Korin Hudson, and Kelly Williamson.

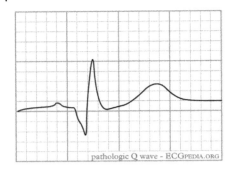

Figure 4.6.1 Example of a pathologic Q wave. Not the complete absence of a preceding upward deflecting R wave, as well as the depth and width of the Q wave. *Source:* Image reproduced with permission from http://ECGpedia.org

Firm consensus for the defining characteristics of "pathologic" Q waves has been elusive, but in general they are defined by a width of at least 0.03 seconds, or at least 0.02 seconds in leads V1–V3 [6] (Figure 4.6.1).

While the ECG may be useful in diagnosing cardiogenic shock due to acute ischemic cardiomyopathy or other forms of heart failure, it is important to remember its limitations as a diagnostic modality in this instance. For instance, patients experiencing an acute myocardial infarction may not demonstrate clear ECG findings of ischemia. Further, a recent meta-analysis of heart failure patients in the emergency department showed that electrocardiographic findings "lack discriminatory value in making or excluding the diagnosis of acute heart failure in ED patients" [7]. Thus, while the ECG may assist in diagnosing cardiomyopathy as a cause for shock in a patient in the emergency department, its use alone is not definitive.

Arrhythmias

The ECG may be of more assistance in diagnosing patients in cardiogenic shock due primarily to an arrhythmia. Patients in shock may display a variety of arrhythmias, and the clinician must decide whether the arrhythmia is a result of the shock state or whether it may be the primary driver; these patients must be aggressively treated with either pharmacologic or electrical cardioversion.

Atrial fibrillation, defined by disorganized depolarization within the atria, may be accompanied by a slow, normal, or rapid ventricular rate, and can result from, or be exacerbated by, a myriad of causes, including hypertensive heart disease, alcohol intoxication (the "holiday heart" phenomenon), pulmonary embolism, or catecholamine surge. Patients with chronic atrial fibrillation may be triggered into rapid ventricular response (RVR) for any number of reasons, including dehydration, infection, hemorrhage, or heart failure. Atrial fibrillation on the ECG

is characterized by an irregularly irregular QRS rhythm, lack of P waves, and presence of fibrillatory waves, which contributes to the lack of an isoelectric baseline. Since the origin of the rhythm is the atrium, the QRS complex is generally narrow (<120 msec) unless aberrancy (either a block in conduction or an accessory pathway) is present. In the context of atrial fibrillation, RVR is defined by a ventricular rate greater than 100 beats per minute (bpm). The rate of atrial fibrillation is rarely greater than 170 bpm, and a faster rate should prompt consideration for the presence of an accessory pathway. One other phenomenon of note that occurs in the context of atrial fibrillation is Ashman phenomenon. This refers to an aberrantly conducted beat, often with the morphology of a right bundle branch block (RBBB), which occurs because of the inconsistent heart rate present in atrial fibrillation that result in changes to the refractory period. Thus, when a long R-R cycle with a longer refractory period is followed by a shorter R-R cycle, the following beat is likely to exhibit this kind of aberrant conduction (Figures 4.6.2 and 4.6.3).

The patient in shock may also exhibit an atrioventricular block on the ECG. These present in many varieties, some of which are relatively benign and others which convey serious pathology. First-degree AV block, the most innocuous, consists of a prolonged PR interval greater than 200 msec. This finding can be a normal variant, but can also result from increased vagal tone, electrolyte disturbances, AV nodal blocking agents, or inferior MI. The QRS interval remains normal, no beats are dropped, and no treatment is indicated. While first-degree AV block may be noted on the ECG of a patient in shock, it is not a contributing factor (Figure 4.6.4).

Second-degree AV block exists in two different types: Type 1, also known as Wenckebach, and Type 2. Second-degree AV block is overall characterized by dropped beats, meaning sinus P waves that do not propagate to QRS complexes. Absent other pathology, the QRS duration remains normal. In the case of Wenckebach, the PR interval appears to lengthen between successive beats until a beat is dropped, and then the cycle resets itself. This pattern tends to occur at a regular interval, most often with 2–4 P-QRS pairs followed by a lone P wave with a "dropped" (nonexistent) QRS complex. The cycle begins again and the same number of P-QRS pairs generally appear prior to the next dropped beat. These cycles also illustrate another feature associated with Wenckebach, that of RP/PR reciprocity, meaning that as the distance between the R wave and P wave becomes shorter, the following PR interval becomes longer until an impulse is dropped and the cycle restarts. In most cases, this condition is thought to arise from a problem within the AV node, though other anatomic locations for the lesion are possible [8]. The Wenckebach phenomenon can be associated with acute inferior MI, toxicity from

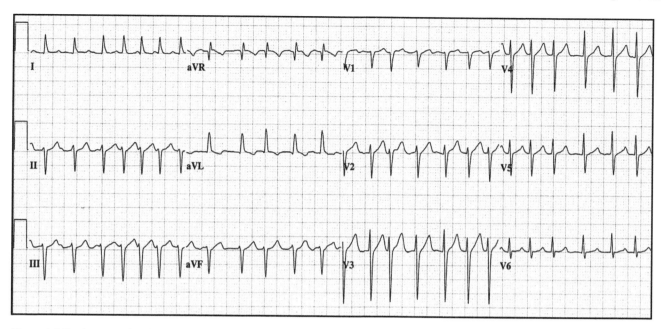

Figure 4.6.2 An example of atrial fibrillation with rapid ventricular response. Note the lack of P waves, the irregularly irregular rhythm and the rate greater than 100 bpm. *Source:* Image reproduced with permission from http://floatnurse-mike.blogspot.com.

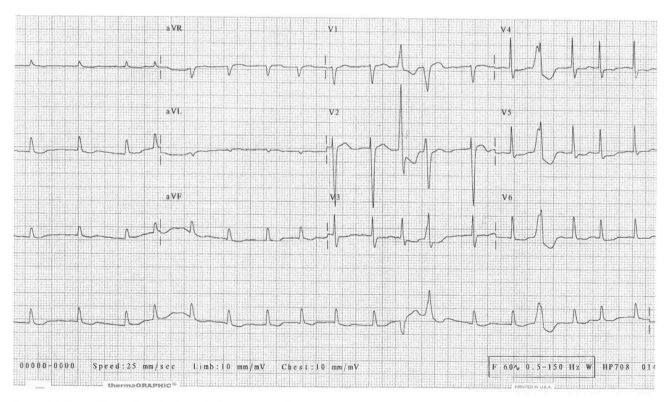

Figure 4.6.3 An illustration of Ashman's phenomenon. Note the aberrant beats that appear 12th and 15th in the rhythm strip with wider QRS complex, following a PVC (in the case of the 12th) and an abrupt change in the R-R interval (in the case of the 15th). *Source:* Image reproduced with permission from http://emedicine.medscape.com.

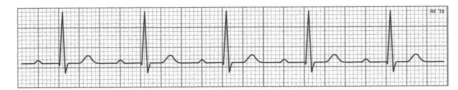

Figure 4.6.4 First-degree AV block. Note the prolonged PR interval (greater than 200 msec), measured from the beginning of the P wave to the beginning of the R wave. *Source:* Image reproduced with permission from Richard Klabunde PhD, and http://cvphysiology.com.

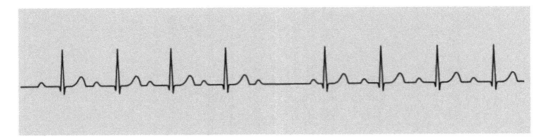

Figure 4.6.5 Second-degree AV block type 1 (Wenckebach). Note the lengthening PR interval followed by a non-conducted P wave (also termed a *dropped beat*). *Source:* Image reproduced with permission from http://ECGpedia.org.

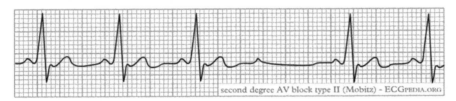

Figure 4.6.6 Second-degree AV block type 2. Note the constant PR interval and nonconducted P waves. *Source:* Image reproduced with permission from http://ECGpedia.org.

digoxin or beta blockers, or inflammatory problems affecting the myocardium and heart valves. For the patient in shock, a finding of Wenckebach on the ECG should prompt further investigation into these etiologies, though the ECG abnormality itself generally requires no treatment (Figure 4.6.5).

The presence of second-degree AV block type 2 is a more concerning finding. ECG features for this diagnosis include a constant PR interval with intermittently "dropped beats," or nonconducted impulses. In addition to the constant PR interval, the PP and RR intervals are also constant. In the absence of aberrant conduction or escape beats, the QRS complex remains narrow (<120 msec). The pathology, though, is most often anatomically located inferior to the AV node, so the possibility of disruptions in normal His-Purkinje conduction resulting in aberrancy does exist. Second-degree AV block type 2 can arise due to an anterior MI, autoimmune, or inflammatory conditions, cardiac surgery, hyperkalemia, or drugs causing AV nodal blockade. There is no effective pharmacologic treatment, and many of these patients will require a pacemaker. For a patient who presents in shock associated with this ECG finding, the clinician should provide immediate transcutaneous or transvenous pacing. Even stable patients require close monitoring and consultation with cardiology (Figure 4.6.6).

Third-degree, or complete, AV block represents the most severe form, as there is no relationship between P wave and the QRS complex. Thus, the ECG will demonstrate complete *AV dissociation,* in which P waves are not conducted and QRS complexes arise due to an escape rhythm. As AV dissociation may exist in entities other than complete heart block, including a primary junctional or ventricular rhythm, clinicians may misdiagnose the rhythm abnormality on a single ECG, and a longer rhythm strip may be required to make a firm diagnosis. This condition shares many of the same causes as the two types of second-degree heart block, including MI, structural heart disease including fibrosis of the cardiac conduction system (Lenegre-Lev disease), and various inflammatory conditions. The treatment for third-degree AV block includes emergent pacing for unstable patients, including those with hypotension or evidence of alterations in end-organ perfusion (Figure 4.6.7).

The patient in shock may also present with an arrhythmia of ventricular origin, including ventricular tachycardia (VT), a broad category of arrhythmias that share the features

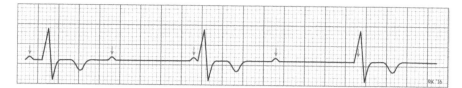

Figure 4.6.7 Third-degree, or complete, AV block. Note the lack of relationship between P waves and QRS complexes, with a ventricular escape pattern (wide QRS complex, rate < 40 bpm). *Source:* Image reproduced with permission from Richard Klabunde PhD, and http://cvphysiology.com.

of a wide QRS and a ventricular rate of greater than 100 bpm. A rhythm can be definitively classified as VT only if it originates at or below the bundle of His. Decision rules to distinguish VT from other causes of wide complex tachycardia have been proposed and examined, and the various underlying etiologies are listed in Table 4.6.1 [9].

The rule proposed by Brugada et al. suggests examining the ECG for the following features that are consistent with VT:

1) Absence of an RS complex in all precordial leads
2) R to S interval >100 msec in one precordial lead
3) Atrioventricular dissociation
4) Morphology criteria for VT present both in precordial leads V1–V2 and V6

If any of these are found on the ECG, then the diagnosis of VT is established [10]. While this rule was found in the original derivation to possess a sensitivity of 99% and a specificity of 96.5%, subsequent investigations have not reproduced such excellent test characteristics, and many clinicians understandably find these rules difficult to remember. A simpler algorithm, proposed by Griffith et al., directs the clinician to search for signs of typical right or left bundle branch block (RBBB or LBBB) in patients with wide complex tachycardia. If those are present, then the diagnosis of supraVT can be presumed, but if not, then VT must be assumed by default [11]. Put another way, QRS morphologies that are not consistent with a bundle branch block are likely to represent VT [9].

VT may present in either a monomorphic or polymorphic form. Monomorphic VT is most commonly associated with ischemic heart disease, and there is a consistent appearance of the QRS complexes on the ECG; it must consist of at least three consecutive beats to be considered VT, and must last at least 30 seconds to be considered *sustained* (less than 30 seconds

being considered *unsustained*). Monomorphic VT most commonly demonstrates a rate of 150–200 bpm, but can occur with slower rates. Polymorphic VT is characterized by multiple foci with QRS complexes of various forms. This may result from QT prolongation, and in this case, typically gives rise to torsades de pointes (TdP), which is considered a type of polymorphic VT (Figures 4.6.8 and 4.6.9).

For patients in shock, the diagnosis of a wide complex tachycardia should prompt immediate intervention. In the case of a patient in shock with VT who has maintained a pulse, the immediate treatment is synchronized cardioversion. In fact, the aforementioned distinction between supraventricular tachycardia and VTs clinically irrelevant for such a patient as both conditions in an unstable patient should prompt immediate cardioversion. Previously, it had been suggested to start with 50–100 J and increase in 50 J increments in the case of failure, yet many practitioners now advocate for starting at a higher energy, such as 100–200 J, in order to ameliorate the need for repeated, painful shocks. VT is also one of the two rhythms that responds to unsynchronized defibrillation in the case of cardiac arrest, as discussed in chapter 1 in this section. Patients who are more stable can be treated with antiarrythmic agents such as amiodarone, lidocaine, or procainamide as well as by correcting any underlying problems leading to the arrhythmia, such as electrolyte abnormalities, cardiac ischemia, or hypoxia.

Obstructive Shock

Massive Pulmonary Embolism

There has been previous debate in the literature questioning the utility of the ECG in the diagnosis of pulmonary emboli [12–14]. However, more recent studies suggest that ECG findings can both support the diagnosis of a clinically significant pulmonary embolus (PE) in our patients and help predict the development of shock in those same individuals [15]. Table 4.6.2 lists several ECG findings found to be significant predictors of cardiovascular collapse and poor outcome in patients with massive PE [16]. When recognized in a timely fashion these findings can be used to drive further confirmatory testing in a more aggressive fashion such that

Table 4.6.1 Causes of wide-complex tachycardia.

- Ventricular rhythm origin (e.g. ventricular tachycardia)
- Bundle-branch block (e.g. RBBB or LBBB)
- Rate-related bundle branch block or delay (abrupt changes in rate affect the refractory period of the His-Perkinje system)
- Accessory pathway (e.g. Wolff-Parkinson-White syndrome)

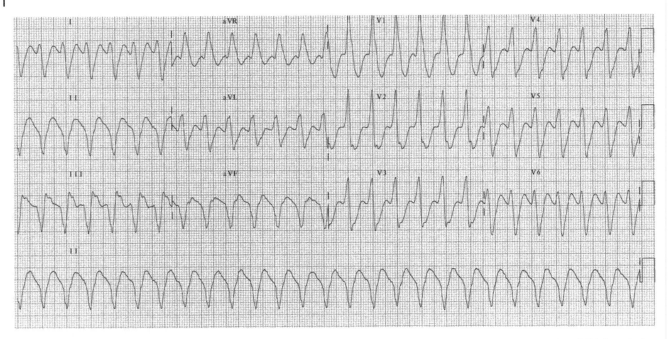

Figure 4.6.8 Monomorphic ventricular tachycardia. Note the significantly widened QRS complexes, some evidence of AV dissociation with superimposed P waves in aVF, rate of approximately 150 bpm and lack of LBBB or RBBB morphology. *Source:* Image reproduced with permission from http://lifeinthefastlane.com.

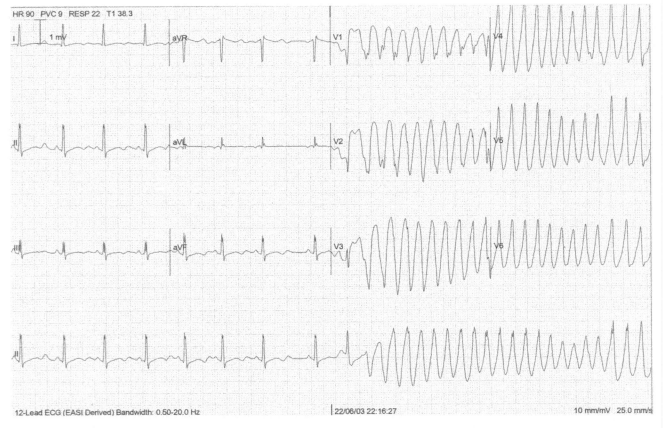

Figure 4.6.9 Polymorphic ventricular tachycardia, specifically torsades de pointes. This ECG illustrates the genesis of the dysrhythmia, as a prolonged QT gives rise to an "R on T" phenomenon, leading to torsades. Note the variation in the QRS complex following the initiation of the rhythm halfway through the electrocardiogram. *Source:* Image reproduced with permission from http://lifeinthefastlane.com.

Table 4.6.2 ECG findings associated with shock in pulmonary embolus.

ECG Findings
Pulse > 100
S1Q3T3
Complete RBBB
T-wave inversion in V1–V4
ST-segment elevation in aVR
Atrial fibrillation

interventions, including anticoagulation with heparin and thrombolysis with tissue plasminogen activator (TPA), could be implemented earlier, thereby reducing the morbidity and mortality associated with this condition.

It is easiest to remember the ECG findings associated with clinically significant PE if one recalls the pathophysiology behind these changes. Pulmonary emboli produce an increase in peripheral vascular resistance by obstructing pulmonary arterial flow, which results in an increase in pulmonary arterial pressures and resultant right ventricular failure. The ECG reflects this right ventricular strain (referred to classically as cor pulmonale) due to the delayed depolarization of the right ventricle, seen as complete or

incomplete RBBB. Figure 4.6.10 demonstrates the typical findings of RBBB that reflect this delay with widening of the QRS complex, an RVR' pattern in V1–V3 (M pattern), and the wide-slurred S wave accompanying this in the lateral leads (W pattern). ST depression and T-wave inversion in the right precordial leads (V1–V3) may also be seen in RBBB. Sometimes rather than an RSR' pattern in V1, there may be a broad monophasic R wave or a qR complex.

While certainly neither sensitive nor specific for PE, the S1Q3T3 pattern is classically associated with this diagnosis and was first described in 1935 [17]. The S wave in lead I signifies a complete or more often incomplete RBBB as mentioned previously. Figure 4.6.11 depicts this finding as well as the Q wave, slight ST elevation, and inverted T wave in lead III that are also due to the pressure and volume overload of the right ventricle causing repolarization abnormalities. While this pattern is classically associated with PE, it is not specific as it can occur in any scenario with acute right ventricular strain, including acute bronchospasm, pneumothorax, and other acute lung disorders.

Figure 4.6.12 depicts the ECG of a 23-year-old male who presented after an episode of syncope with severe respiratory distress. Note the RBBB with a wide QRS, tall R wave in V1, RSR' in leads V1–V3, and deep T-wave inversions in V1–V3. The presentation was so severe that widespread ischemia

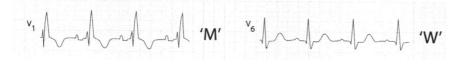

Figure 4.6.10 Diagnostic findings of RBBB. *Source:* Image reproduced with permission from http://lifeinthefastlane.com.

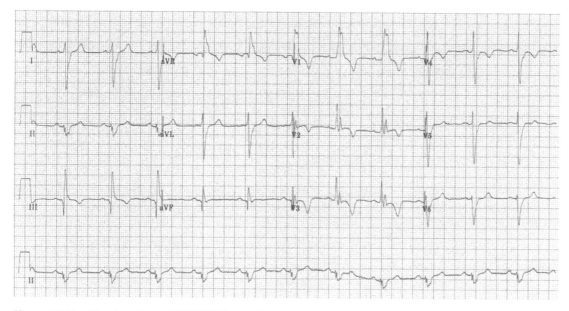

Figure 4.6.11 Classic pattern of S1Q3T3. *Source:* Image reproduced with permission from http://lifeinthefastlane.com.

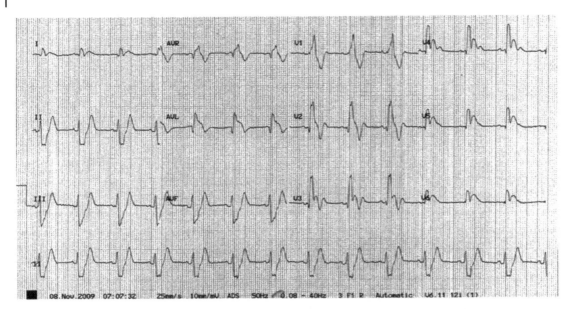

Figure 4.6.12 RBBB with a wide QRS, tall R wave in V1, RSR' in leads V1–V3, and deep T-wave inversions in V1–V3 in a patient with syncope and pulmonary embolism. Image reproduced with permission from http://lifeinthefastlane.com.

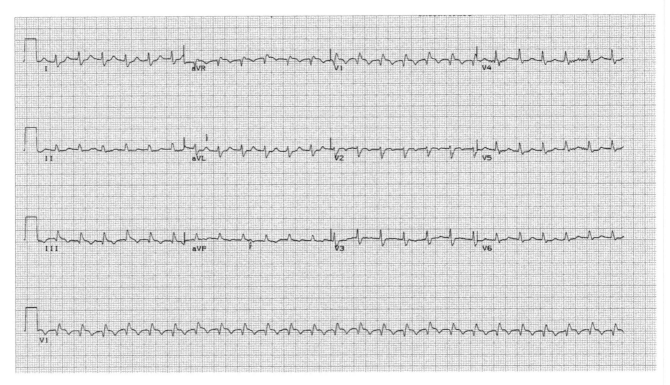

Figure 4.6.13 Sinus tachycardia, classic S1Q3T3 pattern, T-wave inversions in V1 and V2, and findings of RBBB (widened QRS, prominent R wave in V1, and wide-slurred S wave in I, aVL, V5–V6) in a patient with pulmonary embolism. Image reproduced with permission from http://ecglibrary.com.

occurred with ST-segment elevation developing in the lateral leads with reciprocal ST depression evident inferiorly.

Figure 4.6.13 is the ECG of a 40-year-old female presenting with pleuritic chest pain. Note the presence of sinus tachycardia, the classic S1Q3T3 pattern, T-wave inversions in V1 and V2, and findings of RBBB (widened QRS, prominent R wave in V1, and wide-slurred S wave in I, aVL, V5–V6).

Cardiac Tamponade

Cardiac tamponade is the other major cause of obstructive shock. The accumulating pericardial fluid in this condition compresses the heart resulting in decreased stroke volume and the development of sinus tachycardia as the heart rate increases to maintain cardiac output. Other associated ECG findings include low-voltage QRS complexes, related to the disruption of electrical conduction by pericardial fluid [18], and electrical alternans, resulting from the movement of the heart within a pericardial effusion (Figure 4.6.14). In one study authors reviewed the records of approximately 200 subjects with pericardial effusions to determine the sensitivity, specificity, and predictive values of low-voltage QRS complexes, sinus tachycardia, and electrical alternans in the diagnosis of cardiac tamponade [18]. See Table 4.6.3 for a summary of the value of these findings in detecting cardiac tamponade in the ECG.

Distributive Shock

Distributive shock refers to any medical condition resulting in abnormal distribution of blood flow in the smallest blood vessels that lead to an inadequate supply of blood to the body's tissues and organs. This phenomenon may occur when the peripheral vasculature is unable to support adequate central venous return or when cardiac function is unable to support normal stroke volume or heart

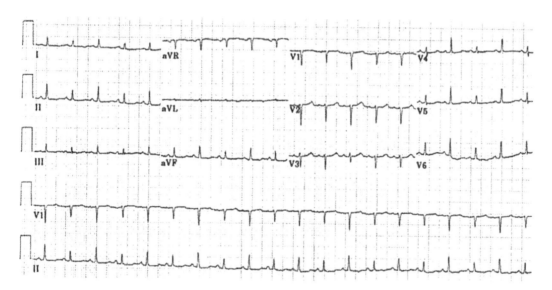

Figure 4.6.14 Electrical alternans. *Source:* Image reproduced with permission from http://lifeinthefastlane.com.

Table 4.6.3 ECG findings and their value in diagnosing cardiac tamponade.

	Sensitivity	Specificity	PPV	NPV	OR (95% CI)
Low QRS voltage	56%	74%	81%	46%	3.7 (1.65–8.30)
Sinus tachycardia	76%	60%	79%	56%	4.9 (2.22–10.80)
Electrical alternans	23%	98%	95%	39%	12.3 (1.58–95.17)
Any of the above	89%	47%	77%	69%	7.3 (2.9–18.1)
All of the above	8%	100%	100%	36%	

rate; some conditions cause decreased cardiac output through a combination of the two. We will cover several major causes of this form of shock, while certain other conditions resulting in distributive shock such as anaphylaxis and acute toxic ingestion are covered elsewhere in the text.

Hypothermia

Hypothermia is defined by a body core temperature <35 °C. As body temperature decreases, cardiovascular function also declines, manifested as slowed conduction velocity and decreased heart rate. The ECG displays these changes with sequential development of bradycardia, prolongation of PR, QRS, and QT intervals (though not necessarily in any specific order), and development of heart block. Though the underlying mechanism is unclear, the development of an Osborn or J wave (Figure 4.6.15) is another common ECG finding in this condition. While the most specific ECG finding in hypothermia and often thought to be pathognomonic for this condition, it has also been documented in patients with hypercalcemia, major CNS insults, and as a *drug effect* [19]. These waves appear as a positive deflection at the end of the QRS complex and are most apparent in the left lateral chest leads; the size of these waves often correlates with the degree of hypothermia.

The ventricular dysrhythmias that constitute the most common cause of death in hypothermia often develop after hypotension and the previously mentioned ECG findings have already occurred [19].

Thyrotoxicosis

Thyrotoxicosis, also referred to as thyroid storm, may result in shock as high levels of triiodothyronine (T3) overstimulate the atria, causing tachyarrhythmia [19] and decreased PVR [20]. Common ECG findings in this condition include sinus tachycardia, atrial fibrillation, and high-voltage QRS complexes. Supraventricular arrhythmias including premature atrial beats, paroxysmal supraventricular tachycardia, multifocal atrial tachycardia, and atrial flutter also occur frequently. Atrial fibrillation is the most common sustained tachyarrhythmia, occurring in about 20% of cases. Males, elderly patients, patients with a particularly high concentration of thyroid hormone, and patients with left atrial enlargement or other intrinsic heart disease are most at risk for developing

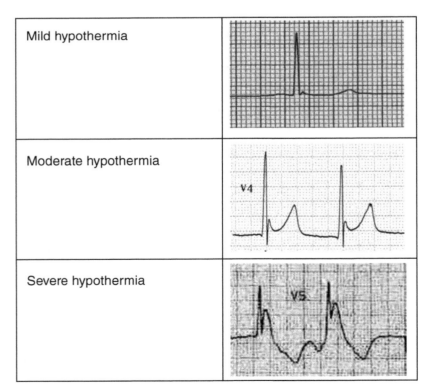

Mild hypothermia	
Moderate hypothermia	
Severe hypothermia	

Figure 4.6.15 Osborne or "J" waves at varying degrees of hypothermia. *Source:* Image reproduced with permission from http://lifeinthefastlane.com.

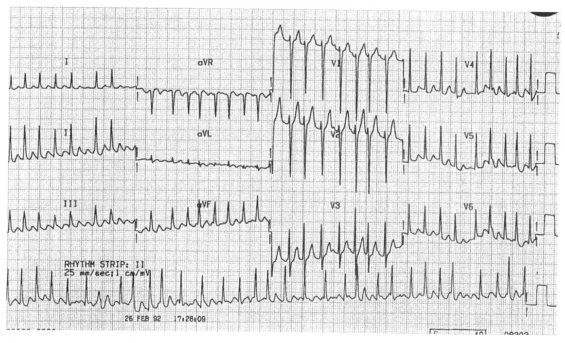

Figure 4.6.16 Atrial fibrillation with RVR accompanied by high-voltage QRS complexes in a patient with thyrotoxicosis. Image reproduced with permission from http://lifeinthefastlane.com.

atrial fibrillation; patients developing atrial fibrillation with RVR in thyrotoxicosis are refractory to cardioversion but often revert spontaneously to sinus rhythm once a euthyroid state is achieved [19]. Figure 4.6.16 depicts the 12-lead ECG of a patient in a-fib with RVR accompanied by high-voltage QRS complexes.

Additional ECG findings associated with thyroid storm include nonspecific ST segment and T-wave changes, ventricular arrhythmias, and ventricular extra-systoles, likely related to strain from high-output heart failure. Of note, while thyrotoxic patients have two or three times more premature ventricular contractions (PVCs) than euthyroid patients, ventricular arrhythmias occur in this condition far less frequently than atrial arrhythmias [19].

Myxedema Coma

Myxedema coma describes an extreme state of hypothy-roidism where the body's metabolic rate is dramatically slowed; from a cardiovascular standpoint, this results in decreased heart rate, decreased cardiac contractility, slowed electrical conduction, increased peripheral vascu-lar resistance, and the possible development of a pericar-dial effusion [19]. These changes may relate to the effects of decreased levels of T3 and T4 on the myocardium, including decreased chronotropy and ionotropy. Most

commonly, sinus bradycardia, QT prolongation, and widespread T-wave flattening or inversion (without accom-panying ST-segment deviation) occur, though low-voltage QRS complexes, heart block, intraventricular conduction delays, and ventricular extrasystoles may also be seen [19]. While uncommon, large pericardial effusions related to this condition can produce electrical alternans as well. The ECG of a 79-year-old male patient presenting with unde-tectable levels of T4 and markedly elevated TSH can be seen below in Figure 4.6.17a. Figure 4.6.17b depicts the ECG of the same patient with resolution of bradycardia and T-wave inversion occurring after thyroid hormone replacement.

Neurogenic Shock

Traditionally, the term *neurogenic shock* refers to spinal cord injury-mediated hypotension, though actually refers to hypotension resulting from insults to either the brain or spinal cord. The prevalence of this condition may have previously been underestimated as it was attributed to other etiologies of shock; some studies suggest that these insults may be primarily responsible for hypotension in up to 19% of blunt trauma patients (6% spinal cord injury-related, 13% brain injury-related) [20].

In spinal cord injury (SCI), the disruption of sympathetic pathways results in parasympathetic predominance and

(a)

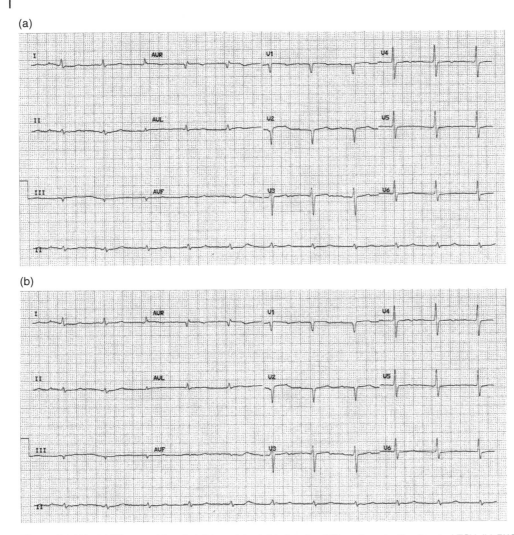

(b)

Figure 4.6.17 (a) 79 year old male with undetectable levels of T4 and markedly elevated TSH. (b) EKG of the same patient with resolution of bradycardia and T-wave inversion occurring after thyroid hormone replacement. Image reproduced with permission from http://lifeinthefastlane.com.

the subsequent development of bradycardia and hypotension with loss of vasomotor tone and decreased cardiac output. There is disagreement on the specific parameters that define this form of neurogenic shock, as well as whether it can occur with SCI below the level of T6, the lowest level at which there is innervation of the heart (though case reports of this presentation in isolated lumbar spine injuries have been published) [21–24]. Though ECG changes might result from ischemia developing as a complication from neurogenic shock, bradycardia appears to be the predominant finding. While nonspecific, the identification of bradycardia in a trauma patient, who would otherwise be suspected to have tachycardia secondary to hypovolemia, pain, and stress, can be a valuable clue to the presence of this rare condition [25] and associated SCI.

Shock can also develop in response to the rapid increases in intracranial pressure that can occur with conditions such as massive subarachnoid hemorrhage (SAH) and acute traumatic intracranial bleeding of any type [26]. Similar to SCI, this phenomenon is related to disruption of sympathetic responses based on injury to sympathetic regulatory centers within the brain. These changes also affect the myocardium and ECG abnormalities are noted in more than 50% of cases in multiple studies of SAH [27, 28]. Though nonspecific, the subsequent development of QTc prolongation and ST depression has been shown to accompany increasing neurogenic pulmonary edema and heralded circulatory collapse in these patients [27]. T-wave inversions are most commonly seen with CNS abnormalities and can

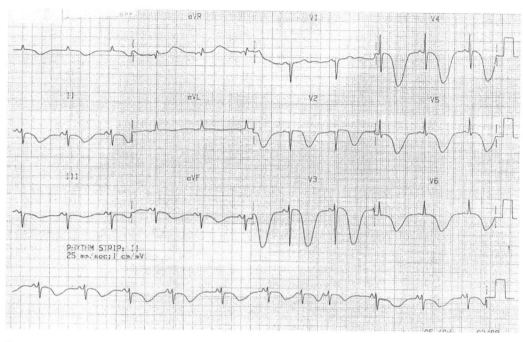

Figure 4.6.18 Widespread "cerebral T waves" as well as QT prolongation. Image reproduced with permission from http://lifeinthefastlane.com.

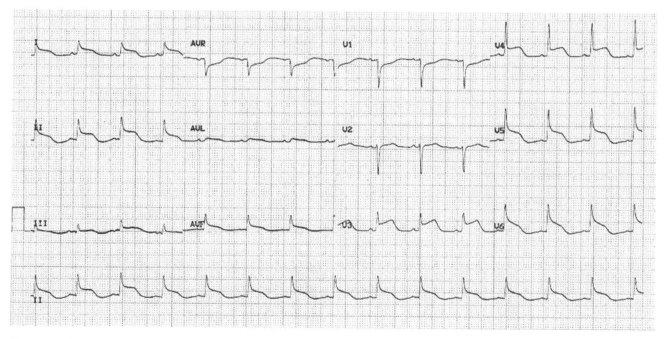

Figure 4.6.19 18 year old female with severe traumatic brain injury and elevated intracranial pressure. Note the widespread STE with a pericarditis-like morphology and absence of reciprocal change (except in aVR and V1). Image reproduced with permission from http://lifeinthefastlane.com.

often be accompanied by ST-segment elevation (STE) of less than 3 mm, U waves of any polarity, and QT prolongation often greater than 60% of normal value [29]. Note the widespread "cerebral T waves" in Figure 4.6.18 as well as the QT prolongation. Figure 4.6.19 demonstrates the ECG of a previously healthy 18-year-old girl with severe traumatic brain injury and massively raised intracranial pressure (30–40 mmHg). Note the widespread STE with a pericarditis-like morphology and no reciprocal change (except in aVR and V1). She had no cardiac injury to explain the STE and the ST segments normalized as the intracranial pressure came under control.

Systemic Inflammatory Response Syndrome (SIRS)

The most common cause of distributive shock encountered in the emergency department is sepsis or infection accompanied by SIRS. The development of vasodilation, increased vascular permeability, and cardiac dysfunction leads to increasing heart rate with falling blood pressure. Sinus tachycardia is the most common electrocardiographic finding; in those predisposed to development of arrhythmias or ischemia, atrial fibrillation with RVR or ischemic changes including ST segment depression may be seen as well. It is important to note that SIRS occurs in several other conditions, including pancreatitis, burns, trauma, ischemia, hemorrhage, pulmonary embolism, and anaphylaxis, among others. These conditions may also demonstrate the same nonspecific ECG findings.

Hypovolemic Shock

This last form of shock occurs in the setting of either dehydration from excessive urinary or fecal output, decreased oral intake, hyperthermia without fluid replacement, as well as hemorrhage of any kind. Sinus tachycardia and atrial fibrillation with RVR are the most common findings with this condition. As the heart rate increases to compensate for decreased stroke volume, the increased work of the heart can result in myocardial ischemia, particularly in those with underlying coronary artery disease. ST-segment depression and T-wave inversion can be seen with this strain and often resolve as heart rate decreases with volume replacement.

Summary

In summary, patients presenting in shock from a variety of causes may show important ECG findings that can signal the cause of shock and assist the clinician in determining care. Figure 4.6.20 is a flowsheet diagramming the important findings that may lead to such diagnostic insight. Precise management will always require clinical judgment, but the ECG can provide helpful clues.

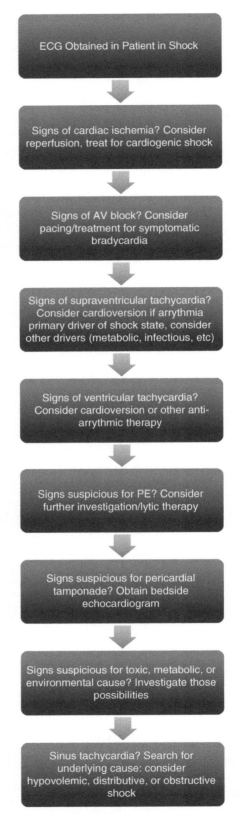

Figure 4.6.20 Approach to patient in shock with ECG findings.

References

1 White, H.D., Palmeri, S.T., Sleeper, L.A. et al. (2004). Electrocardiographic findings in cardiogenic shock, risk prediction, and the effects of emergency revascularization: results from the SHOCK trial. *Am. Heart J.* 148 (5): 810–817.

2 Greig, D., Austin, P., Zhou, L. et al. (2014). Ischemic electrocardiographic abnormalities and prognosis in decompensated heart failure. *Circ. Heart Fail.* 7: 986–993.

3 McMurray, J., Adamopoulos, S., Anker, S. et al. (2012). ESC guidelines for the diagnosis and treatment of acute and chronic heart failure 2012: the task force for the diagnosis and treatment of acute and chronic heart failure 2012 of the European Society of Cardiology. *Eur. Heart J.* 33 (14): 1787–1847.

4 Vaclavik, J., Spinar, J., Vindis, D. et al. (2014). ECG in patients with acute heart failure can predict in-hospital and long-term mortality. *Intern. Emerg. Med.* 9: 283–291.

5 Khan, N., Goode, K., Cleland, J. et al. (2007). Prevalance of ECG abnormalities in an international survey of patients with suspected or confirmed heart failure at death or discharge. *Eur. J. Heart Fail.* 9: 491–501.

6 Antman, E., Bassand, J.P., Klein, W. et al. (2000). Myocardial infarction redefined – a consensus document of the joint European Society of Cardiology/American College of Cardiology committee for the redefinition of myocardial infarction. *J. Am. Coll. Cardiol.* 36 (3): 959–969.

7 Martindale, J., Wakai, A., Collins, S. et al. (2016). Diagnosing acute heart failure in the emergency department: a systematic review and meta-analysis. *Acad. Emerg. Med.* 23: 223–242.

8 Cabeen, W.R., Roberts, N.K., and Child, J.S. (1978). Recognition of the Wenckebach phenomenon. *West. J. Med.* 129 (6): 521–526.

9 Brugada, P., Brugada, J., Mont, L. et al. (1991). A new approach to the differential diagnosis of a regular tachycardia with a wide QRS complex. *Circulation* 83 (5): 1649–1659.

10 Griffith, M.J., Garratt, C.J., Mounsey, P., and Camm, A.J. (1994). Ventricular tachycardia as default diagnosis in broad complex tachycardia. *Lancet* 343 (8894): 386–388.

11 Stahmer, S. and Cowan, R. (2006). Tachydysrhythmias. *Emerg. Med. Clin. North Am.* 24: 11–40.

12 Rodger, M., Maropoulos, D., Turek, M. et al. (2000). Diagnostic value of the electrocardiogram in suspected pulmonary embolism. *Am. J. Cardiol.* 86: 807–809.

13 Ferrari, E., Imbert, A., Chevalier, T. et al. (1997). The ECG in pulmonary embolism* predictive value of negative T waves in precordial Leads-80 case reports. *Chest* 111: 537–543.

14 Chan, T.C., Vilke, G.M., Pollack, M., and Brady, W.J. (2001). Electrocardiographic manifestations: pulmonary embolism. *J. Emerg. Med.* 21: 263–270.

15 Geibel, A., Zehender, M., Kasper, M. et al. (2005). Prognostic value of the ECG on admission in patients with acute major pulmonary embolism. *Eur. Respir. J.* 25: 843–848.

16 Shopp, J.D., Stewart, L.K., Emmett, T.W., and Kline, J.A. (2015). Findings from 12-lead electrocardiography that predict circulatory shock from pulmonary embolism: systematic review and meta-analysis. *Acad. Emerg. Med.* 22: 1127–1137.

17 McGinn, S. and White, P.D. (1935). Acute cor pulmonale resulting from pulmonary embolism its clinical recognition. *JAMA* 104: 1473–1480.

18 Argula, R.G., Negi, S.I., Banchs, J. et al. (2015). Role of a 12-Lead electrocardiogram in the diagnosis of cardiac Tamponade as diagnosed by transthoracic echocardiography in patients with malignant pericardial effusion. *Clin. Cardiol.* 38: 139–144.

19 Slovis, C. and Jenkins, R. (2002). ABC of clinical electrocardiography: conditions not primarily affecting the heart. *BMJ* 324: 1320–1323.

20 Mahoney, M.D., Biffl, W.L., Harrington, D.T. et al. (2003). Isolated brain injury as a cause of hypotension in the blunt trauma patient. *J. Trauma* 55: 1065–1069.

21 Hagen, E.M., Faerestrand, S., Hoff, J.M. et al. (2011). Cardiovascular and urological dysfunction in spinal cord injury. *Acta Neurol. Scand. Suppl.* 124: 71–78.

22 Zahra, M., Samdani, A., Piggott, K. et al. (2010). Acute changes in systemic hemodynamics and serum vasopressin after complete cervical spinal cord injury in piglets. *Neurocrit. Care.* 13: 132–140.

23 Alexander, M.S., Biering-Sorensen, F., Bodner, D. et al. (2009). International standards to document remaining autonomic function after spinal cord injury. *Spinal Cord* 47: 36–43.

24 Fox, A.D. (2014). Assessment and treatment of spinal cord injuries and neurogenic shock. *JEMS* 39: 64–67.

25 Taylor, M.P., Wrenn, P., and O'Donnell, A.D. (2017). Presentation of neurogenic shock within the emergency department. *Emerg. Med. J.* 34: 157–162.

26 Cushing, H. (1902). Some experimental and clinical observations concerning states of increased intracranial pressure. *Am J Med Sci* 124: 375–400.

27 Kerro, A., Woods, T., and Chang, J.J. (2017). Neurogenic stunned myocardium in subarachnoid hemorrhage. *J. Crit. Care* 38: 27–34.

28 Zhang, L. and Qi, S. (2016). Electrocardiographic abnormalities predict adverse clinical outcomes in patients with subarachnoid Hemorrhage. *J. Stroke Cerebrovasc. Dis.* 25: 2653–2659.

29 Perron, A.D. and Brady, W.J. (2000). Electrocardiographic manifestations of CNS events. *Am. J. Emerg. Med.* 18: 715–720.

7

The Patient with Overdose

Ashley Pastore[1] and Andrea Carlson[2,3]

[1] *Emergency Physician, Ochsner Medical Center, New Orleans, LA, USA*
[2] *Advocate Christ Medical Center Emergency Medicine Residency, Chicago, IL, USA*
[3] *Department of Emergency Medicine, University of Illinois at Chicago, Chicago, IL, USA*

Introduction

Nearly 200 deaths occur daily in the United States as a result of drug and alcohol-induced exposures [1]. Because cardiotoxicity is a well-recognized complication of many toxins, the role of the electrocardiogram (ECG) in the diagnosis and management of poisoning has been extensively investigated. Many qualities of electrocardiography make this modality a useful diagnostic aid: it is inexpensive, portable, non-invasive, and painless. Immediate results are obtained that can suggest specific toxin exposure, allowing for timely therapeutic intervention. Additionally, many ECG derangements show prognostic value. Certain findings (ectopy, QTc >500 ms, nonsinus rhythm, and findings of ischemia/infarction) in the setting of poisoning are highly predictive of adverse cardiovascular events [2]. While the absence of ECG findings does not reliably exclude toxin exposure, routine use of ECG is recommended in the initial investigation and management of poisoned patients along with available history, physical exam, and laboratory findings.

Approach to the ECG in the Poisoned Patient

When analyzing the ECG in a patient with suspected or confirmed toxic exposure, a systematic approach is important. Careful, stepwise attention to each component of the ECG can uncover subtle clues concerning the toxicity. Assessment of heart rate is a logical first step. Sinus tachycardia can be associated with specific toxins (Table 4.7.1), or may be a surrogate marker of other physiologic stress

(e.g. hypoxia, hypoglycemia). Likewise, sinus bradycardia also proposes a discrete list of toxins (Table 4.7.2).

In addition to heart rate, dysrhythmia may suggest a specific toxin or may reflect a secondary process (e.g. acidosis, electrolyte disturbance). For instance, patients with methylxanthine toxicity are prone to the development of supraventricular tachycardia (SVT), while drugs and toxins that block the atrioventricular (AV) node manifest varying degrees of heart block or ventricular dysrhythmias.

Recognizing certain morphological abnormalities on the ECG can also lead toward the correct diagnosis. The P wave is a manifestation of atrial depolarization; a normal P wave has duration of 80–110 milliseconds (ms) and is less than 0.25 mV in amplitude. In certain conditions, such as left atrial enlargement, the P wave becomes "notched" as atrial depolarization is prolonged. In toxicology, this widened, "notching" effect has been classically ascribed to quinidine, but abnormalities of P-wave morphology may also be caused by hyperkalemia, or by drugs that depress automaticity, such as alpha antagonists or calcium channel blockers (CCBs).

The PR interval is defined as the interval from the onset of the P wave to the start of the QRS complex, reflecting conduction through the AV node and normally lasting between 120 and 200 ms. The PR interval can become prolonged due to increased vagal tone or increased sympathetic tone, resulting in various degrees of AV block. Many drugs prolong the PR interval by affecting AV nodal conduction [3] (Table 4.7.3).

The QRS complex represents depolarization of the ventricles, with a duration typically less than 120 msec. Drug-induced QRS prolongation represents slowed conduction

Electrocardiogram in Clinical Medicine, First Edition. Edited by William J. Brady, Michael J. Lipinski, Andrew E. Darby, Michael C. Bond, Nathan P. Charlton, Korin Hudson, and Kelly Williamson.

Table 4.7.1 Common drugs and toxins that cause tachycardia.

Amphetamines	Ephedrine
Antihistamines	Epinephrine
Beta agonists (Albuterol, Salmeterol)	Nicotine
Caffeine	Phencyclidine (PCP)
Cocaine	Pseudoephedrine
Cyclic antidepressants	Theophylline

Table 4.7.2 Common drugs and toxins that cause bradycardia.

Baclofen	Gamma-hydroxybutyric acid (GHB)
Beta-adrenergic receptor blockers	Imidazolines
Calcium channel blockers	*Clitocybe, Inocybe spp* mushrooms (Muscarine)
Carbamates	Opioids
Cardiac glycosides	Organophosphates
Ciguatera toxin	Physostigmine
Clonidine	Sedative-hypnotics

Table 4.7.3 Drugs affecting the PR interval.

Adenosine

Amiodarone

Arsenic trioxide

Beta blockers

Calcium channel blockers

Clonidine

Digoxin

Mefloquine

Opioids

Pregabalin

Protease inhibitors (atazanavir, saquinavir, etc.)

Sedative-hypnotics

Table 4.7.4 Drugs causing QRS prolongation.

Amantadine	Flecainide
Bupropion	Phenothiazines
Carbamazepine	Procainamide
Cocaine	Propafenone
Diphenhydramine	Propranolol
Disopyramide	Tricyclic antidepressants
Doxylamine	Venlafaxine

due to sodium channel blockade [4]. See Table 4.7.4 for a list of drugs and toxins causing QRS prolongation.

The QT interval, defined as the time from the onset of the Q wave to the termination of the T wave, represents the total time of depolarization and repolarization of the ventricles. As QT interval length is inversely proportional to heart rate, the corrected QT interval (QTc) is calculated for more reliable comparison of the interval: the QTc duration should be less than 440 ms in men and 460 ms in women. Blockage of potassium efflux channels delays the termination of Phase 2 of the action potential of the ventricular myocyte and prolongs the QT interval (Figure 4.7.2). A QTc interval greater than 500 ms increases the risk of polymorphic ventricular tachycardia/torsades de pointes (TdP) (Figure 4.7.3). The risk of arrhythmia with QT prolonging drugs is highly variable and unpredictable, even when nonpharmacologic risk factors are considered (Table 4.7.5).

The ST segment is the flat, isoelectric section between the end of the S wave and the beginning of the T wave, representing the interval between ventricular depolarization and repolarization. ST-segment elevation or depression is concerning for myocardial ischemia or infarction, yet may also be disrupted as a secondary effect of intoxication (Table 4.7.6). Cocaine

Table 4.7.5 Drugs that prolong the QT interval.

ACE Inhibitors	Dofetilide	Methadone
Amantadine	Donepezil	Moxifloxacin
Amiodarone	Dronedarone	Olanzapine
Amphetamines	Droperidol	Ondansetron
Anagrelide	Erythromycin	Organophosphates
Arsenic trioxide	Escitalopram	Pentamidine
Azithromycin	Flecainide	Pimozide
Bupropion	Fluconazole	Procainamide
Chloral Hydrate	Haloperidol	Propafenone
Chloroquine	Hydroxychloroquine	Propofol
Chlorpromazine	Ibutilide	Quetiapine
Cilostazol	Itraconazole	Quinidine
Ciprofloxacin	Ketoconazole	Risperidone
Citalopram	Levofloxacin	Sotalol
Clarithromycin	Lithium	Thioridazine
Cocaine	Loperamide	Trimethoprim/ sulfamethoxazole
Cyclic antidepressants	Loratidine	Vandetanib
Diphenhydramine	Lidocaine	Venlafaxine
Disopyramide	Mesoridazine	Ziprasidone

Table 4.7.6 Drugs causing ST-segment change.

Amphetamines
Cellular asphyxiants (hydrogen cyanide, hydrogen sulfide, and carbon monoxide)
Cocaine
Digoxin
Ergotamine
Sympathomimetics (ephedrine, methylphenidate, etc.)

toxicity is a well-described precipitant of myocardial infarction [5]. Another well-described ST-segment change associated with drug toxicity is the "scooping" pattern attributed to digitalis glycosides.

The T wave follows the QRS complex, and it is a representation of ventricular repolarization. A normal T wave is <5 mm amplitude in limb leads, and <15 mm in precordial leads. T-wave changes in overdose are secondary effects, generally from hyperkalemia or myocardial ischemia.

The U wave is a small deflection immediately after the T wave, typically in the same direction. The U wave is most commonly associated with severe hypokalemia or hypomagnesemia, but rarely it can be related to exposure to digoxin (Figure 4.7.4), lithium, methylxanthines, phenothiazines (thioridazine), class IA antiarrhythmics (quinidine, procainamide), and class III antiarrhythmics (sotalol, amiodarone).

Classic Toxicology ECGs

Cardiac Glycosides

Digoxin is a cardiac glycoside frequently used to treat atrial fibrillation, atrial flutter, and heart failure. It reversibly binds to the α-subunit of the Na+/K+ ATPase pump in the cardiac myocyte, impairing sodium and potassium exchange. The rising intracellular sodium concentration reverses the sodium-calcium exchange pump, which leads to an increase in the intracellular calcium concentration and increased calcium release from the sarcoplasmic reticulum during each action potential. The net effect is increased inotropy of the heart.

Digoxin has a narrow therapeutic index, and due to the drug's dependence on adequate renal function for proper elimination, the potential for significant toxicity from both acute and chronic exposure is significant (Figure 4.7.5). In 2015, cardiac glycoside exposures accounted for >2500 calls to US Poison Control Centers [6]. Nearly every dysrhythmia has been reported in the setting of digoxin poisoning; intoxication can lead to sinoatrial or AV-nodal

block, sometimes in combination with tachycardia. These effects are intensified by concomitant hypokalemia. In profound poisonings, ventricular tachycardia or ventricular fibrillation may develop.

Bidirectional ventricular tachycardia is a rare presentation of severe digoxin toxicity, characterized by a beat-to-beat alternation of the frontal QRS axis (Figure 4.7.6). The QRS axis shifts 180° from left to right with each beat, or alternates between left and right bundle-branch block.

Noncardiac clinical manifestations of digoxin toxicity are nonspecific, though most often gastrointestinal and neurological in nature. Patients may complain of loss of appetite, nausea/vomiting, or abdominal pain. Confusion and hallucinations may be present and incorrectly ascribed to psychiatric illness or dementia. Visual disturbances, when present, may more specifically suggest digoxin toxicity, particularly if aberrations of color vision (yellow, green) are present.

Laboratory findings in acute digoxin overdose include hyperkalemia and elevated digoxin serum concentration; the degree of hyperkalemia is a prognostic indicator of mortality [7]. Renal failure or insufficiency is another common laboratory finding and reflects decreased drug clearance.

Elevated serum digoxin concentrations should be clinically correlated in order to differentiate true digoxin toxicity from other causes of illness [8]. When interpreting the laboratory results, it is essential to consider whether the measured value reflects a steady-state level as serum concentrations drawn within six hours of ingestion may be misleadingly elevated due to incomplete drug distribution.

Initial management of digoxin toxicity involves stabilization, decontamination, administration of digoxin-specific antibody fragment therapy, and supportive care. While atropine is indicated for bradycardia/dysrhythmias, pacing is of limited utility. Tachydysrhythmias may be treated with beta blockers and aggressive management of ventricular tachycardia or ventricular fibrillation with cardioversion or defibrillation as necessary. Potassium and magnesium abnormalities should be corrected. Classically, calcium has been thought to be contraindicated in treating the hyperkalemia of digoxin toxicity, as the "stone heart" theory posited that this could impair adequate myocardial relaxation. However, recent studies have shown no clinical evidence for this theory [9].

Antidotal therapy for digoxin is purified digoxin-specific antibody Fab fragments (trade name Digibind®). This therapy is indicated for cardiac arrest or significant ventricular dysrhythmia in known digoxin overdose, bradydysrhythmias unresponsive to atropine, hyperkalemia >5.5 mEq/l,

Table 4.7.7   ECG findings with therapeutic digoxin use.

ST depression with "scooped out" appearance of the ST segment
Flat, negative, or biphasic T wave
Shortened QT interval
Increased U-wave amplitude
Prolonged PR interval
Sinus bradycardia

serum digoxin concentration >10 ng/ml (steady state) or >15 ng/ml at any time, ingestion >10 mg in an adult, or when combination CCB/digoxin overdose is suspected. Patients with digoxin toxicity should be admitted to the intensive care setting for close monitoring of electrolytes and their cardiac rhythm (Table 4.7.7).

Drug-Induced SVT

SVT is a tachydysrhythmia originating from an ectopic focus in the atria or AV junction. The tachycardia is generally narrow-complex, although the QRS may be widened in the presence of a bundle-branch block, with a rate typically around 150 bpm. Because methylxanthines (caffeine, theophylline) are potent adenosine receptor antagonists, even high doses of adenosine may fail to convert SVT in the setting of overdose. For this reason, benzodiazepines are recommended as first line treatment of SVT caused by methylxanthines, as they reduce sympathetic outflow and catecholamine release. Second-line treatment includes CCBs such as diltiazem or verapamil. This approach differs from treatment of nontoxicologically mediated SVT, which relies on vagal maneuvers, adenosine, CCBs, beta blockers, amiodarone, and cardioversion. Sympathomimetic overdose leading to SVT is also treated with benzodiazepines (Figure 4.7.7).

Brugada Pattern

Brugada syndrome, as described in Chapter 4 of this section is a hereditary condition affecting sodium channels, which can lead to arrhythmias and sudden cardiac death. A "Brugada pattern" on ECG consists of ST elevation and partial right bundle branch block (RBBB) in V1–V2 with a characteristic "coved" morphology (Figure 4.7.8). Various toxins and drugs have been shown to mimic this pattern, even when the patient does not possess the underlying syndrome (Table 4.7.8). Most reports of Brugada pattern in the setting of intoxication are in association with sodium channel blockers including cocaine,

Table 4.7.8   Drugs and toxins associated with Brugada pattern on ECG.

Cannabis sp.	Nicotine
Carbon monoxide	Nitrates
Cocaine	Phenothiazines
Diphenhydramine	Phosphides
Ethanol	Propafenone
Flecainide	Propranolol
Ketamine	Tramadol
Lamotrigine	Tricyclic antidepressants
Lithium	*Taxus sp.*

flecainide, propafenone, phenothiazines, diphenhydramine, propranolol, and tricyclic antidepressants (TCAs) [10], though alcohol, lithium, and ketamine have also been shown to manifest a Brugada pattern [11]. When caused by a toxin, the ECG pattern is often transient, though it may be associated with hypotension. Management involves treating the underlying toxin.

Tricyclics Antidepressants

TCAs are used in the treatment of mood and neurological disorders. Although their use has declined in recent years in favor of SSRIs, they remain a significant cause of fatal ingestion due to severe cardiac and neurological toxicity.

TCAs have a rapid onset of action, with toxic effects occurring within one to two hours of overdose. The early clinical presentation of a TCA overdose is an anticholinergic toxidrome, manifesting as hypotension, tachycardia, hyperthermia, mydriasis, dry skin and mucous membranes, hypoactive bowel sounds, and urinary retention. Toxic effects on the central nervous system include confusion, agitation, mania, delirium, dystonia, tremor, myoclonus, impaired memory, sedation, coma, and seizures.

The cardiovascular effects of TCA overdose may be profound, including life-threatening arrhythmia in patients with significant overdose. Toxic effects on the cardiovascular system are mediated by blockade of several receptors, most notably myocardial fast sodium channels and potassium channels. In addition, the toxic effect of TCAs is mediated by direct myocardial depression, GABA/Cl-channel blockade, and blockade at histamine, muscarinic, and α1- and α2-adenergic receptors (Figure 7.4.9).

There are several characteristic ECG changes associated with TCA overdose. Slowed Phase 0 depolarization results manifest as QRS prolongation, right axis deviation, and a RBBB pattern. Delayed repolarization and Phase 4 depolarization

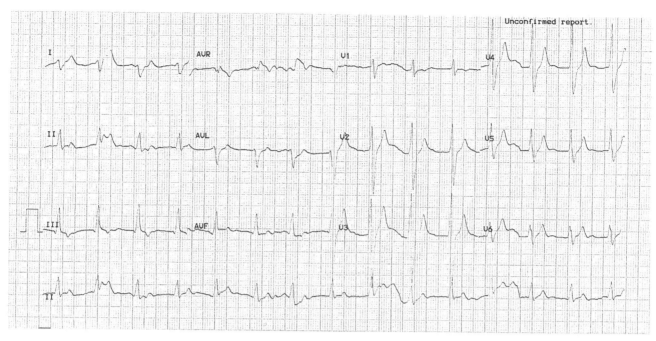

Figure 4.7.1 Sodium channel blockade causing QRS prolongation in carbamazepine overdose. *Source:* Image reproduced with permission from http://lifeinthefastlane.com.

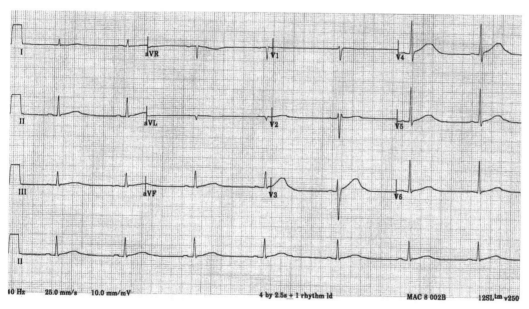

Figure 4.7.2 QT prolongation and bradycardia from sotalol toxicity. *Source:* Image reproduced with permission from http://lifeinthefastlane.com.

leads to QTc prolongation. The duration of the QRS complex is also important: a QRS >100 ms is predictive of seizures, and a QRS >160 msec is predictive of ventricular arrhythmias. A terminal R wave ≥3 mm amplitude in lead aVR also predicts seizures and arrhythmias in the setting of TCA toxicity [12].

The primary antidote in the management of TCA-induced cardiotoxicity is sodium bicarbonate, which works to alkalinize the serum to decrease circulating free drug and provide a sodium gradient to overcome sodium channel blockade (Figure 4.7.1) [13]. Indications for sodium bicarbonate administration include QRS prolongation >100 ms,

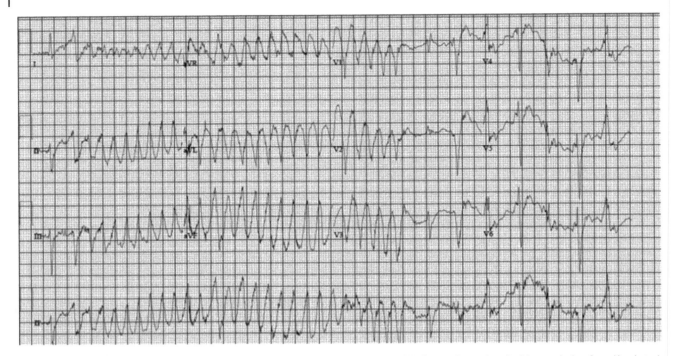

Figure 4.7.3 Torsades de pointes in a patient with a fatal overdose of citalopram [14]. *Source:* Reproduced with permission from Kraai et al.

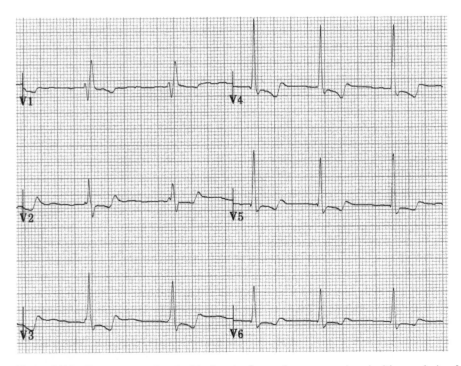

Figure 4.7.4 U waves associated with digoxin. *Source:* Image reproduced with permission from http://lifeinthefastlane.com.

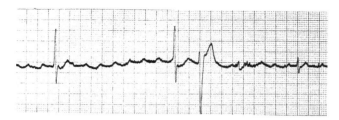

Figure 4.7.5 Atrial tachycardia with block in digoxin toxicity. *Source:* Image reproduced with permission from life http://lifeinthefastlane.com.

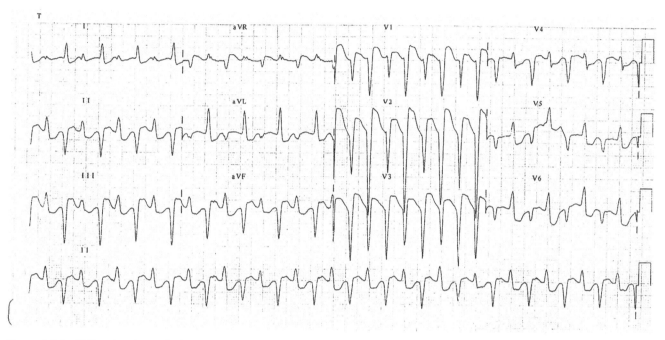

Figure 4.7.6 Bidirectional ventricular tachycardia. *Source:* Image reproduced with permission from http://lifeinthefastlane.com.

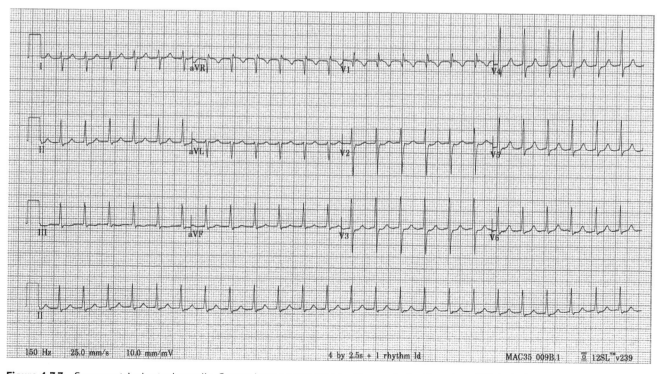

Figure 4.7.7 Supraventricular tachycardia. *Source:* Image reproduced with permission from http://lifeinthefastlane.com.

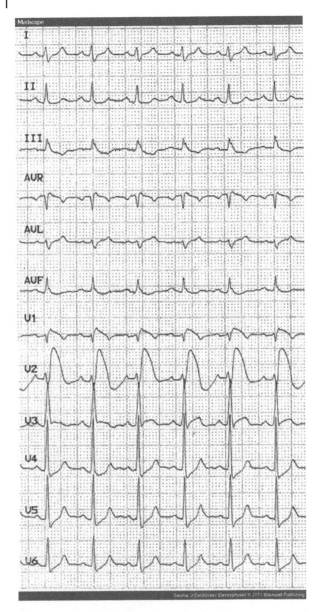

Figure 4.7.8 Coved ST elevation in a Brugada-like pattern in a patient with high plasma levels of ketamine [12]. *Source:* Image reproduced with permission from Rollin et al.

marked acidosis, refractory hypotension, and cardiac arrest. Administer IV sodium bicarbonate 100 mEq (1–2 mEq/kg). Repeat every one to two minutes until blood pressure improves and QRS complexes narrow. Serial ECGs with computer-measured intervals may detect subtle response that could be otherwise missed. If arrhythmias persist despite bicarbonate administration, the use of lidocaine is recommended [15]. Class 1A and 1C antiarrhythmics are contraindicated, as they can worsen cardiotoxicity.

Patients remaining asymptomatic for six hours post-ingestion are appropriate for medical clearance. Isolated persistent tachycardia greater than 120 bpm or a QTc >480 ms are indications for 24-hour admission to observe for progression of symptoms. Signs of significant cardio-vascular or neurological toxicity are an indication for close cardiac monitoring in the intensive care unit. Notably, sinus tachycardia may persist for up to one week following ingestion.

Calcium Channel Blockers

CCBs antagonize L-type voltage sensitive slow calcium channels in cardiac myocytes, leading to decreased intracellular calcium. In turn, this results in negative inotropy leading to myocardial depression, negative chronotropy leading to sinus bradycardia, and negative dromotropy leading to AV node blockade. Severe CCB overdose is highly lethal, and early and aggressive treatment is imperative.

Onset of CCB toxicity is typically within one to two hours of ingestion, but may be delayed in the case of sustained-release drug preparations. Early in CCB overdose, the ECG may simply show bradycardia and/or first degree AV block. As toxicity progresses, hypotension, and more profound AV nodal blockade ensues (Figure 4.7.10). High-grade AV block in CCB is notoriously difficult to treat, with pacing attempts frequently showing failure to capture, and the rhythm may eventually deteriorate to asystole.

Treatment involves fluid resuscitation and administration of calcium as a temporizing measure. Atropine is often ineffective for CCB-induced bradycardia but may be tried. Glucagon, which bypasses the blocked receptor and initiates a cyclic AMP-mediated cascade that allows calcium influx into the cardiac myocyte, has been proposed as a treatment for CCB overdose due to its success in beta blocker overdose. However, evidence of its efficacy for this purpose is limited [16]. The growing body of evidence behind high-dose insulin euglycemic therapy (HIET) has led to its recommendation for early use in CCB overdose [17]. Epinephrine is the favored choice for vasopressor support, as it will counteract hypotension with vasoconstriction and greatest inotropic effect. Finally, intralipid administration may be considered in refractory cases, as CCBs are lipid soluble; however, intralipid use for this indication has not shown clear mortality benefit in studies.

Patients with ingestions of CCBs clearly confirmed to be immediate release preparations may be medically cleared if remaining asymptomatic with reassuring ECG tracings throughout six hours of observation. Symptomatic patients

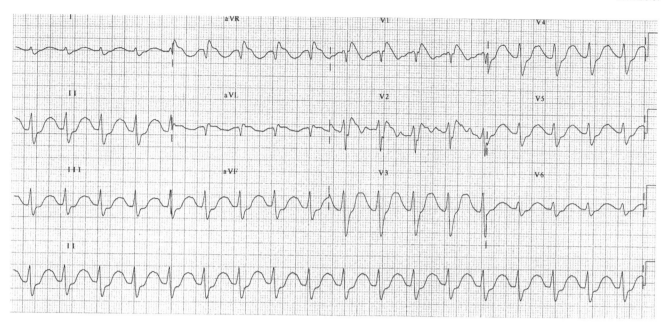

Figure 4.7.9 TCA overdose causing tachycardia, QRS widening, and terminal R wave in aVR. *Source:* Image reproduced with permission from http://lifeinthefastlane.com.

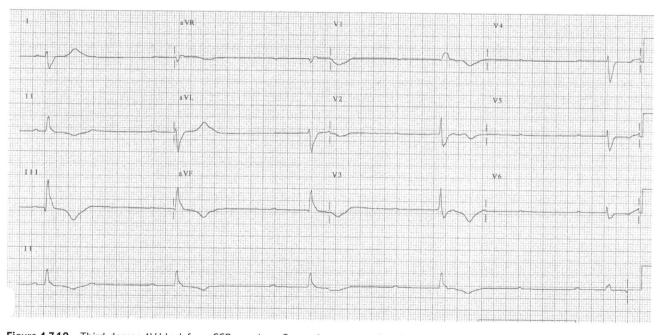

Figure 4.7.10 Third-degree AV block from CCB overdose. *Source:* Image reproduced with permission from http://lifeinthefastlane.com.

with immediate release CCB overdose should be admitted to an ICU setting for close monitoring. If a sustained released formulation is the suspected ingestant, or if the formulation cannot be confirmed, judicious admission for 24 hours of monitoring is recommended due to risk of delayed toxicity.

Conclusion

Given its wide availability and immediate results, the ECG is an essential diagnostic tool in the time-sensitive management of patients with suspected overdose and can also provide important prognostic information. QTc prolongation

>500 ms is an independent predictor for in-hospital adverse cardiovascular events after acute overdose, which when combined with one or more other predictors (serum bicarbonate <20 meq/l, prior cardiac disease) has a 90.9% positive predictive value [18]. Similarly, QT prolongation, ventricular ectopy, any nonsinus rhythm, and evidence of ischemia on the initial ECG are strongly associated with adverse cardiovascular events [19]. The ECG thereby is critical as both a diagnostic tool as well as an instrument that may assist in predicting the patient's course and long-term outcome, and allow for early arrangement of resources and appropriate disposition.

References

1 Centers for Disease Control and Prevention (2010). *Wide-Ranging Online Data for Epidemiologic Research (WONDER Database)*. Atlanta, GA: US Department of Health and Human Services, CDC. Available at http://wonder.cdc.gov. Accessed April 2, 2017.

2 Manini, A.F., Nair, A.P., Vendanthan, R. et al. (2017 Feb 3). Validation of the prognostic utility of the electrocardiogram for acute drug overdose. *J. Am. Heart Assoc.* 6: e004320.

3 Nada, A., Gintant, G.A., Kleiman, R. et al. (2013). The evaluation and management of drug effects on cardiac conduction (PR and QRS intervals) in clinical development. *Am. Heart J.* 165 (4): 489–500.

4 Li, E., Esterly, J., Pohl, S. et al. (2010). Drug-induced QT interval prolongation: considerations for clinicians. *Pharmacotherapy* 30 (7): 684–701.

5 Hoffman, R.S. and Hollander, J.E. (1996). Thrombolytic therapy and cocaine-induced myocardial infarction. *Am. J. Emerg. Med.* 14: 693–695.

6 Mowry, J.B., Spyker, D.A., Brooks, D.E. et al. (2016). 2015 annual report of the American Association of Poison Control Centers' National Poison Data System (NPDS): 33rd annual report. *Clin. Toxicol.* 54 (10): 924–1109.

7 Israelit, S.H., Strizevsky, A., and Raviv, B. (2012). ST elevation myocardial infarction in a young patient after ingestion of caffeinated energy drink and ecstasy. *World J Emerg Med* 3 (4): 305–307.

8 Kanji, S. and MacLean, R. (2012 Oct). Cardiac glycoside toxicity: more than 200 years and counting. *Crit. Care Clin.* 28 (4): 527–535.

9 Levine, M., Nikkanen, H., and Pallin, D.J. (2011 Jan). The effects of intravenous calcium in patients with digoxin toxicity. *J. Emerg. Med.* 40 (1): 41–46.

10 Yap, Y.G., Behr, E.R., and Camm, J. (2009). Drug-induced Brugada syndrome. *Europace* 11 (8): 989–994.

11 Rollin, A., Maury, P., Guilbeau-Frugier, C., and Brugada, J. (2011. Jan). Transient ST elevation after ketamine intoxication: a new cause of acquired Brugada ECG pattern. *J. Cardiovasc. Electrophysiol.* 22 (1): 91–94.

12 Liebelt, E.L. and Francis, P.D. (1995). Woolf AD. ECG lead aVr versus QRS complex in predicting seizures and arrhythmia in acute tricyclic antidepressant poisoning. *Ann. Emerg. Med.* 26: 195–201.

13 Bruccoleri, R.E. and Burns, M.M. (2016 Mar). A literature eview of the use of sodium bicarbonate for the treatment of QRS widening. *J. Med. Toxicol.* 12 (1): 121–129.

14 Kraai, E.P. and Seifert, S.A. (2015 Jun). Citalopram Overdose: A Fatal Case. *J. Med. Toxicol.* 11 (2): 232–236.

15 Foianini, A., Wiegand, T., and Benowitz, N. (2010 May). What is the role of lidocaine or phenytoin in tricyclic antidepressant-induced cardiotoxicity? *Clin. Toxicol. (Phila.)* 48 (4): 325–330.

16 Bailey, B. (2003). Glucagon in beta-blocker and calcium channel blocker overdoses: a systematic review. *J. Toxicol. Clin. Toxicol.* 41 (5): 595–602.

17 Engebretson, K.M., Kaczmarek, K., Morgan, J., and Holger, J.S. (2011). High-dose insulin therapy in beta-blocker and calcium channel-blocker poisoning. *Clin. Toxicol.* 49: 277–283.

18 Manini, A.F., Hoffman, R.S., Stimmel, B. et al. (2015). Clinical risk factors for in-hospital adverse cardiovascular events after acute drug overdose. *Acad. Emerg. Med.* 22: 499–507.

19 Yates, C. and Manini, A.F. (2012 May). Utility of the electrocardiogram in drug overdose and poisoning: theoretical considerations and theoretical implications. *Curr. Cardiol. Rev.* 8 (2): 137–151.

Section V

The ECG in Poison, Electrolyte, Metabolic and Environmental Emergencies

1

ECG Diagnosis and Management of the Poisoned Patient

William F. Rushton[1,2] and Christopher P. Holstege[3]

[1] *Department of Emergency Medicine, University of Alabama, Birmingham, AL, USA*
[2] *Regional Poison Control Center of Children's of Alabama, Birmingham, AL, USA*
[3] *Department of Emergency Medicine and Pediatrics, University of Virginia, Charlottesville, VA, USA*

Introduction

The health care provider is no stranger to the poisoned patient. In 2018, there were approximately 2.2 million calls to US poison centers regarding poisoned patients with almost one-third presenting to a health care facility. Cardiovascular drug intoxication was the sixth most common pharmaceutical class reported [1]. However, even in patients who do not ingest cardiovascular medications, cardiac abnormalities are common. One study estimated that almost 70% of poisoned patients had an abnormal electrocardiogram (ECG) [2]. The 12-lead ECG is, therefore, one of the most crucial tools in evaluating the poisoned patient. Combined with the rhythm strip, ECGs help diagnose, dictate management, and reflect signs of end organ toxicity. This chapter will discuss the various applications of the ECG in caring for the poisoned patient.

Cardiac Action Potential

The application of the ECG in toxicology begins with understanding the principles of the cardiac action potential and how it is affected by different xenobiotics. The action potential begins with phase 0 as rapid voltage sensitive sodium (Na^+) channels (I_{na+}) open in response to a stimulus or intrinsic pacemaker activity, resulting in depolarization from the resting membrane potential of $-90\,mv$ (Figure 5.1.1). This sodium influx, which leads to a rapid upstroke of the cardiac action potential, is directly responsible for the QRS interval on the ECG. Phase 1 begins as the transient outward potassium current (I_{to}) causes a partial repolarization and the fast-acting sodium channels close. Inward depolarizing calcium channel (I_{ca}) currents are balanced by outward potassium efflux channels (I_{ks}), thus creating the plateau phase (phase 2) that subsequently results in cardiac myocyte contraction. The L-type calcium channels close in phase 3, while the I_{ks} current continues; this results in a net repolarization and recruits other delayed rectifier potassium channels (I_{kr}), returning the resting membrane potential to $-90\,mv$. Phase 3 is represented on the ECG as the QT interval. Phase 4 is the resting period for the cell where sodium, potassium, and calcium are all pumped against their electrochemical gradients by an ATPase dependent process [3].

Tachycardia in the Poisoned Patient

Multiple xenobiotics are implicated in causing tachycardia in the poisoned patient (Table 5.1.1). Sinus tachycardia is the most common rhythm disturbance. Xenobiotics that excite the sympathetic nervous system cause tachycardia by stimulating catecholamine surges and directly activating B1-adrenergic receptors. Plants and pharmaceuticals with anticholinergic properties can exacerbate tachycardia by inhibiting the parasympathetic vagal tone on the sinoatrial node, thereby allowing the majority of the heart's stimulus to originate from the sympathetic nervous system. Other toxidromes, including serotonin syndrome, neuroleptic malignant syndrome, and malignant hyperthermia, can cause autonomic instability resulting in tachycardia. Surprisingly, some drugs that are classically thought to cause bradycardia can result in an increase in heart rate. For instance, cholinergic medications such as organophosphates and nicotinic agonists may initially stimulate the sympathetic nervous system before exhibiting a greater effect at the parasympathetic system. Multiple

Electrocardiogram in Clinical Medicine, First Edition. Edited by William J. Brady, Michael J. Lipinski, Andrew E. Darby,
Michael C. Bond, Nathan P. Charlton, Korin Hudson, and Kelly Williamson.
© 2021 John Wiley & Sons Ltd. Published 2021 by John Wiley & Sons Ltd.

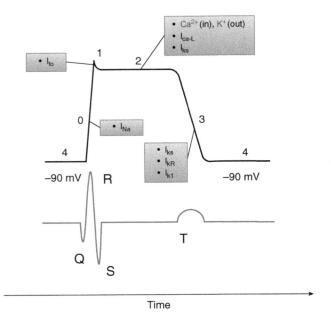

Figure 5.1.1 Cardiac action potential.

patients with sympathomimetic syndrome generally will demonstrate mydriasis, hypertension, and agitation in addition to tachycardia. On the other hand, those poisoned with an anticholinergic xenobiotic will have tachycardia along with mydriasis, dry axilla, absent bowel sounds, and urinary retention. Serotonin syndrome patients often present not only with tachycardia but also with altered mental status, hyperreflexia, and inducible clonus.

The tachycardia encountered with xenobiotics should be considered as one sign of the overall intoxication. Intravenous fluids are generally indicated to help establish preload. Primary treatment is focused on managing the underlying pathophysiology and not just correcting numbers. For example, tachycardia caused by adrenergic hyperactivity from a stimulant such as cocaine should be treated with a benzodiazepine. Treating a tachycardic patient intoxicated on a stimulant with a beta adrenergic blocker can have disastrous effects; depending on the cause, an increased heart rate in a poisoned patient may be crucial to maintaining cardiac output [5].

xenobiotics that cause peripheral vasodilatation can also be expected to cause reflex tachycardia as the heart attempts to increase output to compensate for the decrease in systemic vascular resistance.

Certain classes of xenobiotics are well known to cause ventricular tachydysrhythmias. Rhythm changes may be precipitated by catecholamine excess released by sympathomimetic drugs [4]. Caffeine and theophylline poisoning can predispose to arrhythmias by exaggerating the myocyte response to electrical and neurohormonal stimulation [5]. Halogenated hydrocarbons have also been implicated in propagating unstable ventricular rhythms by sensitizing the cardiac membrane to circulating catecholamines [6].

The physical exam can augment the diagnostic aid of an ECG in a poisoned patient with tachycardia. For example,

Bradycardia

Unlike tachycardia, the toxin-induced differential for bradycardia is much more concise (Table 5.1.2). These xenobitoics largely slow the heart rate by either decreasing the sympathetic tone or increasing the parasympathetic tone. At the sinoatrial (SA) node, several xenobiotics can directly antagonize the sympathetic response such as B1-adrenergic blockers. Alpha-2 adrenergic agonists, certain sedative hypnotics, baclofen, and opioids can also decrease activity of the sympathetic nervous system leading to bradycardia. Cardiac steroids such as digoxin increase the vagal tone to the SA and atrioventricular (AV) node resulting in bradycardia or heart block

Table 5.1.1 Classes of drugs that can cause tachycardia.

Classes of drugs that cause tachycardia
Acetylcholinesterase inhibitors[a]
Alpha-2 adrenergic antagonists
Cardiac glycosides[a]
Halogenated hydrocarbons
Methylxanthines
Muscarinic antagonists (anticholinergic)
Nicotinic agonists[a]
Serotonergic xenobiotics
Sympathomimetics

[a] These drugs can cause both tachycardia and bradycardia.

Table 5.1.2 Classes of drugs that can cause bradycardia.

Classes of drugs that cause bradycardia
Acetylcholinesterase inhibitors[a]
Alpha-2 adrenergic agonists
B-adrenergic antagonists
Calcium channel blockers
Cardiac glycosides[a]
GABA- B agonists
Nicotinic agonists[a]
Opioids

[a] These drugs can cause both tachycardia and bradycardia.

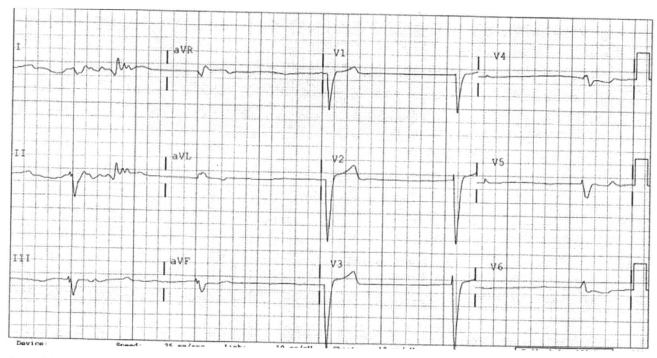

Figure 5.1.2 Junctional bradydysrhythmia in a digoxin poisoned patient. Notice lack of discernable P waves before QRS complex.

(Figure 5.1.2). Similarly, organophosphates, carbamates, and clitocybe mushrooms all stimulate the muscarinic receptors at the SV node, mimicking parasympathetic stimulation and leading to bradycardia. Non-dihydropyridine calcium channel blockers, such as verapamil and diltiazem, can inhibit the L-type calcium channel from opening. This mechanism slows the recovery in both the sinoatrial and AV node and ultimately decreases the heart rate (Figure 5.1.3) [7].

Other physical exam findings can also help narrow the differential in the bradycardic poisoned patient. For example, bradycardia with miosis can be seen with alpha-2 adrenergic agonists, opioids, and cholinergic xenobiotics. Bradycardia associated with marked diaphoresis, bronchorrhea, bronchoconstriction, diarrhea, and vomiting would indicate toxicity by an acetylcholinesterase inhibitor. Bradycardia with loss of P waves and associated hypotension, decreased mental status, and hyperglycemia may indicate calcium channel blocker toxicity.

Treatment of toxin-induced bradycardia is generally supportive and should be directed at maintaining adequate tissue perfusion and not a target heart rate. When monitoring perfusion, careful attention should be paid to mental status, urine output, and acid–base status. Atropine and electrical pacing may be attempted but are of limited benefit in numerous toxicities [8–10]. Several recent studies have supported the use of glucagon, calcium, and high-dose insulin therapy with toxicity from beta adrenergic antagonists and calcium

channel blockers [10, 11]. These therapies, however, should be used with caution, and consultation with a medical toxicologist is advised.

QRS Prolongation

A plethora of xenobiotics cause severe cardiotoxicity through antagonism at the cardiac sodium channel (Table 5.1.3). These xenobitoics bind the cardiac sodium channel in the inactivated or activated phase and slow recovery of these channels. This decreases the amount of sodium per unit time entering the cell [12]. One model demonstrates that these toxins exert their effect through physical blockade of the inner opening of the channel pore [13]. By exerting their influence on this channel, these toxins can effectively prolong phase 0 of the cardiac action potential. This pathophysiology manifests itself on an ECG by a prolongation of the QRS interval [14]. The magnitude of a xenobitoic's sodium channel blockade is rate dependent, with a higher percentage of sodium channels being blocked as the heart rate increases [15, 16]. Since the QRS duration depends on the number of sodium channels poisoned, worsening tachycardia precipitates further widening of the interval.

Interpretation of the QRS segment can be challenging. Generally a widened QRS is defined as greater than 120 ms; however, any QRS greater than 100 ms could represent a potentially poisoned patient and one at risk for ventricular

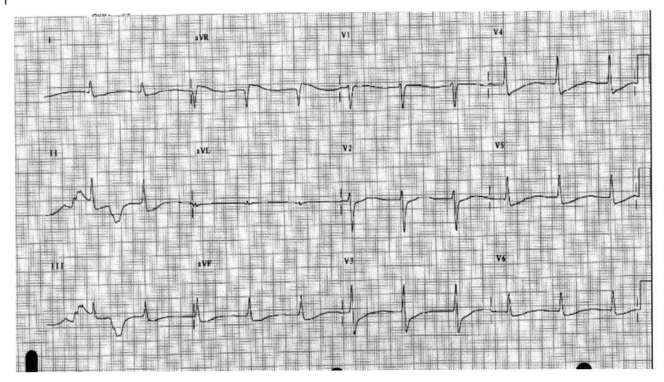

Figure 5.1.3 Bradydysrhythmia with a junctional rhythm associated with a calcium channel blocker toxicity. Notice absence of P waves as the SA node is not active in severe nondihydropyridine calcium channel blocker toxicity.

dysrhythmia [17]. In the setting of a cardiac sodium channel blocker, conduction to the right side of the heart is preferentially impaired resulting in a rightward shift of the terminal 40 ms of the complex. This is often demonstrated on the ECG as an "S" wave in both leads I and aVL and an "R" wave in lead aVR (Figures 5.1.4 and 5.1.5) [18]. Often, the morphology may resemble a right bundle branch block (RBBB). With severe toxicity, distinguishing between a supraventricular and ventricular rhythm may be impossible (Figure 5.1.6) [17, 19]. While this sodium channel binding pattern was initially described in tricyclic antidepressant (TCA) poisoning, it has been validated as representative of all cardiac sodium channel blocking xenobiotics [20]. QRS prolongation has been proposed as a surrogate marker for impending ventricular arrhythmia and negative inotropy, but studies are not definitive [16]. The duration of QRS prolongation can also be used to judge the severity of the systemic toxicity and guide management. One retrospective poison center study of patients with TCA ingestion demonstrated no seizures or dysrhythmias in patients with QRS length under 100 ms, a moderate risk of seizures in those with a QRS from 100 to 160 ms, and a moderate risk of both seizures and dysrhythmias with a QRS greater than 160 ms [21].

Table 5.1.3 Sodium channel blocking drugs (not all inclusive).

Sodium channel blocking drugs	
Amantadine	Cyclic antidepressants
Carbamazepine	Amitriptyline
Chloroquine	Amoxapine
Class IA antidysrhythmics	Desipramine
Disopyramide	Doxepin
Quinidine	Imipramine
Procainamide	Nortriptyline
Quinine	Maprotiline
Class IC antidysrhythmics	Diphenhydramine
Encainide	Hydroxychloroquine
Flecainide	Loxapine
Propafenone	Orphenadrine
Cocaine	Phenothiazines
Propranolol	Mesoridazine
Verapamil	Thioridazine
Diltiazem	Propoxyphene

(a)

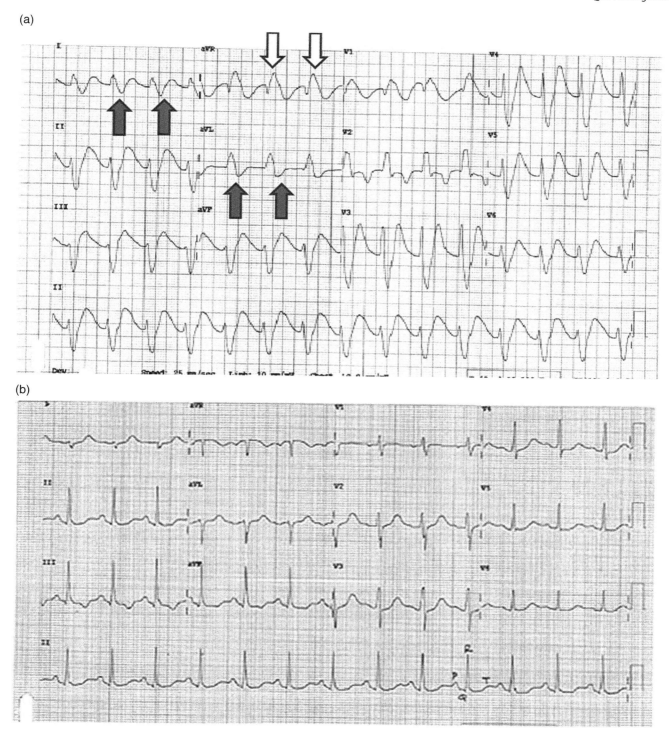

(b)

Figure 5.1.4 Patient who overdosed on a cardiac sodium channel blocking agent. (a) In the first ECG, notice the prolonged QRS (224 ms) with a prominent R′ in aVR (outlined arrows) and deep S waves in I and aVL (solid arrows). This is indicative of terminal 40 ms delay. (b) The second ECG is the same patient after 200 meq of sodium bicarbonate. Notice the narrowing of the QRS interval.

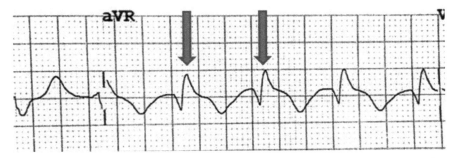

Figure 5.1.5 Prominent R′ in lead aVR (arrows) in a patient after a severe amitriptyline overdose.

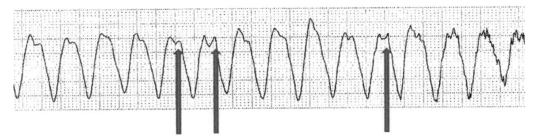

Figure 5.1.6 Sinus tachycardia in lead II in a diphenhydramine overdose; the widened QRS can give the appearance of ventricular tachycardia. However, P waves (shown on the arrows) remain discernible suggesting that this is a sinus rhythm.

Regardless of the xenobiotic involved, sodium bicarbonate is the treatment of choice for QRS prolongation in the poisoned patient. While older studies suggested that protein binding was increased in the presence of alkalosis, the primary mechanism has now been demonstrated to be decreased sodium channel binding by the toxin. Sodium bicarbonate also has the advantage of increasing the sodium ion concentration, favoring the movement of sodium across cell membranes [16]. Multiple studies initially performed in TCA models, and now extrapolated to other cardiac sodium channel antagonists, have demonstrated improvement of inotropy and stabilization of the cardiac myocyte with sodium bicarbonate (Figure 5.1.4). Therefore, sodium bicarbonate may be used as therapy for both wide complex tachydysrhythmias and hypotension in the setting of a sodium channel antagonist [16, 20, 22]. The typical adult dose is 1–2 meq/kg intravenously. It is reasonable to administer sodium bicarbonate boluses in patients with a markedly widened QRS interval, hemodynamic instability, and dysrhythmias, while an infusion may be started in more stable patients. Worsening acidosis, such as that caused by seizures, can be extremely dangerous and increase the risk of dysrhythmia in patients poisoned with a cardiac sodium channel blocking agent. Administration of sodium bicarbonate can help mitigate this risk. Various studies have also evaluated hypertonic

saline and lidocaine in animal models; however, no large scale human trials demonstrate a clear benefit [22–24]. Other class I anti- dysrhythmics, calcium channel blockers, and beta adrenergic antagonists should be avoided due to their propensity to exacerbate an already stressed conduction system, leading to decreased cardiac output [20, 22]. In the presence of a nonperfusing rhythm such as ventricular fibrillation or pulseless ventricular tachycardia, unsynchronized electrical defibrillation should be first-line therapy.

QT Prolongation

Multiple medications, potentially up to 3% of all drugs, have been implicated in QT interval prolongation (Table 5.1.4). These xenobiotics vary in their ability to increase the interval. For instance, several drugs have caused severe QT interval prolongation in therapeutic dosing and have subsequently been removed from the market, while other drugs only manifest QT prolongation in severe overdose [19]. Some pharmaceuticals, such as sotalol, a class III antiarrhythmic, take advantage of this mechanism for their therapeutic effect. Of all the drug classes, the antipsychotic medications are the most frequently implicated.

Table 5.1.4 Potassium efflux channel blocking drugs (not all inclusive).

Potassium efflux channel blocking drugs	
Antihistamines	Class III antidysrhythmics
Astemizole	Amiodarone
Diphenhydramine	Dofetilide
Loratidine	Ibutilide
Terfenadine	Sotalol
Antipsychotics	Cyclic antidepressants
Chlorpromazine	Amitriptyline
Droperidol	Amoxapine
Haloperidol	Desipramine
Mesoridazine	Doxepin
Pimozide	Imipramine
Quetiapine	Nortriptyline
Risperidone	Maprotiline
Thioridazine	Fluoroquinolones
Ziprasidone	Ciprofloxacin
Arsenic trioxide	Gatifloxacin
Bepridil	Levofloxacin
Chloroquine	Moxifloxacin
Cisapride	Sparfloxacin
Citalopram	Halofantrine
Class IA antidysrhythmics	Hydroxychloroquine
Disopyramide	Levomethadyl
Quinidine	Macrolides
Procainamide	Clarithromycin
Class IC antidysrhythmics	Erythromycin
Encainide	Pentamidine
Flecainide	Quinine
Moricizine	Tacrolimus
Propafenone	Venlafaxine

The QT interval represents the duration of ventricular systole and phase 3 of the cardiac action potential (Figure 5.1.1). Blockade of the outward potassium rectifier current (I_{kr}) delays repolarization and prolongs the action potential (Figure 5.1.7). Unfortunately, delaying repolarization can activate an inward depolarization current that can lead to early after-depolarization (EAD). EADs can precipitate a polymorphic ventricular tachycardia known as torsades de pointes (TdP) [25]. Bradycardia increases the risk of TdP as slower heart rates prolong the action potential, thereby lengthening the time available for an EAD to occur [26].

Interpretation of the QT interval can also be difficult. Although there are multiple formulas designed to standardize the QT interval, they may not be accurate in tachycardia or bradycardia. The most commonly used method of correction is Bazett's formula ($QTc = QT/\sqrt{RR}$). Risks of dysrhythmias have most commonly been associated with a QTc interval greater than 500 ms; however, a patient's risk is varied and is further dependent on individual patient characteristics and other co-ingestions [19, 25]. Furthermore, abnormal T waves and the introduction of U waves that can accompany blockage of the potassium rectifying channel hinder accurate measurement of the interval.

First-line therapy for a prolonged QTc interval is immediate treatment of any systemic factors, including electrolyte imbalances, hypoxia, and removal of the offending xenobiotic. Patients should receive frequent cardiac interval monitoring. Intravenous treatment of magnesium sulfate (1–2 g in the adult patient) is the initial pharmacologic intervention both for TdP and a prolonged QT interval [25]. Several authors recommend maintaining serum potassium in the high normal range (4.5–5 mmol/l) [25, 27]. As tachycardia shortens the action potential, overdrive pacing up to 100–120 beats per minute is often effective at terminating TdP. Options for overdrive pacing include both electrical and through pharmacologic means such as isoprotenerol [27]. As with cardiac sodium channel blocking toxicity, all nonperfusing rhythms should be treated with standard ACLS protocol.

Electrolyte abnormalities leading to QT prolongation include hypomagnesemia, hypokalemia, and hypocalcemia [28]. It is important to remember that xenobiotics that cause these electrolyte abnormalities, such as hydrofluoric acid, toluene, and sympathomimetics, can then lead to QT prolongation. Treatment of the underlying electrolyte disorder should be the primary therapy.

Conclusion

ECG changes in the poisoned patient are common and present the health care practitioner with diagnostic aids to the etiology of the exposure. In the unstable patient, the ECG can further direct care by demonstrating what portions of the cardiac action potential are being impeded. For every poisoned and intoxicated patient, careful evaluation of the heart rate, QRS, and the QT interval should be undertaken and therapies applied appropriately. With a basic understanding of the drug interactions at the cardiac receptors and their associated ECG changes, a prudent health care practitioner can stabilize, diagnose, and manage the cardiotoxic manifestations of most xenobiotics.

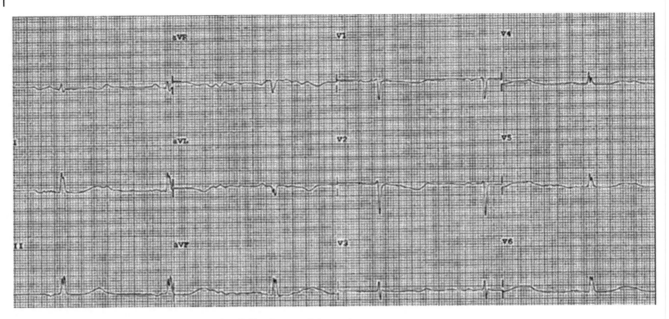

Figure 5.1.7 Severe QT interval prolongation following sotalol overdose.

References

1 Gummin, D.D., Mowry, J.B., Spyker, D.A. et al. (2019). 2018 Annual Report of the American Association of Poison Control Centers' National Poison Data System (NPDS): 36th Annual Report. *Clin Toxicol.* 57(12): 1220–1413.

2 Homer, A., Brady, W.J., and Holstege, C. (2005 Sept.). *The Association of Toxins and ECG Abnormality in Poisoned Patients.* Nice, France: Mediterranean Emergency Medicine Congress.

3 Delk, C., Holstege, C.P., and Brady, W.J. (2007). Electrocardiographic abnormalities associated with poisoning. *Am. J. Emerg. Med.* 25 (6): 672–687.

4 Schwartz, A.B., Janzen, D., Jones, R.T., and Boyle, W. (1989). Electrocardiographic and hemodynamic effects of intravenous cocaine in awake and anesthetized dogs. *J. Electrocardiol.* 22 (2): 159–166.

5 Holstege, C.P., Hunter, Y., Baer, A.B. et al. (2003). Massive caffeine overdose requiring vasopressin infusion and hemodialysis. *J. Toxicol. Clin. Toxicol.* 41 (7): 1003–1007.

6 Mullin, L.S., Azar, A., Reinhardt, C.F. et al. (1972). Halogenated hydrocarbon- induced cardiac arrhythmias associated with release of endogenous epinephrine. *Am. Ind. Hyg. Assoc. J.* 33 (6): 389–396.

7 DeWitt, C.R. and Waksman, J.C. (2004). Pharmacology, pathophysiology and management of calcium channel blocker and beta-blocker toxicity. *Toxicol. Rev.* 23 (4): 223–238.

8 Siddiqi, T.A., Hill, J., Huckleberry, Y., and Parthasarathy, S. (2013). Non-cardiogenic pulmonary edema and life-threatening shock due to calcium channel blocker overdose and its management: a case report and a clinical review. *Respir. Care* 59 (2): e15–e21.

9 Shepherd, G. and Klein-Schwartz, W. (2005). High-dose insulin therapy for calcium-channel blocker overdose. *Ann. Pharmacother.* 39 (5): 923–930.

10 Engebretsen, K.M., Kaczmarek, K.M., Morgan, J., and Holger, J.S. (2011). High-dose insulin therapy in beta-blocker and calcium channel-blocker poisoning. *Clin. Toxicol.* 49 (4): 277–283.

11 Holger, J.S., Stellpflug, S.J., Cole, J.B. et al. (2011). High-dose insulin: a consecutive case series in toxin-induced cardiogenic shock. *Clin. Toxicol.* 49 (7): 653–658.

12 Kolecki, P.F. and Curry, S.C. (1997). Poisoning by sodium channel blocking agents. *Crit. Care Clin.* 13 (4): 829–848.

13 Keating, M.T. and Sanguinetti, M.C. (2001). Molecular and cellular mechanisms of cardiac arrhythmias. *Cell* 104 (4): 569–580.

14 Phillips, K., Luk, A., Soor, G.S. et al. (2009). Cocaine cardiotoxicity; a review of the pathophysiology, pathology, and treatment options. *Am. J. Cardiovasc. Drugs* 9 (3): 177–196.

15 Wood, D.M., Dargan, P.I., and Hoffman, R.S. (2009). Management of cocaine-induced cardiac arrhythmias due to cardiac ion channel dysfunction. *Clin. Toxicol.* 47 (1): 14–23.

16 Seger, D.L. (2006). A critical reconsideration of the clinical effects and treatment recommendations for sodium channel blocking drug cardiotoxicity. *Toxicol. Rev.* 25 (4): 283–296.

17 Brady, W.J. and Skiles, J. (1999). Wide QRS complex tachycardia: ECG differential diagnosis. *Am. J. Emerg. Med.* 17 (4): 376–381.

18 Niemann, J.T., Bessen, H.A., Rothstein, R.J., and Laks, M.M. (1986). Electrocardiographic criteria for tricyclic antidepressant cardiotoxicity. *Am. J. Cardiol.* 57 (13): 1154–1159.

19 Holstege, C.P., Eldridge, D.L., and Rowden, A.K. (2006). ECG manifestations: the poisoned patient. *Emerg. Med. Clin. North Am.* 24 (1): 159–178.

20 Hoffman, R.S. (2010). Treatment of patients with cocaine-induced arrhythmias: bringing the bench to the bedside. *Br. J. Clin. Pharmacol.* 69 (5): 448–457.

21 Boehnert, M.T. and Lovejoy, F.H. (1985). Value of the QRS duration versus the serum drug level in predicting seizures and ventriculararrhythmias after an acute overdose of tricyclic antidepressants. *N. Engl. J. Med.* 313 (8): 474–479.

22 Winecoff, A.P., Hariman, R.J., Grawe, J.J. et al. (1994). Reversal of the electrocardiographic effects of cocaine by lidocaine. Part 1. Comparison with sodium bicarbonate and quinidine. *Pharmacotherapy* 14 (6): 698–703.

23 McCabe, J.L., Cobaugh, D.J., Menegazzi, J.J., and Fata, J. (1998). Experimental tricyclic antidepressant toxicity: a randomized, controlled comparison ofhypertonic saline solution, sodium bicarbonate, and hyperventilation. *Ann. Emerg. Med.* 32 (3): 329–333.

24 Foianini, A., Joseph Wiegand, T., and Benowitz, N. (2010). What is the role of lidocaine or phenytoin in tricyclic antidepressant-induced cardiotoxicity? *Clin. Toxicol.* 48 (4): 325–330.

25 Yap, Y.G. and Camm, A.J. (2003). Drug induced QT prolongation and torsades de pointes. *Heart* 89 (11): 1363–1367.

26 Hondeghem, L.M. and Snyders, D.J. (1990). Class III antiarrhythmic agents have a lot of potential but a long way to go. Reduced effectiveness and dangers of reverse use dependence. *Circulation* 81 (2): 686–690.

27 Gupta, A., Lawrence, A.T., Krishnan, K. et al. (2007). Current concepts in the mechanisms and management of drug-induced QT prolongation and torsade de pointes. *Am. Heart J.* 53 (6): 891–899.

28 Holstege, C.P., Baer, A., and Brady, W.J. (2005). The electrocardiographic toxidrome: the ECG presentation of hydrofluoric acid ingestion. *Am. J. Emerg. Med.* 23 (2): 171–176.

2

The Use of the ECG in the Poisoned Patient

The "Rule-out Ingestion" Strategy

Heather A. Borek[1] and Lewis S. Hardison[2,3]

[1] Division of Medical Toxicology, Department of Emergency Medicine, University of Virginia, Charlottesville, VA, USA
[2] College of Pharmacy, University of South Carolina, Columbia, SC, USA
[3] Department of Emergency Medicine, Prisma Health Richland Hospital, Columbia, SC, USA

Introduction

In 2018 there were a total of 2 211 678 substances with associated human exposure reported to the American Association of Poison Control Centers (AAPCC) [1]. Analgesics, sedatives/hypnotics/antipsychotics, cardiovascular drugs, and antihistamines make up 4 of the top 10 substance categories involved in human exposures. These same agents also represent the four most common substance categories with the greatest rate of increasing exposure [1]. Unfortunately, when evaluating these exposures, patient histories are often unreliable. Parents may be uncertain as to which medication in the pill planner the child was exposed. A patient who is truly suicidal may minimize the substances or amounts ingested to facilitate the suicide attempt; alternatively, some patients may overexaggerate the circumstances of an overdose. Therefore, clinicians treating these patient populations must gather historical clues from other sources. Often this consists of eyewitness history by friends or family members, or gathering a list of substances to which the patient may have been exposed (patient's or family members' medications). There is also a greater reliance on physical examination and ancillary testing, making laboratory testing and electrocardiogram (ECG) assessment crucial to proper evaluation.

The diagnosis and management of the poisoned patient can challenge even the most experienced clinician. In addition, the clinician is often tasked to medically clear the poisoned patient before psychiatric care. A significant amount of data must be gathered in order to safely and efficiently medically clear a patient who is possibly poisoned. Among other things, vital signs and laboratory values should be normal, and the ECG, including rate, rhythm, and morphology should be normal.

Cardiovascular complications are a common cause of morbidity and mortality in the poisoned patient. Even outside of the cardiovascular drug class, drug-induced abnormalities on the 12-lead ECG are common [2]. The clinician can, therefore, use the ECG to help guide evaluation and management of the poisoned patient. This chapter will discuss the use of the ECG in the poisoned patient, and how specifically it can assist in ruling in or ruling out toxicity.

Background

When using the ECG to help "rule out" ingestion, it is helpful to think about the potential cardiovascular effects of each specific agent that was possibly ingested. Xenobiotics affecting the heart can cause rate, rhythm, and conduction disturbances on the ECG. For instance, beta blockers can lead to bradycardia, while agents that affect sodium influx or potassium efflux from the myocyte can cause QRS and QT interval prolongation, respectively. A patient who is suspected of beta-blocker ingestion, but has an ECG that reveals sinus tachycardia during monitoring should alert the clinician that significant beta-blocker toxicity is unlikely or that a different agent may be involved. Conversely, if an agent such as clonidine is ingested and the patient has signs of bradycardia and an atrioventricular (AV) block on ECG, then the ECG findings may be helpful in supporting the suspected toxicity.

Rate

When evaluating the ECG, altered heart rate is a common initial indicator of potential toxicity, and all patients with altered heart rate in the setting of a potential poisoning

Electrocardiogram in Clinical Medicine, First Edition. Edited by William J. Brady, Michael J. Lipinski, Andrew E. Darby, Michael C. Bond, Nathan P. Charlton, Korin Hudson, and Kelly Williamson.
© 2021 John Wiley & Sons Ltd. Published 2021 by John Wiley & Sons Ltd.

should be considered to have drug effect. When discussing heart rate, it is useful to start by taking a closer look at the autonomic nervous system, which is divided into the sympathetic and parasympathetic systems. By understanding the innervation of the autonomic nervous system, one can predict the effects that will be seen clinically after ingestion. Norepinephrine and epinephrine, which are the sympathetic nervous system's primary neurotransmitters, are responsible for causing mydriasis, vasoconstriction, and tachycardia. Stimulation of the parasympathetic nervous system results in miosis, lacrimation, salivation, bronchorrhea, bronchospasm, and bradycardia. Therefore, agents that stimulate the sympathetic nervous system or those that block the parasympathetic system are expected to result in tachycardia. Conversely, agents that block the sympathetic nervous system or those that stimulate the parasympathetic system are expected to cause bradycardia.

Tachycardia is a telling, but nonspecific, feature on the ECG that reflects a potential toxic ingestion. A variety of agents can cause tachycardia. Sympathomimetic substances such as cocaine or amphetamines stimulate adrenergic receptors resulting in tachycardia. This hyperstimulation may also cause ischemia, especially in the older population or those at risk for coronary artery disease or vasospasm. Ischemic changes, such as ST segment elevations or depressions and T-wave inversions, may be noted on the ECG of a sympathomimetic poisoned patient (Figure 5.2.1).

A variety of other agents can also cause tachycardia. Anticholinergic agents induce tachycardia as part of their toxidrome. In combination with clinical examination findings such as mydriasis, hallucinations, dry mucous membranes, and urinary retention, an ECG revealing sinus tachycardia in a suspected anticholinergic-poisoned patient helps to support the diagnosis. Antidepressants such as selective serotonin reuptake inhibitors (SSRIs) may cause sinus tachycardia, especially in the setting of serotonergic excess or serotonin syndrome. A patient who overdosed on an SSRI who is exhibiting clonus, mydriasis, diaphoresis, hyperreflexia, hyperthermia, altered mental status, and increased bowel motility will also likely have sinus tachycardia as part of the constellation of serotonergic effects. Serotonin-norepinephrine reuptake inhibitor (SNRI) poisoning with agents such as duloxetine or venlafaxine also commonly results in tachycardia, due to both serotonergic effects and sympathomimetic effects resulting from excess norepinephrine.

Numerous agents are known to cause bradycardia in both therapeutic use and toxicity. Opioids and benzodiazepines, as well as other sedatives, can result in bradycardia due to their profound sedative effects. Centrally acting alpha-2 adrenergic agonists decrease sympathetic outflow resulting in bradycardia and hypotension. Two other agents that commonly result in bradycardia are beta blockers and calcium channel blockers. Beta-blocker toxicity would be expected to exhibit signs of sinus bradycardia with concomitant hypotension. Centrally acting calcium channel blockers are also known to cause bradycardia and hypotension; although, the dihydropyridine class may cause hypotension and tachycardia due to peripheral vasodilatory effects.

Unfortunately, ingestions do not typically involve a single agent. The clinical picture is often mixed, with effects from multiple agents acting synergistically or antagonistically.

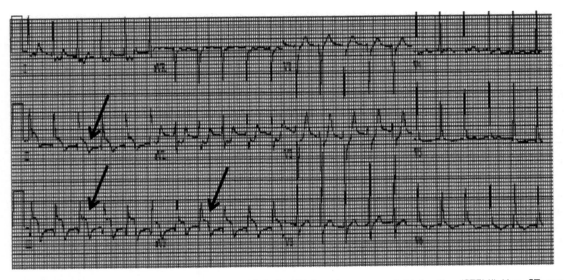

Figure 5.2.1 ECG showing sinus tachycardia and inferior ST elevation myocardial infarction (STEMI). Note ST segment elevations in leads II, III, and aVF (arrows).

For example, a patient with a sympathomimetic ingestion may not exhibit the same degree of tachycardia if the patient is also taking a beta blocker, or coingested a sedative, such as a benzodiazepine. Anticholinergic agents may delay gastrointestinal motility, prolonging absorption, and therefore prolonging or augmenting the toxicity of other ingested agents. In addition, certain agents may also have multiple mechanisms of action. For example, tricyclic antidepressants (TCAs) are alpha-adrenergic receptor blockers, anticholinergic, and have effects on biogenic amines, such as norepinephrine and serotonin. These mechanisms all contribute to the tachycardia seen in TCA poisoning.

Tachycardia and bradycardia are signs of potential xenobiotic-induced cardiac or autonomic dysfunction and should prompt further evaluation. The clinician should not medically clear the patient unless these features can otherwise be explained.

Rhythm

Following an impulse from the sinoatrial (SA) node through atrial conducting fibers, the AV node relays the impulse into the ventricles to allow for complete emptying of the atrium. This process is represented on the ECG as the PR interval. Consequently, xenobiotics that delay atrial electrical impulse or increase the refractory nature of the AV node can increase the PR interval. Cardiac steroids increase vagal tone and prolong the AV refractory period. Cholinergic xenobiotics directly stimulate the muscarinic receptors, thereby also increasing the refractory state of the AV node. Beta-adrenergic antagonists and nondihydropyridine calcium channel blockers alter the influx of calcium through L-type calcium channels into AV nodal cells. All can result in sinus bradycardia with PR interval prolongation; on the ECG, the presence of a P wave preceding each QRS complex is expected (Figure 5.2.2).

Excitation of the sinus node is mediated primarily by calcium ion influx rather than sodium channels [3]. Consequently, centrally acting calcium channel blockers, such as verapamil and diltiazem, may cause a loss of P waves preceding each QRS complex, as the impulse from the sinus node is affected by calcium channel blockade. The loss of the sinus node input causes the development of a junctional rhythm on ECG, and can be suggestive of calcium channel blocker toxicity (Figure 5.2.3).

Although these findings are expected based on mechanisms of action, a variety of ECG findings can be seen

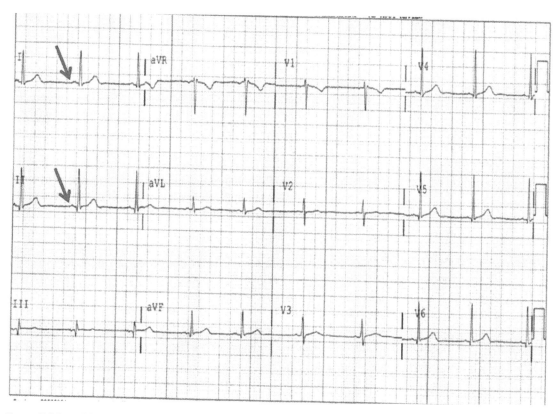

Figure 5.2.2 ECG of a patient with beta-blocker toxicity. Note the sinus bradycardia with a P wave preceding each QRS complex (arrow). The PR interval is normal in this example.

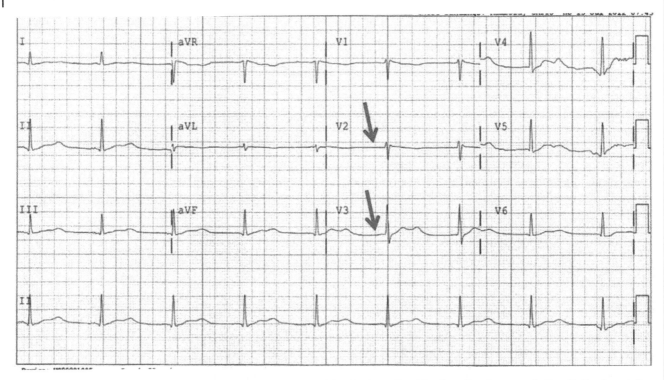

Figure 5.2.3 ECG of a patient with calcium channel blocker toxicity. Bradycardia with a junctional escape rhythm. Notice how a P wave does not directly precede each QRS in the following ECG (arrow).

clinically. For example, sinus bradycardia, junctional escape rhythms, idioventricular rhythms, and complete heart block have been reported with significant calcium channel blocker toxicity [4]. Likewise, beta-blocker toxicity may result in sinus bradycardia, sinus pauses, junctional rhythms, or AV blocks. Clinicians should be aware of the presence or absence of P waves and the PR interval, particularly those with bradycardia, as these can be clues to a potential xenobiotic toxicity.

Morphology of the Cardiac Action Potential and the ECG

In order to understand the more subtle ECG changes associated with various agents, one must first understand the action potential of the cardiac myocyte and how this is reflected on the ECG tracing (see Figure 5.2.1 and Section 5, Chapter 1).

In its resting state, the myocardial cell membrane is impermeable to sodium (Na+). The sodium/potassium ATPase actively pumps three sodium ions out of the cardiac cells while pumping in two potassium ions in order to maintain a negative resting membrane potential. With depolarization, there is a rapid opening of Na+ channels leading to an influx of Na+ ions (phase 0). This rapid influx of Na+ causes the rapid upstroke of the cardiac

action potential that is conducted through the ventricles, directly reflective of the beginning of the QRS interval on the ECG. Phase 1, beginning at the peak of the action potential, represents the closure of Na+ channels and the activation of the transient outward potassium channels. This is followed by the plateau phase (phase 2) in which calcium influx occurs and myocardial contraction continues. Phase 3 of the action potential represents the end of the cardiac cycle, which results in closure of the Ca+ channels and opening of the *delayed rectifier* potassium efflux channels, resulting in repolarization. The potassium efflux from the myocardial cell during phase 3 of the action potential is represented by the QT interval on the ECG. The cell then returns to its resting membrane state (phase 4), maintained by the sodium-potassium ATPase. For additional review of the cardiac action potential, please refer to Section 5, Chapter 1.

QRS Interval Prolongation

Many xenobiotics are capable of prolonging the QRS interval (Table 5.2.1). When a sodium channel blocking agent is present, there is a prolongation of phase 0 of the action potential as less sodium per unit time is entering the cell; changes can be seen with the duration and axis of the QRS complex. In the general patient population, a QRS interval of 120 ms is used to define a bundle branch block. However, in the setting of a poisoned patient, a QRS >100 ms may be indicative of sodium channel blocker toxicity. Medications that block sodium channels such as TCAs and Vaughan-William Class IA (e.g. procainamide, quinidine) and IC (e.g. flecainide, propafenone) antidysrhythmics cause a delay in the influx of sodium during phase 0. This delay is represented by the less-pronounced slope of phase 0 causing a prolongation of the QRS complex on the ECG (Figure 5.2.4).

Interestingly, Class IB antidysrhythmics such as lidocaine and phenytoin also exert their effects on sodium channels but do not result in QRS prolongation. This is due to the fact that IB agents bind the sodium channels in the inactivated state and are not active during phase 0 of the action potential. Table 5.2.1 lists common agents causing sodium channel blockade and QRS prolongation.

The QRS duration and morphology can be used by the clinician to both diagnose and predict toxicity. Much of the literature related to drug-induced QRS prolongation stems from experience with TCAs, however, this information is often extrapolated to other sodium channel blocking agents as well. Sodium channel blockers such as TCAs not only cause widening of the QRS interval, but they display a specific pattern of widening and other changes on the ECG. The changes that are often described are widening and right axis deviation of the terminal 40 ms of the QRS complex, resulting in an R wave in lead aVR and an S wave in leads I and aVL (Figure 5.2.4) [5–7]. When these changes occur, even when subtle, the clinician should be suspicious for a TCA or other sodium channel blocker toxicity.

Table 5.2.1 Examples of sodium channel blocking agents, not all inclusive.

QRS prolonging agents (Na+ channel blockers)	
Amantadine	Cyclic
Carbamazepine	antidepressants
Chloroquine	Diltiazem
Class IA antiarrhythmics	Diphenhydramine
– Disopyramide	Hydroxychloroquine
– Quinidine	Loxapine
– Procainamide	Orphenadrine
Class IC antiarrhythmics	Phenothiazines
– Encainanide	– Medoridazine
– Flecainide	– Thioridazine
– Propafenone	Propanolol
Cocaine	Propoxyphene
	Quinine
	Verapamil

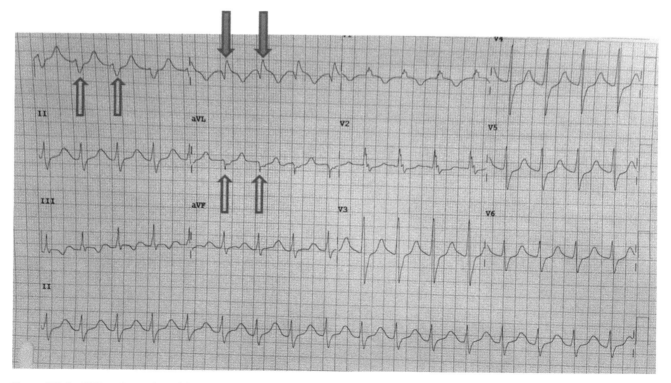

Figure 5.2.4 QRS prolongation with terminal 40 ms delay as represented by an R wave in lead aVR (solid arrow) and an S wave in leads I and aVL (hollow arrow). This is suggestive of the presence of a cardiac sodium channel blocker.

An early ECG with QRS alteration, even if the patient is otherwise asymptomatic, can be suggestions of impending toxicity. In TCA poisoning, QRS prolongation not only places the patient at risk for cardiovascular compromise, but the degree of QRS prolongation also portends a poor prognosis due to other effects of TCAs. One study by Boehnert et al. showed that in TCA poisoned patients with a QRS duration less than 100 ms, no patients developed seizures. However, in this study, a QRS interval greater than 100 ms was associated with a 30% incidence of seizures and QRS interval greater than 160 ms was associated with a 50% risk of ventricular dysrhythmias [5].

Given the morbidity and mortality associated with TCA overdoses, it is imperative to identify toxicity as early as possible in the clinical course. Cardiotoxicity is the main contributor to serious illness and death from cyclic antidepressants. The most common dysrhythmia following a TCA overdose is sinus tachycardia and this finding is expected in patients with significant toxicity [4]. The ECG may be the most useful tool in evaluating a patient with a cyclic antidepressant overdose. Generally, it is expected that symptoms of a TCA poisoning will manifest within six hours of ingestion. While this may not be the peak of toxicity, clinical and electrocardiographic findings are likely to manifest approximately within that time frame. If a patient presents immediately after a suspected TCA ingestion, or other agent causing QRS prolongation on the ECG, it is important to monitor for clinical findings of toxicity as well as ECG changes, and frequent reassessments are imperative. In a suspected TCA ingestion, ECGs should generally be performed at least hourly on stable patients, for a minimum of six hours following ingestion. ECGs may need to be performed more frequently in deteriorating or unstable patients. If the patient's mental status and physical examination findings are normal without any findings on ECG after a six hours observation period, it is unlikely that a significant TCA ingestion has occurred; in many cases, patients with a normal mental status, normal vital signs and normal set of comprehensive laboratory values can then be medically cleared for evaluation by a psychiatrist.

Sodium channel blockers are a diverse group of drugs. Depending on the time since ingestion, QRS widening might not yet have developed and, therefore, a normal ECG early after ingestion, may not rule out toxicity. Most immediate release sodium channel blocking agents would be expected to show signs of toxicity (either clinically on vital signs or physical examination, or on the ECG) within 6 hours. However, due to the rise in extended release products and the diversity of these agents, the authors recommend consultation with a regional poison control center prior to medical clearance of the patient.

Following overdose of a sodium channel blocking agent, the ECG can also be used to monitor response to therapy. Sodium bicarbonate should be given in cases of suspected sodium channel blocker poisonings that manifest a widened QRS (>100 ms) or hypotension. Both the sodium load and the alkalosis are beneficial to improve contractility and function of the heart. It is important to note that administering sodium bicarbonate in a patient with sodium channel blocker toxicity should result in narrowing of the QRS, therefore, the authors recommend repeating an ECG five minutes after the bolus to reassess the QRS and response to therapy. The recommended sodium bicarbonate dose is 1–2 mEq/kg bolus, and this can be repeated every 3–5 minutes until the QRS narrows and/or hemodynamics improve.

In evaluating the poisoned patient, not all patients who present with a QRS duration >100 ms will be poisoned. In the setting of a potential poisoning, a QRS interval greater than 100 ms should be considered abnormal and should prompt further investigation to see if a conduction disturbance was present on a prior ECG. If the QRS is prolonged greater than 100 ms without evidence of prior conduction delay, in most instances 1–2 meq/kg of sodium bicarbonate can be given intravenously to evaluate the response. Significant QRS interval narrowing following the administration of sodium bicarbonate can be a clue to poisoning with a sodium channel blocker. If there is no improvement, this could be suggestive of an underlying conduction delay. It is also important to repeat an ECG to make sure the QRS is not further widening prior to clearing the patient.

QTc Interval Prolongation

QT interval prolongation can occur for a variety of reasons, including congenital abnormalities and electrolyte disturbances, however, there are many xenobiotics that can also produce QT interval prolongation. Consequently, when evaluating an ECG with QT interval prolongation, drug effect, including polypharmacy or acute poisoning, should be on the differential diagnosis. In addition, QT interval prolongation in the patient with altered mental status could be suggestive of poisoning.

The QT interval is commonly prolonged in cardiotoxic ingestions secondary to the effects on cardiac potassium efflux channels. The QT interval is representative of ventricular systole. Changes to phase 2 or phase 3 of the action potential will cause changes in the QT interval duration. When the QT interval is prolonged, the heart is at risk for ventricular dysrhythmias. This occurs because the cardiac myocytes do not all return to resting potential at the same time; some myocytes remain in the refractory period while others are in a relative refractory period and are capable of firing again. When this occurs, "early after-depolarizations" may be triggered, resulting in premature ventricular contractions, ventricular tachycardia, ventricular fibrillation, or torsades de pointes (polymorphic ventricular tachycardia) [2, 5, 7, 8]. As the QT interval varies with heart rate, when evaluating the QT interval a value corrected for heart rate (QTc) is used. There are various formulas for calculating the QTc from the ECG, including Bazett's formula [QTc (ms) = QT(ms) ÷ $\sqrt{RR}$ interval (ms)] and Fridericia's formula [QTc = QT ÷ $\sqrt[3]{RR}$ interval(ms)], which is thought to be more accurate at higher heart rates. A normal QTc interval is considered to be <450 ms for men and <460 ms for women [8]. A QTc greater than 500 ms is generally considered to signify an increased risk for ventricular dysrhythmia.

QTc prolongation is not only a sign of acute poisoning, but also of toxicity from therapeutic doses of QT prolonging agents or from polypharmacy. Psychiatrists often assess a baseline ECG to assess for QTc prolongation prior to initiation of antipsychotic agents that may prolong the QT interval at therapeutic doses. Table 5.2.2 lists agents that are commonly associated with QTc interval prolongation.

Timing

The time since ingestion is an important factor when assessing a poisoned patient. Substances must go through phases of absorption, distribution, and elimination; the clinical findings will often vary, depending on the stage. For example, if a patient overdoses on a lethal dose of a TCA, the patient will be asymptomatic for a short time until absorption and some distribution can occur. Similarly, a patient in the recovery phase of a TCA overdose may still have supratherapeutic concentrations of the drug in the body, but the tissue burden is decreased and the patient may no longer be exhibiting clinical findings of toxicity. Furthermore, as medication ingestions are a dynamic process, different symptoms may manifest based on the phase of toxicity. For example, clonidine, a centrally acting alpha-2 agonist, generally causes hypotension and bradycardia in overdose. However, immediately after ingestion clonidine can stimulate peripheral adrenergic receptors (prior to its centrally acting inhibitory effects) and may, for a brief period, result in hypertension [4]. It is, therefore, important to continue to monitor the ECG during the course of the ingestion. In addition, an ECG should be obtained following resolution of systemic symptoms to assure resolution of any ECG abnormalities.

Table 5.2.2 Sample of QTc prolonging agents. Not all inclusive.

QTc Prolonging Agents (K+ efflux blockers)

Antihistamines	Class III antiarrhythmics
– Astemizole	– Amiodarone
– Diphenhydramine	– Dofetilide
– Loratidine	– Ibutilide
– Terfenadine	– Sotalol
Antipsychotics	Cyclic antidepressants
– Chlorpromazine	– Amitriptiline
– Droperidol	– Amoxapine
– Haloperidol	– Desipramine
– Mesoridazine	– Doxepin
– Pimozide	– Imipramine
– Quetiapine	– Nortriptyline
– Risperidone	– Maprotiline
– Thioridazine	Erythromycin
– Ziprasidone	Fluoroquinolones
Arsenic trioxide	– Ciprofloxacin
Beperidil	– Gatifloxacin
Chloroquine	– Levofloxacin
Citalopram	– Moxifloxicin
Clarithromycin	– Parfloxacin
Class IA antiarrhythmics	Halofantrine
– Disopyramide	Hydroxychloroquine
– Quinidine	Levomethadyl
– Procainamide	Methadone
Class IC antiarrhythmics	Pentamidine
– Encainide	Quinine
– Flecainide	Tacrolimus
– Moricizine	Venlafaxine
– Propafenone	

Certain agents may have active metabolites that need to be considered when medically clearing a poisoned patient. As formation of the metabolites depends on the xenobiotic's half-life, toxicity can take longer to develop in overdose due to the altered toxicokinetics. For example, citalopram, an SSRI that can cause serotonin syndrome, is generally considered more cardiotoxic than other SSRIs. It is known to cause QTc prolongation and torsades de pointes, which can present in a delayed fashion. Citalopram is metabolized to desmethylcitalopram and subsequently didesmethylcitalopram, which has been associated with QT prolongation in animal studies [9]. If a practitioner were to medically clear a patient after a standard 4- to 6-hour period of observation, they would be putting that patient at risk for cardiotoxicity in a setting that would be ill-equipped to deliver proper treatment. A pharmacokinetic-pharmacodynamic modeling study published in 2006 recommended a minimum of 13 hours of monitoring after citalopram overdose. The study found that if the QT interval was normal at 13 hours post dose, the risk of developing future QT prolongation was less than 1% [10].

It is known that pharmacokinetic data are not directly applicable to the overdose patient population. This is because pharmacokinetic profiles (time of onset, elimination half-lives, etc.) are typically obtained in a controlled patient population at therapeutic doses. Xenobiotics behave differently at supratherapeutic levels, often in an unpredictable fashion. Clinicians must use multiple resources, including pharmacokinetic and toxicokinetic data (if available), along with clinical experience and reports in the literature to determine reasonable recommendations. Often, a period of 6 hours of observation is recommended after an overdose. This number is somewhat arbitrary, but for many immediate release substances, one would expect initial signs of drug effect to manifest within such a time frame. Typically, observation periods are prolonged in extended release products. As a greater number of extended release products become available, the clinician's job becomes more difficult until overdose data on each specific product become available. As an example, in an adult, the pharmacokinetic date for immediate release verapamil notes a time of onset of 1–2 hours [11]. If a margin of safety multiplier of 3 is used, that extends observation to a 6-hour period. If the same multiplier is used for an extended release verapamil product with a predicted onset of 4–5 hours [12], then the minimum observation time of 15 hours would result. This example is used not to specifically guide the management of verapamil poisoning (as many practitioners would advocate overnight monitoring, even for an immediate release product), but to illustrate that extended release products should warrant extended periods of observation before medically clearing a patient.

The Undifferentiated Patient

Emergency medicine practitioners are often tasked with managing undifferentiated patients; for example the patient that presents in an altered mental state of an unclear etiology. In addition to infection, trauma, metabolic, or neurologic causes of altered mentation, toxicologic etiologies are frequently in the differential. In these situations, evaluating for toxidromes may help differentiate and guide treatment. For example, a young person that presents in a comatose state with track marks on the arm, miosis, respiratory depression, and decreased bowel sounds may raise suspicion for opioid toxicity. Improvement in mental status with naloxone dosing may further raise the clinician's suspicion for opioid poisoning.

The ECG is also a useful tool in evaluating the undifferentiated patient. As mentioned in prior paragraphs, new onset QRS and QTc prolongation in the patient with altered mental status should give the clinical some suspicion of poisoning. Tachycardia with QRS prolongation suggests a possible sympathomimetic or anticholinergic agent that is also a sodium channel blocker. Bradycardia suggests a sedative or cardioactive drug such as a beta blocker or calcium channel blocker. In the setting of QRS prolongation, particularly in the hypotensive patient, it is reasonable to give a trial of 1–2 mg/kg of sodium bicarbonate IV. If narrowing of the QRS occurs within 5–10 minutes, this is suggestive of the presence of a sodium channel blocker. QTc prolongation may also be suggestive of drug toxicity; unfortunately, treatment with magnesium may not narrow the QTc interval as bicarbonate does with the QRS.

Other incidental findings may also be useful in helping to diagnose an undifferentiated patient. Digoxin inhibits conduction through the SA and AV nodes, which often results in bradycardia and PR interval prolongation. It also increases intracellular calcium, resulting in irritability of the ventricular; this may results in PVCs or other ventricular tachydysrhythmias. The increased calcium can result in a shortened QT interval as well as scooping of the ST segments due to changes in repolarization. *Digitalis effect* refers to the PR prolongation and the scooping of the ST segments (Figure 5.2.5). This finding is not necessarily indicative of digoxin toxicity, but if seen on the ECG, it could provide further information to the clinician as to the patient's history.

Conclusion

Many times when a younger person presents with altered mental status, a toxicologic etiology is high on the clinician's differential. The physical exam, ancillary lab testing, and ECG may help guide the practitioner toward, or away from, that initial impression. Unfortunately, the ECG cannot definitively rule in or rule out poisoning. Consequently, the authors caution the practitioner to maintain a broad differential diagnosis. Cases of infectious encephalitis, seizures, strokes, and paraneoplastic syndromes, among others, are likely to have some features that overlap with toxidromes.

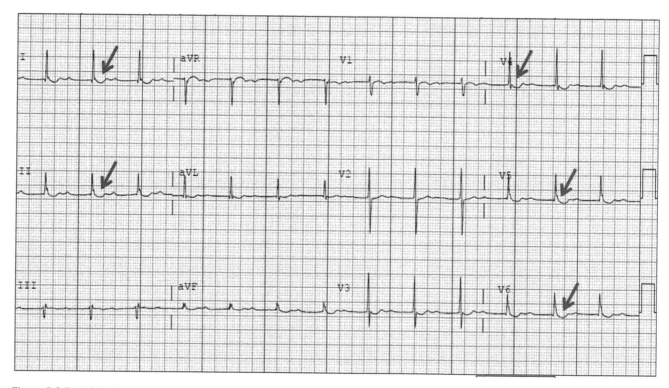

Figure 5.2.5 ECG of a patient on therapeutic digoxin. Notice scooping of the ST segments in leads I, II, V3–V6 (arrows).

Most toxic ingestions have good outcomes with appropriate supportive care. This includes protecting the airway, maintaining adequate circulation, treating QRS or QT prolongation, and closely monitoring the patient.

Fortunately, the ECG, including rate, rhythm and morphology can suggest the presence of certain classes of toxin and may help guide management of the poisoned patient.

References

1 Gummin, D.D., Mowry, J.B., Spyker, D.A. et al. (2019). 2018 Annual Report of the American Association of Poison Control Centers' National Poison Data System (NPDS): 36th Annual Report. *Clin Toxicol.* 57(12): 1220–1413.

2 Holstege, C.P., Eldridge, D.L., and Rowden, A.K. (2006). ECG manifestations: the poisoned patient. *Emerg. Med. Clin. North Am.* 24: 159–177.

3 Clancy, C. (2011). Electrophysiologic and electrocardiographic principles. In: *Goldfrank's Toxicologic Emergencies*, 9e (eds. L.S. Nelson, N.A. Lewis, M.A. Howland, et al.), 314. McGraw Hill.

4 DeRoos, F.J. (2011). Calcium channel blockers. In: *Goldfrank's Toxicologic Emergencies*, 9e (eds. L.S. Nelson, N.A. Lewis, M.A. Howland, et al.), 884. McGraw Hill.

5 Boehnert, M.T. and Lovejoy, F.H. (1985). Value of the QRS duration versus the serum drug level in predicting seizures and ventricular arrhythmias after an acute overdose of tricyclic antidepressants. *N. Engl. J. Med.* 313: 474–479.

6 Holstege, C.P. and Borek, H.A. (2012). Toxidromes. *Crit. Care Clin.* 28: 479–498.

7 Lawrence, D.T., Bechtel, L., Walsh, J.P., and Holstege, C.P. (2007). The evaluation and management of acute poisoning emergencies. *Minerva Med.* 98: 543–568.

8 Moss, A.J. (2003). Long QT syndrome. *JAMA* 289: 2041–2044.

9 Boeck, V., Fredricson, O.K., and Svendsen, O. (1982). Studies on acute toxicity and drug levels of citalopram in the dog. *Acta Pharmacol. Toxicol.* 50: 169–174.

10 Isbister, G.K., Friberg, L.E., and Duffull, S.B. (2006). Application of pharmacokinetic-pharmacodynamic modelling in management of QT abnormalities after citalopram overdose. *Intensive Care Med.* 32 (7): 1060–1065.

11 Searle & Co. (1997). Product Information: Calan(R), verapamil HCl. Skokie, IL.

12 Neutel, J.M., Alderman, M., Anders, R.J., and Weber, M.A. (1996). Novel delivery system for verapamil designed to achieve maximal blood pressure control during the early morning. *Am. Heart J.* 132: 1202–1206.

3

The ECG and Electrolyte Abnormalities

Justin Rizer[1], Joshua D. King[2], and Nathan P. Charlton[1]

[1]*Division of Medical Toxicology, Department of Emergency Medicine, University of Virginia, Charlottesville, VA, USA*
[2]*University of Maryland, Maryland Poison Center, Baltimore, MD, USA*

Introduction

Cardiac electrical activity depends on transmembrane ionic gradients and the time-and voltage-dependent alterations of their conductance. Electrolyte imbalances affect all phases of the cardiac cycle action potential by shifting potentials across cellular membranes. The most common electrolyte abnormalities affecting the electrocardiogram include disturbances of potassium, calcium, and magnesium. These changes have a range of manifestations on the electrocardiogram from incidental, superficial findings, to life-threatening dysrhythmias. This chapter will review important aspects of electrolyte abnormalities individually, but it is prudent to point out that electrolyte homeostasis is a dynamic relationship and abnormalities of these ions may have impacts on others as well.

Calcium

Calcium exists as a nearly inexhaustible reservoir in skeletal bones stored as hydroxyapatite and has a diverse role in cellular regulatory mechanisms. In the heart, the most prominent effect of calcium on the cardiac action potential is exhibited during phase 2 (plateau) [1]. Ionized calcium is the necessary portion for normal physiologic processes. Of the approximately 1–2 kg of calcium in the body, less than 1% resides in the extracellular and intracellular compartments, of which most is located intracellularly. Plasma calcium distribution is about 40% ionized, 40% protein bound, and about 10% bound to anions (i.e. phosphate, carbonate, citrate, etc.) [2]. The reference range of serum calcium concentrations vary among laboratories but generally is 8.7–10.4 mg/dl, with ionized calcium concentrations normally ranging from 4.5–5.5 mg/dl [3]. Plasma calcium concentrations are tightly regulated and rapid transmembrane shifts are possible through voltage-sensitive channels. Alkalemia increases calcium protein binding, which decreases ionized calcium; whereas an acidic environment decreases binding to albumin, increasing ionized calcium.

Hypocalcemia

Background

Hypocalcemia is frequently encountered in hospitalized patients, and is particularly common in the critical care setting [4]. The most common cause of hypocalcemia is a low serum albumin concentration, which can result from myriad conditions including malnutrition, sepsis, and cirrhosis. Chronic renal failure and hypoparathyroidism are also classic causes of hypocalcemia. Hypocalcemia can cause a variety of symptoms such as numbness and paresthesias, muscle cramps, carpopedal spasm, cardiac irritability, and seizures. Hypomagnesemia is also frequently encountered concurrently with hypocalcemia [4–6].

ECG Findings

Within the cardiovascular system, hypocalcemia is known to cause lengthening of the QTc interval and impaired myocardial contractility [5]. In the setting of hypocalcemia, phase 2 of the cardiac action potential is prolonged causing calcium ion channels to remain open for a longer period, allowing a late calcium inflow and the formation of early after-depolarizations [1, 7]. This predisposes to ventricular dysrhythmias, such as torsades de pointes (TdP). However,

Electrocardiogram in Clinical Medicine, First Edition. Edited by William J. Brady, Michael J. Lipinski, Andrew E. Darby, Michael C. Bond, Nathan P. Charlton, Korin Hudson, and Kelly Williamson.

while electrocardiographic conduction disturbances are common, serious dysrhythmias are infrequent and develop more frequently with other simultaneous co-morbidities [2]. Congenital long QT syndromes are associated with atrial tachydysrhythmias, so there is some consideration that acquired QT prolongation, such as from hypocalcemia, may also predispose to atrial dysrhythmias, but the data are limited [5]. Decreased myocardial contractility secondary to hypocalcemia can lead to heart failure, hypotension, and angina.

Treatment

Parenteral calcium is indicated for the treatment of associated severe symptoms and life-threatening dysrhythmias. Options for intravenous calcium replacement are calcium gluconate and calcium chloride: 10 ml of 10% calcium gluconate contains 90 mg elemental calcium, whereas 10 ml of 10% calcium chloride contains 272 mg elemental calcium. Calcium gluconate can be given through peripheral IVs, while calcium chloride should only be administered via central line. 10 ml of 10% calcium gluconate calcium gluconate is expected to raise serum calcium concentration by approximately 0.5 mg/dl. Acute cardiomyopathies resulting from hypocalcemia are most often reversible with calcium replacement and vitamin D supplementation [6]. It is prudent to correct other associated electrolyte abnormalities as well.

Hypercalcemia

Background

Plasma calcium concentrations are regulated by complex interaction and feedback of parathyroid hormone, calcitriol, and calcitonin. Hyperparathyroidism is the most common cause of hypercalcemia with malignancy being another common source [3]. Hypercalcemia resulting from malignancy often results in rapidly rising levels, whereas hyperparathyroidism may cause mild, even asymptomatic hypercalcemia over the course of years. Common, noncardiac, clinical effects of hypercalcemia include nausea, constipation, lethargy, weakness, confusion, and renal stones. Serum calcium concentrations greater than 15 mg/dl are considered to be a medical emergency necessitating aggressive treatment.

ECG Findings

Intuitively, hypercalcemia manifestations on the electrocardiogram are the opposite of that of hypocalcemia, resulting in an abnormally shortened QTc interval [2]. An elevated extracellular calcium concentration has a stabilizing effect on the membrane, increasing the extent of depolarization needed to initiate an action potential. Severe hypercalcemia, which is more frequently witnessed in paraneoplastic syndromes and intentional ingestions, can manifest as Osborn (J waves) waves and ST segment elevation on the electrocardiogram. However, the relationship among hypercalcemia and J point and ST segment elevation has been described primarily in case reports and case series [8]. The presence of a J wave, or early repolarization, is characterized by an elevation at the junction between the end of the QRS complex and the beginning of the ST segment (J point) in a 12-lead electrocardiogram [9]. It has been associated with an increased risk of ventricular irritability and ventricular fibrillation. Hypothermia should also be considered with the presence of J point elevation. The two may be difficult to differentiate based on ECG appearance alone. Bradycardia and hypothermia on vital signs would point toward hypothermia as the etiology, whereas hypercalcemia is more likely to have a normal temperature and heart rate. The ST-segment elevation has a scooped appearance and does not seem to be a mimicker of an ST-segment elevation myocardial infarction (STEMI). A variety of conditions can manifest as nonspecific ST changes; so these findings are neither sensitive nor specific for hypercalcemia.

Treatment

Treatment is based on clinical signs, although an absolute level of >14 mg/dl may warrant empiric therapy, even in an asymptomatic patient. It is not advised to base treatment on ECG findings alone, as these findings may be nonspecific and several other clinical factors are important to consider prior to providing a specific therapy. The mainstays of treatment are volume repletion with intravenous fluids and bisphosphonate agents that inhibit osteoclastic bone resorption. Volume depletion tends to exacerbate hypercalcemia so appropriate volume resuscitation with isotonic solutions is an effective initial short-term therapy. The administration of loop diuretics may play an adjunctive role; however, special attention must be paid to the patient's volume status, as well as other potential electrolyte disturbances.

Magnesium

Approximately one-third of the 21–28 g of magnesium contained in the human body is located in the intracellular compartment, making it the second-most abundant intracellular cation. Only about 1% of total body magnesium resides extracellularly. The overwhelming majority of magnesium is stored intracellularly, with the predominant portion distributed in the bone. The majority of plasma magnesium is ionized, with approximately 20% being protein-bound. Magnesium is an essential cofactor for hundreds of enzymatic reactions in the body including ATP formation and metabolism of protein, carbohydrates, and fat. Despite such large body stores, an ongoing dietary intake of 300–400 mg/day is required to maintain normal levels, which are 1.7–2.1 mg/dl [2, 10]. While food processing and cooking practices may deplete magnesium content, it is ubiquitous in nature and is especially plentiful in green vegetables, cereals, grains, nuts, legumes, and chocolate. Magnesium acts as a powerful membrane stabilizing agent and is the standard therapy for TdP. In the treatment of TdP, while magnesium does not shorten the QT interval itself, it is a cofactor for the sodium-potassium ATPase channel in cardiac myocytes, it increases intracellular potassium, which hyperpolarizes the cell to make it less excitable, and competes with calcium in entering the cell.

Hypomagnesemia

Background

A broad variety of clinical conditions can lead to low plasma magnesium concentrations, such as decreased intake, redistribution, gastrointestinal losses, and renal losses. Hypokalemia is a common concurrent event with hypomagnesemia, occurring in up to 60% of patients. Both conditions may be a consequence of the same process (such as diuretics or GI fluid losses), but low serum magnesium also stimulates intrinsic renal potassium excretion, leading to increased potassium loss and making potassium repletion much less effective. Severe hypomagnesemia can result in hypocalcemia as well. Low serum magnesium impairs normal calcium exchange and also leads to decreased release of PTH, both of which contribute to low serum calcium levels [11]. Hypomagnesemia is often not an isolated electrolyte abnormality, so the ECG changes found are likely a multifactorial cause of complex electrolyte abnormality interplay [12].

ECG Findings

Deficiency in magnesium was once thought to have no clinical significance on cardiac action, but is now recognized to cause dysrhythmias [1, 2, 13]. The primary abnormality recognized on the ECG is a prolonged QTc interval. A variety of ECG changes, such as atrial ectopy, ventricular ectopy, and atrial tachydysrhythmias have been documented in the context of low serum magnesium; however, this is often confounded with other simultaneous electrolyte disturbances. Therefore, the degree to which specific conduction disturbances can be attributed solely to hypomagnesemia remains controversial. While the treatment of TdP includes magnesium supplementation, TdP has been reported in the context of both normal and low serum magnesium levels. Patients with magnesium deficiency may also be predisposed to digoxin-associated dysrhythmias since both digoxin and low magnesium act to inhibit the sodium-potassium ATPase channel [12]. While not a direct cause of ECG change, magnesium deficiency may predispose to coronary artery disease (CAD), which can ultimately lead to myocardial infarction including STEMI.

Treatment

Intravenous magnesium is highly effective in terminating TdP [14]. A rapid IV bolus over 15 minutes of 2 g magnesium sulfate (4 ml of 50% solution mixed with D5W to a total volume of 10 ml or more), in conjunction with standard ACLS, is standard emergency treatment, regardless of whether the patient has normal or low levels of serum magnesium. In the situation of ectopy and other atrial tachydysrhythmias, correction of serum magnesium, as well as concurrent correction of other electrolyte abnormalities, is often effective at achieving rhythm control. Several studies, including the MAGIC trial [15], have looked at the administration of IV magnesium for the treatment of acute myocardial infarction with mixed results. Currently, the routine use of magnesium supplementation for myocardial infarction is not standard, but consideration of the patient's magnesium status should be taken into account and corrected if concentrations are low in order to help optimize cardiac function.

Hypermagnesemia

Hypermagnesemia is an uncommon condition, and concentrations resulting in ECG changes are even more rare, with most causes resulting from iatrogenic or intentional exposure to excess magnesium salts. By blocking calcium channels and neuromuscular transmission, hypermagnesemia can manifest with nausea, vomiting, loss of deep tendon reflexes, and muscle weakness [12]. Serum magnesium levels of 5–10 mg/dl can cause nonspecific intraventricular conduction delay and QTc interval lengthening. Atrioventricular block may be seen at concentrations greater than 9 mg/dl. Asystole and cardiac arrest have been reported with serum concentrations greater than 14 mg/dl, however, magnesium concentrations this high are most often due to iatrogenic injury or intentional ingestion of magnesium salts [16]. Few cases have been reported in which patient's survived with levels greater than 18 mg/dl. Management of severely elevated serum magnesium is complex but involves administration of IVF and IV calcium, with the potential for use of hemodialysis.

Potassium

Potassium is the primary intracellular cation and is maintained in a narrow homeostatic range of 3.5–5.0 mEq/l. It is vital for regulating the normal electrical activity of the heart. The potassium ion gradient across the cardiac cell membrane is the most important factor in establishing the −90 mV resting membrane potential, so even small alterations in extracellular concentration may lead to profound effects on myocyte electrophysiologic function [17]. The electric gradient is maintained by sodium-potassium adenosine triphosphatase (Na+/K +− ATPase) pumps in the cell membrane, which actively transport potassium into and sodium out of the cell. Alterations in serum potassium levels can have impressive effects on cardiac myocyte conduction, which can lead to electrocardiographic changes. While ECG aberrations may not always accompany potassium abnormalities, the ECG is a useful clinical tool for gauging the severity of potassium abnormalities.

Hyperkalemia

Background

Hyperkalemia is defined as a serum potassium concentration greater 5.5 mEq/l in adults (this level is age dependent among pediatric population). Under normal conditions, approximately 90% of potassium is excreted in the urine, so it is not surprising that renal failure is the most common cause of hyperkalemia. Other causes of hyperkalemia include excessive intake, shifts from intracellular to extracellular space, and other mechanisms of impaired excretion [18]. Increased extracellular potassium reduces myocardial excitability, with depression of both pacemaking and conducting tissues.

Hyperkalemia is a common clinical condition that can induce potentially life-threatening cardiac dysrhythmias. Because potential delays exist in the determination of serum potassium, the clinician's ability to recognize electrocardiographic manifestations of hyperkalemia is essential for early diagnosis and empiric treatment.

ECG Findings

The ECG is crucial in the management of hyperkalemia and is sometimes the first sign of pathology. In the emergency

Table 5.3.1 ECG abnormalities associated with hyperkalemia.

Serum potassium level	Expected ECG abnormality
Mild hyperkalemia 5.5–6.5 mEq/l	Tall, "peaked" T waves (narrow base, precordial leads)
Moderate hyperkalemia 6.5–8.0 mEq/l	Peaked T waves Prolonged PR interval Decreased amplitude of P waves Widened QRS complex
Severe hyperkalemia >8.0 mEq/l	Absence of P waves Intraventricular blocks Progressive widening of WRS complex Sinoventricular rhythm, aka "sine wave" Ventricular fibrillation, asystole

department setting, initial ECG has fairly poor sensitivity of about 35–45%, but good specificity (85–90%) of making the diagnosis of hyperkalemia [19]. Hyperkalemia typically follows a predictable progression of electrocardiographic changes relative to the serum potassium level (Table 5.3.1). Increasing extracellular potassium results in a decrease in the resting cardiac myocyte membrane potential. As potassium levels rise, this resting membrane potential gradually becomes less negative. This change causes a slowing of impulse conduction through the myocardium as well as a prolongation of the depolarization phase of the cardiac action potential [17]. Phase 0 velocity is slowed (Figure 5.3.1). Peaked T waves in the precordial leads are among the most common and the most frequently recognized findings on the ECG [2, 20] (Figure 5.3.2). This is the earliest electrocardiographic change and is described as symmetrically narrow, tall, and pointed.

With higher levels of serum potassium, cardiac conduction between myocytes is suppressed. Atrial tissue is

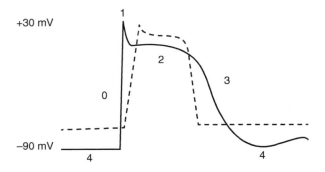

Figure 5.3.1 Cardiac action potential, normal (solid line) and after exposure to sodium channel blocker (dotted line).

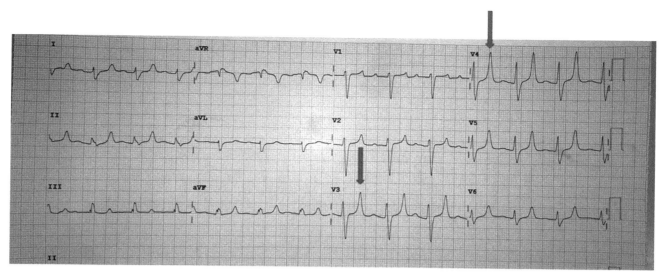

Figure 5.3.2 Peaked T waves (solid arrows), the most common finding of hyperkalemia.

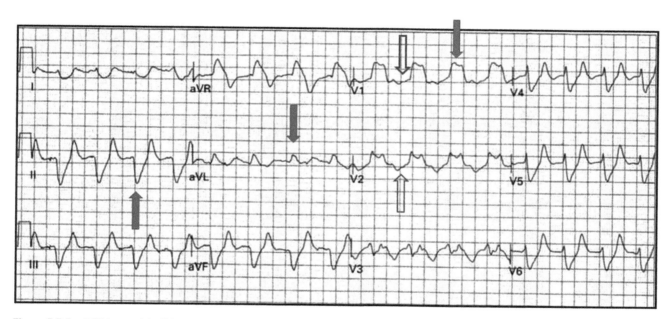

Figure 5.3.3 QRS interval (solid arrows) and PR widening (hollow arrows) consistent with worsening hyperkalemia.

sensitive to these changes will manifest with the P-wave flattening, widening, and it may eventually disappear altogether. Both the PR segment and QRS interval increases (Figure 5.3.3). Severe hyperkalemia can eventually result in a wide array of conduction deficits from high-degree AV block to fascicular blocks to bundle branch blocks [2, 19, 20]. Escape beats can also be encountered in this setting. Intraventricular conduction disturbance may also cause a shift in the QRS complex axis. Sine wave appearance of the ECG is a preterminal event that requires immediate treatment [2, 20]. (Figure 5.3.4) This occurs as a result of the markedly prolonged QRS fusing with the T wave, producing

the slurred sinusoidal shape. Ventricular fibrillation, asystole, and PEA are all possible consequences of severely elevated serum potassium. While the above ECG changes have been described in the classic progression from mild to severe hyperkalemia, it should be noted that changes do not always occur in order, and patients may jump from peaked T waves to a sine wave without having manifested the other classic sequential changes.

Elevated potassium can also produce electrocardiographic changes that may mimic an acute myocardial infarction pattern. ST segment elevation can be widespread, but is more frequently observed to be localized

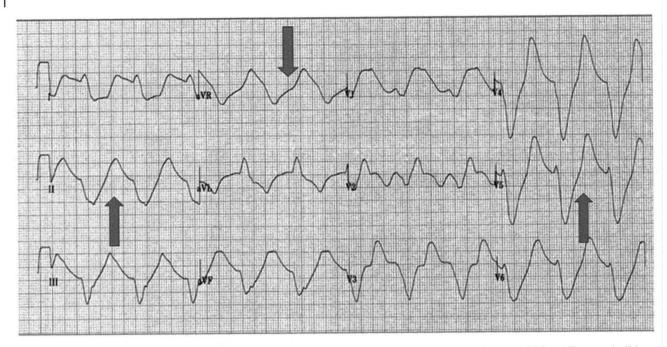

Figure 5.3.4 Hyperkalemia transitioning to a sine wave pattern. Notice lack of clear transitions between QRS and T waves (solid arrows).

to the inferior leads (II, III, aVF) [20]. The absence of Q waves and reciprocal changes, as well as patient history, can help differentiate the two causes of this finding. In addition, there are reports of ST-segment depression and T-wave inversion in the setting of hyperkalemia, which can also be seen in myocardial ischemia [20]. However, these findings are less frequently encountered than those previously described, and resolve after appropriate hyperkalemia management.

Treatment

Patients with suspected or known hyperkalemia require continuous cardiac monitoring and IV access. The degree of aggressiveness of treatment for hyperkalemia depends on the rapidity of rise, absolute serum concentration, and evidence of clinical toxicity; patients with a faster rise in concentration, higher total level, and greater evidence of cardiotoxicity warrant more aggressive management strategies. Ideally, laboratory data are available to help guide treatment, but frequently physicians must initiate management decisions based on clinical scenario alone. While only a mild elevation with no ECG changes may not warrant pharmacologic intervention, treatment is recommended for serum potassium levels greater than 6.5 mEq/l, regardless of ECG findings [17]. Treatment can be broken down into three categories: membrane stabilization, promoting intracellular influx, and removal from the body.

Stabilization of the cardiac cellular membranes with calcium is the initial treatment of hyperkalemia. Calcium effectively "restores" the depolarization energy required by shifting the threshold potential to a less negative value. Hyperkalemia makes the resting potential less negative thereby reducing the amount of millivolts of depolarization required to reach the threshold potential. By moving the threshold potential, calcium returns the myocyte excitability back to normal. Calcium also reverses the myocyte depression of atrial tissue (specifically in the SA and AV node) by increasing the electrochemical gradient across the myocyte, which enhances impulse propagation. The hyperkalemia-induced resting membrane potential change is counteracted by the calcium-induced threshold potential change: 10 ml of a 10% solution calcium gluconate can be given through peripheral IV over 2–10 minutes. Its effects are seen almost immediately and the duration of effect is approximately 30–60 minutes [17]. Calcium chloride can also be considered; however, its use is typically restricted to central venous lines due to the higher concentration of elemental calcium potentially causing peripheral vein sclerosis.

Shifting excess extracellular potassium into cells is the next target of treatment. While these therapies are temporary, they can help bridge the patient to definitive care. Insulin is used to lower potassium by stimulating the Na-K ATPase pump, which moves potassium ions intracellularly. This effect is independent of insulin's effect on serum glucose. Typical dosing is 10 units of intravenous regular insulin followed by 50 ml of 50% dextrose to help prevent hypoglycemia. Onset is within 10–20 minutes and remains for approximately 1 hour and is expected to lower serum potassium by about 0.5–1.0 mEq/l. Inhaled beta agonists stimulate beta-2 receptors which also activate the Na-K ATPase channel in a manner that is similar and additive to insulin. Higher doses (10–20 mg) of inhaled nebulized albuterol can be used and show effects within minutes of administration. Duration of beta agonist effect ranges from one to two hours. Sodium bicarbonate is a controversial therapy, but has shown some effectiveness in hyperkalemic patients who are acidemic. The therapy has limited to no benefit in the nonacidemic patient. Sodium bicarb shifts potassium into cells by raising blood pH and taking advantage of the hydrogen-potassium exchanger.

Final goals of treatment are removal of excess potassium from the body. Cation exchange resins such as sodium polystyrene sulfonate (SPS) have been used for the treatment of hyperkalemia for decades. SPS may take up to 24 hours to see effect and must be administered either orally or rectally, so its use in emergent treatment is quite limited [17]. Also, more recent evidence suggests that SPS may not be beneficial and may actually increase risk of colonic necrosis [19]. Patriomer is an orally administered binding agent approved in 2015 that works in the distal colon. Studies showed a significant reduction in serum potassium after 4 weeks of therapy and no serious adverse events have been associated with its use [21]. Hemodialysis is the quickest, most efficient way to remove total body potassium. However, due to the time, expense, and invasive nature of this procedure, hemodialysis is typically reserved for patients with end-stage renal disease already on dialysis or those with truly life-threatening hyperkalemia.

Hypokalemia

Background

Hypokalemia is common, and is possibly the electrolyte disorder most frequently associated with dysrhythmias. Hypokalemia may be caused by renal loss of potassium, loss of potassium outside the kidneys (e.g. GI tract), or shifts of potassium from plasma to the intracellular space. Some common causes include renal losses, diuretics, vomiting, diarrhea, insulin, and alkali therapy.

Hypokalemia predisposes the patient to developing of a number of dysrhythmias. Milder dysrhythmias caused by hypokalemia include premature atrial and ventricular contractions and sinus bradycardia. However, more serious dysrhythmias may arise in the setting of hypokalemia, including atrioventricular block, a variety of supraventricular tachycardias including atrial and junctional tachycardias, ventricular tachycardia (both monomorphic and polymorphic, such as TdP), and ventricular fibrillation.

The degree of hypokalemia worsens the frequency and severity of dysrhythmias [22]. Potassium levels ≤3.0 mEq/l have been associated with a doubling of the risk of ventricular dysrrhythmias [23]. Hypokalemia may also increase the risk of dysrhythmias in patients with other prodysrhythmic factors, such as increased beta-adrenergic activity, systolic heart failure, cardiac ischemia, certain medications (e.g. digoxin), and other electrolyte disorders (e.g. hypomagnesemia) [24]. Furthermore, patients who have prodysrhythmic conditions such as congestive heart failure often have concomitant hypokalemia, especially in older populations [22].

In addition, hypomagnesemia is often concomitantly associated with hypokalemia; in most cases, patients with hypokalemia should have evaluation of their serum magnesium levels, particularly if potassium levels are low despite potassium repletion.

ECG Findings

Characteristic ECG changes from hypokalemia include ST segment depression, prolongation of the QT interval, flattening of T waves, and the appearance of U waves, small waves immediately following the T wave (Figure 5.3.5). Of these changes, U waves are thought to be most specific for hypokalemia, and may be most common [25, 26].

While U waves are not specific to hypokalemia, they are classically associated with low serum potassium levels. The causes of U waves are not known; proposed causes include mechanical relaxation of the ventricular wall, delayed repolarization of Purkinje fibers, and prolonged regional repolarization of a portion of the myocardium. It is not known how hypokalemia may lead to the development of U waves, but treatment of hypokalemia leads to resolution of U waves in nearly all patients [24, 27]. U waves seem to be the most common ECG finding in hypokalemia, but are still present in less than one-third of all patients [26].

During cardiac repolarization, hypokalemia principally leads to an electrochemical gradient less favorable toward repolarization; as a result, the resting membrane potential is hyperpolarized. In the cardiac conduction system, the repolarization phase is prolonged, leading to a prolongation of the QT interval (Figure 5.3.6) [27]. Chronic hypokalemia leads to decreased expression of the inward rectifying potassium channels, which also contributes to development of a long QT interval. Despite these mechanisms, long QT intervals are relatively uncommon in severe hypokalemia (perhaps less than 10% of all patients), and

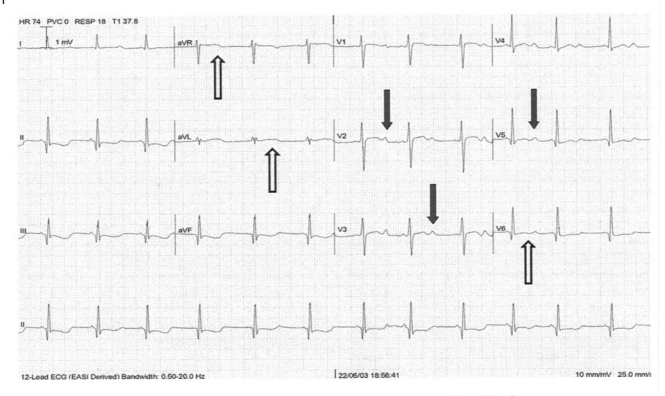

Figure 5.3.5 T-wave flattening (hollow arrows) and U waves (solid arrows) consistent with hypokalemia.

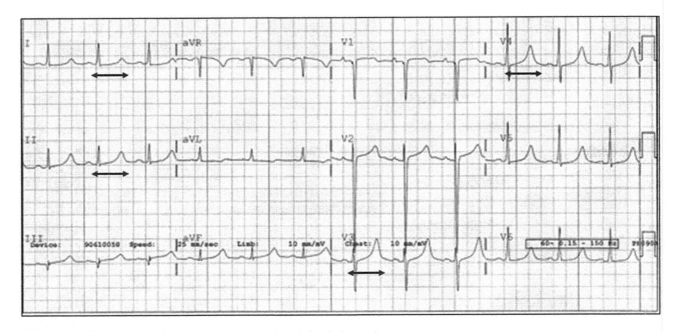

Figure 5.3.6 QT interval prolongation secondary to hypokalemia (arrows).

are less often seen than ST depression, U waves, and T wave flattening (Figure 5.3.4) [26].

The relative hyperpolarization in the cardiac membrane potential induced by chronic hypokalemia leads to an increase in the number of fast sodium channels available for depolarization. As a result, recurrence of excitability may occur at earlier time points during repolarization [27]. This may explain how hypokalemia leads to development of multiple types of atrial and ventricular dysrhythmias, most commonly premature contractions and various tachydysrhythmias.

The mechanisms behind the development of ST-segment depression and flattening of T waves are not precisely known. These changes have been ascribed to decreased conduction throughout the myocardium, reduced excitability from membrane hyperpolarization, and nonuniform depolarization of cardiac myocytes. These findings are not found uniformly – in fact, they are present in a minority of patients with severe hypokalemia, likely less than one-third of all patients [26].

Treatment

Due to the danger of rapidly increasing serum potassium levels in a short period of time, treatment of hypokalemia is generally accomplished over hours. While hypokalemia from renal and extrarenal losses are treated the same way – by replacing potassium – hypokalemia caused by intracellular shifts is ideally treated by directly addressing the cause of intracellular shifting. Special note should be made of conditions causing dramatic intracellular shifts of potassium, such as hypokalemic periodic paralysis, thyrotoxic periodic paralysis, and barium poisoning – these may

all cause potassium levels to drop below 2 mEq/l and can cause life-threatening paralysis and dysrhythmias. While administration of potassium is usually required in these cases, very frequent monitoring of serum potassium levels should be performed as resolution of intracellular shifts may lead to inadvertent hyperkalemia if repletion is aggressive.

A useful "rule of thumb" for mild hypokalemia is that administration of 10 mEq of potassium to most adults will raise their potassium levels by 0.1 mEq/l; this does not apply to very large adults, children, or in the setting of moderate–severe hypokalemia, where intracellular losses of potassium may be severe. For patients who are not critically ill and able to take enteral intake, oral administration of potassium is typically faster and less complex than intravenous administration. Most adults can be safely administered up to 40 mEq oral potassium per hour or up to 20 mEq intravenous potassium per hour (as potassium is irritating to the veins, more than 10 mEq of intravenous potassium per hour usually requires a central line).

ECG changes due to hypokalemia typically resolve with restoration of serum potassium levels to normal. While this may also apply to dysrhythmias caused by hypokalemia, more serious dysrhythmias such as supraventricular tachycardias, ventricular tachycardia, and ventricular fibrillation should be treated urgently or emergently rather than waiting for normalization of serum potassium. Repletion of potassium in patients with conditions such as acute myocardial infarction or systolic heart failure that predispose to arrhythmias in the setting of hypokalemia is commonly carried out to a goal potassium level of 4.0 mEq/l or above, as patients with potassium levels lower than this may be at increased risk for arrhythmias [28, 29].

References

1 Surawicz, B. (1967). Relationship between electrocardiogram and electrolytes. *American Heart Journal* 73 (6): 814–834.

2 Diercks, D.B., Shumaik, G.M., Harrigan, R.A. et al. (2004). Electrocardiographic manifestations: electrolyte abnormalities. *The Journal of Emergency Medicine* 27 (2): 153–160.

3 Levine, B.A. and Williams, R.J.P. (1982). Calcium binding to proteins and other large biological anion centers. In: *Calcium and Cell Function* (ed. W.Y. Cheung), 1–38. New York, NY: Academic Press.

4 Carlstedt, F. and Lind, L. (2001). Hypocalcemic syndromes. *Critical Care Clinics* 17: 139–153.

5 Nijjer, S., Ghosh, A., and Dubrey, S. (2010). Hypocalcemia, long QT interval and atrial arrhythmias. *BMJ Case Reports* https://doi.org/10.1136/bcr.08.2009.2216.

6 Brushinsky, D.A. and Monk, R.D. (1998). Electrolyte quintet: calcium. *Lancet* 352: 306–311.

7 El-Sherif, N. and Turitto, G. (2011). Electrolyte disorders and arrhythmogenesis. *Cardiology Journal* 18 (3): 233–245.

8 Sonoda, K., Watanabe, H., Hisamatsu, T. et al. (2016 Jan). High frequency of early repolarization and Brugada-type electrocardiograms in Hypercalcemia. *Annals of Noninvasive Electrocardiology* 21 (1): 30–40.

9 Otero, J. and Lenihan, D.J. (2000). The "Normothermic" Osborn wave induced by severe hypercalcemia. *Texas Heart Institute Journal* 27 (3): 316–317.

10 Glasdam, S.M., Glasdam, S., and Peters, G.H. (2016). The importance of magnesium in the human body: a systematic literature review. *Advances in Clinical Chemistry* 73: 169–193.

11 Rude, R.K., Oldham, S.B., and Singer, F.R. (1976 May). Functional hypoparathyroidism and parathyroid hormone end-organ resistance in human magnesium deficiency. *Clinical Endocrinology* 5 (3): 209–224.

12 Agus, Z.S. and Morad, M. (1991). Modulation of cardiac ion channels by magnesium. *Annual Review of Physiology* 53: 299–307.

13 Khan, A.M., Lubitz, S.A., Sullivan, L.M. et al. (2013 Jan 1). Low serum magnesium and the development of atrial fibrillation in the community: the Framingham heart study. *Circulation* 127 (1): 33–38.

14 American Heart Association (2000). Part 6: Advanced cardiovascular life support: section 5: pharmacology I: agents for arrhythmias. *Circulation* 102 (8 Suppl): I112–I128.

15 Magnesium in Coronaries (MAGIC) Trial Investigators (2002 Oct 19). Early administration of intravenous magnesium to high-risk patients with acute myocardial infarction in the magnesium in coronaries (MAGIC) trial: a randomised controlled trial. *Lancet* 360 (9341): 1189–1196.

16 Tofil, N.M., Benner, K.W., and Winkler, M.K. (February 2005). Fatal Hypermagnesemia caused by an Epsom salt enema: a case illustration. *Southern Medical Journal* 98 (2): 253–256.

17 Parham, W.A., Mehdirad, A.A., Biermann, K.M., and Fredman, C.S. (2006). Hyperkalemia revisited. *Texas Heart Institute Journal* 33: 40–47.

18 Einhorn, L.M., Zhan, M., Hsu, V.D. et al. (2009 June 22). The frequency of hyperkalemia and its significance in chronic kidney disease. *Archives of Internal Medicine* 169 (12): 1156–1162.

19 Pepin, J. and Shields, C. (February 2012). Advances in diagnosis and management of hypokalemic and hyperkalemic emergencies. *Emergency Medicine Practice* 14 (2): 1–20.

20 Mattu, A., Brady, J., and Robinson, D. (October 2000). Electrocardiographic manifestations of Hyperkalemia. *American Journal of Emergency Medicine* 18 (6): 721–729.

21 Chaitman, M., Dixit, D., and Bridgeman, M. (2016 Jan). Potassium-binding agents for the clinical management of hyperkalemia. *P and T* 41 (1): 43–50.

22 Guo, H., Lee, J.D., Ueda, T. et al. (2005). Different clinical features, biochemical profiles, echocardiographic and electrocardiographic findings in older and younger patients with idiopathic dilated cardiomyopathy. *Acta Cardiologica* 60: 27–31.

23 Siegel, D., Hulley, S.B., Black, D.M. et al. (1992). Diuretics, serum and intracellular electrolyte levels, and ventricular arrhythmias in hypertensive men. *JAMA* 267: 1083.

24 Rautaharju, P.M. (2015). The riddle of the mechanism of generation of the U wave. Is the long search over? *Journal of Electrocardiology* 48: 33–34.

25 Diercks, D.B., Shumaik, G.M., Harrigan, R.A. et al. (2004). Electrocardiographic manifestations: electrolyte abnormalities. *The Journal of Emergency Medicine* 27 (2): 153–160.

26 Marti, G., Schwarz, C., Leichtle, A.B. et al. (2014 Feb). Etiology and symptoms of severe hypokalemia in emergency department patients. *European Journal of Emergency Medicine* 21 (1): 46–51.

27 Osadchii, O.E. (2010). Mechanisms of hypokalemia-induced ventricular arrhythmogenicity. *Fundamental & Clinical Pharmacology* 24: 547–559.

28 Duke, M. (1978). Thiazide-induced hypokalemia: association with acute myocardial infarction and ventricular fibrillation. *JAMA* 239: 43–45.

29 Cohn, J.N., Kowey, P.R., Whelton, P.K., and Prisant, L.M. (2000 Sep 11). New guidelines for potassium replacement in clinical practice: a contemporary review by the National Council on Potassium in Clinical Practice. *Archives of Internal Medicine* 160 (16): 2429–2436.

4

The ECG and Metabolic Abnormalities

George F. Glass[1], Amita Sudhir[1], and Amit Anil Kumar Pandit[2]

[1] *Department of Emergency Medicine, University of Virginia, Charlottesville, VA, USA*
[2] *Department of Emergency Medicine, University of Mississippi Medical Center, Jackson, MS, USA*

Introduction Metabolic Disturbances and the ECG

The ECG may provide useful information in the management of systemic metabolic disturbance including alterations of pH and glucose metabolism. The savvy clinician should be aware of these changes and implications behind these changes to better evaluate and treat patients with metabolic disturbances.

ECG Findings During Acute Complications of Diabetes Mellitus

The electrocardiogram is a critical adjunct in the management of diabetic emergencies and can inform patient care during acute episodes of hypo- and hyperglycemia. Not only can the ECG give clues as to the cause of hyperglycemia (e.g. stress induced by an ST-elevation myocardial infarction) but it can also give clues to body potassium stores and even volume status.

Hyperglycemia and DKA

ECG changes in hyperglycemia and diabetic ketoacidosis (DKA) have long been recognized and are most often a manifestation of associated electrolyte disarray and metabolic acidosis. Acidosis occurs due to ketogenesis and subsequent accumulation of acetoacetic and beta-hydroxybutyric acids. Electrolyte abnormalities are compounded by the accompanying glucose-induced osmotic diuresis. Serum potassium levels are often elevated due to acidosis despite total body depletion of potassium [1]. Many of the ECG manifestations of DKA are a result of this elevation of serum potassium.

The ECG changes of hyperkalemia are well established and thought to occur due to myocardial conduction abnormalities and changes in myocyte resting potential [2]. These changes generally progress with degree of hyperkalemia: mild hyperkalemia is associated with the common symmetric "tented" or "peaked" T-waves best seen in II, III, and V2–V4, whereas further elevations result in ablation of the P wave, QRS prolongation and eventual development of a sinoventricular or "sine-wave" appearance [3] (Figure 5.4.1). Further elevations of potassium may result in terminal ventricular fibrillation or asystole. Also, while ECG manifestations of hyperkalemia are common, they may not always correlate with the degree of disarray and case reports of extreme hyperkalemia (>9.0 mEq/l) without subsequent ECG changes exist [4].

Another ECG pattern seen in DKA is comprised of ST-segment elevation mimicking ischemia, also known as a "pseudoinfarction" pattern. Initially reported as another manifestation of DKA-associated hyperkalemia [5, 6], case reports describe ST elevation (STE) in isolated inferior, anterior, and lateral distributions mimicking myocardial infarction (Figure 5.4.2). Management of this pattern is complicated by the fact that myocardial infarction can often be a precipitating factor in DKA [7]. DKA-associated pseudoinfarction most frequently presents with STE in V1–V3 or V4 with associated RBBB and left anterior fascicular block and resolve with standard treatment of DKA and hyperkalemia [5]. Rapid laboratory evaluation including cardiac biomarkers can aid in correct diagnosis. Cardiac

Electrocardiogram in Clinical Medicine, First Edition. Edited by William J. Brady, Michael J. Lipinski, Andrew E. Darby, Michael C. Bond, Nathan P. Charlton, Korin Hudson, and Kelly Williamson.

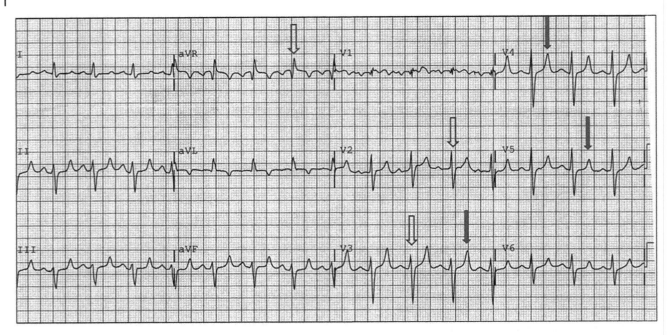

Figure 5.4.1 Peaked T waves (solid arrows) and mild QRS prolongation (hollow arrows) from hyperkalemia in DKA.

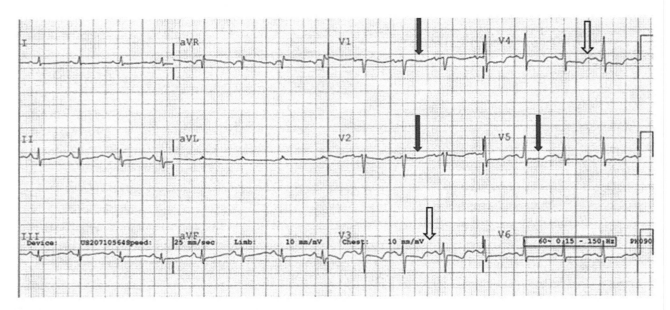

Figure 5.4.2 DKA with hypokalemia. Flattened T waves in lateral precordial leads (solid arrow) and U waves best seen in leads V3 and V4 (hollow arrows).

biomarkers are usually not elevated; however, there have been reports of mild elevations of CK-MB and troponin (up to two times the upper limit of normal) [8].

The ECG changes of pseudoinfarction seem to be caused by metabolic or electrolyte disarray rather than coronary vessel-induced ischemia, as they have been described in patients with concomitant or subsequent normal cardiac angiography [6, 8]. Similar changes have also been reported in patients with renal failure-induced hyperkalemia [9] and hepato-renal syndrome [10]. A single case

of DKA-associated pseudoinfarction pattern with simultaneous normokalemia (4.4 mEq/l) has also been reported, raising the possibility that ECG changes are induced by a relative serum-to-intracellular potassium mismatch due to intracellular depletion, or another non-potassium mediated mechanism altogether [11].

Prolonged DKA with profound osmotic diuresis may eventually result in hypokalemia secondary to total body potassium depletion. Severe hypokalemia may result in ECG changes, most commonly including ST depression,

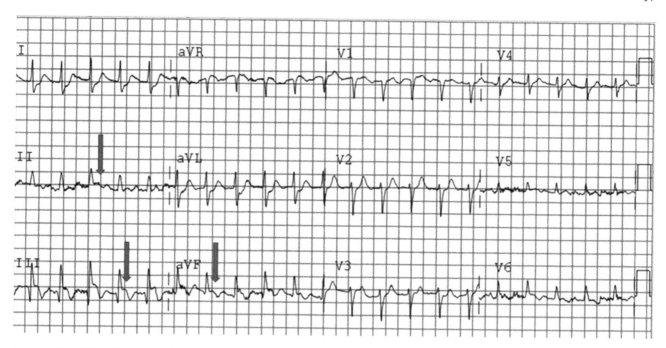

Figure 5.4.3 DKA with sinus tachycardia and ST segment elevations in II, III, and aVF (arrows).

decreased T-wave amplitude, and QTc prolongation [12] (Figure 5.4.3). QTc prolongation that reverses with standard hyperglycemia therapy has also been demonstrated in pediatric patients with DKA [13]. This prolongation was independent of potassium levels and positively associated with the degree of anion gap elevation, implicating a possible link between QTc prolongation and degree of ketosis. The authors cite previously described evidence of QTc prolongation in alcoholic ketoacidosis and ketogenic diets as evidence of a purported link [14–16].

Hypoglycemia

Hypoglycemic episodes (serum glucose <70 mg/dl) are common among patients with both Type I and Type II diabetes mellitus and are associated with adverse cardiac events (both infarction and dysrhythmias) [17]. Several mechanisms have been proposed for these findings.

Hypoglycemia induces endogenous catecholamine release resulting in increased myocardial oxygen demand. An association between symptomatic hypoglycemic episodes and electrocardiographic evidence of ischemia (both ST depressions and elevations) has been shown in patients with known coronary artery disease undergoing continuous ECG monitoring [18]. Other ischemic ECG changes have also been noted in patients presenting with hypoglycemia, including junctional rhythm with deep ST depressions, which resolved with euglycemia [19], and new LBBB pattern associated with significant cardiac marker elevation consistent with acute infarction [20].

In addition to having pro-ischemic effects, there is evidence that hypoglycemia may be directly dysrythmogenic. One study of 18 previously healthy patients demonstrated that induction of hyperinsulinemic hypoglycemia was associated with the development of a significant increase in QTc (399 ms ± 4 to 429 ms ± 7) and decreased in T-wave amplitude (0.55 mV ± 0.08 to 0.20 mV ± 0.05) [21]. A similar study of 15 patients with diabetes mellitus demonstrated an even greater magnitude of QTc prolongation occurring with hypoglycemia among this population [22]. Serial nocturnal ECGs of pediatric patients with Type 1 DM have demonstrated an association between nocturnal hypoglycemic events with prolonged QTc (>440 ms) independent of age, diabetes duration, or HbA1c levels [23]. Fatal dysrhythmia due to prolonged QTc has subsequently been proposed as a potential mechanism for sudden unexplained death in type 1 diabetes, or the "dead in bed" syndrome [24].

Disturbances Due to Alterations of pH

In vitro animal models have demonstrated that the influence of bicarbonate, CO_2 levels, and pH on the electrical activity of isolated heart muscle is limited [25]; however, pH disturbances are often accompanied by electrolyte derangements. The complex *in vivo* response to acidosis may influence cardiac conduction through alteration of catecholamine response or other more complex and incompletely understood pathways [26]. The direct effects of particular electrolyte abnormalities are discussed elsewhere; however, notable electrocardiographic changes observed in particular patterns of pH disturbance are discussed below.

Metabolic Acidosis

Metabolic acidosis, defined as acidosis due to depletion of serum bicarbonate, has little direct association with cardiac dysrhythmia. Although it has been demonstrated to be associated with decreased myocyte contractility in animal models [27], echocardiography of patients with severe diabetic acidosis (pH < 7.1) has demonstrated no change in overall cardiac contractility [28]. Rhythm disturbances in lactic acidosis are generally not seen apart from those associated with electrolyte or other associated abnormality [29], and acidosis is not predictive of ventricular dysrhythmia following myocardial infarction [30]. Dysrhythmias were also not observed in human subjects with mild metabolic acidosis (pH of 7.3) induced by infusion of hydrochloric acid [31]. One study has observed tall, symmetric T-waves in normokalemic patients with metabolic acidosis and resolution following correction of acidosis; however, the clinical implications of this finding are unclear [32].

Some case reports of rhythm disturbance associated with metabolic acidosis exist, however, they are complicated by associated hypoxia and other metabolic disturbances. A single reported case of severe metformin-induced lactic acidosis (pH 6.7, lactic acid 18 mmol/l) was associated with extreme bradycardia and complete AV block (HR 30); however, the patient was also hypothermic and hypotensive [33]. Another case series of 26 patients evaluated for carbon monoxide poisoning demonstrated that most subsequent ECG changes (ST elevation, depression, and T-wave inversion) were associated with acute coronary ischemia and elevated troponin. Other dysrhythmias were rarely observed and were relatively benign (sinus brady- and tachycardia) [34].

Metabolic Alkalosis

Metabolic alkalosis, or persistent elevation of serum bicarbonate secondary to metabolic disarray, is a manifestation of an underlying condition that initiates and maintains alkalosis. Initiation is normally attained through gain of serum alkali, such as the milk alkali syndrome, versus loss of hydrogen ions, as is seen in alkalosis secondary to vomiting. Acute alkalosis is normally rapidly corrected by renal clearance of bicarbonate and respiratory compensation. Sustained or profound alkalosis is normally only achieved with concomitant impairment of renal bicarbonate excretion, most often associated with chloride depletion, potassium depletion reduced GFR and volume contraction [35].

ECG changes in the setting of metabolic alkalosis are thought to be primarily due to underlying hypokalemia, usually secondary to renal losses compounded by the intracellular shift of potassium stores. ECG changes normally occur when potassium concentration reaches level less than 2.7 mmol/l. These changes may include decreased T-wave amplitude, ST depression, U waves, QT prolongation (comprised mostly of QU prolongation – true QT prolongation is associated with concomitant hypomagnesemia putting patients at risk for torsades and other ventricular dysrhythmias) [12]. Wide complex tachycardia had been reported in cases of severe alkalosis (pH > 7.55) with associated hypokalemia (<2.0 mEq/l) due to excessive bicarbonate ingestion for gastrointestinal associated pain [36, 37]. These were successfully treated with either electrical cardioversion or lidocaine with resolution of ventricular tachycardia. One patient continued to have shortened PR-interval and frequent PVCs and fusion beats on 12-lead ECG; however, these eventually resolved with correction of the alkalosis, potassium repletion, and administration of normal saline [36].

Respiratory Acidosis

Respiratory acidosis, a decrease in pH due to retention of carbon dioxide, is frequently encountered and can either be due to hypoventilation syndromes (COPD, obesity-hypoventilation syndrome, or sleep apnea), acute apnea due to cardiac or pulmonary arrest or neurologic trauma, or less frequently iatrogenic (apnea due to sedation). Of these, the strongest association between respiratory depression and dysrhythmia is seen among patients with obstructive sleep apnea. In contrast, case reports of arrhythmia associated with sedation are most frequently linked to the use of arrythmogenic agents [38], and ECG changes associated with COPD are likely due to underlying long-term anatomic and physiologic changes [39].

One study of 400 patients with sleep apnea demonstrated incidence of associated dysrhythmia during apneic episodes in nearly 50% of subjects. The most frequent observed ECG changes were frequent PVCs (20%), sinus pause (11%), and sinus bradycardia (<30 bpm for greater than 10s, 7%). Nonsustained ventricular tachycardia was observed in 3% of patients, and Mobitz type I and II blocks in 5% and 3% of patients, respectively. Other smaller studies have demonstrated similar dysrhythmia rates [40]. Transient ST depressions have also been described during periods of apnea.

These depressions are postulated to be due to catecholamine surge associated with awakening from apnea, as they were independent of hypoxia, improved or ablated with positive-pressure ventilation, and were not associated with an increased rate of inducible ischemia on cardiac stress testing [41]. Alarmingly, these findings seem to coincide with an increased risk of sudden cardiac death during normal sleeping hours (midnight – 6 a.m.) in patients with OSA compared to the general population [42].

Respiratory Alkalosis

Sustained respiratory alkalosis is rare and usually associated with mechanical ventilation at a higher than normal respiratory rate. Associated ECG changes are seldom seen; however, two cases of atrioventricular junctional rhythm with associated hypotension (both at pH > 7.6) and one case of associated sinus tachycardia have been reported [43]. In the cases of junctional rhythm, control was attempted with pharmacologic agents (atropine, lidocaine, diphenylhydantion, and IV potassium) without success. The first case was notable for only a relatively minor case of hypokalemia (3.5 mEq/l), whereas the second patient had a serum potassium of 2.5 mEq/l and was also confounded by prior administration of digoxin. In both cases, return of normally conducting P waves and resolution of hypotension was observed following correction of the alkalosis through reduction of the ventilatory rate.

Other Metabolic Conditions

The ECG in Hypothyroidism

Clinically apparent hypothyroidism may include many cardiac manifestations including decreased contractility, narrow pulse pressure, and mild diastolic hypertension. Myxedema coma is the most extreme complication of overt hypothyroidism. The ECG may demonstrate the triad of bradycardia, low voltage, and T-wave inversions or flattening usually without ST segment changes [44]. Significant hypothyroidism has also been demonstrated to prolong the QT interval, predisposing to ventricular dysrhythmias, including torsades de pointes, especially in patients with underlying ischemic heart disease [45].

The ECG in Hyperthyroidism

The ECG in thyrotoxicosis most often demonstrates sinus tachycardia, increased electrical amplitude in all leads, or atrial fibrillation. Sinus tachycardia is seen in nearly all patients with hyperthyroidism and is considered characteristic for the disease. Atrial fibrillation is a common manifestation with prevalence of nearly 14% in overt hyperthyroidism compared to 2.3% of the general population [46]. Treatment of the underlying disease usually results in return to sinus rhythm within 2–3 months [47].

The ECG in Mitochondrial Disease

The cardiac manifestations of mitochondrial deletion are still undergoing study, but may be variable by subtype. Early research indicates that mitochondrial DNA deletion may predispose patients to conduction abnormalities, including AV conduction disturbances, QT prolongation, and heart block [48]. Nucleotide substitutions may predispose to cardiac hypertrophy or cardiomyopathy, resulting in LVH pattern on ECG [48]. Abnormal EKG findings in these patients may prompt cardiologist evaluation and patients may benefit from pacemaker-defibrillator placement.

In conclusion, ECG abnormalities found in states of metabolic derangement often reflect the results of specific associated electrolyte abnormalities, but may also represent general myocardial dysfunction. The clinician should be aware of the potential for ECG changes in patients with metabolic disarray, and treat both the underlying cause as well as any dangerous electrolyte abnormalities such as hyperkalemia. Patients with significant metabolic problems should receive cardiac monitoring until resolution of the underlying etiology.

References

1 Foster, D.W. and McGarry, J.D. (1983). The metabolic derangements and treatment of diabetic ketoacidosis. *N. Engl. J. Med.* 309: 159–169.

2 Dittrich, K.L. and Walls, R.M. (1986). Hyperkalemia: ECG manifestations and clinical considerations. *J. Emerg. Med.* 4: 449–455.

3 Mattu, A., Brady, W.J., and Robinson, D.A. (2000). Electrocardiographic manifestations of hyperkalemia. *Am. J. Emerg. Med.* 18: 721–729.

4 Szerlip, H.M., Weiss, J., and Singer, I. (1986). Profound hyperkalemia without electrocardiographic manifestations. *Am. J. Kidney Dis.* 7: 461–465.

5 Simon, B.C. (1988). Pseudomyocardial infarction and hyperkalemia: a case report and subject review. *J. Emerg. Med.* 6: 511–515.

6 Ziakas, A., Basagiannis, C., and Stiliadis, I. (2010). Pseudoinfarction pattern in a patient with hyperkalemia, diabetic ketoacidosis and normal coronary vessels: a case report. *J. Med. Case Rep.* 4 (115).

7 Delaney, M.F., Zisman, A., and Kettyle, W.M. (2000). Diabetic ketoacidosis and hyperglycemic hyperosmolar nonketotic syndrome. *Endocrinol. Metab. Clin. N. Am.* 29: 683–705.

8 Moller, N., Foss, A.C.H., Gravholt, C.H. et al. (2005). Myocardial injury with biomarker elevation in diabetic ketoacidosis. *J. Diabetes Complicat.* 19: 361–363.

9 Levine, H.D., Wanzer, S.H., and Merrill, J.P. (1956). Dialyzable currents of injury in potassium intoxication resembling acute myocardial infarction or pericarditis. *Circulation* 13: 29–36.

10 Gonzáles-Vargas-Machuca, M.F., Arizón-Muñoz, J.M., and Villa-Gil-Ortega, M. (2011). Pseudo inferior myocardial infarction pattern caused by hyperkalemia. *Rev. Esp. Cardiol. Engl. Ed.* 64: 416.

11 Aksakal, E., Ulus, T., Bayram, E., and Duman, H. (2009). Acute inferior pseudoinfarction pattern in a patient with normokalemia and diabetic ketoacidosis. *Am. J. Emerg. Med.* 27: 251.e3–251.e5.

12 Slovis, C. and Jenkins, R. (2002). Conditions not primarily affecting the heart. *BMJ* 324: 1320–1323.

13 Kuppermann, N., Park, J., Glatter, K. et al. (2008). Prolonged qt interval corrected for heart rate during diabetic ketoacidosis in children. *Arch. Pediatr. Adolesc. Med.* 162: 544–549.

14 Fisler, J.S. (1992). Cardiac effects of starvation and semistarvation diets: safety and mechanisms of action. *Am. J. Clin. Nutr.* 56: 230S–234S.

15 Denmark, L.N. (1993). The investigation of beta-hydroxybutyrate as a marker for sudden death due to hypoglycemia in alcoholics. *Forensic Sci. Int.* 62: 225–232.

16 Best, T.H., Franz, D.N., Gilbert, D.L. et al. (2000). Cardiac complications in pediatric patients on the ketogenic diet. *Neurology* 54: 2328–2330.

17 Desouza, C.V., Bolli, G.B., and Fonseca, V. (2010). Hypoglycemia, diabetes, and cardiovascular events. *Diabetes Care* 33: 1389–1394.

18 Desouza, C., Salazar, H., Cheong, B. et al. (2003). Association of hypoglycemia and cardiac ischemia: a study based on continuous monitoring. *Diabetes Care* 26: 1485–1489.

19 Markel, A., Keidar, S., and Yasin, K. (1994). Hypoglycaemia-induced ischaemic ECG changes. *Presse Méd. Paris Fr.* 1983 (23): 78–79.

20 Mahajan, V.V., Dogra, V., Pargal, I., and Singh, N. (2012). Silent myocardial infarction during hypoglycemic coma. *Indian J. Endocrinol. Metab.* 16: 139–140.

21 Laitinen, T. et al. (2008). Electrocardiographic alterations during hyperinsulinemic hypoglycemia in healthy subjects. *Ann. Noninvasive Electrocardiol.* 13: 97–105.

22 Marques, J.L. et al. (1997). Altered ventricular repolarization during hypoglycaemia in patients with diabetes. *Diabet. Med. J. Br. Diabet. Assoc.* 14: 648–654.

23 Murphy, N.P., Ford-Adams, M.E., Ong, K.K. et al. (2004). Prolonged cardiac repolarisation during spontaneous nocturnal hypoglycaemia in children and adolescents with type 1 diabetes. *Diabetologia* 47: 1940–1947.

24 Heller, S.R. (2002). Abnormalities of the electrocardiogram during hypoglycaemia: the cause of the dead in bed syndrome? *Int. J. Clin. Pract. Suppl.*: 27–32.

25 Williams, E.M.V. (1955). The individual effects of CO2, bicarbonate and pH on the electrical and mechanical activity of isolated rabbit auricles. *J. Physiol.* 129: 90–110.

26 Kidney International – Abstract of article (1972). The effects of acid-base disturbances on cardiovascular and pulmonary function. *Kidney Int.* 1: 375–389.

27 He, C., Sl, F., Ar, M. et al. (1975). Depression of human myocardial contractility with 'respiratory' and 'metabolic' acidosis. *Surgery* 77: 427–432.

28 Does bicarbonate therapy improve the management of severe di …: Critical Care Medicine. http://journals.lww.com/ccmjournal/Fulltext/1999/12000/Does_bicarbonate_therapy_improve_the_management_of.14.aspx

29 Forsythe, S.M. and Schmidt, G.A. (2000). Sodium bicarbonate for the treatment of lactic acidosis. *Chest* 117: 260–267.

30 Pilcher, J. and Nagle, R.E. (1971). Acid-base imbalance and arrhythmias after myocardial infarction. *Br. Heart J.* 33: 526–532.

31 Reid, J.A., Enson, Y., Harvey, R.M., and Ferrer, M.I. (1965). The effect of variations in blood pH upon the electrocardiogram in man. *Circulation* 31: 369–373.

32 Dreyfuss, D. et al. (1989). Tall T waves during metabolic acidosis without hyperkalemia: a prospective study. *Crit. Care Med.* 17: 404–408.

33 Silvestre, J., Carvalho, S., Mendes, V. et al. (2007). Metformin-induced lactic acidosis: a case series. *J. Med. Case Rep.* 1: 126.

34 Maready, E. Jr., Holstege, C., Brady, W., and Baer, A. (2004). Electrocardiographic abnormality in carbon monoxide–poisoned patients. *Ann. Emerg. Med.* 44: S92.

35 Levinsky, N. (1991). *Harrison's Principals of Internal Medicine*, 294. McGraw-Hill.

36 Fitzgibbons, L.J. and Snoey, E.R. (1999). Severe metabolic alkalosis due to baking soda ingestion: case reports of two

patients with unsuspected antacid overdose. *J. Emerg. Med.* 17: 57–61.

37 Al-Abri, S.A. and Olson, K.R. (2013). Baking soda can settle the stomach but upset the heart: case files of the medical toxicology fellowship at the University of California, San Francisco. *J. Med. Toxicol.* 9: 255–258.

38 Pershad, J., Palmisano, P., and Nichols, M. (1999). Chloral hydrate: the good and the bad. *Pediatr. Emerg. Care* 15: 432–435.

39 Harrigan, R.A. and Jones, K. (2002). Conditions affecting the right side of the heart. *BMJ* 324: 1201–1204.

40 Miller, W.P. (1982). Cardiac arrhythmias and conduction disturbances in the sleep apnea syndrome: prevalence and significance. *Am. J. Med.* 73: 317–321.

41 Hanly, P., Sasson, Z., Zuberi, N., and Lunn, K. (1993). ST-segment depression during sleep in obstructive sleep apnea. *Am. J. Cardiol.* 71: 1341–1345.

42 Gami, A.S., Howard, D.E., Olson, E.J., and Somers, V.K. (2005). Day–night pattern of sudden death in obstructive sleep apnea. *N. Engl. J. Med.* 352: 1206–1214.

43 Lawson, N.W., Butler, G.H., and Ray, C.T. (1973). Alkalosis and cardiac arrhythmias. *Anesth. Analg.* 52: 951–962.

44 Wagner, G.S. and Marriott, H.J.L. (2013). *Marriott's Practical Electrocardiography*. LWW.

45 Fredlund, B.O. and Olsson, S.B. (1983). Long QT interval and ventricular tachycardia of 'torsade de pointe' type in hypothyroidism. *Acta Med. Scand.* 213: 231–235.

46 Klein, I. (2005). *Braunwald's Heart Disease: A Textbook of Cardiovascular Medicine 2051–2065*. W.B. Saunders.

47 Nakazawa, H., Lythall, D.A., Noh, J. et al. (2000). Is there a place for the late cardioversion of atrial fibrillation? A long-term follow-up study of patients with post-thyrotoxic atrial fibrillation. *Eur. Heart J.* 21: 327–333.

48 Anan, R., Nakagawa, M., Miyata, M. et al. (1995). Cardiac involvement in mitochondrial diseases a study on 17 patients with documented mitochondrial DNA defects. *Circulation* 91: 955–961.

5

The ECG in Environmental Urgencies and Emergencies

Heather T. Lounsbury[1] and Seth O. Althoff[2]

[1]*Department of Emergency Medicine, University of Virginia, Charlottesville, VA, USA*
[2]*Grandview Hospital, Sellersville, PA, USA*

Introduction

Environmental emergencies encompass a broad range of medical conditions. Most people equate environmental emergencies with the wilderness; however, a large majority of these conditions occur in the chronically ill, in or near their homes. A significant number of hypothermia and hyperthermia cases occur in the elderly during extreme fluctuations in ambient temperature. For example, approximately 600 deaths occur annually from primary hypothermia in the United States. Half of those occur in patients 65 years and older [1]. Clinicians can use the ECG to help diagnose and manage some environmental emergencies. This chapter will cover environmental emergencies that have unique or specific electrocardiogram (ECG) findings.

Hypothermia

Background

Each year there are approximately 600 deaths in the United States attributed to primary hypothermia, which is classified as accidental, suicidal, or homicidal. Secondary hypothermia is usually considered a natural complication of systemic disorders, trauma, drug abuse, and sepsis. The true incidence of secondary hypothermia is unknown, because these deaths are likely attributed to the underlying medical condition. Most cases occur in elderly patients over the age of 65 in an urban setting. Not all of these cases occur in locations that would be considered extremely cold; in one survey evaluating cases of accidental hypothermia, 69 out of 428 occurred in Florida [1].

Hypothermia is defined as a core body temperature <35 °C (<95 °F), which is further categorized into mild, moderate, and severe. Mild hypothermia occurs from 35–32 °C (95–89.6 °F), during which the patient is considered to be in an excitation phase. In this temperature range, the patient's physiologic responses are stimulated and their heart rate, blood pressure, and cardiac output will increase. As the temperature drops into the moderate hypothermia range from 32–29 °C (89.6–85.2 °F), the patient's physiologic responses will slow and they will enter the adynamic stage. The blood pressure, heart rate, and cardiac output will all begin to decrease throughout this stage. Severe hypothermia is categorized as any temperature <29 °C (85.2 °F). Below 29 °C (85.2 °F) the patient's body temperature will cool to that of the ambient temperature [1, 2].

ECG Finding

Hypothermia has profound and various effects on the ECG. Because of the irritability of the myocardium and the effects of hypothermia on the conduction system, almost any dysrhythmia can be seen: from atrial fibrillation/flutter to atrioventricular blocks, premature ventricular contractions (PVCs), T-wave inversions, and nodal rhythms.

As the patient's temperature falls into mild hypothermia, the patient will initially develop sinus tachycardia. Following the initial tachycardia, there is an incremental decrease in heart rate of approximately 50% at 28 °C (82.4 °F) [1]. This sinus bradycardia is a result of the decrease in spontaneous repolarization of the pacemaker cells (Figure 5.5.1). Due to cold-induced changes within metabolic parameters on pH, oxygen, and electrolytes, there can be various changes within the cardiac conduction system, leading to prolongation of the PR, QRS, and QTC intervals (Figure 5.5.2).

Electrocardiogram in Clinical Medicine, First Edition. Edited by William J. Brady, Michael J. Lipinski, Andrew E. Darby, Michael C. Bond, Nathan P. Charlton, Korin Hudson, and Kelly Williamson.

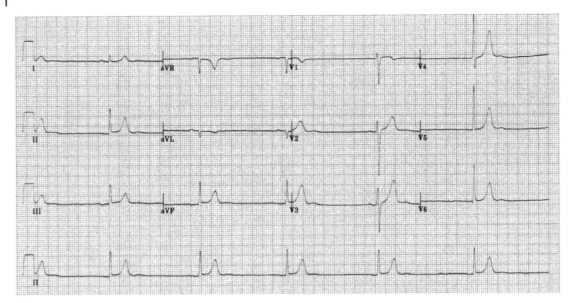

Figure 5.5.1 Sinus bradycardia due to impairment in spontaneous repolarization of pacemaker cells. Notice P waves before every QRS complex. *Source:* used with permission from http://lifeinthefastlane.com/ecg-library/basics/hypothermia.

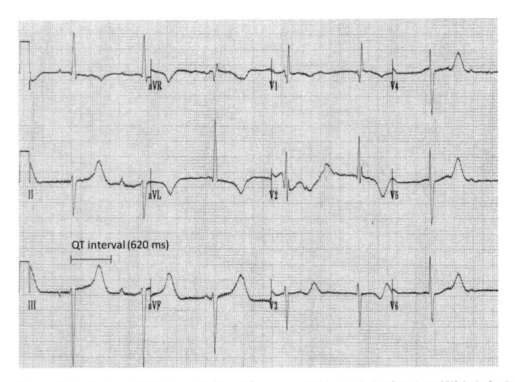

QT interval (620 ms)

Figure 5.5.2 Prolonged QTC interval (620 ms). *Source:* used with permission from http://lifeinthefastlane.com/ecg-library/basics/hypothermia.

Typically, dysrhythmias start to occur around 32.2 °C (90 °F). The risk for ventricular fibrillation and asystole increases as the patient progresses into severe hypothermia, and may spontaneously occur below 25 °C (77 °F) [1]. Although almost any dysrhythmia can be encountered, the typical progression is from sinus bradycardia to atrial fibrillation with a slow ventricular response (Figure 5.5.3),

to ventricular fibrillation (Figure 5.5.4), and ultimately asystole [2].

The classic ECG finding in hypothermia is the Osborne or J wave. The J wave, or *camel-hump sign*, is a positive deflection that occurs at the junction of the QRS complex and the beginning of the ST segment take-off (Figure 5.5.5a–c). J waves can occur at any temperature below 32.3 °C (90 °F),

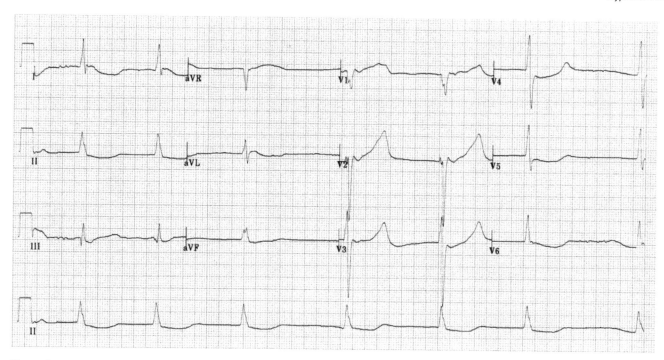

Figure 5.5.3 Atrial fibrillation with slow ventricular response. Note the lack of defined P waves. *Source:* used with permission from http://lifeinthefastlane.com/ecg-library/basics/hypothermia.

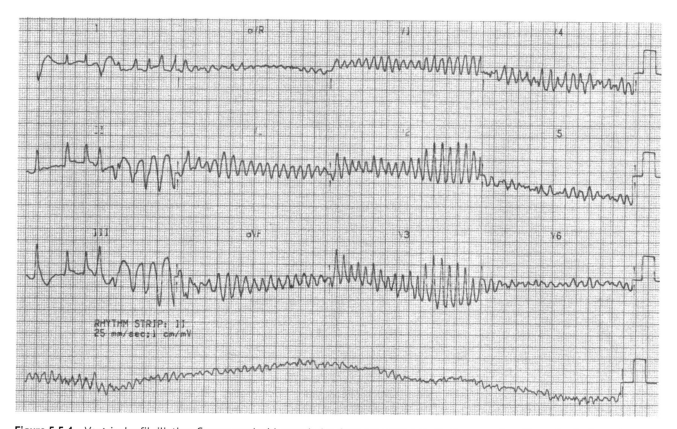

Figure 5.5.4 Ventricular fibrillation. *Source:* used with permission from http://lifeinthefastlane.com/ecg-library/basics/hypothermia.

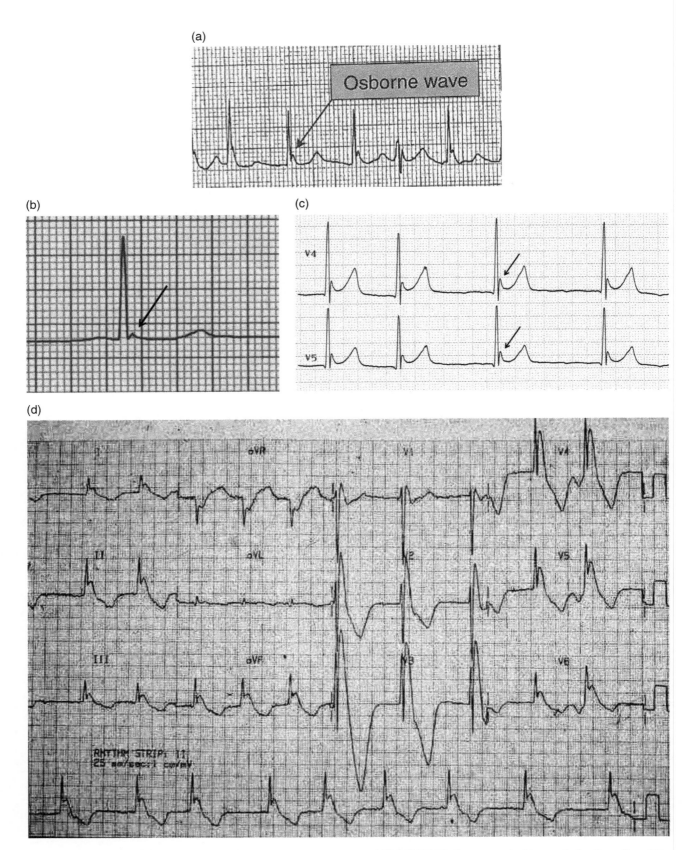

Figure 5.5.5 Osborne, or J, waves: (a) Osborne wave at a temperature of 32.2 °C (90 °F). *Source:* used with permission from Chan [3]; (b) Subtle Osborne wave (red arrow). *Source:* used with permission from http://lifeinthefastlane.com/ecg-library/basics/hypothermia; (c) Osborne wave in moderate hypothermia 30 °C (86 °F) (red arrows). *Source:* used with permission from http://lifeinthefastlane.com/ecg-library/basics/hypothermia; (d) Osborne wave in Severe hypothermia. *Source:* used with permission from http://lifeinthefastlane.com/ecg-library/basics/hypothermia.

and are best appreciated in leads II and V6. The size of the J wave increases as the core body temperature decreases (Figure 5.5.5d). J waves are not pathognomonic of hypothermia and can be found in patients with central nervous system lesions, sepsis, and cardiac ischemia [1].

Treatment

The initial treatment is the same as in any other emergency, ABCs: airway, breathing, circulation. After that, the care is twofold. First, patients must be transported with as little manipulation as possible because the myocardium is extremely irritable, and any manipulation may precipitate ventricular fibrillation. Second, the patient needs to be rewarmed.

There are three categories of rewarming; passive, active external, and active core rewarming. How fast and with which specific technique is not clearly defined. Passive warming involves removing the patient from the environment, removing all wet clothing, drying the patient, and applying a blanket or other dry insulating material. This can typically be accomplished in those patients who are awake, stable, and healthy as an intact thermoregulatory system is required for passive rewarming to be effective [2].

Active external rewarming involves the application of exogenous heat to the patient through warm water immersion, heating blankets, radiant heat, or forced air. Active rewarming should be implemented in those patients who have cardiac instability, core temperature <32.2 °C (90 °F), or patients who likely do not have intact thermoregulatory systems and who fail to rewarm with passive techniques [1].

Active core rewarming includes all of the following: inhalation rewarming, heated IV fluids, GI tract lavage, peritoneal lavage, pleural lavage, mediastinal lavage, arteriovenous rewarming, and cardiopulmonary bypass [2]. The indications for each of these warming mechanisms are beyond the scope of discussion for this chapter.

The treatments for the various dysrhythmias that occur while the patient is hypothermic are typically ineffective. Interventions such as atropine and transcutaneous pacing are typically ineffective for bradydysrhythmias, and transcutaneous pacing may precipitate v-fib. Bretylium may be beneficial in patients in v-fib; however, it is uncommonly supplied at most hospitals. The unstable patient should be actively warmed, which may in itself stop the dysrhythmia or may aide the utility of more standard ACLS (advanced cardiovascular life support) treatments [1]. Classically, due to reports of full neurologic recovery following prolonged arrest in hypothermic patients, "the patient is not dead until warm and dead." In most cases, resuscitation efforts should be continued until the patient's core temperature is at least 30–32 °C (86–89.6 °F) [2].

Lightning Strikes

Background

It is estimated that lightning strikes cause roughly 50–300 deaths in North America each year [4]. However, approximately 90% of lightning-strike victims survive. Most of the victims die from sudden cardiac death as a result of direct depolarization of the myocardium causing asystole [5]. However, secondary cardiac arrest may also occur, as spontaneous cardiac activity may resume following asystole but respiratory centers may be disrupted, leading to a subsequent hypoxic arrest.

Lightning can strike in several different ways. A *direct* strike, as it implies, is when the electrical discharge directly strikes the victim. A *side flash*, or *splash*, injury occurs when lightning strikes a nearby object and current traverses through the air, striking the victim. This type of injury may affect several victims at once. Another form of injury that may occur is called a *contact* strike, in which current is passed from an object the victim is holding, for example a telephone, to the ground. Similar to a *contact* strike is *ground current*. This occurs when lightning strikes the ground and is then transmitted to the victim. At times current flows upward from the ground toward the sky in what is called an *upward streamer*, which has also been implicated in causing a fatal injury [5].

Lightning injuries are significantly different from other, generator-produced, high-voltage exposures in both the injuries that occur and their treatment. Lightning injuries occur instantaneously, causing a flashover, whereas generator-produced high voltage has a prolonged exposure. Therefore, lightning strike victims suffer less severe thermal injuries both externally and internally. They also do not typically experience rhabdomyolysis or compartment syndrome. Patients may sustain cerebral contusions, tympanic membrane rupture, and peripheral neuropathies either from the lightning strike or its blast effect [6]. When a patient is brought in who was found unresponsive or confused, it may be difficult to determine if it was secondary to a lightning strike. The best clue may be in the history from emergency medical services (EMS).

ECG Findings

The ECG findings that can occur in those patients who survive a lightning strike exposure can be highly variable. Most commonly, the patient will present with sinus tachycardia. Patients have been reported to present with both atrial (most commonly atrial fibrillation) as well as ventricular arrhythmias [5]. Other ECG findings that have *been reported are T-wave inversions, nonspecific ST-segment* changes, ST-segment elevation consistent with ischemia, a prolonged QTc interval, and a late transition of R-wave progression (Figure 5.5.6). These findings may not initially be present, but may occur 24–48 hours after the primary event. It is speculated that the pathophysiology of these finding is related to a combination of direct injury from the strike, possible coronary artery vasospasm, and contusion from the blast effect [8]. Victims may demonstrate some signs of myocardial injury with an elevation of cardiac enzymes. Patients have also developed pericardial effusions and acquired Takotsubo cardiomyopathy [7].

Treatment

As previously mentioned, even if the victim suffers a cardiac arrest from the initial strike, they may survive if intrinsic pacers resume cardiac activity. Therefore, lightning strikes present a direct contradiction to normal triage guidelines for a multiple casualty scenario. Typically, in normal mass-casualty situations dead persons are bypassed in search for those who are injured but may benefit from resuscitation. In lightning strikes, however, one should attempt to "resuscitate the dead" to prevent secondary arrest in those patients with continued respiratory arrest [5].

The cardiovascular effects that result, such as cardiomyopathy, ischemic changes with enzyme leak, and pericardial effusions should be managed expectantly. In the case of Takotsubo cardiomyopathy, with severe cardiac dysfunction and subsequent cardiogenic shock, initiation of vasopressors, inotropes, and intra-aortic balloon pump (IABP) have been reported [9–11]. Most of these changes will resolve and typically not cause any long-term sequela. If the patient develops a dysrhythmia, the indications for standard antidysrhythmic agents remains the same as per ACLS guidelines [6].

There are a few other unique injuries that occur from lightning strikes, including cataracts, tympanic membrane rupture, vasomotor spasm, pupillary dilatation, heat-induced coagulation of the cerebral cortex, seizures, and cutaneous burns. Some patients may present with pale, cool extremities and no palpable pulse. This is theorized to be secondary to extreme vasoconstriction and will resolve over time. Several burns are associated with lightning strikes, but the Lichtenberg figures are pathognomonic and consist of a feathering or ferning pattern [5].

There is also a significant neuropsychological affect in lightning strike victims. For example, they may develop posttraumatic stress disorder, sleep disturbances, anxiety,

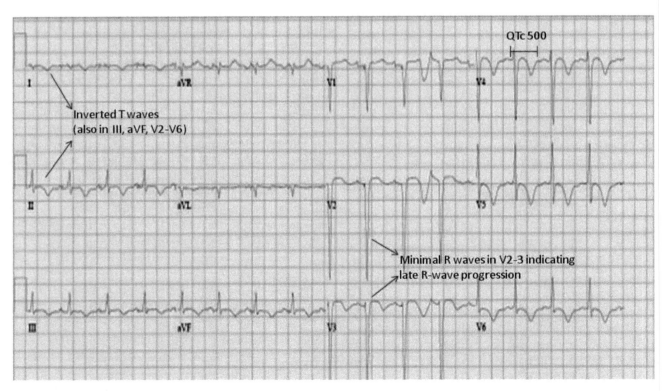

Figure 5.5.6 A 27-year-old male presenting 24 hours after a lightning strike injury: sinus rhythm at 98 bpm, T-wave inversion in the precordial and limb leads, late transition shift, rS pattern in leads I and aVL, and long QT interval (QTc = 500 ms) [7].

and memory deficits. For this reason, these patients should be referred to support groups upon discharge [6].

Underwater Submersion

Background

Submersion in water, particularly of the face, for any amount of time is known to elicit the "diving response," which consists of bradycardia and increased peripheral vascular resistance. These reflexes are mediated by increased parasympathetic as well as sympathetic nervous system activity. Apnea and facial immersion stimulating the trigeminal nerve are responsible for stimulating these increases in activity [12]. A practical use of this reflex in the emergency department is that facial immersion in cold water can be used to break supraventricular tachycardia (SVT) in children; the immersion stimulates the vagus nerve without requiring any voluntary action by the patient, and this increased vagal activity slows or breaks the SVT. In well-trained breath-hold divers, the bradycardia, hypoxia, and hypercapnea can be profound. Heart rates of as low as 20–30 bpm have been documented, with SpO_2 of 50–60% also noted in a different study [13, 14].

ECG Findings

Usually, only insignificant arrhythmias have been documented with breath-hold dives, including multiple premature atrial contractions (PACs) and PVCs. In one study in which trained breath-hold divers were monitored with ECG, 75% of subjects demonstrated some sort of dysrhythmia [14]. These included PACs, PVCs, intermittent bundle branch blocks, and bigeminy. These dysrhythmias were noted to occur just prior to surfacing and had maximal occurrence just after surfacing when the apnea was broken. In another study of ECG changes in trainees undergoing a simulated escape from a submerged helicopter, similar dysrhythmias were noted with an underwater time of less than 10 seconds, suggesting that arrhythmias are not dependent on the time of submersion [15].

These dysrhythmias are thought to become clinically significant in the setting of underlying cardiac disease or congenital heart conditions. One important group includes those with congenital channelopathies manifesting as a long QT interval on their baseline ECG (long QT syndrome, or LQTS) (Figure 5.5.2). LQTS is a hereditary mutation in one of many genes that code for cardiac potassium channels. There are three categories of LQTS: LQTS1, where cardiac events usually occur during exercise, and classically submersion or swimming; LQTS2, where events

occur during emotional stress or with sudden auditory stimulus (e.g. an alarm); and LQTS3, where events typically occur during sleep. The long QT interval seen on ECG represents delayed or prolonged return to resting state of the myocardium. This delay in repolarization makes it more likely that some parts of the myocardium may not be refractory to another action potential. An errant action potential (or early afterdepolarization), may then be perpetuated in an area of the ventricle that is in a different phase of the cardiac cycle than those cells around it, causing a PVC on ECG. When the neighboring cells are able to be depolarized again, they will begin to conduct the action potential from the cells that were depolarized prior. This cycle of neighboring cells depolarizing each other at slightly different times results in ventricular tachycardia (VT) and/or torsades de pointes (Figure 5.5.7) [16].

Another congenital channelopathy that is phenotypically similar to LQTS1 in that it causes sudden cardiac death with submersion is called catecholaminergic polymorphic ventricular tachycardia (CPVT). The gene affected by CVPT is thought to encode for a cardiac sodium channel, though this entity is of relatively recent discovery and has fewer genes elucidated than LQTS. Unfortunately, CPVT does not have any apparent changes on resting ECG the way LQTS does, and, therefore, usually goes undiagnosed until a cardiac event occurs. The mechanism of arrhythmia in CPVT is somewhat different than LQTS; errant PVC or PACs are caused by delayed afterdepolarizations, or depolarizations that occur after the refractory period is over. The exact mechanism of how these types of depolarizations cause arrhythmia is poorly understood [16].

Treatment

Those with pulseless VT or fibrillation should be defibrillated immediately. Additional treatment of torsade de pointes can include IV magnesium and/or overdrive pacing. VT with a pulse in a patient with known or suspected congenital heart disease should be managed in close consultation with a cardiologist, as treatments are controversial and can be quite different from other causes of VT. However, the patient with congenital channelopathy who presents while still in VT is a very rare occurrence; they more likely will present after successful resuscitation following a prehospital cardiac event.

It is important to obtain an ECG on any patient who arrives in the emergency department after near-drowning to assess for LQTS. Long-term management of LQTS and CPVT includes beta blockade, which decreases the incidence of PVC/PACs. ICD implantation may also be indicated, and should be accomplished prior to hospital

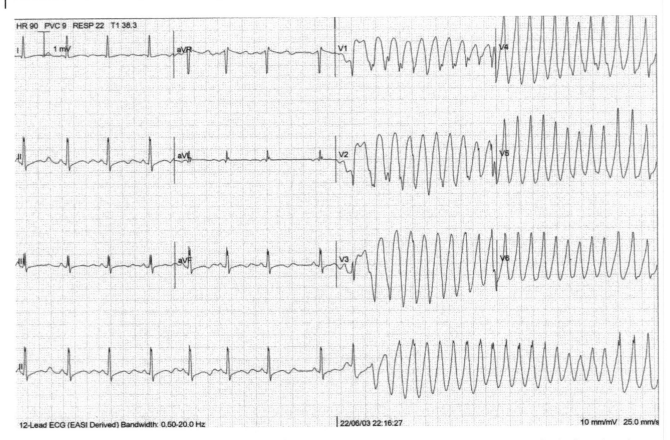

HR 90 PVC 9 RESP 22 T1 38.3

12-Lead ECG (EASI Derived) Bandwidth: 0.50-20.0 Hz   22/06/03 22:16:27   10 mm/mV 25.0 mm/s

Figure 5.5.7 Torsade de pointes. *Source:* used with permission from http://lifeinthefastlane.com/ecg-library/basics/hypothermia.

discharge from any near-drowning or sentinel cardiac event in those with genetic conduction abnormalities. Electrophysiologic testing may be required to uncover a channelopathy. The diagnosis can be essential not only for the patient but also their family members, who should subsequently be offered testing and treatment, if appropriate, prior to any life-threatening event.

Heat Stroke

Background

Heat illnesses are particularly common in the general population and range on a spectrum from heat rash and heat exhaustion to heat stroke. Heat stroke is defined as a core body temperature >40 °C and altered mental status [17]. Mortality approaches 100% in untreated patients. The cardiovascular system is often the first to be affected by a heat insult, as a main thermoregulatory mechanism is dilatation of cutaneous blood vessels and loss of volume through sweating; this dilatation requires a significant increase in heart rate in order to maintain

cardiac output [17]. This increase in heart rate is often not sustainable or even mountable in those with significant underlying cardiac morbidities such as congestive heart failure or coronary artery disease. Even in those with structurally normal hearts, heat stress capable of causing heat stroke can cause significant cardiovascular changes in addition to altered mental status, seizure, and coma.

ECG Findings

On ECG the presence of ST elevations has been well documented in heat stroke. One case report noted territorial ST elevations in the lateral precordial leads (Figure 5.5.8) with associated echocardiographic abnormalities in the form of left ventricular systolic dysfunction with regional wall motion abnormalities [18]. The patient also demonstrated a mild increase in troponin I levels. The unique part of this case report was that the patient underwent subsequent cardiac catheterization, which demonstrated completely normal coronary arteries. This constellation of territorial ST elevation, echocardiographic abnormalities,

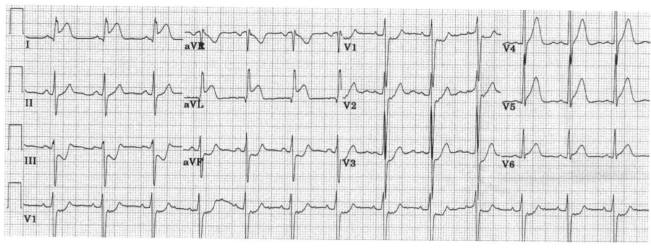

Figure 5.5.8 Lateral STEMI with ST elevation in leads I, aVL, V5, and V6 with reciprocal depression in leads III, aVF, V1, V2, and V3. *Source:* used with permission of http://lifeinthefastlane.com/ecg-library.

and normal coronaries is consistent with stress-induced, or Takotsubo, cardiomyopathy. Previous case reports of ST elevation in heat stroke did not include coronary angiography to ensure that the EKG finding were not due to coronary artery disease. Patients in these other reports were reportedly asymptomatic (i.e. without chest pain, shortness of breath, or other angina equivalent). Unfortunately, true acute coronary syndrome (ACS) can be precipitated by heat stress in those with cardiac risk factors due to the sudden increase in cardiac demand. Takotsubo cardiomyopathy is indistinguishable from true ACS on ECG and echocardiogram; differentiation requires cardiac catheterization. In the above case report, the patient also developed significant cardiogenic shock requiring the placement of an intraaortic balloon pump. This patient's ST elevations and wall motion abnormalities resolved spontaneously as he recovered from his heat stroke.

Another case report describes development of a Brugada ECG pattern secondary to heat stroke [19]. This patient's presenting ECG demonstrated right bundle branch block (RBBB) and coved ST elevations in V1 and V2 (Figure 5.5.9). Brugada syndrome is an autosomal dominant channelopathy involving the cardiac sodium channels [20]. Reduction in sodium channels results in slowed current conduction, predisposing to arrhythmias. The patient in the study did not have any of the genetic mutations associated with Brugada syndrome, but family members did not undergo testing. The theory behind why heat stroke caused this ECG finding is that sodium channels are heat-sensitive and may exhibit enough activity suppression to present as a Brugada pattern in susceptible individuals at high enough temperatures.

The ECG findings in this patient resolved within 24 hours of admission.

Treatment

Treatment of a heat stroke patient involves rapid cooling the patient and supportive care. With regards to the work-up of ST elevation, particularly in a territorial pattern, an echocardiogram should be done as early as possible to evaluate for wall motion abnormalities. This can help predict the likelihood of developing cardiogenic shock. Treatment of cardiogenic shock can be limited to fluid resuscitation, require inotropic agents (dobutamine, norepinephrine, epinephrine), or require more invasive treatments like an IABP.

The decision to take the patient directly to cardiac catheterization from the emergency department is a difficult one in the setting of heat stroke. If a patient has multiple coronary risk factors or known coronary artery disease, it is reasonable to treat as ACS until proven otherwise and involve a cardiologist early in the course. In a younger, previously healthy patient it is likely reasonable to observe for resolution of ST elevation and repeat echocardiograms to monitor any wall motion abnormalities. Of course, at any point in their course, a patient may be taken to cardiac catheterization if they are requiring more aggressive treatments for cardiogenic shock or if ECG abnormalities are not resolving as quickly as anticipated.

Patients with a Brugada ECG pattern or other interval changes suggestive of underlying channelopathy require further electrophysiologic and/or genetic testing prior to leaving the hospital to determine need for defibrillator placement.

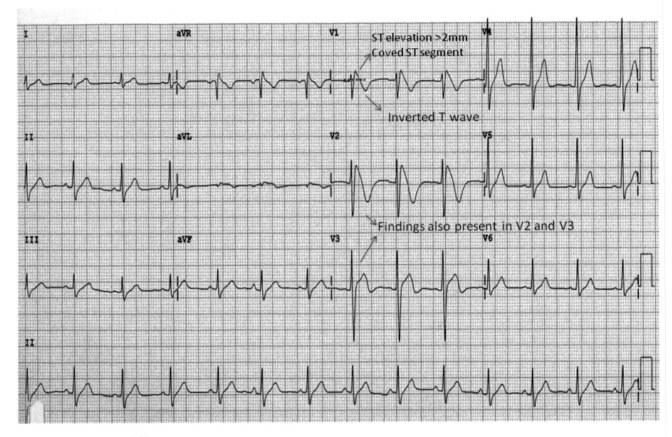

Figure 5.5.9 Brugada ECG pattern.

Conclusion

While rare, environmental emergencies, including lightning strikes, heat stroke, and near-drowning, can have significant cardiac consequences for patients. These consequences can be more severe based on underlying cardiac abnormalities or predisposing factors that the patient and clinician may or may not be aware of. More common situations such as hypothermia, ranging from mild to severe, have more well-known cardiac dysfunction associated with them. The ECG can be a crucial piece of information for the clinician in patients who have knowingly experienced an environmental emergency or even in undifferentiated patients at risk for an environmental exposure. A patient's treatment and/or disposition and follow-up requirements may be significantly affected by findings on their presenting ECG, and knowledge of important findings and the ability to triage these findings as serious or benign is imperative for emergency physicians.

References

1 Danzl, D.F. and Hueker, M.R. (2012). Accidental hypothermia. In: *Wilderness Medicine*, 6e (ed. P.S. Auerbach), 135. Elsevier.

2 Bessen, H.A. and Bryan, N. (2011). Hypothermia. In: *Tintinalli's Emergency Medicine: A Comprehensive Study Guide*, 7e (eds. J.E. Tintinalli, J.S. Stapczynski, J.O. Ma, et al.). McGraw-Hill.

3 Chan, T.C., Brady, W., Harrigan, R. et al. (2005). *ECG in Emergency Medicine and Acute Care.*, 309. Maryland Heights, MO: Mosby.

4 O'Keefe, G.M. and Zane, R.D. (2004). Lightning injuries. *Emerg. Med. Clin. North Am.* 22: 369–403.

5 Fish, R.M. (2011). Lightning injuries. In: *Tintinalli's Emergency Medicine: A Comprehensive Study Guide*, 7e

(eds. J.E. Tintinalli, J.S. Stapczynski, J.O. Ma, et al.), 1391–1393. McGraw-Hill.

6 Cooper, M.A., Andrews, C.J., Holle, R.L. et al. (2012). Lightning-related injuries and safety. In: *Wilderness Medicine*, 6e (ed. P.S. Auerbach), 71. Elsevier.

7 McIntyre, W.F., Simpson, C.S., Redfearn, D.P. et al. (2010). The lightning heart: a case report and brief review of the cardiovascular complications of lightning injury. *Indian Pacing Electrophysiol. J.* 10 (9): 429–433.

8 Lichtenberg, R., Dries, D., Ward, K. et al. (1993). Cardiovascular effects of lightning strikes. *J. Am. Coll. Cardiol.* 21 (2): 531–536.

9 Dundon, B.K., Puri, R., Leong, D.P., and Worthley, M.I. (2008). Takotsubo cardiomyopathy following lightning strike. *Emerg. Med. J.* 25 (7): 460–461.

10 Rivera, J., Romero, K.A., Gonzalez-Chon, O. et al. (2007). Severe stunned myocardium after lightning strike. *Crit. Care Med.* 35 (1): 280–285.

11 Slesinger, T.L., Bank, M., Drumheller, B.C. et al. (2010). Immediate cardiac arrest and subsequent development of cardiogenic shock caused by lightning strike. *J. Trauma* 68 (1): E5–E7.

12 Foster, G.E. and Sheel, A.W. (2005). The human diving response, its function, and its control. *Scand. J. Med. Sci. Sports* 15: 3–12.

13 Ferrigno, M., Ferretti, G., Ellis, A. et al. (1997). Cardiovascular changes during deep breath-hold dives in a pressure chamber. *J. Appl. Physiol.* 83: 1282–1290.

14 Hansel, J., Solleder, I., Gfroerer, W. et al. (2009). Hypoxia and cardiac arrhythmias in breath-hold divers during voluntary immersed breath-holds. *Eur. J. Appl. Physiol.* 105: 673–678.

15 Tipton, M.J., Gibbs, P., Brooks, C. et al. (2010). ECG during helicopter underwater escape training. *Aviat. Space Environ. Med.* 81: 399–404.

16 Choi, G., Kopplin, L.J., Tester, D.J. et al. (2004). Spectrum and frequency of cardiac channel defects in swimming-triggered arrhythmia syndromes. *Circulation* 110 (15): 2119–2124.

17 Waters, T.A. and Al-Salamah, M.A. (2011). Heat emergencies. In: *Tintinalli's Emergency Medicine: A Comprehensive Study Guide*, 7e (eds. J.E. Tintinalli, J.S. Stapczynski, J.O. Ma, et al.). 1339–1343. McGraw-Hill.

18 Chen, W.T., Lin, C.H., Hsieh, M.H. et al. (2012). Stress-induced cardiomyopathy caused by heat stroke. *Ann. Emerg. Med.* 60: 63–66.

19 Lacunza, J., San Roman, I., Moreno, S. et al. (2009). Heat stroke, an unusual trigger of Brugada electrocardiogram. *Am. J. Emerg. Med.* 27: 634.e1–634.e3.

20 Crawford, M.H., DiMarco, J.P., and Paulus, W.J. (2010). *Cardiology*, 3e. Elsevier.

Section VI

The ECG in Special Inpatient Groups

1

The ECG-Monitored Patient

Feras Khan

Department of Emergency Medicine, University of Maryland School of Medicine, Baltimore, MD, USA

Introduction

For patients who are hospitalized with conditions requiring telemetry, the electrocardiogram (ECG) is vital in monitoring the delivery of treatment and patients' response to it. Most hospitals have a limited number of telemetry beds, and this continuous monitoring becomes very expensive. Nevertheless, telemetry monitoring tends to be overused, so the astute physician who understands the appropriate use of this advanced technology will be able to contribute to decisions regarding the need for it in various clinical scenarios. This chapter discusses specific indications for telemetry among patients being monitored and managed on hospital units other than intensive care units (ICUs) and the clinical manifestations, specifically the electrocardiographic manifestations, of specific cardiac conditions.

Clinical Scenarios Requiring Telemetry/Electrocardiographic Monitoring

Implantable Cardioverter-Defibrillator (ICD)/ Pacemaker Firing

Patients who have implanted ICDs tend to have structural heart disease and are at risk of developing arrhythmias. These devices sometimes fire in response to an arrhythmia or erroneously. Electrocardiographic monitoring will indicate what triggered the ICD to fire.

Atrioventricular (AV) Block

Patients who have third-degree AV block with hemodynamic compromise are usually admitted to an ICU for pacing and treatment (Figures 6.1.1–6.1.3). Patients with other types of AV block, including second-degree (Mobitz types I and II), that cause syncope or other issues such as bradycardia need to be monitored for progression and resolution of the arrhythmia. These patients might need permanent pacemakers, depending on the degree of AV block.

Acute Heart Failure

Every heart failure patient who is admitted to the hospital should be monitored with telemetry to detect atrial or ventricular arrhythmias. Occasionally, these patients are on continuous infusions of a pro-arrhythmic medication (e.g. milrinone or dobutamine). Furthermore, other medications given to these patients (e.g. furosemide) can cause electrolyte abnormalities, which can alter the ECG.

Chest Pain Syndrome

There is some debate as to whether patients with low-risk chest pain syndromes require 24-hour telemetry monitoring (Figure 6.1.4) [1]. Nevertheless, any patient who has cardiac risk factors and baseline electrocardiographic abnormalities such as T-wave changes should be monitored on telemetry and have serial ECGs to detect ST-segment changes.

Electrocardiogram in Clinical Medicine, First Edition. Edited by William J. Brady, Michael J. Lipinski, Andrew E. Darby, Michael C. Bond, Nathan P. Charlton, Korin Hudson, and Kelly Williamson.

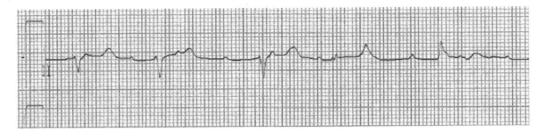

Figure 6.1.1 Third-degree AV block.

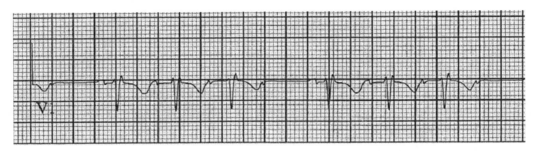

Figure 6.1.2 Mobitz Type 1 block.

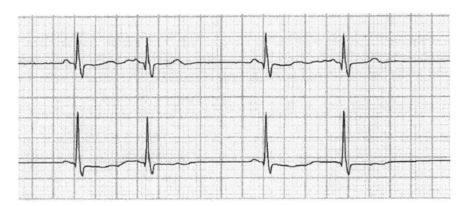

Figure 6.1.3 Mobitz Type 1 block.

Procedures

Cardiac procedures that require cardiac monitoring before and after the intervention are listed in Table 6.1.1.

Syncope

Patients with syncope thought to have a cardiac cause (e.g. arrhythmia or conduction system disease) should be monitored on telemetry. Patients with a history of heart disease such as congestive heart failure have a greater risk of developing an arrhythmia such as ventricular tachycardia or a nonsustained ventricular tachycardia.

Acute Coronary Syndrome (STEMI, Non-STEMI, Unstable Angina)

Patients with acute coronary syndrome should be monitored for ST-segment changes as well as progression of the ECG after treatment (Figure 6.1.5). Reocclusion can occur after primary angioplasty, as can recurrent ischemia or progression of the infarction. All of these can be detected by electrocardiographic monitoring.

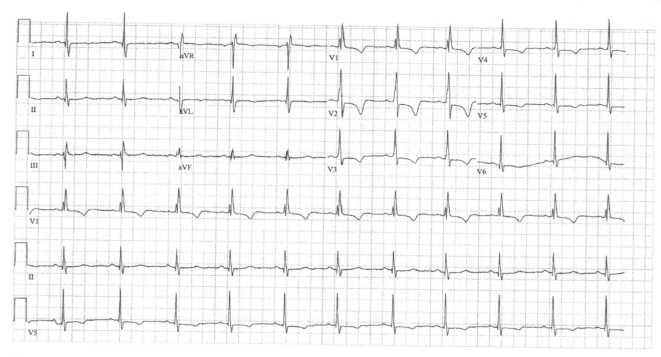

Figure 6.1.4 Chest pain syndrome. T-wave inversions in V1–V5 in a patient who had a NSTEMI.

Table 6.1.1 Procedures requiring electrocardiographic monitoring [1].

Procedure	ECG abnormality
Percutaneous coronary intervention	Bradycardia, tachycardia
Coronary angiography	Bradycardia
Arrhythmia ablation	AV block, QT prolongation, torsades de pointes
Pacemaker implantation	Pacemaker function/capture

Stroke

Patients admitted to the hospital for stroke or stroke-like symptoms should be placed on telemetry monitoring (Figure 6.1.6). These patients are at risk for atrial fibrillation and ST-segment and T-wave abnormalities [2]. Ventricular dysrhythmias are also possible but are rare.

Blood Transfusion

Patients who receive large quantities of blood are at risk of electrolyte abnormalities such as hypocalcemia and hypomagnesemia, which can prolong the QT interval and

lead to arrhythmias [2]. These patients are usually admitted to an ICU, but, no matter where they are treated, they should be on telemetry monitoring during hospitalization.

Atrial Tachyarrhythmias

Patients with atrial fibrillation and flutter with rapid ventricular response require telemetry monitoring to determine if the medications that are being used to treat them are working appropriately (Figure 6.1.7).

Electrolyte Abnormalities

Patients who have severe hyperkalemia (>6.5 mmol/l) need cardiac monitoring (Figures 6.1.8 and 6.1.9). Hyperkalemia can lead to life-threatening arrhythmias such as AV dissociation and bradycardia with QRS widening. These patients require continuous telemetry monitoring while their potassium level is being reduced. Hypokalemia, hypocalcemia, and hypomagnesemia can all prolong the QT interval, so patients with any of these imbalances need continuous monitoring while the respective electrolyte is being replenished. Patients with any of these electrolyte deficiencies can also experience premature ventricular contractions.

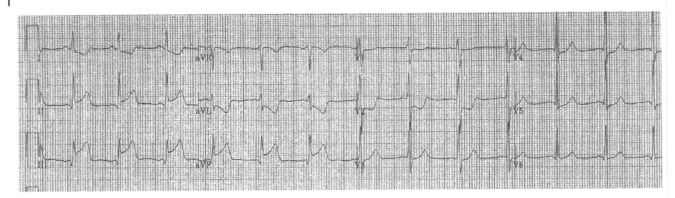

Figure 6.1.5 ST-elevation myocardial infarction in leads II, III, and aVF.

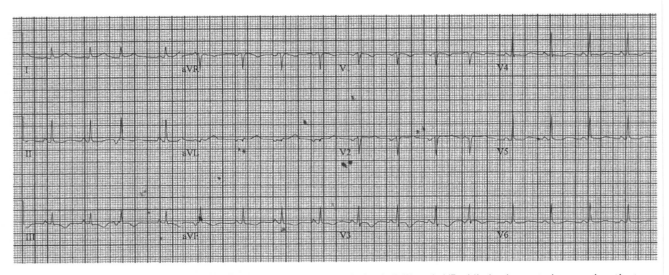

Figure 6.1.6 Acute stroke. This patient developed T-wave inversions in leads II, III, and aVF while having a stroke as an inpatient.

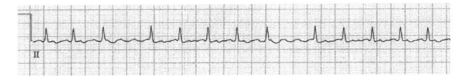

Figure 6.1.7 Atrial flutter with regular narrow QRS complex tachycardia at 150 bpm.

Drug Overdose or Toxicity

Patients who have accidentally or intentionally overdosed on medications that affect cardiac conduction (Table 6.1.2) require electrocardiographic monitoring.

Conclusion

Telemetry and electrocardiographic monitoring are important components of the plan of care for certain hospitalized patients. The flow of information provided by continuous monitoring can help clinicians determine whether patients are improving and guide them to the correct diagnosis. The conditions mentioned in this chapter require attention to the ECG. But after a certain point, patients can be removed from telemetry and electrocardiographic monitoring [3]. In general, if patients have improved and the reason for monitoring the ECG has been resolved or elucidated, the monitoring can be decreased in frequency or discontinued.

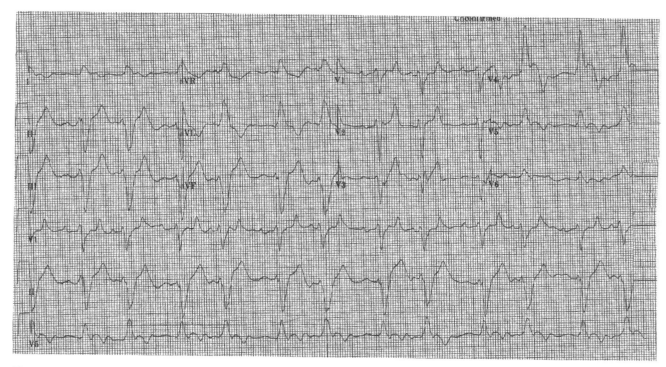

Figure 6.1.8 Hyperkalemia. This patient had an elevated potassium level, leading to a widened QRS interval.

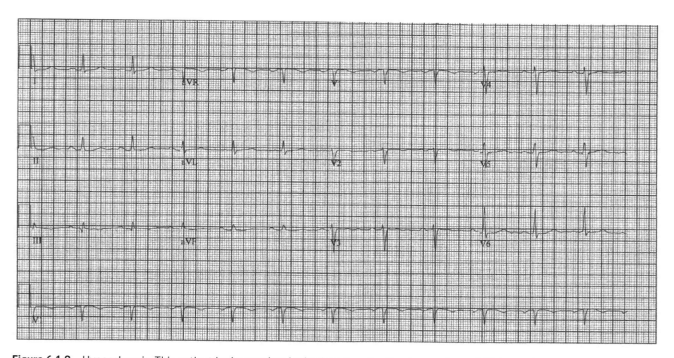

Figure 6.1.9 Hypocalcemia. This patient had a very low ionized calcium, leading to a prolonged QT interval.

Table 6.1.2 Electrocardiographic effects of drug toxicity.

Drugs	Electrocardiographic effects
Digitalis	• Atrial tachycardia • Premature ventricular contractions (PVCs) • Ventricular tachycardia • Sinoatrial arrest • AV block
Beta blockers	• Sinus bradycardia • AV block • AT prolongation
Amiodarone	• AV block • Bradycardia • QT prolongation
Calcium-channel blockers	• Sinus bradycardia • Reflex sinus tachycardia • AV block
Antipsychotics	• QT prolongation
Lithium	• T-wave changes • Sinus node dysfunction
Tricyclic antidepressants	• Sinus tachycardia • Prominent R wave in aVR • Wide QRS complex
Sympathomimetics (e.g. cocaine)	• Tachycardias (SVT, atrial fibrillation) • PVCs • QT prolongation • ST-segment changes

References

1 Drew, B., Califf, R., Funk, M. et al. (2004). Practice standards for electrocardiographic monitoring in hospital settings: an American Heart Association scientific statement from the councils on cardiovascular nursing, clinical cardiology, and cardiovascular disease in the young: endorsed by the International Society of Computerized Electrocardiology and the American Association of Critical-Care Nurses. *Circulation* 110: 2721–2746.

2 Chen, E. and Hollander, J. (2007). When do patients need admission to a telemetry bed? *J. Emerg. Med.* 33: 53–60.

3 Dhillon, S., Rachko, M., Hanon, S. et al. (2009). Telemetry monitoring guidelines for efficient and safe delivery of cardiac rhythm monitoring to noncritical hospital inpatients. *Crit. Pathw. Cardiol.* 8: 125–126.

2

Electrocardiography in the Operating Room

Feras Khan

Department of Emergency Medicine, University of Maryland School of Medicine, Baltimore, MD, USA

Introduction

Arrhythmias are often seen in the operating room (OR), either during a procedure (particularly heart surgery), in response to medications administered during a procedure, or in the postoperative period. They arise in as many as 70% of patients undergoing general anesthesia; the vast majority do not require therapeutic intervention [1].

This chapter describes situations in which careful analysis of the electrocardiogram (ECG) will contribute to decisions regarding treatment. Therapeutic decisions are strengthened by combining the electrocardiographic data with knowledge of the patient's overall clinical condition.

Types of Monitoring

In the OR, patients can be monitored by either three- or five-electrode electrocardiographic setups. The three-electrode system (using leads I, II, and III) allows tracking of the heart rate, can detect ventricular fibrillation, and allows cardioversion. It is inadequate for detecting more complicated arrhythmias such as ventricular tachycardias (VTs) and ST-segment changes. The five-electrode system is typically used in patients who have a higher risk of cardiac arrhythmias. This includes patients with preexisting cardiac disease or risk factors that predispose them to conduction abnormalities. In the five-electrode system, any of the six lead limbs can be monitored as well as a fifth electrode along V1 through V6. This system provides better monitoring for more complicated arrhythmias such as bundle branch blocks and ST-segment changes.

Risks for Arrhythmias in the OR

Several events and circumstances in the OR heighten the risk of electrocardiographic abnormalities (Table 6.2.1). The medications used for induction and intubation, including inhaled anesthetics, can all cause cardiac conduction abnormalities. The process of endotracheal intubation can cause arrhythmias and hypoxia. A variety of procedures can trigger autonomic reflexes, such as bradycardia from vagal nerve stimulation. Central venous cannulation of the internal jugular vein can lead to atrial arrhythmias if the guidewire irritates the myocardium. Direct cardiac manipulation, which is necessary when connecting cardiac bypass equipment, can also induce arrhythmias.

Postoperative Electrocardiographic Abnormalities

In the postoperative period, most abnormalities on the ECG can be traced to hypoxemia, cardiac ischemia, electrolyte disturbances, or drugs that have been given to the patient (Table 6.2.2). Management strategies depend on the patient's hemodynamic state.

Initial Management and ECG Evaluation

Whether in the OR or the postanesthesia care unit (PACU), the initial evaluation for patients with dysrhythmias should start with assessing the clinical picture by

Electrocardiogram in Clinical Medicine, First Edition. Edited by William J. Brady, Michael J. Lipinski, Andrew E. Darby, Michael C. Bond, Nathan P. Charlton, Korin Hudson, and Kelly Williamson.

obtaining vital signs, including heart rate, blood pressure, respiratory rate, pulse oximetry, and temperature. Telemetry and a 12-lead ECG should be obtained to clarify the type of dysrhythmia. For patients who are unstable (hypotensive or unconscious), the decision to use cardioversion in response to tachyarrhythmias should be made quickly. If the patient is hemodynamically stable, there is more time to evaluate the cause of arrhythmias and select the best course of treatment. The next sections review the types of arrhythmias, their causes, and treatment options.

Table 6.2.1 Causes of arrhythmias in the operation room.

- General anesthetics
- Local anesthetics
- Endotracheal intubation
- Preexisting cardiac conditions
- CNS simulation and underlying conditions
- Central line (procedures)
- Direct surgical manipulation of cardiac structures
- Autonomic reflexes

Source: From [2].

Table 6.2.2 Causes of arrhythmias in the postanesthesia care unit.

- Hypoxemia
- Hypercarbia
- Acidosis
- Hypotension
- Electrolyte imbalances
- Mechanical irritation
- Chest tubes
- Pulmonary artery catheter
- Hypothermia
- Myocardial ischemia

Types of Arrhythmias

Bradycardia

Bradycardia is usually caused by sinus node dysfunction. It manifests in several forms [3]:

- Sinus bradycardia (heart rate <60 bpm, P:QRS ratio of 1:1, and normal QRS morphology) (Figures 6.2.1 and 6.2.2)
- Sinus pause
- Sinoatrial block
- Sinus arrest

Causes include increased vagal tone, which can be a response to spinal or epidural anesthesia, laryngoscopy, or surgical intervention [4]. If the patient has poor perfusion or low cardiac output (hypotension), treatment with atropine (0.5–1 mg IV bolus) or a β-agonist such as epinephrine or norepinephrine is usually required.

Complete heart block can be seen in patients with structural heart disease or in acute myocardial infarction. Temporary (transcutaneous or transvenous) pacing might be required in patients with hemodynamic compromise.

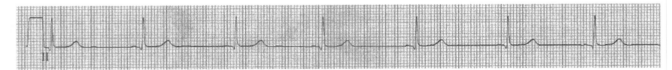

Figure 6.2.1 Sinus bradycardia.

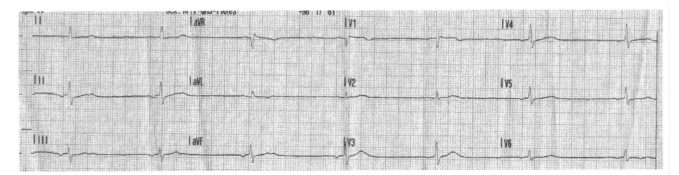

Figure 6.2.2 Sinus bradycardia.

Tachyarrhythmias

The first step in diagnosing a tachyarrhythmia is determining if the rhythm is originating from above the A-V node. Supraventricular arrhythmias (Figures 6.2.3 and 6.2.4) are listed below:

- Sinus tachycardia
- Atrial flutter
- Ectopic atrial tachycardia
- Multifocal atrial tachycardia (MAT)
- Atrial fibrillation
- AV nodal re-entry tachycardias

Ventricular arrhythmias include the following:

- Premature ventricular contractions (PVC)
- VT (Figure 6.2.5)
- Ventricular fibrillation

In general, the ECG should be examined for P waves, rate, morphology, relationship between the P and QRS complexes, and the size of the QRS complex.

Sinus tachycardia (Figure 6.2.6) is a regular rhythm with a P:QRS ratio of 1:1 and a rate greater than 100 beats/min. It is the most common arrhythmia seen in the OR. Common causes of sinus tachycardia are pain, inadequate sedation, hypovolemia, fever, sepsis, and drug side effects. The treatment of sinus tachycardia is aimed at the underlying cause and is generally well tolerated in the short term.

Atrial tachycardia (Figure 6.2.7) is the result of an automatic focus or reentrant pathway originating in the atria. Its P-wave morphology is different from the typical sinus P-wave morphology. This rhythm is commonly the result of atrial irritation or digitalis toxicity. Treatment consists of rate control with a beta blocker or calcium channel blocker.

MAT is a rhythm most often seen in elderly people with significant pulmonary disease. This irregularly irregular rhythm has three or more P-wave morphologies (in a single lead). The causes of MAT are thought to be hypercarbia, hypoxia, ischemia, and electrolyte disturbances. The mainstay of treatment is addressing the underlying cause (pulmonary disease), but beta blockers, calcium channel blockers, and magnesium sulfate have also been used with some success.

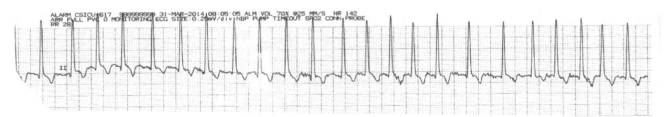

Figure 6.2.3 Supraventricular tachycardia.

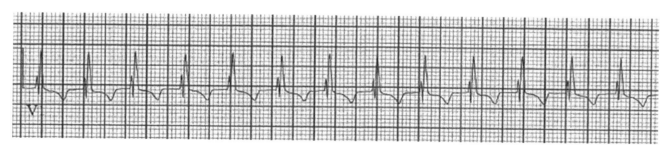

Figure 6.2.4 Supraventricular tachycardia.

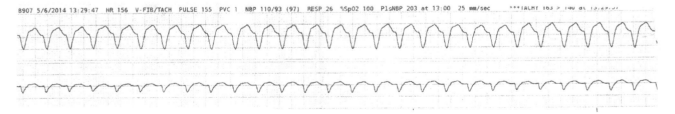

Figure 6.2.5 Ventricular tachycardia.

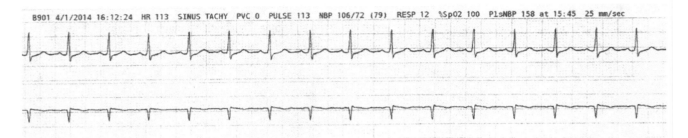

B901 4/1/2014 16:12:24 HR 113 SINUS TACHY PVC 0 PULSE 113 NBP 106/72 (79) RESP 12 %SpO2 100 PlsNBP 158 at 15:45 25 mm/sec

Figure 6.2.6   Sinus tachycardia.

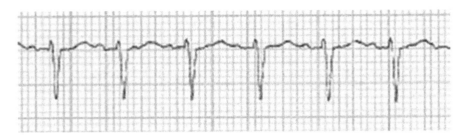

Figure 6.2.7   Atrial tachycardia with inverted P waves as seen in I and aVL.

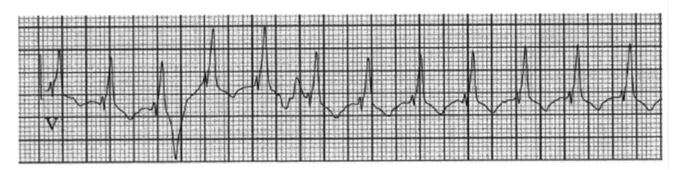

Figure 6.2.8   AV nodal re-entry tachycardia.

Atrioventricular nodal reentry (AVNRT) (Figure 6.2.8) is the result of dual AV nodal pathways with different conduction velocities and refractory periods. Often the P waves are hidden in the QRS complex or they can appear immediately before or after it. Treatment of AVRNT should start with vagal maneuvers or adenosine but might require the cautious use of beta blockers or calcium channel blockers. Unstable patients can be electrically cardioverted.

Atrioventricular reentry tachycardia (AVRT) is similar to AVNRT except that a separate bypass tract is present. The P waves usually follow the QRS complex. Treatment is similar to that for AVNRT: start with vagal maneuvers or adenosine; if they are ineffective, amiodarone, or a beta blocker can be administered. Unstable patients should undergo synchronized cardioversion.

Paroxysmal supraventricular tachycardia (PSVT) (Figure 6.2.9) is a rapid regular rhythm that can occur in an orthodromic or antidromic manner. Orthodromic PSVT is the result of retrograde conduction along a bypass tract and antegrade conduction down the AV node, whereas antidromic PSVT is caused by antegrade accessory pathway conduction with normal retrograde conduction. Antidromic PSVT has a narrow QRS complex unless aberrant conduction is being caused by another block (e.g. right or left bundle branch blocks). Patients with PSVT typically have a heart rate of 140–280 beats/min with a 1:1 P:QRS ratio; it might be difficult to see the P waves because they can be hidden. Common causes of PSVT include hemodynamic changes, medication, and increased autonomic reflexes. Treatment options for orthodromic PSVT include vagal maneuvers, adenosine, amiodarone, overdrive pacing, and cardioversion if the patient is hemodynamically unstable. Treatment for antidromic PSVT consists of procainamide or amiodarone in stable patients, and cardioversion for hemodynamically unstable patients.

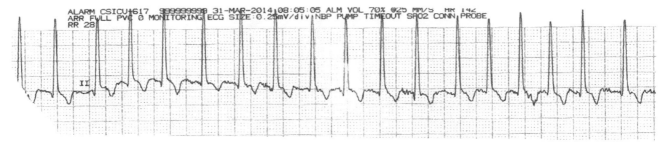

Figure 6.2.9 Paroxysmal supra-ventricular tachycardia.

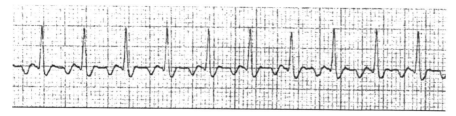

Figure 6.2.10 Atrial flutter with 2:1 block.

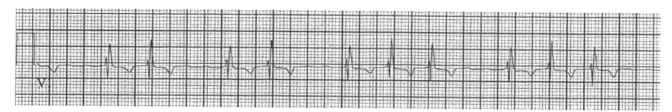

Figure 6.2.11 Atrial flutter with variable block.

Atrial flutter (Figures 6.2.10 and 6.2.11) is one of the most common arrhythmias after cardiac surgery, particularly coronary artery bypass graft or valve replacement surgery. Atrial flutter is a characterized by a regular sawtooth pattern on the ECG with an atrial rate of 250–350 bpm. This is a re-entrant arrhythmia that originates in the right atrium. Although the atria are beating at 300 bpm, a 2:1 block that is typically at the AV node results in a ventricular rate of about 150 bpm. Since the impulses are transmitted through the AV node, the QRS complexes are normal.

Risk factors for atrial flutter include cardiac surgery, advanced age, electrolyte disturbances, congestive heart failure, and chronic obstructive pulmonary disease [5]. Treatment is similar to that for atrial fibrillation, with cardioversion as needed in patients who recently experienced acute atrial flutter (<48 hours). The rate can be controlled with beta blockers, calcium channel blockers, or amiodarone. Patients who are unstable from rapid atrial flutter, as evidenced by shortness of breath, chest pain, hypotension, or dizziness, should be cardioverted immediately.

Atrial fibrillation (Figures 6.2.12–6.2.14) is an irregularly irregular rhythm caused by rapid and irregular atrial activation. This rhythm is characterized by its lack of P waves, a variable heart rate, and narrow QRS complexes. Atrial fibrillation is seen after up to 8% of all noncardiac surgeries and 16–46% of cardiac surgeries [6]. The postoperative causes of atrial fibrillation include atrial distension, inflammation, and volume shifts that affect atrial repolarization. Common risk factors for atrial fibrillation are a history of cardiac surgery, advanced age, electrolyte imbalances, a history of preoperative atrial fibrillation, congestive heart failure, and chronic obstructive pulmonary disease.

Atrial fibrillation can impair cardiac output, lead to demand ischemia of the heart, and result in atrial thrombus formation, which increases the patient's risk of stroke. Current recommendations for treatment are centered on getting the ventricular rate under control. For hemodynamically unstable patients, this can be achieved by synchronized electrical cardioversion. Patients who have been in atrial fibrillation less than 48 hours can undergo elective electrical or chemical cardioversion. If it is unclear how long a patient has been in atrial fibrillation or if it has been more than 48 hours since its onset, the risk of thromboembolism is heightened, so cardioversion should be used after

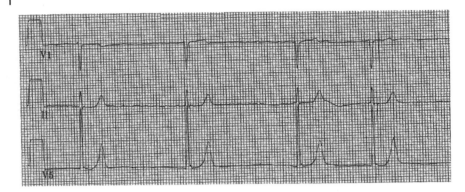

Figure 6.2.12 Atrial fibrillation. This rhythm has a slow response due to excessive beta blockade in a patient with baseline atrial fibrillation.

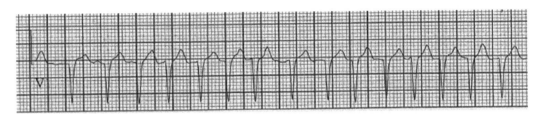

Figure 6.2.13 Atrial fibrillation. The irregular rhythm is caused by rapid and irregular atrial activation, shown here with a rapid ventricular response.

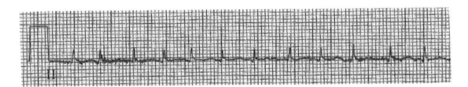

Figure 6.2.14 Atrial fibrillation with a rapid ventricular response.

a period of anticoagulation or after a transesophageal echocardiogram has excluded the presence of an atrial thrombus. Preoperative treatment with amiodarone or a beta blockers can be considered for patients at high risk for atrial fibrillation.

Atrial premature beats or *premature atrial complex (PAC)* originates from parts of the atria other than the sinus node. The PR interval is variable, yielding an irregular rhythm. The P:QRS ratio remains 1:1; however, the P-wave morphology will change depending on the location of the atrial impulse. This is generally a benign rhythm that does not require any treatment.

PVCs are abnormal beats that result in wide (>0.12 s) QRS complexes. Since these are ectopic beats that originate below the AV junction, there are no P waves. PVCs often occur randomly, but if they occur every other beat or every third beat,

they are called bigeminy or trigeminy, respectfully. PVCs are generally benign and do not require treatment.

Nonsustained ventricular tachycardia (NSVT) (Figure 6.2.15) is characterized by three or more *PVCs*. The ventricular rate is greater than 100 beats/min, and episodes typically last less than 30 seconds. The ventricular contractions can be monomorphic or polymorphic. Since the event is not sustained, patients rarely experience hemodynamic compromise and thus do not usually require treatment other than a search for the cause.

Sustained VT (Figures 6.2.16 and 6.2.17) is a re-entrant rhythm that can be monomorphic or polymorphic and result in a rapid (>100 beats/min) heart rate with wide QRS complexes. Common risk factors for VT are existing structural heart disease, coronary artery disease, a history of myocardial infarction, cardiomyopathy, and a history of cardiac surgery.

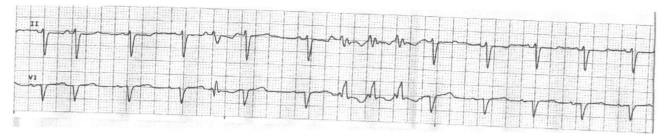

Figure 6.2.15 Nonsustained ventricular tachycardia (NSVT). Three beats of NSVT are seen in this rhythm strip.

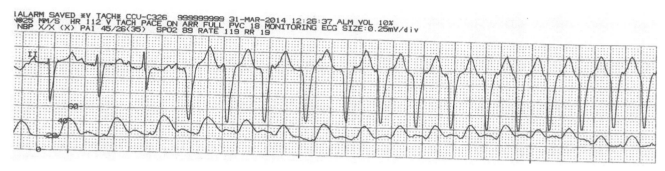

Figure 6.2.16 Ventricular tachycardia as seen in lead II. The bottom waveform is an arterial line waveform.

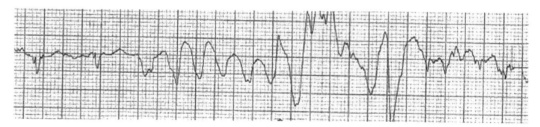

Figure 6.2.17 Ventricular tachycardia develops while obtaining the ECG in the later part of the image.

Sustained and unstable VT should be treated with electrical cardioversion; hemodynamically stable VT can be treated with amiodarone, lidocaine, or procainamide.

Torsades de pointes is a polymorphic VT. Individuals are at greatest risk for it if they have a prolonged QT interval, which can be acquired by the use of certain medications (e.g. anti-arrhythmic agents, azole antifungal drugs, tricyclic antidepressants, and methadone). Other risk factors include hypomagnesemia and hypokalemia.

Ventricular fibrillation is an irregular rhythm that originates from ventricular foci and results in ventricular fasciculations that are variable. No P waves or QRS complexes are associated with this rhythm. In the absence of organized cardiac activity, patients are pulseless.

Common causes of ventricular fibrillation are shock, myocardial ischemia, severe electrolyte imbalances, and

hypothermia. Treatment consists of the initiation of cardiopulmonary resuscitation (CPR) with external asynchronous defibrillation. Current Basic Life Support (BLS) or Advanced Cardiac Life Support (ACLS) protocols from the American Heart Association should be followed. The two interventions that improve outcomes are good quality CPR and early defibrillation with a manual defibrillator or automatic external defibrillator (AED).

Specific Clinical Conditions

Myocardial Ischemia

In patients with minimal risk factors for ischemia, it is common to see postoperative ST-segment changes, which can be caused by electrolyte disturbances, hyperventilation, or anxiety. It is important for the clinician to keep a low level of suspicion for myocardial ischemia. Older patients, those with a history of myocardial infarction, and those with specific risk factors (e.g. hypertension, hyperlipidemia, family history, smoking history, or obesity) should be monitored with postoperative telemetry so that myocardial ischemia can be detected. Myocardial ischemia in the PACU does not manifest as the chest pain that is otherwise typical of this cardiac emergency.

Drug Withdrawal

It is important to obtain a preoperative assessment of the patient's social history. The patient or the clinician might have underestimated the extent of alcohol abuse. Alcohol withdrawal can ensue, sometimes undetected, in the PACU. It presents as sinus tachycardia with accompanying clinical symptoms: shivering, delirium, hallucinations, autonomic instability, seizures, and agitation. Opiate withdrawal should also be considered in patients with cardiac abnormalities that emerge in the postoperative period. A patient might have been on chronic opiate therapy as an outpatient.

Other Causes of Bradydysrhythmias

Anticholinesterase reversal of neuromuscular blockade can cause postanesthetic bradycardia that is usually transient and rarely requires treatment. Bradycardia can also be caused by procedures that cause bowel distension, increased intracranial pressure, or spinal anesthesia (specifically, spinal blocks from T1–T4) [2]. Large doses of anesthetics such as lidocaine or bupivacaine that are inadvertently given for spinal anesthesia can cause profound bradycardia. These cases can be treated with intralipid infusion.

Postoperative Shivering

Shivering is usually caused by hypothermia but can also be seen in patients recovering from general anesthesia. It can lead to sinus tachycardia. Certain induction agents (e.g. propofol) are associated with an increased incidence of shivering [6]. Shivering patients can be treated with external rewarming and meperidine [7].

Electrolyte Disturbances

Hypocalcemia can prolong the QT interval. Hypercalcemia can shorten the QT interval and induce ST-segment changes. Hyperkalemia can lead to progressive changes in the ECG, starting with diffuse peaked T waves and shortening of the QT interval. Further elevations in potassium can lead to widening of the QRS complex and prolongation of the PR interval. The last change to be seen before asystole is a sine wave pattern. Hypokalemia can cause prolongation of the QT interval as well as a characteristic "U" wave after the T wave.

General Anesthetics

An inhaled anesthetic such as halothane or enflurane can produce re-entrant dysrhythmias [2]. In addition, sevoflurane has been found to cause severe bradycardia in infants [8]. The drugs commonly used in anesthesia and their effects on heart rate are listed in Table 6.2.3.

Conclusion

The perioperative setting is a time where the ECG can be very helpful in certain clinical situations. In patients who have dysrhythmias, quickly diagnosing the cause will help the clinician decide on the appropriate treatment. In general, the same dysrhythmias seen in any other acute care clinical setting will be seen in the OR. For the most part, the treatments are the same. The one difference is that most dysrhythmias in the perioperative setting are benign and require minimal treatment. In addition, once the inciting cause has been fixed, most patients return to their inherent cardiac rhythm without long-term consequences.

Table 6.2.3 The effects of common drugs on cardiac conduction.

Drug	Effect
Isoflurane	Ventricular dysrhythmia
Desflurane	Sinus tachycardia
Sevoflurane, halothane, isoflurane	Prolonged QT interval
Ketamine	Sinus tachycardia
Opioids	Sinus bradycardia
Bronchodilators	Sinus tachycardia
Dexmedetomidine	Sinus bradycardia
Propofol	Sinus bradycardia
Succinylcholine	Tachycardia or bradycardia

References

1 Forrest, J., Cahalan, M., Rehder, K. et al. (1990). Multicenter study of general anesthesia. II. Results. *Anesthesiology* 72: 262–268.

2 Miller, R., Eriksson, I.L., and Flesisher, L.A. (2010). *Miller's Anesthesia*, 7e. Elsevier.

3 Hollenberg, S.M. and Dellinger, R.P. (2000). Noncardiac surgery: postoperative arrhythmias. *Crit. Care Med.* 28 (10 suppl): N145–N150.

4 Atlee, J.L. (1997). Perioperative cardiac dysrhythmias: diagnosis and management. *Anesthesiology* 86: 1397–1424.

5 Ellenbogen, K.A., Chung, M.K., Asher, C.R. et al. (1997). Postoperative atrial fibrillation. *Adv. Card. Surg.* 9: 109–130.

6 Buggy, D.J. and Crossley, A.W. (2000). Thermoregulation, mild perioperative hypothermia and post anesthetic shivering. *Br. J. Anaesth.* 84: 615–628.

7 Kurz, A., Ikeda, T., Sessler, D.I. et al. (1997). Meperidine decreases the shivering threshold twice as much as the vasoconstriction threshold. *Anesthesiology* 86: 1046–1054.

8 Green, D.H., Townsend, P., Bagshaw, O. et al. (2000). Nodal rhythm and bradycardia during inhalation induction with sevoflurane in infants: a comparison of incremental and high-concentration techniques. *Br. J. Anaesth.* 85: 368–370.

3

ECG in the ICU Patient

Identification and Treatment of Arrhythmias in the Intensive Care Unit

Feras Khan

Department of Emergency Medicine, University of Maryland School of Medicine, Baltimore, MD, USA

Introduction

The intensive care unit (ICU) is designed to meet the needs of critically ill patients requiring aggressive clinical care and continuous monitoring. Telemetry monitoring is the standard of care for all patients admitted to an ICU. Changes in telemetry readings and heart rate can be the first signs that a patient's clinical status is deteriorating. Occasionally, patients are admitted to the ICU specifically to manage a malignant arrhythmia. In addition, medications given in the ICU can cause a variety of arrhythmias. This chapter describes the most common arrhythmias seen in the ICU and presents strategies for their basic treatment.

Common Dysrhythmias in the ICU

Bradydysrhythmias

Severe bradycardias that require emergent treatment are rare in the ICU. The more common dysrhythmias that warrant clinical intervention are discussed in this section.

Sinus bradycardia (Figures 6.3.1 and 6.3.2) is a regular rhythm with a ventricular rate less than 60 beats per minute (bpm). The heart rate is set by the sinus node and transmitted through the AV node, so the P:QRS ratio is 1:1 and the QRS complex is narrow. Sinus bradycardia is typically a benign rhythm in a hemodynamically stable patient. Treatment is based on the underlying cause (Table 6.3.1). If the patient becomes hemodynamically unstable, atropine should be administered and transcutaneous or transvenous pacing should be attempted.

Junctional rhythm (Figures 6.3.3 and 6.3.4) is an escape rhythm that typically starts at the AV node (the junction). It produces a regular, narrow complex ventricular rate of 45–60 bpm. If the patient is hemodynamically stable, then no treatment is necessary. Otherwise, transcutaneous, or transvenous pacing may be required.

Third-degree AV block (Figure 6.3.5) occurs when there is no relationship between the atrial contractions (P waves) and ventricular contractions (QRS complex), typically because of an electrical block below the AV node. Causes of third-degree heart block are presented in Table 6.3.2. Most patients with this arrhythmia require treatment with transcutaneous or transvenous pacing until a permanent pacemaker can be placed.

Sinoventricular rhythm can be seen in patients with severe hyperkalemia and is indicated by delayed conduction between the atria and the ventricles. Typically, P waves are absent and the QRS complexes are wide, with a rate less than 60 bpm. The more bizarre the appearance of the complex appearance, the more hyperkalemia should be suspected. Treatment consists of correcting the hyperkalemia with intravenous administration of calcium, insulin, and dextrose. Albuterol nebulizers can also help shift potassium out of the extracellular space. Ultimately, potassium removal can be aided with loop diuretics, sodium polystyrene, and dialysis.

Tachydysrhythmias

Tachycardia (heart rate >100 bpm) is the most common arrhythmia seen in the ICU. These accelerated rhythms can cause hemodynamic instability, so the clinician must be adept at recognizing and treating them.

Electrocardiogram in Clinical Medicine, First Edition. Edited by William J. Brady, Michael J. Lipinski, Andrew E. Darby, Michael C. Bond, Nathan P. Charlton, Korin Hudson, and Kelly Williamson.

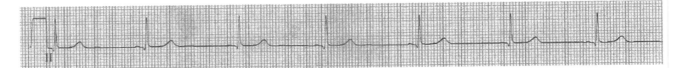

Figure 6.3.1 Sinus bradycardia.

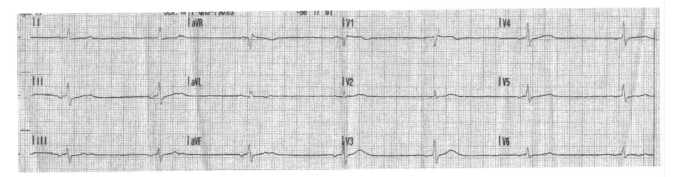

Figure 6.3.2 Sinus bradycardia.

Table 6.3.1 Causes of sinus bradycardia in ICU patients.

- Physiologic
- Beta blockers
- Calcium-channel blockers
- Sleep apnea
- Elevated intracranial pressure
- Increased vagal tone (endotracheal suctioning)
- Sedatives (opioids, dexmedetomidine)
- Hypothermia
- Hypothyroidism
- Digoxin

Tachycardia has three causes:

- Increased automaticity – faster depolarization of cardiac cells from one of the main conduction sites
- Reentry – two distinct pathways allow conduction
- Triggered activity – an ectopic source of conduction

Supraventricular tachycardias (SVTs) originate above the AV node and have a narrow QRS complex. Ventricular tachycardias (VTs), originating below the AV node, have a wider QRS complex.

The narrow complex tachycardias are sinus tachycardia, atrial tachycardia, AV nodal reentry tachycardia, atrial flutter, and atrial fibrillation. The wide complex tachycardias are VT and SVT with aberrancy.

SVTs originate above the AV node and have a narrow QRS complex. The narrow complex tachycardias are sinus tachycardia, atrial tachycardia, AV nodal reentry tachycardia, atrial flutter, and atrial fibrillation. Wide complex tachycardias consist of VT and SVT with aberrancy. These rhythms do not use the normal conduction pathways so have a wider QRS complex.

Sinus tachycardia (Figure 6.3.6) is a regular rhythm with a P:QRS ratio of 1:1. It is the most common arrhythmia seen in the ICU setting. Common causes of sinus tachycardia include pain, inadequate sedation, hypovolemia, fever, sepsis, and drug side effects. Treatment is aimed at the underlying cause, and sinus tachycardia is generally well tolerated in the short term.

Atrial fibrillation (Figures 6.3.7–6.3.9) is an irregularly irregular rhythm caused by rapid and irregular atrial activations. This rhythm is characterized by its lack of P waves, a variable heart rate, and narrow QRS complexes. Atrial fibrillation is seen after up to 8% of noncardiac surgeries and after 16–46% of cardiac surgeries [1]. Postoperative atrial fibrillation can be caused by atrial distension, inflammation, and volume shifts that affect atrial repolarization [2]. Risk factors are a history of cardiac surgery, advanced age, electrolyte imbalances, preoperative atrial fibrillation, congestive heart failure, and chronic obstructive pulmonary disease.

Atrial fibrillation can impair cardiac output, lead to demand ischemia of the heart, and result in atrial thrombus formation, increasing the patient's risk of stroke. Treatment recommendations center on getting the ventricular rate under control. For hemodynamically unstable patients, rate control can be attempted with synchronized electrical cardioversion. Patients who have been in atrial fibrillation less than 48 hours can undergo elective electrical or chemical cardioversion. If it is unclear how long the patient has been in atrial fibrillation or if it has been more than 48 hours since its onset, the patient is at higher risk for

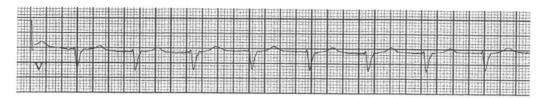

Figure 6.3.3 Accelerated junctional rhythm. This ECG has a higher rate than a traditional junctional rhythm.

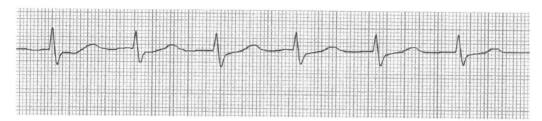

Figure 6.3.4 Junctional bradycardia in V4 rhythm strip.

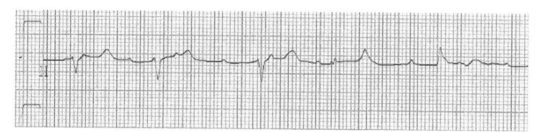

Figure 6.3.5 Third-degree AV block.

Table 6.3.2 Causes of third-degree heart block.

- Medications (beta blockers, calcium-channel blockers)
- Myocardial infarction
- Anti-arrhythmics
- Myocarditis
- Lyme disease
- Amyloidosis
- Sarcoidosis
- Rheumatic fever
- Aortic valve surgery

thromboembolism and should be cardioverted after a period of anticoagulation or after a transesophageal echocardiogram has excluded the presence of an atrial thrombus. Ventricular rate control is often obtained by blocking the AV node with β-blockers, calcium-channel blockers, amiodarone, procainamide, or digoxin.

Atrial tachycardia (Figures 6.3.10 and 6.3.11) is the result of an automatic focus or re-entrant pathway originating in the atria. The associated P-wave morphology will be different from the typical sinus P-wave morphology, usually a result of atrial irritation or digitalis toxicity. Treatment

for this rhythm consists of rate control with beta blockers or calcium-channel blockers.

Multi-focal atrial tachycardia (MAT) is most often seen in elderly people with significant pulmonary disease. This irregularly irregular rhythm has three or more P-wave morphologies (in a single lead). The causes of MAT are thought to be hypercarbia, hypoxia, ischemia, and electrolyte disturbances. The mainstay of treatment is to address the underlying cause (pulmonary disease). Beta blockers, calcium-channel blockers, and magnesium sulfate have been used with some success.

Atrioventricular nodal reentry (AVNRT) (Figure 6.3.12) is the result of dual AV nodal pathways with different conduction velocities and refractory periods. The P waves are often hidden in the QRS complex, or they can appear immediately before or after it. Treatment of AVRNT should start with vagal maneuvers or adenosine but might require the cautious use of beta blockers or calcium-channel blockers. Unstable patients can be electrically cardioverted.

Atrioventricular reentry tachycardia (AVRT) is similar to AVNRT, except that a separate bypass tract is present. The P waves usually follow the QRS complex. Treatment is similar to that for AVNRT, i.e. starting with vagal

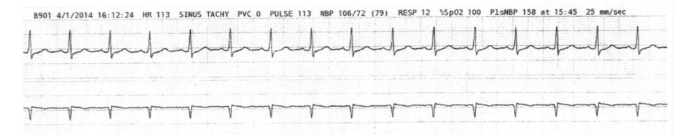

B901 4/1/2014 16:12:24 HR 113 SINUS TACHY PVC 0 PULSE 113 NBP 106/72 (79) RESP 12 %SpO2 100 PlsNBP 158 at 15:45 25 mm/sec

Figure 6.3.6 Sinus tachycardia.

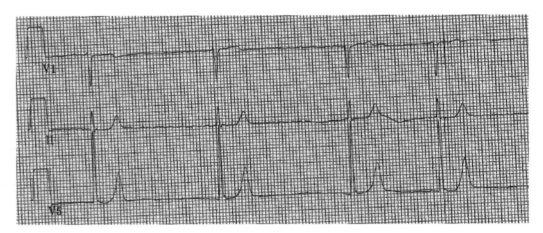

Figure 6.3.7 Atrial fibrillation. This rhythm has a slow response due to excessive beta blockade in a patient with baseline atrial fibrillation.

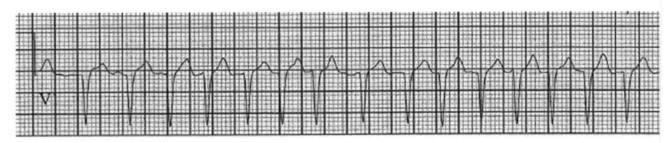

Figure 6.3.8 Atrial fibrillation with a rapid ventricular response.

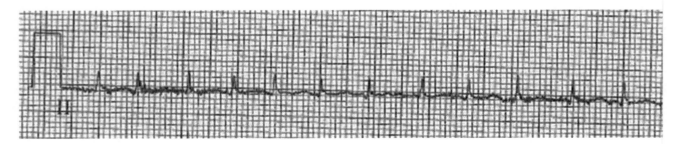

Figure 6.3.9 Atrial fibrillation with a rapid ventricular response.

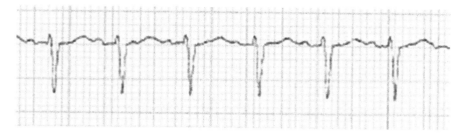

Figure 6.3.10 Atrial tachycardia with inverted P waves as seen in I and aVL.

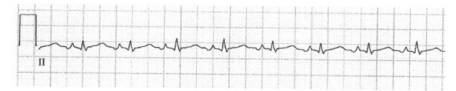

Figure 6.3.11 Atrial tachycardia.

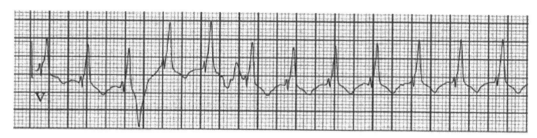

Figure 6.3.12 AV nodal reentry tachycardia.

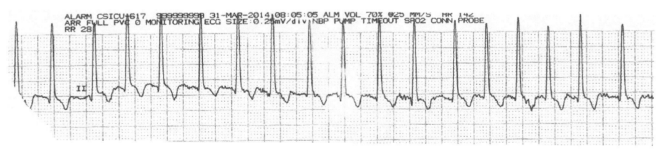

Figure 6.3.13 Paroxysmal supraventricular tachycardia.

maneuvers or adenosine; if those are ineffective, amiodarone, or beta blockers can be used. In the unstable patient, synchronized cardioversion should be performed.

Paroxysmal supraventricular tachycardia (PSVT) (Figure 6.3.13) is a rapid regular rhythm that can occur in an orthodromic or antidromic manner. Orthodromic PSVT is the result of a retrograde conduction along a bypass tract and antegrade conduction down the AV node, whereas antidromic PSVT is caused by an antegrade accessory pathway conduction with normal retrograde conduction. Antidromic PSVT has a narrow QRS complex unless another block (e.g. a right or left bundle branch block) is

causing aberrant conduction. Patients with PSVT typically have a heart rate of 140–280 bpm with a P:QRS ratio of 1:1, though it might be difficult to see the P waves because they can be hidden. Common causes of PSVT include hemodynamic changes, medication, and increased autonomic reflexes.

It's not clear which treatment applies to hemodynamically unstable patients. I'll insert a possible revision following the sentence. Treatment for orthodromic PSVT includes vagal maneuvers, adenosine, amiodarone, and overdrive pacing for stable patients and cardioversion if the patient is hemodynamically unstable. Treatment for antidromic PSVT consists of procainamide or amiodarone in stable patients and cardioversion for hemodynamically unstable patients.

Atrial flutter (Figures 6.3.14 and 6.3.15) is one of the most common arrhythmias after cardiac surgery, particularly after coronary artery bypass graft or valve replacement surgery. Atrial flutter is a characterized by a regular sawtooth pattern on the ECG, with an atrial rate of 250–350 bpm. This is a re-entrant arrhythmia that originates in the right atrium. Though the atria are beating at 300 bpm, a typical 2:1 block at the AV node results in a ventricular rate around 150 bpm. Since the impulses are transmitted through the AV node, the QRS complexes are normal.

Risk factors for atrial flutter include cardiac surgery, advanced age, electrolyte disturbances, congestive heart failure, and chronic obstructive pulmonary disease [3]. Treatment is similar to that for atrial fibrillation, with cardioversion as needed in patients with recent acute atrial flutter (lasting <48 hours). The rate can be controlled with beta blockers, calcium-channel blockers, or amiodarone. Patients who are unstable from rapid atrial flutter, as evidenced by shortness of breath, chest pain, hypotension, or dizziness, should undergo cardioversion immediately.

Nonsustained ventricular tachycardia (NSVT) (Figures 6.3.16 and 6.3.17) is characterized by three or more premature

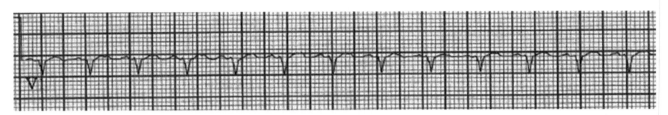

Figure 6.3.14   Atrial flutter with 2:1 block.

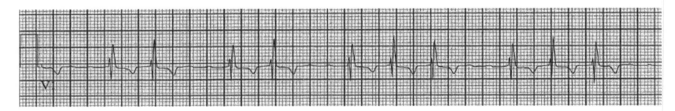

Figure 6.3.15   Atrial flutter with variable block.

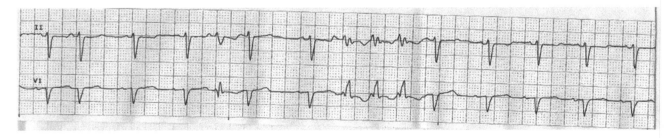

Figure 6.3.16   Non-sustained ventricular tachycardia (NSVT). Three beats of NSVT are seen in this rhythm strip.

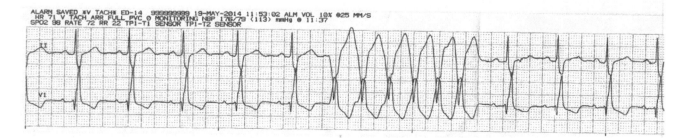

Figure 6.3.17   NSVT. Six beats of NSVT are seen in this rhythm strip.

ventricular contractions (PVCs). The ventricular rate is greater than 100 bpm and typically lasts less than 30 seconds. The ventricular contractions can be monomorphic or polymorphic. Since the event is not sustained, patients rarely experience any hemodynamic compromise. Common causes of NSVT are presented in Table 6.3.3. Most patients with this

Table 6.3.3 Causes of NSVT/SVT in ICU patients.

- Hypoxemia
- Hypercarbia
- Acidosis
- Hypotension
- Electrolyte imbalances
- Mechanical irritation
- Pulmonary artery catheter/central line
- Chest tube
- Hypothermia
- Myocardial ischemia

rhythm do not require treatment, but its cause should be sought and addressed.

Sustained *VT* (Figures 6.3.18–6.3.20), a re-entrant rhythm that can be monomorphic or polymorphic, produces a rapid (>100 bpm) heart rate with wide QRS complexes. Common risk factors for VT are structural heart disease, coronary artery disease, a history of myocardial infarction, cardiomyopathy, and a history of cardiac surgery. Sustained and unstable VT should be treated with electrical cardioversion, while hemodynamically stable VT can be treated with amiodarone, lidocaine, or procainamide.

Torsades de pointes is a polymorphic VT. Individuals are at greatest risk if they have a prolonged QT interval, which can be acquired by the use of certain medications (e.g. antiarrhythmic agents, azole antifungal drugs, tricyclic antidepressants, and methadone). Other risk factors include hypomagnesemia and hypokalemia. Torsades de pointes can be difficult to treat. All patients with this rhythm

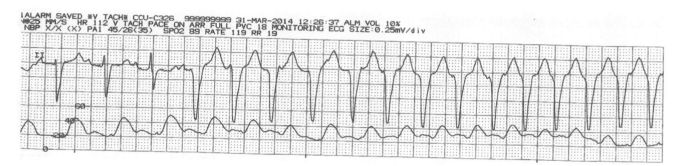

Figure 6.3.18 Ventricular tachycardia as seen in Lead II. The bottom waveform is an arterial line waveform.

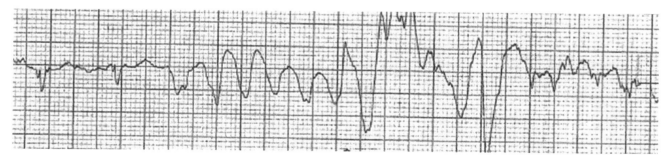

Figure 6.3.19 Ventricular tachycardia develops while obtaining the ECG in the later part of the image.

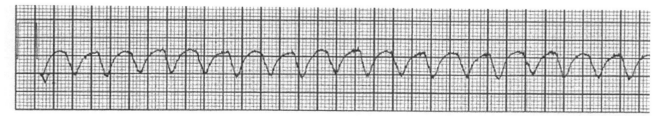

Figure 6.3.20 Ventricular tachycardia.

should be given magnesium sulfate. Temporary overdrive pacing via transcutaneous or transvenous pacemakers has been successful in terminating this rhythm and therefore should be attempted.

Ventricular fibrillation is an irregular rhythm that originates from ventricular foci and results in ventricular fasciculations that vary. P waves and QRS complexes are absent. Since there is no organized cardiac activity, patients are pulseless. Common causes of ventricular fibrillation are shock, myocardial ischemia, severe electrolyte imbalances, and hypothermia. Treatment consists of the initiation of cardiopulmonary resuscitation (CPR) with external asynchronous defibrillation. Current basic life support (BLS) and advanced cardiac life support (ACLS) protocols from the American Heart Association should be followed. The two interventions that have been proven to improve outcomes are good-quality CPR and early defibrillation with a manual defibrillator or automatic external defibrillator (AED).

Other Common Electrocardiographic Findings

Atrial premature beats (also called *premature atrial complex [PAC]*) (Figure 6.3.21) originate from parts of the atria other than the sinus node. The PR interval is variable, yielding an irregular rhythm. The P:QRS ratio remains 1:1; however, the P-wave morphology changes depending on the location of the atrial impulse. This is generally a benign rhythm that does not require treatment.

PVCs (Figure 6.3.22) are abnormal beats that result in wide (>0.12 second) QRS complexes. Since these are ectopic beats that originate from below the AV junction, P waves are absent. PVCs often occur randomly. If they occur every other beat or every third beat, they are called bigeminy or trigeminy, respectfully. PVCs are generally benign and do not require treatment.

The Effect of Vasopressors on Cardiac Conduction

A variety of vasopressors can be administered to ICU patients in shock. The next few sections review the most commonly used vasopressors and their potential adverse effects on cardiac conduction.

Epinephrine, Norepinephrine, and Dopamine

Epinephrine is a mixed α- and β-agonist that increases blood pressure by vasoconstriction and increased cardiac output. It is used commonly in patients with cardiogenic, septic, or anaphylactic shock. Norepinephrine is an α_1- and β_1-agonist that also increases blood pressure using vasoconstriction. It has inotropic effects as well, but to a lesser degree than epinephrine. It is most often used in patients with distributive forms of shock. Dopamine is an α- and β-adrenergic agonist

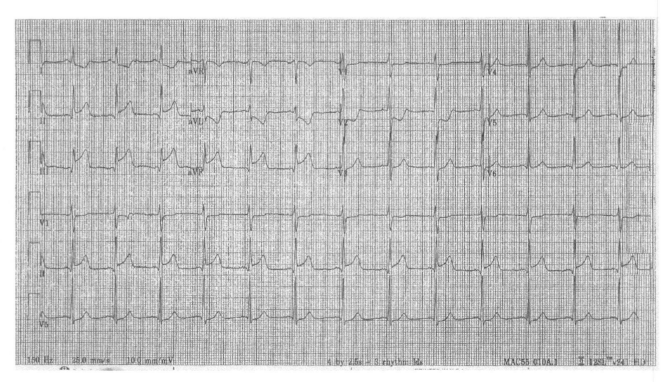

Figure 6.3.21 ST-elevation myocardial infarction in leads II, III, and aVF.

in addition to a stimulant of dopaminergic receptors, DA_1, and DA_2. The β effects are seen in the 3–10 µg/kg/min range of dosage. It is also a vasoconstrictor at higher doses, with more of an α agonist effect. Patients' responses vary to different doses of dopamine, which limits the drug's use.

Each of these agents can cause tachyarrhythmias, including sinus tachycardia, atrial fibrillation, and SVT. These arrhythmias are usually preceded by an increasing amount of PVCs or premature atrial contractions (PACs). Increasing doses of these medications can increase the frequency of these events. In general, these agents are relatively safe but should be reserved for situations of shock in which increasing perfusion is more important than the chance of arrhythmia [4]. Dopamine, in particular, has been found to cause relatively more arrhythmias, which limits its use; it is being used less frequently, specifically for septic shock [5].

Dobutamine

Dobutamine has mainly β-agonist effects. It has $β_1$-agonism that causes positive inotropic effects and $β_2$-effects that cause a vasodilatory action. This leads to increased cardiac output and decreased systemic vascular resistance. It has been found to cause both VTs and ventricular fibrillation, though rarely [6]. It should not be given to patients with a history of ventricular tachyarrhythmias.

Phenylephrine

Phenylephrine is an $α_1$-adrenergic agonist that is used in patients with vasodilatory shock. It increases blood pressure through its effect on systemic vascular resistance. In relation to other vasoactive medications, phenylephrine can decrease heart rate, but it usually does not lead to profound bradycardia [7].

Milrinone

Milrinone is a phosphodiesterase III inhibiter that increases intracellular calcium stores, inducing an inotropic effect that improves cardiac output. However, it can lead to an overload of intracellular calcium, which can cause ventricular tachyarryhthmias secondary to an increase in myocardial oxygen demand [3].

Consequences of Anti-Arrhythmic Medications

Table 6.3.4 lists the anti-arrhythmic drugs most often used in the ICU and the arrhythmias that each agent can cause.

Table 6.3.4 Anti-arrhythmic drugs and their potential cardiac effects.

Drug	Effect
Sotalol	Bradycardia
Procainamide	QT prolongation
Propafenone	Bradycardia
Flecainide	Bradycardia

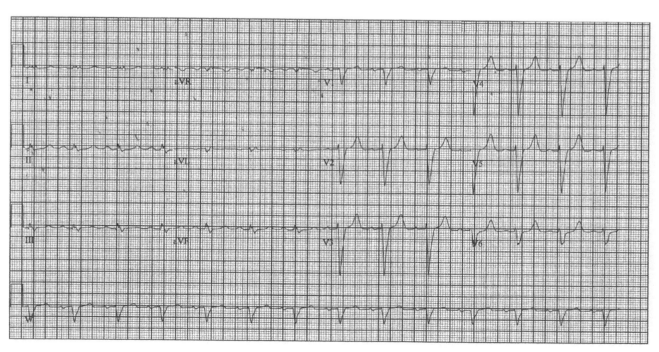

Figure 6.3.22 Left bundle branch block.

Arrhythmias Induced by Central Line Placement

The placement of a central line can cause atrial arrhythmias such as SVT and PACs. Ventricular ectopy might also be seen, usually in response to overinsertion of the guidewire [8]. These rhythms tend to be self-limited and resolve when the guidewire is pulled back or removed. Swan-Ganz catheters can also cause arrhythmias, e.g. VT or SVT. PVCs are the most commonly seen arrhythmia. NSVT can be seen when the catheter is located in the right ventricle and resolves when it is pulled back or advanced into the pulmonary artery [9]. The ECG might show transient right bundle branch block (RBBB) when the catheter is in the pulmonary artery [9].

Specific Clinical Conditions

Cardiac Arrest

Patients who have return of spontaneous circulation after cardiac arrest are at increased risk for arrhythmias and need continuous ECG/telemetry monitoring in the ICU. During this period, the cause of the arrest (e.g. VT, hyperkalemia, QT prolongation, or ST-elevation myocardial infarction) might be revealed (Figure 6.3.21). These patients are usually being managed according to hypothermia protocols, which can also lead to arrhythmias, including sinus bradycardia.

Myocardial Infarction

Patients who have had pharmacologic or interventional treatment for ST-elevation myocardial infarction are at risk for reperfusion arrhythmias, including accelerated idioventricular rhythm.

Cardiac Surgery

Patients who have had coronary artery bypass grafting or valvular surgery are at risk of developing postoperative atrial fibrillation. Risk factors include advanced age, history of atrial fibrillation, valvular disease, and lack of beta blockers prior to surgery [10].

Myocarditis

In the United States, myocarditis is usually caused by a viral infection, but, worldwide, the most common cause is Chagas disease [11]. Occasionally, this syndrome becomes so severe as to cause acute decompensated heart failure, necessitating ICU admission. Typical electrocardiographic findings include sinus tachycardia, bundle branch blocks (Figures 6.3.22 and 6.3.23), and atrioventricular conduction delays leading to complete heart block [12].

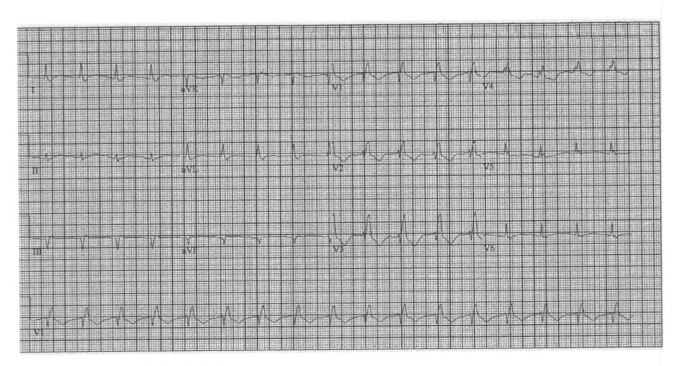

Figure 6.3.23 Right bundle branch block.

Endocarditis

Endocarditis can produce cardiac conduction abnormalities such as AV block and bundle branch blocks. Third-degree block can be seen in patients with paravalvular disease such as abscess formation [13]. These patients might need permanent pacemaker placement.

Left Ventricular Assist Device Arrhythmias

VTs are common in patients with left ventricular assist devices (LVADs) and can be caused by suction events, myocardial fibrosis, or electrical remodeling after implantation [14]. To stabilize the rhythm, the amount of fluid being administered, as well as the settings of the device, can be adjusted. If those modifications are not successful, then the administration of a medication such as amiodarone or a beta blocker should be considered.

Pulmonary Embolism

Patients who have massive or submassive pulmonary embolism are usually admitted to an ICU. The possible electrocardiographic findings in these patients [15], caused by right ventricular strain and dilation [16], are listed below:

- Sinus tachycardia
- Right bundle branch block
- Right axis deviation
- Right ventricular strain pattern with T-wave inversions in V1 through V4 and the inferior leads (II, III, aVF) (Figure 6.3.24)
- $S_IQ_{III}T_{III}$ with an S wave in lead I, a Q wave in lead III, and T-wave inversion in III

Pericardial Effusion

Patients with a large pericardial effusion are admitted to the ICU for management of the hypotension caused by hemodynamic compromise. ECGs from these patients will show low voltage, tachycardia, electrical alternans, and sinus tachycardia (Figure 6.3.25). Electrical alternans shows a variation in the magnitude of the ECG complex.

Hyperthyroidism and Hypothyroidism

Patients with severe hypothyroidism have bradycardia and low voltage [17]. In contrast, tachycardia is usually seen in patients with thyroid storm stemming from high levels of thyroid hormone [18].

Hypothermia

Specific electrocardiographic changes are associated with accidental hypothermia. Ventricular fibrillation, asystole,

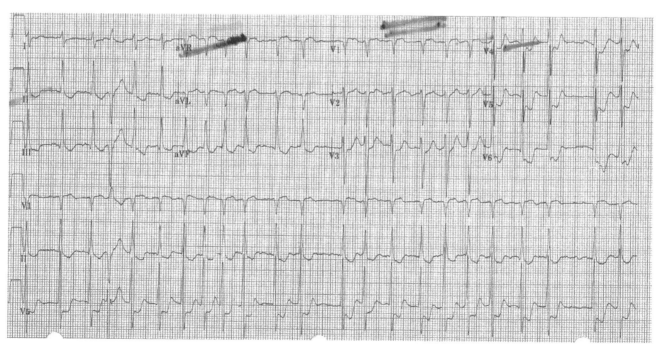

Figure 6.3.24 Atrial fibrillation with a rapid ventricular response with T-wave inversions in II, II, aVF, V4–V6, in a patient with a large pulmonary embolism.

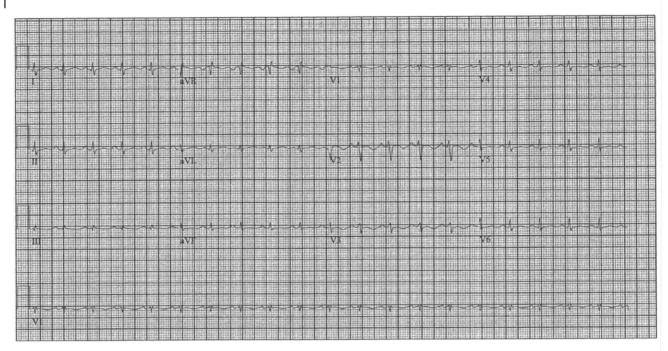

Figure 6.3.25 Low electrical voltage in all leads as seen in a patient with a large pericardial effusion.

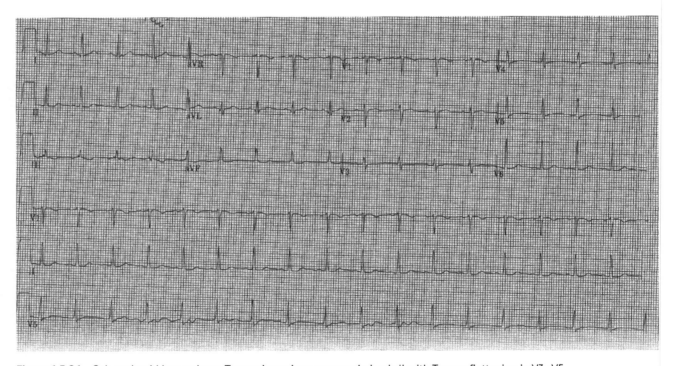

Figure 6.3.26 Subarachnoid hemorrhage. T-wave inversions are seen in leads II with T-wave flattening in V3–V5.

and severe bradycardia are all seen in patients with hypothermia and usually resolve with rewarming measures. When the body temperature falls below 25 °C, Osborn or "J" waves will appear as an extra deflection between the QRS complex and ST segment [19].

Subarachnoid Hemorrhage

Patients with subarachnoid hemorrhage (SAH) can experience atrial fibrillation and atrial flutter [20]. ST-segment changes are routinely seen in patients with SAH (Figure 6.3.26). For the vast majority of patients, these arrhythmias are self-limiting but have been associated with a higher mortality rate [20].

Conclusion

The ECG is an important tool for monitoring critically ill patients with arrhythmias. Those arrhythmias can be primary disorders, or they can arise in response to medical interventions for other conditions. By understanding the information that is captured by ECGs, and combining it with clinical examination findings, the critical care clinician can make informed decisions regarding adjustments in current treatment and subsequent therapeutic goals.

References

1 Miller, R. et al. (2010). *Miller's Anesthesia*, 7e. Elsevier.
2 Ellenbogen, K.A., Chung, M.K., Asher, C.R., and Wood, M.A. (1997). Postoperative atrial fibrillation. *Adv. Card. Surg.* 9: 109–130.
3 Herget-Rosenthal, S., Saner, F., and Chawla, L. (2008). Approach to hemodynamic shock and vasopressors. *Clin. J. Am. Soc. Nephrol.* 3: 546–553.
4 Tisdale, J.E., Patel, R., Webb, C. et al. (1995). Electrophysiologic and proarrhythmic effects of intravenous inotropic agents. *Prog. Cardiovasc. Dis.* 38: 167–180.
5 De Backer, D., Aldecoa, C., Njimi, H., and Vincent, J.L. (2012). Dopamine versus norepinephrine in the treatment of septic shock: a meta-analysis. *Crit. Care Med.* 40: 725–730.
6 Bigi, I., Partesana, N., Verzoni, A. et al. (1995). Incidence and correlates of complex ventricular arrhythmias during dobutamine stress echocardiography after acute myocardial infarction. *Eur. Heart J.* 16: 1819–1824.
7 Morelli, A., Lange, M., Ertmer, C. et al. (2008). Short-term effects of phenylephrine on systemic and regional hemodynamics in patients with septic shock: a crossover pilot study. *Shock* 29: 446–451.
8 Stuart, R.K., Shikora, S.A., Akerman, P. et al. (1990). Incidence of arrhythmia with central venous catheter insertion and exchange. *JPEN J. Parenter. Enteral Nutr.* 14: 152–155.
9 Evans, D.C., Doraiswamy, V.A., Prosciak, M.P. et al. (2009). Complications associated with pulmonary artery catheters: a comprehensive clinical review. *Scand. J. Surg.* 98: 199–208.
10 Asher, C.R., Miller, D.P., Grimm, R.A. et al. (1998). Analysis of risk factors for development of atrial fibrillation early after cardiac valvular surgery. *Am. J. Cardiol.* 82: 892–895.
11 Feldman, A.M. and McNamara, D. (2000). Myocarditis. *N. Engl. J. Med.* 343: 1388–1398.
12 Nakashima, H., Honda, Y., and Katayama, T. (1994). Serial electrocardiographic findings in acute myocarditis. *Intern. Med.* 33: 659–666.
13 Meine, T.J., Nettles, R.E., Anderson, D.J. et al. (2001). Cardiac conduction abnormalities in endocarditis defined by the Duke criteria. *Am. Heart J.* 142: 280–285.
14 Pedrotty, D.M., Rame, J.E., and Margulies, K.B. (2013). Management of ventricular arrhythmias in patients with ventricular assist devices. *Curr. Opin. Cardiol.* 28: 360–368.
15 McGinn, S. and White, P.D. (1935). Acute cor pulmonale resulting from pulmonary embolism: its clinical recognition. *JAMA* 104: 1473.
16 Chan, T., Brady, W., Harrigan, R. et al. (2005). Pulmonary embolism. In: *ECG in Emergency Medicine and Acute Care* (eds. T. Chan, W. Brady, R. Harrigan, et al.). Philadelphia: Elsevier Mosby.
17 Vela, B.S. and Crawford, M.H. (1995). Endocrinology and the heart. In: *Current Diagnosis and Treatment in Cardiology* (ed. M.H. Crawford), 411–427. New York: Lange Medical Books.
18 Chipkin, S. (1994). Lipoprotein metabolism and coronary artery disease. In: *Diagnostic Atlas of the Heart* (ed. J.S. Alpert), 503–516. New York: Raven Press.
19 Chou, T.C. (1991). *Electrocardiography in Clinical Practice*, 3e, 503–508. Philadelphia: WB Saunders.
20 Frontera, J.A., Parra, A., Shimbo, D. et al. (2008). Cardiac arrhythmias after subarachnoid hemorrhage: risk factors and impact on outcome. *Cerebrovasc. Dis.* 26: 71–78.

4

The ECG in Patients with Implanted Cardiac Devices

Ali Farzad[1], Benjamin J. Lawner[2], and Tu Carol Nguyen[2]

[1] *Department of Emergency Medicine, Baylor University Medical Center, Dallas, TX, USA*
[2] *Department of Emergency Medicine, University of Maryland School of Medicine, Baltimore, MD, USA*

Implanted cardiac devices have revolutionized the treatment of life-threatening dysrhythmias and end-stage cardiac failure refractory to medical therapy. Today's acute care clinicians are tasked with caring for patients with complex medical histories, some of whom have had cardiac devices implanted for a wide and growing range of indications. A multitude of cardiac devices, and multiple different generations of each type, have been created as manufacturers attempt to optimize size, safety, and effectiveness. The level of expertise required to care for patients with these devices might be overwhelming to most clinicians. Moreover, all of the devices are susceptible to complications, malfunction, and failure. Fortunately, proficiency in rapid and thorough interpretation of the electrocardiogram (ECG) can be exceptionally useful in the acute management of patients with implanted devices, some of whom are critically ill. In this chapter, we discuss select implanted cardiac devices – pacemakers, implantable cardioverter defibrillators, and left ventricular assist devices (LVADs). The goal is to educate clinicians regarding the basic components of each device, the expected normal and abnormal associated electrocardiographic findings, and the initial management steps when abnormalities arise.

Basics of Pacemakers

With advances in technology and an aging population, acute care clinicians are seeing increasing numbers of patients with implanted cardiac pacemakers. The list of indications for permanent cardiac pacemaker placement is also growing (Table 6.4.1) [1, 2]. Modern pacemakers have

significantly evolved in function, capability, and effectiveness [3–5]. Depending on the indication for placement, pacemakers may pace the atria, the ventricle, or both sequentially. Sensing of either atrial or ventricular activity is possible, and sensing can trigger or inhibit pacer activity [3–5].

Pacemakers consist of a pulse generator and single or multiple electrical leads that are implanted into the myocardium or coronary sinus tract. The pulse generator consists of circuitry that can detect and analyze the native rhythm and produce electrical output as necessary [3, 6]. The pulse generators are typically powered by a lithium battery and can last upwards of 10 years after implantation [6]. The pacemaker also has a reed switch, which can be used to inactivate the sensing system through an externally placed magnet [6]. Placement of a magnet on the chest activates the reed switch, causing asynchronous pacing (pacing regardless of the patient's underlying rhythm at the programmed rate), and removal of the magnet allows the pacemaker to resume its sensing function [6].

A five-letter coding system is used to describe the various pacemaker modes (Tables 6.4.2 and 6.4.3) [7]. The first letter describes the chamber(s) of the heart that is *paced* (A = atrium; V = ventricle; D = dual [both atrium and ventricle]); the second letter denotes the chamber that is *sensed*; and the third letter indicates the *response* to sensing function (I = inhibited by a sensed event; T = triggered by a sensed event; D = dual [I and T]). If the device has no programmable or anti-tachycardia functions, the last two letters can be left off the code (e.g. DDDOO or DDD) [3, 6, 7]. Although modern pacemakers are fairly reliable, the acute care clinician must be sufficiently familiar with the management of life-threatening malfunction and

Electrocardiogram in Clinical Medicine, First Edition. Edited by William J. Brady, Michael J. Lipinski, Andrew E. Darby, Michael C. Bond, Nathan P. Charlton, Korin Hudson, and Kelly Williamson.
© 2021 John Wiley & Sons Ltd. Published 2021 by John Wiley & Sons Ltd.

Table 6.4.1 Indications for pacing.

Bradycardia due to sinus and AV node dysfunction
- Sinus node dysfunction
- Acquired AV block in adults
- Chronic bifascicular block
- AV block associated with acute MI
- Hypersensitive carotid sinus syndrome
- Neurocardiogenic syncope

Prevention and termination of arrhythmias
- Atrial arrhythmias
- Long QT syndrome
- Atrial fibrillation

Specific conditions
- Cardiac transplantation
- Neuromuscular diseases
- Sleep apnea syndrome
- Cardiac sarcoidosis
- Children, adolescents, and patients with congenital heart disease

Hemodynamic indications
- Cardiac resynchronization therapy
- Obstructive hypertrophic cardiomyopathy

Pacemakers are usually implanted to treat symptomatic bradycardia and various types of heart blocks. This table lists the most common indications for cardiac pacing. For more detailed indications and recommendations [1].

complications associated with the device. Expertise and familiarity with the interpretation of the 12-lead ECG are essential to both the evaluation of normal pacemaker function and the diagnosis of pacemaker malfunction and its complications.

Electrocardiographic Findings in Normally Functioning Pacemakers

The electrocardiographic findings in patients with pacemakers depend on the pacing mode, the location of the pacing leads, the device's pacing thresholds, and the presence of native electrical activity [8]. Normally functioning pacemakers that are actively pacing produce small "pacing spikes," which are usually evident on the surface ECG (Figure 6.4.1). These low-amplitude spikes are short in duration (usually 2 ms) and might be difficult to see in every lead. Amplitude and visibility depend on the position and type of lead. Bipolar leads (I, II, III) typically convey smaller spacing spikes compared with unipolar leads (aVR, aVL, aVF, and V1–V6); hence, the pacer spikes in bipolar leads can be difficult to visualize [2, 3].

Atrial pacing leads are typically implanted in the appendage of the right atrium. Atrial pacing spikes should be visualized just before the P wave (Figure 6.4.2). The morphology of the P wave depends on the exact placement of the atrial lead, but paced P waves usually have normal axis and morphology [2, 8]. In contrast, right ventricular paced QRS complexes have abnormal axis and morphology because the pacing lead is placed in the apex of the right ventricle. Unlike normal native conduction, the paced right ventricle depolarizes and contracts from right to left, causing QRS morphology similar to that of a left bundle branch block (LBBB), with prolongation of the QRS interval (Figure 6.4.3) [2, 3, 8–10]. In the precordial leads (V1–V6), the altered ventricular conduction from a paced right ventricle causes wide and negative QS or rS complexes with poor R-wave progression (Figure 6.4.3). QS complexes are seen commonly in leads II, III, and aVF, whereas a large R wave typically is seen in the high lateral leads (I and aVL) (Figure 6.4.3) [2, 8]. Apically placed ventricular pacing leads also cause contraction from apex to base, yielding leftward deviation of the QRS axis. When a pacing lead is implanted toward the right ventricular outflow tract, depolarization occurs from base to apex, resulting in right axis deviation [2]. Occasionally, patients have epicardial rather than intracardiac pacemaker leads. If the ventricular epicardial lead is placed over the left ventricle, the ventricular paced pattern is that of a right bundle branch block (RBBB) [2].

Table 6.4.2 The revised NASPE/BPEG generic code for antibradycardia pacing [7].

I	II	III	IV	V
Chamber(s) Paced	Chamber(s) Sensed	Response to Sensing	Rate Modulation	Multisite Pacing
O = None	O = None	O = None	O = None	O = None
A = Atrium	A = Atrium	T = Triggered	R = Rate Modulation	A = Atrium
V = ventricle	V = ventricle	I = Inhibited		V = ventricle
D = Dual (A + V)	D = Dual (A + V)	D = Dual (T + I)		D = Dual (A + V)

Table 6.4.3 Examples of the revised NASPE/BPEG generic code.

Code	Meaning
VOO, VOOO, or VOOOO	Asynchronous ventricular pacing; no sensing, rate modulation, or multisite pacing.
VVIRV	Ventricular inhibitory pacing with rate modulation and multisite ventricular pacing (i.e. biventricular pacing or more than one pacing site in one ventricle). This mode is often used in patients with heart failure, chronic atrial fibrillation, and intraventricular conduction delay.
AAI, AAIO, or AAIOO	Atrial pacing inhibited by sensed spontaneous atrial depolarizations; no rate modulation or multisite pacing.
AAT, AATO, or AATOO	Atrial pacing with atrial outputs elicited without delay on atrial sensing during the alert period outside the pulse generator's refractory period (used primarily as a diagnostic mode to determine exactly when atrial depolarizations are sensed); no rate modulation or multisite pacing.
AATOA	Atrial pacing with atrial outputs elicited without delay on atrial sensing during the alert period outside the pulse generator's refractory period, without rate modulation but with multisite atrial pacing (i.e. biatrial pacing, more than one pacing site in one atrium, or both features).
DDD, DDDO, or DDDOO	Dual-chamber pacing (normally inhibited by atrial or ventricular sensing during the alert portion of the VA interval or by ventricular sensing during the alert portion of the AV interval, and with ventricular pacing triggered after a programmed PV interval by atrial sensing during the alert portion of the VA interval); no rate modulation or multisite pacing.
DDI, DDIO, or DDIOO	Dual-chamber pacing without atrium synchronous ventricular pacing (atrial sensing merely cancels the pending atrial output without affecting escape timing); no rate modulation or multisite pacing.
DDDR or DDDRO	Dual chamber, adaptive-rate pacing; no multisite pacing.
DDDRA	Dual chamber, adaptive-rate pacing with multisite atrial pacing (i.e. biatrial pacing, more than one pacing site in one atrium, or both features).
DDDOV	Dual-chamber pacing without rate modulation, but with multisite pacing (i.e. biventricular pacing, more than one pacing site in one ventricle, or both features).
DDDRD	Dual-chamber pacing with rate modulation and multisite pacing both in the atrium (i.e. biatrial pacing, pacing in more than one site in one atrium, or both features) and the ventricle (i.e. biventricular pacing, pacing in more than one site in one ventricle, or both features).

Although the ventricular placement of the pacing leads determines QRS axis and morphology (RV pacing = LBBB morphology, LV pacing = RBBB morphology), the corresponding ST segments and T waves should be discordant to the QRS complex. In paced rhythms, the major QRS vector is expected to be opposite the vector of the ST segment/T-wave complex (Figure 6.4.4). This is referred to as the "rule of appropriate discordance" and is a normal and expected finding (Figure 6.4.5) [2, 3, 8–10]. Acute care providers most commonly encounter AAIR, VVIR, DDD, DDDR pacemakers and backup pacing modes for defibrillator devices [2]. Examples of single-chamber and dual-chamber demand pacing are presented in Figures 6.4.6 through 6.4.8.

Electrocardiographic Findings in Abnormally Functioning Pacemakers

Detection of pacemaker malfunction and failure can be challenging. The clinical presentation varies widely, ranging from nonspecific clinical symptoms with subtle or absent electrocardiographic changes to obvious symptomatic bradycardia and dangerous pacemaker-induced tachycardias. Malfunction can be caused by a wide variety of reasons, including changes to underlying native rhythms, metabolic derangements, and equipment failure.

The clinician should attempt to obtain as much information as possible about the cardiac device and its implantation. Patients are given identification cards that indicate the manufacturer, model number, and type of device. The pacemaker itself has a radiopaque code that can be identified by a dedicated chest radiograph, and it is possible to identify the pacing mode using the surface ECG [4, 6, 11]. This information can be used to contact the manufacturer of the device when necessary. Table 6.4.4 provides contact information for the major companies that produce and service pacemakers/ICDs.

Physical examination should first include a review of vital signs, as malfunction in the pacemaker-dependent patient can lead to clinical instability. The implant site should be examined for signs of infection, erosion, migration, or trauma. Assessment of apical pulses and their

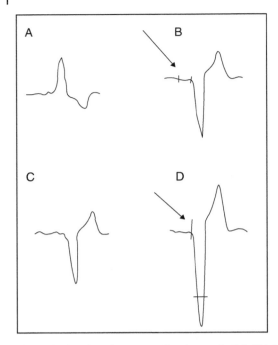

Figure 6.4.1 Note the pacer spikes (arrows in B & D) initiating atrial and ventricular depolarizations. The QRS complexes are all wide. **(A)** A monophasic R wave follows the rule of appropriate discordance. The QRS complex is positive, and the corresponding ST segment is depressed below the baseline with an inverted T wave. **(B, C,** and **D).** All have negative QRS complexes, accompanied by elevated ST segments with upright T waves. They all follow the rule of appropriate discordance. (*Source:* Image modified from Figure 33.3 (i) in [3].)

correlation to distal pulses permits judgments about mechanical capture and appropriate pacer function. Physical findings of significance include jugular venous distension, which may be a sign of tamponade or pacemaker syndrome; cannon A waves, which can signal atrioventricular (AV) dyssynchrony; and signs of diaphragmatic or skeletal muscle stimulation, which might indicate lead dislodgement [4]. Attention to volume status, metabolic derangements, and comorbid diseases can help identify common conditions (e.g. acidosis, hyperkalemia, hypokalemia, hypoxia, and cardiac ischemia) that predispose a pacemaker to complications [3, 6]. Careful and methodical interpretation of the ECG is critical, as the diagnostic accuracy of computer-based interpretation is variable and particularly prone to error in patients with pacemakers [12, 13].

Problems with Sensing

Problems with the sensing function include failure to sense, undersensing, and oversensing. Failure to sense usually is caused by increased resistance within the pacemaker circuit (pulse generator failure [battery], lead malfunction [dislodgement], fibrosis at the lead-tissue interface, or electrolyte abnormalities) [3, 5]. Undersensing occurs when the pacemaker fails to detect native cardiac activity and will result in asynchronous pacing that competes with the intrinsic rhythm [3, 6]. Undersensing may be caused by changes to the native rhythm (e.g. new

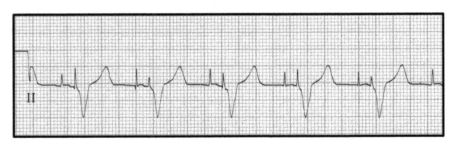

Figure 6.4.2 Atrial (before the p wave) and ventricular (before the QRS complex) pacing spikes showing appropriate pacing and capture. (*Source:* Image used with permission by Dr. Edward Burns from the Life in the Fastlane ECG Library [8].)

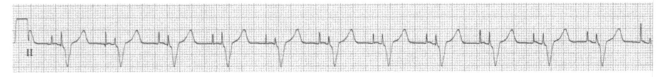

Figure 6.4.3 AV sequential pacing. There is 100% atrial capture (small P waves are seen following each atrial pacing spike) and 100% ventricular capture (QRS complex follows each ventricular pacing spike). QRS complexes are broad with a LBBB morphology and left axis deviation, indicating the presence of a pacing electrode in the apex of the right ventricle. (*Source:* Image used with permission by Dr. Edward Burns from the Life in the Fastlane ECG library [8], Example.)

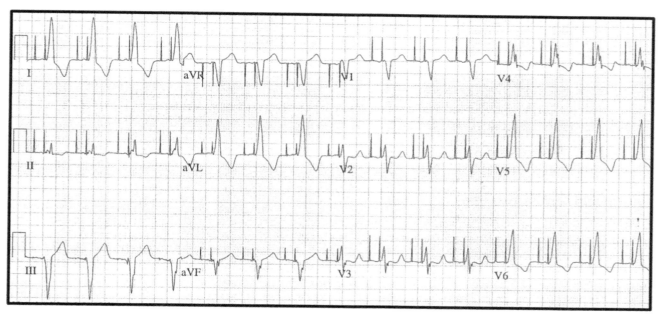

Figure 6.4.4 Another example of AV sequential pacing. Note the obvious atrial and ventricular pacing spikes. There is complete capture off both atrial and ventricular paced beats. The QRS complexes are widened, with a LBBB morphology that is consistent with right ventricular placement of the ventricular pacing lead. The QRS complexes are "appropriately discordant" to the ST segment/T wave complexes. (*Source:* Image used with permission by Dr. Edward Burns from the Life in the Fastlane ECG library [8], Example 4.)

Figure 6.4.5 The rule of appropriate discordance is shown here, illustrating the normal relationship of the major, terminal portion of the QRS complex and the initial ST-segment T wave. (*Source:* Image modified from Figure 33.3 (ii) in [3].)

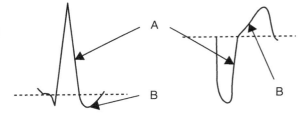

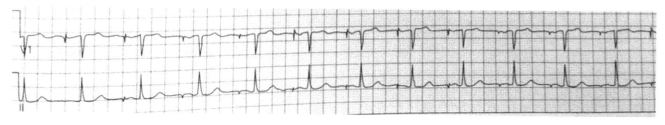

Figure 6.4.6 Typical ECG produced by complete AAI pacing. The AAI pacemaker (useful in patients with sinus node dysfunction and intact AV node conduction) paces and senses the atrium and can inhibit pacing activity when it senses appropriate spontaneous atrial activity. (*Source:* Image from Figure 33.4 in [3].)

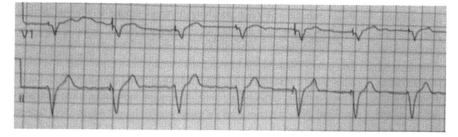

Figure 6.4.7 Typical ECG produced by complete VVI pacing. VVI pacemaker (useful in patients with chronic atrial fibrillation or flutter) paces and senses the ventricle and can inhibit pacing activity when a QRS complex is not sensed within a predefined interval. (*Source:* Image from Figure 33.5 in [3].)

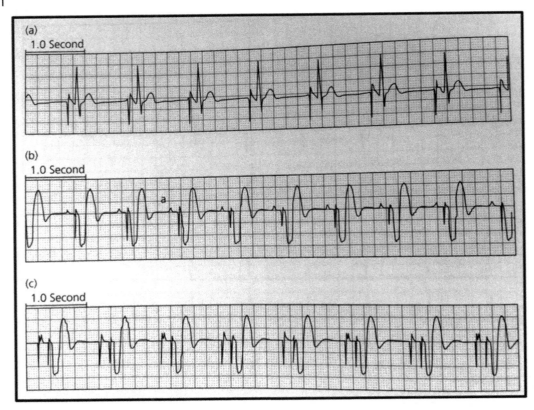

Figure 6.4.8 Rhythm strips produced by DDD pacing. (a) Atrial pacing with native ventricular activity (ventricle not paced) and intact AV conduction. (b) Atrial sensing of native p waves, and subsequent ventricular pacing. (c) Atrial and ventricular pacing. (*Source:* Image from Figure 33.6 in [3].)

Table 6.4.4 Phone numbers for technical support from the major manufacturers of pacemakers and ICDs.

Company	Phone Number
Medtronic	800-MEDTRONIC (800-633-8766)
Guidant	800-CARDIAC (800-227-3422)
St Jude Medical	800-722-3774

bundle branch blocks, premature ventricular contractions, ventricular tachydysrrhythmias), or problems with the device itself (programing, poor lead contact, battery failure, or exit block) [2, 3, 5, 9, 10, 14]. Undersensing can be difficult to detect because it has often has no obvious ECG findings [2]. Pacer spikes might or might not be visible, so the clinician must attempt to deduce if sensing and response are appropriate. However, the presence of pacing spikes within native QRS complexes suggests undersensing (Figures 6.4.9 and 6.4.10) [2, 3, 9, 10, 14].

Oversensing occurs when electrical signals are mistaken as native cardiac activity and pacing is inhibited inappropriately. These signals can come from large P, T, or U waves and/or surrounding skeletal muscle activity. Problems with lead contact (wire fracture, lead dislodgement, or loose connection to pulse generator) and overly sensitive or inappropriately programmed pacemaker parameters can also cause oversensing [3, 5, 9, 10, 14]. Bedside attempts to reproduce oversensing from skeletal muscle activity can be performed by having the patient contract his or her rectus and pectoralis muscles while a surface ECG is recorded [2]. Magnet placement over the pacemaker will disable sensing functions and allow assessment of capture, which may also be useful in certain clinical scenarios (Figure 6.4.11) [2, 3]. In patients with dual-chamber pacemakers, crosstalk oversensing (stimulus from one chamber sensed by another chamber's sensors as its own impulse) can also lead to inadequate pacing [5]. Ultimately, the inappropriate sensing signals might or might not be seen on the surface ECG, and reprogramming of the pacemaker is usually required to correct oversensing [2, 3, 9, 10, 14].

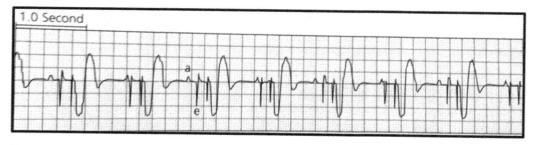

Figure 6.4.9 Rhythm strip produced by atrial undersensing in a patient with a DDD pacemaker. The native atrial events (a) are not sensed. If sensing were occurring, atrial pacing would be inhibited. (*Source:* Image from Figure 33.8 in [3].)

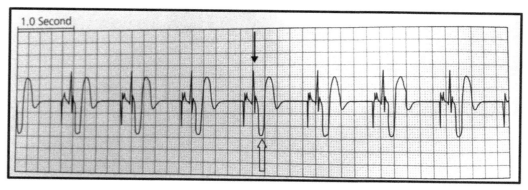

Figure 6.4.10 Rhythm strip produced by ventricular undersensing in a patient with a DDD pacemaker. The native ventricular events are not sensed. Native, upright, narrow QRS complex (*narrow arrow*) occurs soon after each atrial stimulus but is not being sensed. Ventricular pacing (*wide arrow*) occurs before ventricular repolarization of the native beat occurs. (*Source:* Image from Figure 33.9 in [3].)

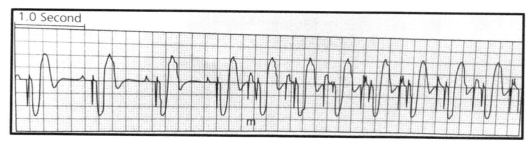

Figure 6.4.11 Placement of magnet inhibits sensing and reverts the pacemaker to asynchronous pacing. The magnet allows assessment of capture (but not sensing). The first four beats show native atrial activity inhibiting atrial pacing and triggering ventricular pacing. When the magnet is placed (*m*), atrial sensing is halted and asynchronous atrial and ventricular pacing occurs. This represents DOO pacing. (*Source:* Image from Figure 33.7 in [3].)

Problems with Pacing

Pacemaker failure is caused by a failure to pace (stimulus not generated) and/or a failure to capture (stimulus does not result in myocardial depolarization) in a situation in which pacing should occur. Oversensing is the most common cause of failure to pace, although problems with lead contact (wire fracture, dislodgement, trauma, or loose connections) and interference (e.g. MRI) can also be contributing factors [2, 3, 9, 10, 14]. Failure to pace results in absent pacer spikes where the spikes would be expected. If the patient's native heart rate is above the preprogrammed

pacing threshold, no pacing activity is expected and failure to pace or capture cannot be recognized. Placement of a magnet can help in assessment of pacer function in this situation, by temporarily halting sensing functions and initiating asynchronous pacing [2, 3, 9, 10, 14]. Failure to pace in patients with dual-chambered devices can be isolated to specific atrial or ventricular leads [2].

In failure of capture, the ECG typically shows a packing spike without evidence of capture and myocardial depolarization (Figures 6.4.12 and 6.4.13). Cardiac ischemia, electrolyte disturbance, and exit block are important causes

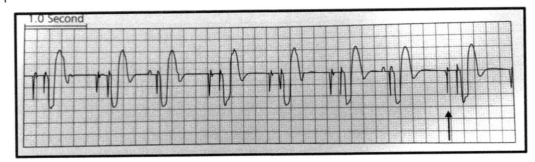

Figure 6.4.12 Failure of atrial capture. Atrial and ventricular pacing spikes are visible, but only the ventricular stimuli are capturing. There are no P waves following the atrial spikes (*arrow*). (*Source:* Image from Figure 33.10 in [3].)

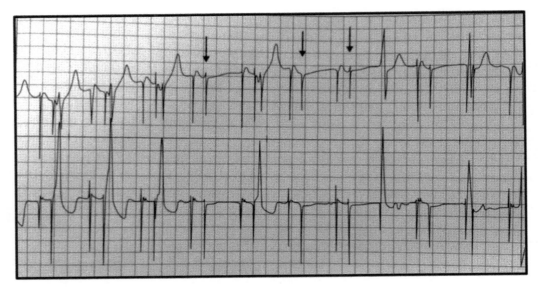

Figure 6.4.13 DDD pacing with intermittent loss of ventricular capture (*arrow*). A junctional escape beat (*J*) follows the third loss of capture event. In the next-to-last beat, a junctional escape beat is bracketed by two pacing spikes as a form of safety pacing. Rather than inhibiting ventricular pacing (and risk having no ventricular output if the sensed event were not truly a native ventricular depolarization), the AV interval is shortened and a paced output(s) occurs. (*Source:* Image from Figure 33.11 in [3].)

of failure to capture that should be considered. Exit block can be caused by maturation of tissues at the electrode–myocardium interface in the weeks following implantation or by tissue damage resulting from external cardiac defibrillation [2]. Failure to capture can also be caused by inadequate energy generation from a depleted battery or inappropriate programming [2, 3, 5]. Moreover, lead displacement with or without cardiac perforation by pacer leads should be considered. Cardiac perforation although rare, is suggested by the visualization of the pacer tip lying outside the heart on chest radiograph, and electrocardiographic indications of a paced complex and a new RBBB pattern (recall that RV pacing is expected to cause LBBB morphology) [3, 5]. Manipulation and rotation (accidental or deliberate) of the implanted pulse generator (Twiddler's syndrome) can result in diaphragmatic or brachial plexus pacing (e.g. arm twitching) as the pacemaker lead is

dislodged from the myocardium [3, 5, 14]. Failure to pace and failure to capture will both result in decreased or completely absent pacemaker function, and dependent patients often present with symptoms of lightheadedness, palpitations, or syncope [3, 5].

Pacemaker-Associated Dysrhythmias

Several types of pacemaker-associated dysrhythmias can occur, including pacemaker-mediated tachycardia (PMT), sensor-induced tachycardia, runaway pacemaker, and pacemaker-mediated AV block. These phenomena typically occur in people with dual-chamber pacemakers [3, 5].

PMT, also called endless-loop tachycardia, is a re-entry dysrhythmia that can occur in patients with some dual-chamber pacemakers (DDD or VAT) [2, 3]. The pacemaker itself acts as part of a re-entry circuit that can continuously pace the ventricle at a rate of 160–180 bpm [2]. Fortunately, the maximum rate of PMT is limited by the maximum tracking rate of the pacemaker. Advances in programming of newer pacemakers have allowed recognition and termination of PMT and are expected to decrease its incidence [2, 3]. The tachycardia is typically initiated by a properly timed PVC or paced beat that conducts retrograde via the AV node (or an accessory pathway, if present) to the atrium. The pacemaker acts as the anterograde conductor, and ventriculo-atrial (VA) conduction forms the retrograde limb of this incessant reentry arrhythmia [2, 3]. The ECG will typically show a regular, ventricular paced tachycardia at or less than the maximum upper rate of the pacemaker (Figure 6.4.14) [2, 3]. Acute treatment consists of applying a magnet to turn off sensing and turn to an asynchronous mode of pacing that breaks the circuit [3].

Modern pacemakers are programmed to allow the heart rate to increase in response to physiologic stimuli such as exercise and tachypnea. Sensor-induced tachycardias occur when pacemakers capable of rate-modulation inappropriately pace when stimulated by non-physiologic parameters [2, 3]. Any distracting stimuli (vibrations, limb movement, loud noises, hyperventilation, or electrocautery [e.g. during surgery]) can initiate the tachycardia [3, 14]. The ECG typically shows a paced tachycardia that does not exceed the pacemaker's upper rate limit [2]. These are typically benign and can be terminated with application of a magnet or cessation of the inciting event [3].

Runaway pacemaker, a potentially life-threatening malfunction of older-generation pacemakers, is caused by component failure [2]. The pacemaker delivers inappropriately rapid stimuli up to 400 bpm, potentially inducing ventricular tachycardia or fibrillation [2, 3, 14]. The ECG typically shows a paced ventricular tachycardia that often exceeds the expected maximum upper limit of older pacemakers (Figures 6.4.15 and 6.4.16). Modern pacemakers have a programmed upper rate limit that prevents this complication. Application of a magnet might induce a slower pacing rate temporarily until interrogation and reprogramming can be achieved. If this fails, emergency surgical intervention might be necessary to disconnect or sever the pacemaker leads [2, 5].

Pacemaker syndrome is a constellation of signs and symptoms caused by loss of AV synchrony and retrograde

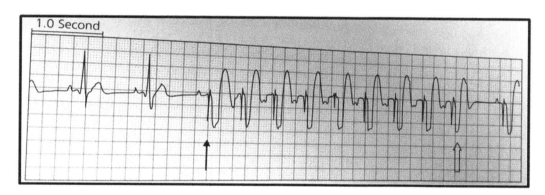

Figure 6.4.14 Pacemaker-mediated tachycardia (PMT). The third QRS complex is a paced beat (*narrow arrow*) and causes a retrograde P wave that triggers a run of PMT. In this case, the pacemaker detects the PMT and, in the penultimate beat (*wide arrow*), temporarily lengthens the PVARP[preventing atrial sensing of the retrograde P wave and breaking the re-entrant loop. (*Source:* Image from Figure 33.12 in [3].)

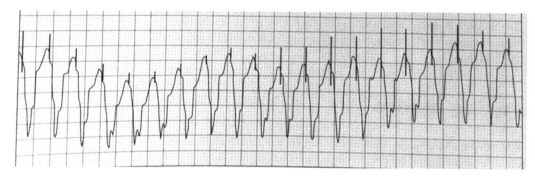

Figure 6.4.15 Runaway pacemaker. (*Source:* Image from Figure 33.2 in [3].)

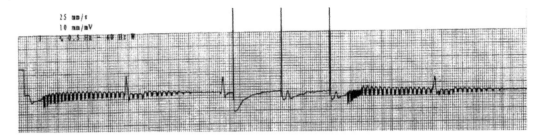

Figure 6.4.16 Paroxysms of rapid pacing spikes at 2000 bpm with decreasing amplitude and rate. These low-amplitude spikes fail to excite the ventricle. The underlying rhythm is atrial flutter with third-degree AV block and a ventricular escape rhythm at 30 bpm. Three pacing spikes are seen at 60 bpm in VOO mode, the first of which has failure to capture. (*Source:* Image used with permission by Dr. Edward Burns from the Life in the Fastlane ECG library [10], Example 3.)

VA conduction, caused by suboptimal pacing modes or programming [5]. Improper timing of atrial and ventricular contractions can cause a decrease of more than 20 mmHg in the systolic blood pressure during the change from a native to a paced rhythm [2]. Symptoms are vague and nonspecific (dyspnea, dizziness, fatigue, orthopnea, and confusion). The diagnosis cannot be made from the ECG alone, but, in the appropriate clinical situation, a lack of AV synchrony is suggestive (Figure 6.4.17) [3]. Device interrogation and programming play a key role in determining the pacemaker mode's contribution to symptoms.

Pseudomalfunction

Pseudomalfunction occurs when the clinician mistakenly expects the pacemaker to be triggering when it is appropriately inactive [2]. Pacemakers have a number of normal adaptive responses that can be interpreted on the ECG as malfunctions. Pacing can also occur without visible pacemaker spikes on the surface ECG, making the diagnosis of true malfunction very difficult and sometimes impossible, depending on the underlying native rhythm. [2, 3]. A common example of pseudomalfunction is the second-degree AV block that can occur with a normally functioning DDD pacemaker (Figure 6.4.18). Clinicians should rely on the patient's symptoms to guide management and, when they are concerned, should have a low threshold for consulting specialists to facilitate pacemaker interrogation and testing.

Key Points: Electrocardiographic Clues to Pacemaker Malfunction

- Missing or absent pacemaker spikes
- Excessive artifact or signal noise
- Hemodynamically significant bradycardias or heart blocks
- Persistently paced tachydysrhythmias

Electrocardiographic Diagnosis of Acute Myocardial Infarction in the Presence of a Paced Rhythm

It is challenging, but possible to diagnose acute myocardial infarction (AMI) in patients with paced rhythms. These patients are usually elderly and at high risk for coronary

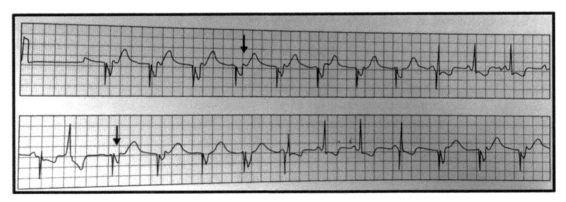

Figure 6.4.17 ECG from a patient with symptoms consistent with pacemaker syndrome. Note the presence of retrograde ventricular to atrial conduction (*arrows*). Inverted P waves occur after the QRS complex, suggesting AV dyssynchrony. (*Source:* Image from Figure 33.14 in [3].)

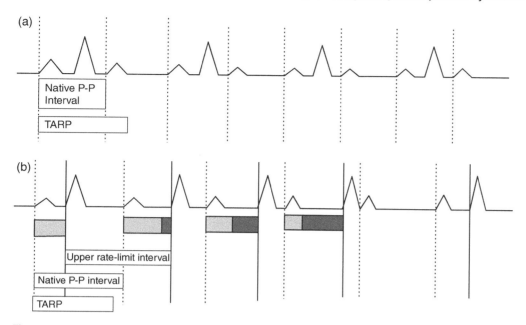

Figure 6.4.18 Pseudo-malfunction. AV block schematic for normally functioning DDD pacemaker. (a) Sinus rate increases such that the native P-P interval is shorter than the total atrial refractory period (TARP). Every other P wave occurs within the TARP and the paced QRS complex is dropped, resulting in a 2 : 1 AV block. (b) In this case, the native P-P interval is shorter than the preset upper rate-limit interval (minimum cardiac cycle duration for maximum pacemaker rate) but still longer than the TARP. The pacemaker detects atrial activity but cannot release its ventricular stimulus faster than the upper limit, resulting in a progressive lengthening of the PR interval until a ventricular beat is dropped (Wenckebach). (*Source:* Image from Figure 33.13 in [3].)

artery disease. Unfortunately, their paced rhythms cause ST-segment and T-wave changes that limit the diagnostic value and reliability of their ECG, causing delays in therapies [15–17]. As in patients with LBBB, paced rhythms can be expected to follow the rule of appropriate discordance, as discussed previously.

Several authors have attempted to characterize diagnostic ischemic changes on ECGs in patients with LBBB and paced rhythms. Based on GUSTO trial data, Sgarbossa et al. identified three electrocardiographic criteria that, although insensitive, are highly specific for the diagnosis of AMI in paced rhythms (Table 6.4.5) [16]. In the appropriate clinical scenario, the presence of any one of these ST patterns in any single lead is highly specific for AMI and the need for emergent cardiac catheterization. Of the three, ST-segment elevation ≥5 mm, is the most specific criterion in patients with paced rhythms [16, 17]. Smith et al. have since hypothesized that replacement of the absolute ST-elevation measurement of ≥5 mm, with an ST/S ratio less than 0.25, might improve the diagnostic utility of the rule [18, 19]. This brings attention to an important fact: the smaller the S wave, the more significant any relative ST-segment elevation [18, 19]. Awareness about the specificity of these criteria, along with careful interpretation of ECGs, might lead to early recognition of STEMI in this high-risk patient population.

Table 6.4.5 Sgarbossa criteria.

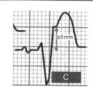	• Discordant STE > 5 mm in leads with a predominantly negative QRS • A ratio of STE to S-wave amplitude of 0.25 or more
	• Concordant STE > 1 mm in leads with a predominantly positive QRS
	• Concordant STD > 1 mm in leads V1, V2, and V3

The presence of any one of these ST patterns in a paced ventricular rhythm is highly suggestive of STEMI and the need for emergent cardiac catheterization, in the appropriate clinical context. The criterion that is most specific for STEMI in this table is discordant STE > 5 mm in leads with a predominantly negative QRS complex. Smith and associates modified these criteria, with substantial improvement in accuracy, by adjusting for proportionality between the degree of ST-segment elevation (STE) and the depth of the S wave [12, 13, 15-17].

Pearl: Paced electrocardiographic morphology should follow the rule of "appropriate discordance." In paced rhythms and LBBB, the QRS complex is in the opposite direction of the ST segment.

Basics of the Implantable Cardioverter Defibrillator

The US Food and Drug Administration approved the automated implantable internal defibrillator for use in 1985. Since its inception as a device of "last resort," the current generation of ICDs has evolved to fulfill more than one therapeutic function. ICD implantation is now considered first-line treatment for patients at risk for life-threatening ventricular dysrhythmia. Modern devices have both pacemaker and anti-dysrhythmic functionality. Device implantation does not significantly "change" the patient's ECG, but the presence of certain historical factors and electrocardiographic findings can clue providers into the presence and function of an automated ICD.

Ventricular Storm

Ventricular dysrhythmias, especially ventricular tachycardia, are observed in association with acute ischemia. Ventricular fibrillation (VF) and tachycardia (VT) are implicated in sudden cardiac death and require prompt treatment with circulatory support and electrical therapy. Recurrent ventricular dysrhythmia, also called *ventricular storm* (VS), has been associated with ICD implantation [20]. The incidence of VS is not precisely known, and the literature describes VS occurring in anywhere from 10% to 20% of patients who receive an ICD [21]. Electrocardiographic findings consistent with VS reveal recurrent bouts of ventricular dysrhythmia that fail to terminate following an appropriately delivered countershock. In a retrospective study, Greene and colleagues found that occurrence of VS was difficult to predict [20]. VS was usually terminated through appropriate shock delivery, anti-tachycardic pacing, and anti-dysrhythmic therapy. The Greene study did not show a link between VS and increased mortality [20]. A 2006 study published in the *European Heart Journal* revealed that patients with chronic renal failure and a decreased left ventricular ejection fraction were more likely to experience VS [21]. The study did not find that VS implied a worsening prognosis.

The persistence of VF or VT following three countershocks alerts the clinician to the presence of electrical storm. Treatment should proceed in accordance with the usual advanced cardiac life support algorithm. However, additional pharmacologic and mechanical therapies deserve consideration in the patient with an ICD. Collaboration with cardiology and electrophysiology colleagues is of prime importance. If specialty resources are not immediately available, consider transfer to a tertiary cardiac care center following patient stabilization. Appropriately delivered shocks in ICD patients should trigger a search for underlying causes of cardiac instability. Ischemia, electrolyte imbalance, and infection can contribute to myocardial irritability. Antitachycardic pacing (ATP) reduces the need for future shocks and may have utility in the setting of "faster" episodes of ventricular tachycardia [22]. Anti-dysrhythmic therapy with amiodarone might also have a role in the treatment of electrical storm. Amiodarone should be used with extreme caution if the tachydysrhythmia is secondary to a prolonged QT interval [22]. A 2000 study published in *Circulation* highlighted the benefits of beta-blockade for patients experiencing VS. It is presumed that medicines such as propanolol mitigate the overwhelming catecholaminergic cascade that accompanies electrical storm. The benefits of beta blockers persisted even in patients with a known, suppressed ejection fraction [23]. Definitive care for patients in VS refractory to pharmacologic and electrical therapy includes general anesthesia, placement of an intra-aortic balloon pump, and ablation of the offending electrical focus [22, 23].

Electrocardiographic Findings after Defibrillation

Post-shock electrocardiographic changes are not unique to the patient with an ICD. Electrocardiographic abnormalities are known to occur following the delivery of biphasic or monophasic defibrillation [24, 25]. Indeed, nonspecific electrocardiographic changes, ST-segment elevation, and ST-segment depression can confound the diagnosis of acute ischemia. Precisely because findings are varied, it is imperative to interpret electrocardiographic findings within the context of the patient presentation. Certainly, ST-segment elevation that occurs in an anatomic distribution raises concern about an AMI. Diffuse ST-segment elevation can suggest stress-induced cardiomyopathy or coronary vasospasm. "Stunned" myocardium is known to occur after defibrillation. Electrical "stunning" appears as gradually resolving ST-segment elevation on the post-shock ECG [24].

Although the mechanism of post-shock electrocardiographic changes is not precisely understood, the loss of signal voltage has been documented in the literature [25]. One possible explanation, featured in a retrospective study by Cuculi and colleagues, linked decreased R-wave amplitude to the myocardial and chest wall edema that occurs following electrical shock delivery [26]. The presence of edema alters myocardial conduction, and the post-shock ECG therefore displays reduced electrical amplitude. Notably, patients with an ICD were used as the control arm for the study. The ECGs obtained from patients with ICDs did not display any voltage loss; however, no ICD patients received external chest compressions or transthoracic defibrillation [26].

Pearl: After defibrillation, ST elevation is often observed in 12-lead ECGs. Look for persistent elevation and changes in an anatomic distribution.

Too Much Noise!

ICDs use sophisticated waveform analysis algorithms to distinguish artifact from dysrhythmia [27]. Electrical activity from muscle groups adjacent to the ICD can provide artifactual input to the device's sensor. Pectoral muscle and diaphragmatic contractions are implicated in the problem of "oversensing." Fortunately, today's devices typically employ bipolar sensing and other technologies that minimize these inputs [27, 28]. Device interrogation, which is beyond the scope of this chapter, is often required to discern the underlying cause of an inappropriate shock. The presence of interference, or noise, on an externally recorded ECG in a patient with an implantable device raises the suspicion of a mechanical problem. Interference from cellular telephones and MRI has been implicated in the presence of ECG noise. Device malfunction is another important cause of ECG noise in the patient with an ICD (Table 6.4.6). Surgical exploration may be necessary to discover the cause of persistent noise that could result in inappropriate shocks [27, 28].

Basics of Left Ventricular Assist Devices

Ventricular assist devices help to support heart function and have various clinical indications as a bridge or transition to definitive therapies. More recently, they have become long-term circulatory support mechanisms [29, 30, 31].

Table 6.4.6 External causes of electrocardiographic noise in patients with implanted cardioverter defibrillators.

- Conductor coil failure
- Insulation breach
- Loose set screw
- Cellular telephones
- Lead fracture
- Lead dislodgement

There are two basic types of VADs: LVADs and right ventricular assist devices (RVADs). Biventricular assist devices (BIVADs) use both types concurrently [29, 31]. For the sake of simplicity, this discussion focuses on LVADs and the effects of the LVAD on the ECG.

First-generation LVADs are pulsatile positive displacement pumps. Second-generation LVADs involve continuous axial or centrifugal flow pump devices. Third-generation devices are designed for optimized durability and are more compact [32]. Their three major components are the inflow cannula, the outflow cannula, and the pump (Figure 6.4.19). The inflow cannula drains blood from the left ventricle into the pump, and the outflow cannula returns blood to the aorta for perfusion throughout the body. A cable (the driveline) connected to the internal unit of the LVAD within the body exits the abdominal skin and then attaches to the external controller, which is worn on a belt. External batteries or a power-based unit provides the power source [32].

There is a lack of literature analyzing the electrocardiographic morphology and changes in individuals with LVADs. Isolated studies have examined ECGs before and after LVAD implantation, demonstrating differences that can be taken into consideration when presented with an individual with one of these devices. LVAD support has immediate and delayed electrophysiological effects on specific intervals. Immediate changes include a decrease in PR, a decrease in QRS, an increase in QT, and an increase in heart-rate-adjusted QTc intervals. With respect to delayed changes, individuals with LVADs show an increase in PR, a decrease in QRS, a decrease in QT, and a decrease in heart-rate-adjusted QTc intervals compared with the respective pre-LVAD implantation intervals (Table 6.4.7, Figure 6.4.20) [33]. Furthermore, since heart failure exhibits QT prolongation, a decreased QT interval reflects the reversal of electrophysiologic remodeling [33].

A retrospective study of individuals with LVADs, treated between 1997 and 2001, showed that those with first-generation devices had an increase in de novo monomorphic ventricular tachycardias after LVAD insertion and no increase in post-LVAD polymorphic ventricular tachycardia or ventricular fibrillation [34]. Another retrospective study, published in 2009, analyzed the incidence of ventricular tachycardia and ventricular fibrillation in 23 patients who received the HeartMate II (a second-generation device) for long-term support. The study showed that ventricular arrhythmias were common, especially in the early postoperative period (within the first four weeks) – half of the patients required treatment [35]. More research is needed to investigate the arrhythmogenicity and the association between LVADs and dysrhythmias. The pathogenesis might be related to the underlying cardiomyopathy, to scar tissue caused by

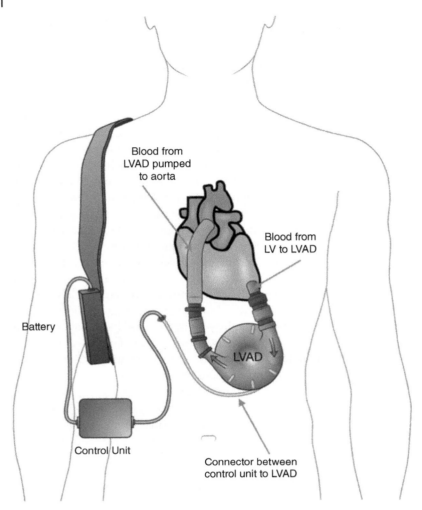

Blood from LVAD pumped to aorta

Blood from LV to LVAD

Battery

LVAD

Control Unit

Connector between control unit to LVAD

Figure 6.4.19 LVAD illustration showing inflow cannula for blood from left ventricle into LVAD, outflow cannula for blood from LVAD into aorta, and driveline as the connector between the LVAD and control unit. (*Source:* Modified image from Madhero88, Wikimedia Commons (CC by SA 3.0)).

Table 6.4.7 Immediate and delayed effects of LVAD implantation on ECG intervals compared with pre-LVAD ECG intervals.

	PR Interval	QRS Interval	QT Interval	HR-Adjusted QTc Interval
Immediate	↓	↓	↑	↑
Delayed	↑	↓	↓	↓

For more information, see [31].

cannula insertions, or to suction events [35]. These studies illustrate how patients with LVADs can present with ventricular arrhythmias. A case report published in 2012 described a patient with a continuous-flow LVAD and an ICD, who presented to the emergency department after sustaining ventricular fibrillation for hours, as evidenced by an ECG [36]. The patient presented with dizziness, was awake and conversant, and was externally defibrillated successfully [36]. An example of an ECG from an individual with an LVAD, who presented in VF and awake, is presented in Figure 6.4.21. These studies suggest that the morphologies of ECGs for individuals with LVADs do not demonstrate definitive characteristics. However, ECGs obtained before and after LVAD implantation show differences in ECG intervals. It is also important to remember that patients with LVAD can have otherwise life-threatening ventricular arrhythmias yet present conscious with nonspecific symptoms. Timely interpretation of the ECG and treatment of underlying ventricular arrhythmias can improve symptoms and optimize device function. It is hoped that ongoing research will further our understanding of how to better recognize abnormalities and more effectively manage these patients.

(a)

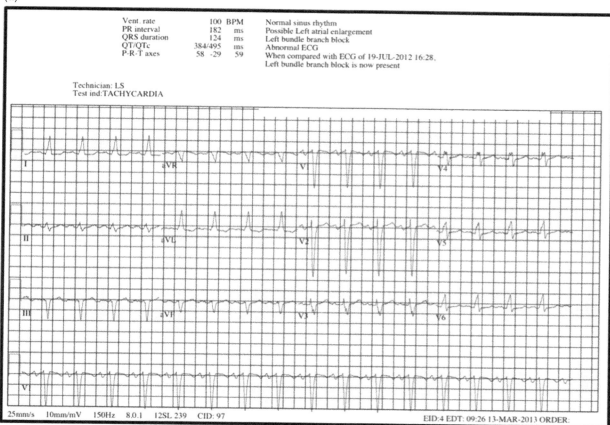

Vent. rate   100   BPM   Normal sinus rhythm
PR interval   182   ms   Possible Left atrial enlargement
QRS duration   124   ms   Left bundle branch block
QT/QTc   384/495   ms   Abnormal ECG
P-R-T axes   58   -29   59   When compared with ECG of 19-JUL-2012 16:28,
                               Left bundle branch block is now present

Technician: LS
Test ind:TACHYCARDIA

25mm/s   10mm/mV   150Hz   8.0.1   12SL 239   CID: 97   EID:4 EDT: 09:26 13-MAR-2013 ORDER:

(b)

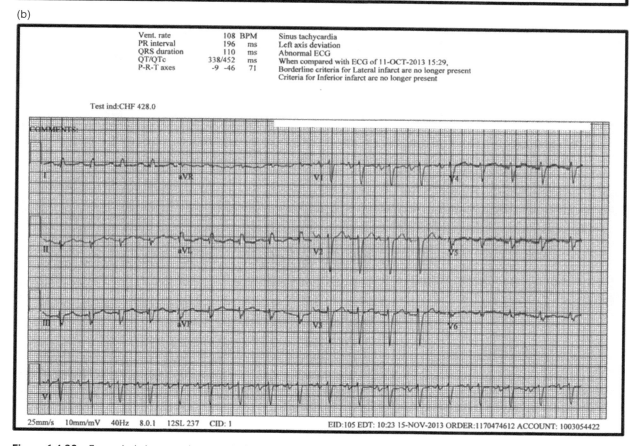

Vent. rate   108   BPM   Sinus tachycardia
PR interval   196   ms   Left axis deviation
QRS duration   110   ms   Abnormal ECG
QT/QTc   338/452   ms   When compared with ECG of 11-OCT-2013 15:29,
P-R-T axes   -9   -46   71   Borderline criteria for Lateral infarct are no longer present
                               Criteria for Inferior infarct are no longer present

Test ind:CHF 428.0

COMMENTS:

25mm/s   10mm/mV   40Hz   8.0.1   12SL 237   CID: 1   EID:105 EDT: 10:23 15-NOV-2013 ORDER:1170474612 ACCOUNT: 1003054422

Figure 6.4.20 Example I shows an increase in PR, a decrease in QRS, a decrease in QT, and a decrease in QTc intervals between the pre-LVAD and delayed post-LVAD intervals. Example II shows a decrease in QRS and an increase in QTc intervals between the pre-LVAD and immediate post-LVAD intervals. A comparison of PR intervals is not noted in Example II, since the immediate post-LVAD ECG did not generate a PR interval. (a) Pre-LVAD. (b) Delayed Post-LVAD. (c) Pre-LVAD (d) Immediate Post-LVAD. These interval changes support the findings in Reference 31. Refer to Table 6.4.7 for a summary of immediate and delayed effects on electrocardiographic interval changes following LVAD implantation. *Source:* Used with permission from Dr. Tu Carol Nguyen.

(c)

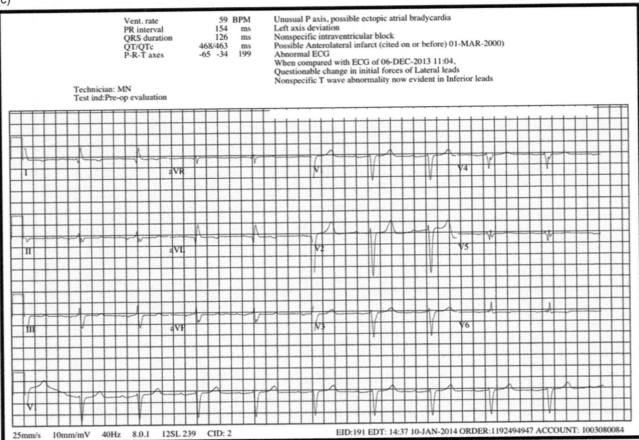

Vent. rate	59	BPM	Unusual P axis, possible ectopic atrial bradycardia
PR interval	154	ms	Left axis deviation
QRS duration	126	ms	Nonspecific intraventricular block
QT/QTc	468/463	ms	Possible Anterolateral infarct (cited on or before) 01-MAR-2000)
P-R-T axes	-65 -34	199	Abnormal ECG

When compared with ECG of 06-DEC-2013 11:04,
Questionable change in initial forces of Lateral leads
Nonspecific T wave abnormality now evident in Inferior leads

Technician: MN
Test ind:Pre-op evaluation

25mm/s   10mm/mV   40Hz   8.0.1   12SL 239   CID: 2   EID:191 EDT: 14:37 10-JAN-2014 ORDER:1192494947 ACCOUNT: 1003080084

(d)

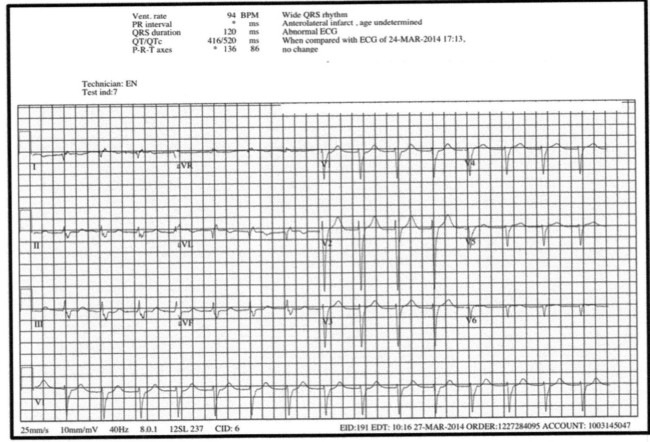

Vent. rate	94	BPM	Wide QRS rhythm
PR interval	*	ms	Anterolateral infarct , age undetermined
QRS duration	120	ms	Abnormal ECG
QT/QTc	416/520	ms	When compared with ECG of 24-MAR-2014 17:13,
P-R-T axes	* 136	86	no change

Technician: EN
Test ind:7

25mm/s   10mm/mV   40Hz   8.0.1   12SL 237   CID: 6   EID:191 EDT: 10:16 27-MAR-2014 ORDER:1227284095 ACCOUNT: 1003145047

Figure 6.4.20   (Continued)

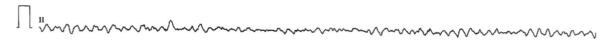

Figure 6.4.21 ECG from a conscious patient with LVAD, showing VF. (*Source:* Image used with permission by Dr. Edward Burns from the Life in the Fastlane ECG library [37]).

References

1 Tracy, C.M., Epstein, A.E., Darbar, D. et al. (2013). 2012 ACCF/AHA/HRS focused update incorporated into the ACCF/AHA/HRS 2008 guidelines for device-based therapy of cardiac rhythm abnormalities. *J. Am. Coll. Cardiol.* 61 (3): e6–e75. https://doi.org/10.1016/j.jacc.2012.11.007.

2 Chan, T.C. and Cardall, T.Y. (2006). Electronic pacemakers. *Emerg. Med. Clin. North Am.* 24 (1): 179–194. https://doi.org/10.1016/j.emc.2005.08.011.

3 Brady, W.J. and Truwit, J.D. (2009). Can the ECG accurately diagnose pacemaker malfunction and/or complication? In: *Critical Decisions in Emergency & Acute Care Electrocardiography*, 284–294. Oxford, UK: Wiley-Blackwell, chapter 33.

4 McMullan, J., Valento, M., Attari, M. et al. (2007). Care of the pacemaker/implantable cardioverter defibrillator patient in the ED. *Am. J. Emerg. Med.* 25 (7): 812–822. https://doi.org/10.1016/j.ajem.2007.02.008.

5 Harper, R.J., Brady, W.J., Perron, A.D., and Mangrum, M. (2001). The paced electrocardiogram: issues for the emergency physician. *Am. J. Emerg. Med.* 19 (7): 551–560. https://doi.org/10.1053/ajem.2001.24486.

6 Sarko, J.A. and Tiffany, B.R. (2000). Cardiac pacemakers: evaluation and management of malfunctions. *Am. J. Emerg. Med.* 18 (4): 435–440. https://doi.org/10.1053/ajem.2000.7351.

7 Bernstein, A.D., Daubert, J.C., Fletcher, R.D. et al. (2002). The revised NASPE/BPEG generic code for antibradycardia, adaptive-rate, and multisite pacing. North American Society of Pacing and Electrophysiology/British Pacing and Electrophysiology Group. *Pacing Clin. Electrophysiol.* 25 (2): 260–264.

8 Burns E. Pacemaker Rhythms – Normal Patterns. Life in the Fastlane ECG Library. http://lifeinthefastlane.com/ecg-library/pacemaker. Accessed March 2014.

9 Surawicz, B. and Knilans, T. (2008). *Chou's Electrocardiography in Clinical Practice*, 6e. Philadelphia: Saunders.

10 Wagner, G.S. (2007). *Marriott's Practical Electrocardiography*, 11e. Philadelphia: Lippincott Williams & Wilkins.

11 Garson, A. (1990). Stepwise approach to the unknown pacemaker ECG. *Am. Heart J.* 119: 924–941.

12 Gulin, M.E. and Datwani, N. (2007). Electrocardiograms with pacemakers: accuracy of computer reading. *J. Electrocardiol.* 40: 144–146.

13 Poon, K., Okin, P.M., and Klingfield, P. (2005). Diagnostic performance of a computer-based ECG rhythm algorithm. *J. Electrocardiol.* 38: 235–238.

14 Burns E. Pacemaker Malfunction. Life in the Fastlane ECG Library. http://lifeinthefastlane.com/ecg-library/pacemaker-malfunction. Accessed March 2014.

15 Sgarbossa, E.B. (1996). Recent advances in the electrocardiographic diagnosis of myocardial infarction: left bundle branch block and pacing. *Pacing Clin. Electrophysiol.* 19 (9): 1370–1379.

16 Sgarbossa, E.B., Pinski, S.L., Gates, K.B., and Wagner, G.S. (1996). Early electrocardiographic diagnosis of acute myocardial infarction in the presence of ventricular paced rhythm. GUSTO-I investigators. *Am. J. Cardiol.* 77 (5): 423–424.

17 Maloy, K.R., Bhat, R., Davis, J. et al. (2010). Sgarbossa criteria are highly specific for acute myocardial infarction with pacemakers. *West. J. Emerg. Med.* 11 (4): 354–357.

18 Smith, S.W., Dodd, K.W., Henry, T.D. et al. (2012). Diagnosis of ST-elevation myocardial infarction in the presence of left bundle branch block with the ST-elevation to S-wave ratio in a modified Sgarbossa rule. *Ann. Emerg. Med.* 60 (6): 766–776. https://doi.org/10.1016/j.annemergmed.2012.07.119.

19 Schaaf, S.G., Tabas, J.A., and Smith, S.W. (2013). A patient with a paced rhythm presenting with chest pain and hypotension. *JAMA Intern. Med.* 173 (22): 2082–2085. https://doi.org/10.1001/jamainternmed.2013.11304.

20 Greene, M., Newman, D., Geist, M. et al. (2000). Is electrical storm in ICD patients the sign of a dying heart? Outcome of patients with clusters of ventricular tachyarrhythmias. *Europace* 2 (3): 263–269. https://doi.org/10.1053/eupc.2000.0104.

21 Brigadeau, F., Kouakam, C., Klug, D. et al. (2006). Clinical predictors and prognostic significance of electrical storm in patients with implantable cardioverter defibrillators. *Eur. Heart J.* 27 (6): 700–707. https://doi.org/10.1093/eurheartj/ehi726.

22 Eifling, M., Razavi, M., and Massumi, A. (2011). The evaluation and management of electrical storm. *Tex. Heart Inst. J.* 38 (2): 111–121.

23 Nademanee, K., Taylor, R., Bailey, W.E. et al. (2000). Treating electrical storm: sympathetic blockade versus advanced cardiac life support-guided therapy. *Circulation* 102 (7): 742–747. https://doi.org/10.1161/01.CIR.102.7.742.

24 Reddy, R.K., Gleva, M.J., Gliner, B.E. et al. (1997). Biphasic transthoracic defibrillation causes fewer ECG ST-segment changes after shock. *Ann. Emerg. Med.* 30 (2): 127–134.

25 Sandroni, C., Sanna, T., Cavallaro, F., and Caricato, A. (2008). Myocardial stunning after successful defibrillation. *Resuscitation* 76 (1): 3–4. https://doi.org/10.1016/j.resuscitation.2007.06.020.

26 Cuculi, F., Kobza, R., and Erne, P. (2007). ECG changes following cardioversion and defibrillation. *Swiss Med. Wkly.* 137 (39–40): 551–555. https://doi.org/10.4414/smw.2007.11759.

27 Scher, D.L. (2004). Troubleshooting pacemakers and implantable cardioverter-defibrillators. *Curr. Opin. Cardiol.* 19 (1): 36–46.

28 Kowalski, M., Ellenbogen, K.A., Wood, M.A., and Friedman, P.L. (2008). Implantable cardiac defibrillator lead failure or myopotential oversensing? An approach to the diagnosis of noise on lead electrograms. *Europace* 10 (8): 914–917. https://doi.org/10.1093/europace/eun167.

29 Cleveland, J.C., Naftel, D.C., Reece, T.B. et al. (2011). Survival after biventricular assist device implantation: an analysis of the interagency registry for mechanically assisted circulatory support database. *J. Heart Lung Transplant.* 30 (8): 862–869.

30 Lietz, K. and Miller, L.W. (2007). Improved survival of patients with end-stage heart failure listed for heart transplantation: analysis of organ procurement and transplantation network/U.S. United Network of Organ Sharing data, 1990 to 2005. *J. Am. Coll. Cardiol.* 50 (13): 1282–1290.

31 McMurray, J.J., Adamopoulos, S., Anker, S.D. et al. (2012). ESC guidelines for the diagnosis and treatment of acute and chronic heart failure 2012: the task force for the diagnosis and treatment of acute and chronic heart failure 2012 of the European Society of Cardiology. Developed in collaboration with the Heart Failure Association (HFA) of the ESC. *Eur. J. Heart Fail.* 14 (8): 803–869.

32 Goldstein, D.J., Oz, M.C., and Rose, E.A. (1998). Implantable left ventricular assist devices. *N. Engl. J. Med.* 339 (21): 1522–1533.

33 Harding, J.D., Piacentino, V., Gaughan, J.P. et al. (2001). Electrophysiological alterations after mechanical circulatory support in patients with advanced cardiac failure. *Circulation* 104 (11): 1241–1247.

34 Ziv, O., Dizon, J., Thosani, A. et al. (2005). Effects of left ventricular assist device therapy on ventricular arrhythmias. *J. Am. Coll. Cardiol.* 45 (9): 1428–1434.

35 Andersen, M., Videbaek, R., Boesgaard, S. et al. (2009). Incidence of ventricular arrhythmias in patients on long-term support with a continuous-flow assist device (HeartMate II). *J. Heart Lung Transplant.* 28 (7): 733–735.

36 Sims, D.B., Rosner, G., Uriel, N. et al. (2012). Twelve hours of sustained ventricular fibrillation supported by a continuous-flow left ventricular assist device. *Pacing Clin. Electrophysiol.* 35 (5): e144–e148.

37 Burns E. Conscious VF. Life in the Fastlane ECG Library. http://lifeinthefastlane.com/conscious-vf. Accessed April 2014.

5

Electrocardiographic Manifestations of Cardiac Transplantation

Semhar Tewelde

Department of Emergency Medicine, University of Maryland School of Medicine, Baltimore, MD, USA

Introduction

South African surgeon Christiaan Barnard applied techniques he learned while studying at Stanford University to perform the first successful cardiac transplant in Cape Town, South Africa, in 1967 [1, 2]. Although cardiac transplantation became achievable, prognosis at the time was poor: patients died soon after the procedure from the body's natural propensity to reject the donor organ. Advances in immunosuppressive therapy over the next 20 years, such as Jean Borel's discovery of cyclosporine, allowed transplantation to be successful well beyond the postoperative period [3]. Today, more than 5000 cardiac transplants are performed annually around the world. The exponential growth in the aging population, especially those with coronary artery disease and heart failure, has increased the demand for transplantation. Furthermore, the progression of transplant medicine has improved recipients' longevity with good quality of life. Thus, practicing clinicians should become familiar with the unique electrocardiographic manifestations of cardiac transplantation.

Cardiac Transplantation

A cardiac allograft can be placed in an orthotopic (natural) or heterotopic (abnormal) position. Orthotropic cardiac transplantation is performed more commonly and favored because of the inherent problems with heterotopic transplantation (e.g. pulmonary compression, difficulty with endomyocardial biopsy, anticoagulation) [4, 5]. An orthotopic transplant involves removal of the recipient's native heart and insertion of the donor heart in its exact place. Surgically, the left atrial anastomosis is performed first, followed by the right atrium and the great vessels

(Figure 6.5.1) [6, 7]. The autonomic denervation of the donor heart that occurs during transplantation causes an increased resting heart rate and reduced heart rate variability in the recipient [8, 9].

Securing the donor heart by suturing it to the remnants of the recipient's atria leads to one of the most common electrocardiographic findings after orthotopic cardiac transplantation – dual P waves. The donor P waves retain their normal amplitude, but the recipient (native) P waves are smaller (Figures 6.5.2 and 6.5.3) [5, 6, 10, 11]. Care should be taken not to misinterpret these dual P waves as an AV block [12]. The suture line between the recipient and donor atria impedes the recipient's electrical impulses from conducting; therefore, only the donor P waves are propagated to the AV node and induce ventricular depolarization. The sinoatrial (SA) nodes from the recipient and donor function independently, leading to variable P-to-P (donor) intervals, known as atrial dissociation [13]. In many cases, the recipient's P waves are not detectable because of their small amplitude, the presence of SA node dysfunction, or preexisting supraventricular tachycardia [14].

Pearl: The electrocardiograms (ECGs) of cardiac transplant patients often show two P waves: one from the recipient and one from the donor. The native P waves have a smaller amplitude and are often not seen at all. Importantly, only the donor P waves are conducted to the AV node.

Another frequent manifestation after orthotopic cardiac transplantation is an intraventricular conduction delay, specifically a complete or incomplete right bundle branch block (Figure 6.5.3) [14–18]. Up to 25% of recipients have been documented as having a left fascicular block (Figure 6.5.2) [10, 14]. Both the cause and significance of these blocks have not been elucidated. Jessen and associates

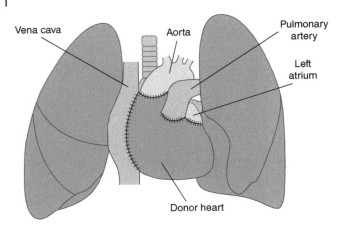

Figure 6.5.1 Donor heart in the orthotopic position. The posterior walls of the native left atrium and the great vessels are retained.

postulated the delays to be secondary to postoperative rotational forces leading to conduction abnormalities [19]. However, Marcus and colleagues, who followed transplant patients for almost a decade, observed that conduction delays developed over time and therefore argued against surgery being their cause [20].

Atrial enlargement is also a common finding (but not as common as dual P waves and conduction delays). During orthotopic transplantation, the recipient's posterior and lateral atrial walls are used to anchor the donor's ventricles, which produces abnormally shaped atria and presumably causes atrial enlargement (Figure 6.5.2) [7, 17, 21]. Pickham et al. calculated that left atrial enlargement was almost twice as common as right atrial enlargement [17]. Other theories of the cause of atrial enlargement suggest cellular rejection, but this connection has not been validated. Ventricular hypertrophy is seen in only a minority of cases and is a nonspecific finding.

Heterotopic heart transplantation is performed rarely, but it is useful in two clinical scenarios: in patients with irreversible pulmonary hypertension and when the donor's heart is too small to support the recipient's circulation. Heterotopic transplants are placed to the right of the native heart. Subsequent ECGs will show two independent dissociated ventricular rhythms (a dual ventricular pattern) (Figure 6.5.4) [22–25]. The polarity of the two rhythms can be unidirectional or bidirectional. If it is bidirectional (QRS complexes are alternating and shifting in axis) two other diagnoses should be excluded – digoxin poisoning and catecholamine induced polymorphic ventricular tachycardia.

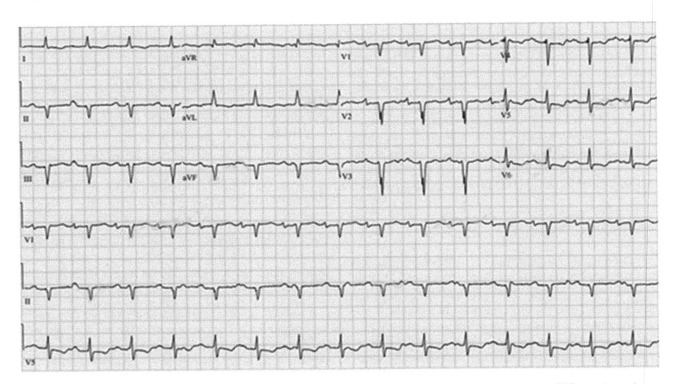

Figure 6.5.2 Orthotopic transplant resulting in dual P waves. The donor's P waves are being conducted to the QRS complexes, but the recipient's slower P waves are nonconducted. Note the small amplitude of the recipient's P waves. A left anterior fascicular block and left atrial enlargement are present. *Source:* From Dual Sinus Nodes – Heart Transplant ECG. Learn the Heart. https://www.healio. com/cardiology/learn-theheart/ecg-review/ecg-archive/dual-sinus-nodes-heart-transplant-ecg. Reprinted with permission from SLACK Incorporated.

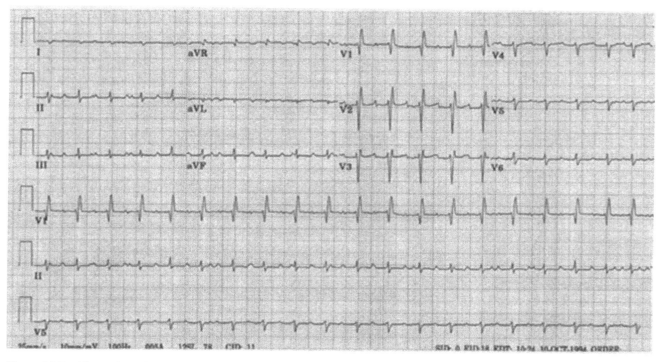

Figure 6.5.3 After orthotopic transplant, dual P waves are seen best in leads II and III. The recipient's nonconducted slower P waves come first, followed by the faster donor P waves, which are conducted to the QRS complexes. Also note the right axis deviation and rSR′ pattern of right bundle branch block (RBBB).

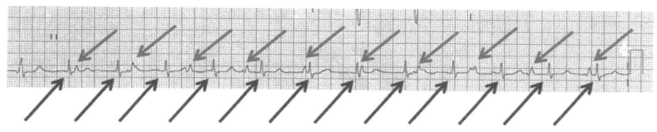

Figure 6.5.4 Heterotopic transplant: unidirectional dual ventricular rhythms (red, donor; purple, recipient).

When an arrhythmia develops in a heterotopic transplant recipient, ECG interpretation is challenging, given the dual conduction. To distinguish between the recipient and donor rhythms, first obtain a standard ECG to observe each rhythm. Then place the precordial leads successively in the dextrocardia position (to the right of the sternum), since that is where the donor heart is positioned. Leads V2R–V6R will represent the donor heart's true rhythm. Case reports of heterotopic transplantation illustrate that ventricular tachycardia and fibrillation (Figure 6.5.5) are more commonly observed in the native heart [10, 18]. When these dysrhythmias occur, they are often better tolerated than those after orthotopic procedures and do not carry the same risk of sudden cardiac death because of preserved cardiac hemodynamics [8].

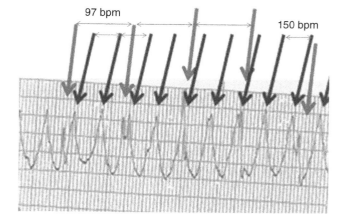

Figure 6.5.5 Heterotopic transplant: unidirectional dual ventricular rhythms (red, donor; blue, recipient). The native heart is displaying ventricular tachycardia.

Pearl: After heterotopic heart transplantations, ventricular fibrillation and tachycardia occur more commonly in the native heart.

Both orthotopic and heterotopic allografts experience conduction disturbances, most often in the immediate postoperative period [18, 26–28]. Typically, the rhythms are transient and resolve on their own [29]. The dysrhythmias most commonly encountered include bradycardia, atrioventricular block, and paroxysmal supraventricular tachycardia [16]. Sinus node dysfunction is infrequent but, when it does occur, permanent pacemaker placement is required [16]. The incidence of atrial fibrillation and flutter is lower after transplantation than after other cardiac operations; their sudden development has been associated with acute rejection [14]. Accelerated atherogenesis occurs after cardiac transplantation and can result in silent myocardial infarctions in up to 40% of recipients [26, 28]. Ventricular dysrhythmias are seen occasionally and are thought to develop as a complication of advanced coronary disease of the donor allograft [26, 28]. Nonspecific ST changes can occur during the immediate postoperative period, and they are classically transient [4, 10, 11, 22]. ST elevations followed by evolutionary ST- and/or T-wave changes are associated with postoperative pericarditis [5, 10, 14].

Conclusion

Advances in cardiac transplantation have greatly expanded the pool of transplant candidates and the length of time their transplants will be functional. Recipients of cardiac transplants, both orthotopic and heterotopic, face unique electrocardiographic manifestations (Table 6.5.1), which the astute clinician will know how to recognize and interpret.

Key Points

1) The transplanted heart is denervated and lacks autonomic control; therefore, an elevated resting heart rate can be expected.

References

1 Barnard, C.N. (1967). The operation. A human cardiac transplant: an interim report of a successful operation performed at Groote Schuur Hospital, Cape Town. *S. Afr. Med. J.* 41 (48): 1271–1274.

2 Barnard, C.N. (1968). Human cardiac transplantation. An evaluation of the first two operations performed at the Groote Schuur Hospital, Cape Town. *Am. J. Cardiol.* 22 (4): 584–596.

Table 6.5.1 Electrocardiographic manifestations of cardiac transplantation.

Increased resting heart rate	
Decreased 24-hour heart rate variability	
Bradydysrhythmias and AV blocks (most common during the postoperative period)	
Supraventricular tachydysrhythmias (most common during the postoperative period)	

Orthotopic	Heterotopic
Dual P waves (donor and recipient)	Dual ventricular rhythms
Intraventricular conduction	Uni/bidirectional tachycardia
Delays; complete or incomplete	Recipient/native dysrhythmias
RBBB	
Hemiblock	
Atrial enlargement	

2) The electrocardiograms (ECGs) of cardiac transplant patients often show dual P waves: one from the recipient and one from the donor.

3) The recipient's atrial remnants might respond to atropine, exercise, and hypotension, but the transplanted atria and ventricles will not exhibit the same response. Therefore, it is possible for a dysrhythmia to be present in one set of atria while a normal rhythm is present in the other, making ECG interpretation challenging.

4) Accelerated atherogenesis is well known to occur after cardiac transplantation. Silent myocardial infarctions occur in 30–40% of recipients.

5) After heterotopic heart transplantations, ventricular fibrillation and tachycardia occur more commonly in the native heart.

6) The role of electrocardiography in the diagnosis of rejection is controversial.

3 Lu, X., Dawson, J., and Borel, J.F. (1996). Effect of cyclosporine and some derivatives on chronic rejection. *Transplant. Proc.* 28 (6): 3152–3153.

4 Copeland, J.G. (1988). Cardiac transplantation. *Curr. Probl. Surg.* 25 (9): 607–672.

5 Miniati, D.N., Robbins, R.C., and Reitz, B.A. (2001). Heart and heart-lung transplantation. In: Heart Disease: A Textbook of

Cardiovascular Medicine (eds. E.Z.D. Braunwald and P. Libby), 615–634. Philadelphia: WB Saunders.

6 Cresci, S., Goldstein, J.A., Cardona, H. et al. (1995). Impaired left atrial function after heart transplantation: disparate contribution of donor and recipient atrial components studied on-line with quantitative echocardiography. *J. Heart Lung Transplant.* 14 (4): 647–653.

7 Stinson, E.B., Schroeder, J.S., Griepp, R.B. et al. (1972). Observations on the behavior of recipient atria after cardiac transplantation in man. *Am. J. Cardiol.* 30 (6): 615–622.

8 Dong, E. Jr., Fowkes, W.C., Hurley, E.J. et al. (1964). Hemodynamic effects of cardiac autotransplantation. *Circulation* 29 (suppl): 77–80.

9 Folino, A.F., Buja, G., Miorelli, M. et al. (1993). Heart rate variability in patients with orthotopic heart transplantation: long-term follow-up. *Clin. Cardiol.* 16 (7): 539–542.

10 Surawicz, B. and Knilans, T. (2001). Diseases of the heart and lungs. In: *Chou's Electrocardiography in Clinical Practice* (eds. B. Surawicz and T. Knilans), 256–309. Philadelphia: WB Saunders.

11 Bexton, R.S., Nathan, A.W., Hellestrand, K.J. et al. (1984). The electrophysiologic characteristics of the transplanted human heart. *Am. Heart J.* 107 (1): 1–7.

12 Butman, S.M., Phibbs, B., Wild, J., and Copeland, J.G. (1990). One heart, two bodies: insight from the transplanted heart and its new electrocardiogram. *Am. J. Cardiol.* 66 (5): 632–635.

13 Cooper, J.A., Saeed, I.M., Moazami, N., and Ewald, G.A. (2007). Images in cardiovascular medicine. Lost P's, but not yet forgotten. *Circulation* 115 (3): e41–e42.

14 Demangone, D. (2006). ECG manifestations: noncoronary heart disease. *Emerg. Med. Clin. North Am.* 24 (1): 113–131.

15 Gao, S.Z., Hunt, S.A., Wiederhold, V., and Schroeder, J.S. (1991). Characteristics of serial electrocardiograms in heart transplant recipients. *Am. Heart J.* 122 (3 Pt 1): 771–774.

16 Golshayan, D., Seydoux, C., Berguer, D.G. et al. (1998). Incidence and prognostic value of electrocardiographic abnormalities after heart transplantation. *Clin. Cardiol.* 21 (9): 680–684.

17 Pickham, D., Hickey, K., Doering, L. et al. (2014). Electrocardiographic abnormalities in the first year after heart transplantation. *J. Electrocardiol.* 47 (2): 135–139.

18 Scott, C.D., Dark, J.H., and McComb, J.M. (1992). Arrhythmias after cardiac transplantation. *Am. J. Cardiol.* 70 (11): 1061–1063.

19 Jessen, M.E., Olivari, M.T., Wait, M.A. et al. (1994). Frequency and significance of right bundle branch block after cardiac transplantation. *Am. J. Cardiol.* 73 (13): 1009–1011.

20 Marcus, G.M., Hoang, K.L., Hunt, S.A. et al. (2006). Prevalence, patterns of development, and prognosis of right bundle branch block in heart transplant recipients. *Am. J. Cardiol.* 98 (9): 1288–1290.

21 Babuty, D., Aupart, M., Casnay, P. et al. (1994). Electrocardiographic and electrophysiologic properties of cardiac allografts. *J. Cardiovasc. Electrophysiol.* 5 (12): 1053–1063.

22 Potenza, D., Vigna, C., Massaro, R. et al. (2008). Double rhythm in double heart. *J. Cardiovasc. Med. (Hagerstown)* 9 (6): 625–627.

23 Tagusari, O., Kormos, R.L., Kawai, A. et al. (1999). Native heart complications after heterotopic heart transplantation: insight into the potential risk of left ventricular assist device. *J. Heart Lung Transplant.* 18 (11): 1111–1119.

24 Vanderheyden, M., de Sutter, J., and Goethals, M. (1999). ECG diagnosis of native heart ventricular tachycardia in a heterotopic heart transplant recipient. *Heart* 81 (3): 323–324.

25 Badheka, A.O., Grover, P.M., Tanawuttiwat, T. et al. (2013). Dual ventricular rhythm. *JAMA Intern. Med.* 173 (13): 1246–1248.

26 Alexopoulos, D., Yusuf, S., Bostock, J. et al. (1988). Ventricular arrhythmias in long term survivors of orthotopic and heterotopic cardiac transplantation. *Br. Heart J.* 59 (6): 648–652.

27 Ali, A., Mehra, M.R., Malik, F.S. et al. (2001). Insights into ventricular repolarization abnormalities in cardiac allograft vasculopathy. *Am. J. Cardiol.* 87 (3): 367–368, A10.

28 Little, R.E., Kay, G.N., Epstein, A.E. et al. (1989). Arrhythmias after orthotopic cardiac transplantation. Prevalence and determinants during initial hospitalization and late follow-up. *Circulation* 80 (5 Pt 2): III140–III146.

29 Jacquet, L., Ziady, G., Stein, K. et al. (1990). Cardiac rhythm disturbances early after orthotopic heart transplantation: prevalence and clinical importance of the observed abnormalities. *J. Am. Coll. Cardiol.* 16 (4): 832–837.

Section VII

Electrocardiographic Differential Diagnosis

1

Abnormalities of the P Wave and PR Interval

Matthew Borloz

Department of Emergency Medicine, Carilion Clinic, Virginia Tech Carilion School of Medicine, Roanoke, VA, USA

The Normal P Wave

The P wave represents atrial depolarization, as well as the start of the cardiac electrical cycle. Atrial activation is normally initiated in or immediately around the sinoatrial (SA) node in the superior right atrium and proceeds toward the left atrium and the atrioventricular (AV) node. The duration of the normal P wave is less than 0.12 seconds (s), and the amplitude should be no greater than 0.25 millivolts (mV) in the frontal-plane leads and 0.15 mV in the transverse-plane leads.

The normal frontal-plane P-wave axis may be anywhere between 0 and +75° but typically ranges from +45 to +60°. The normal P wave is always positive in leads I and II and is usually positive in lead aVF. It is always negative in lead aVR. Regarding the transverse-plane leads, the P wave is typically biphasic in the right precordial leads (i.e. V1 and sometimes V2). The initial positive deflection represents right atrial activation and is followed by a negative deflection, as left atrial activation dominates the terminal portion of the wave and proceeds away from surface leads V1 and V2. The remainder of the precordial leads should display a positive P wave.

The Abnormal P Wave

Atrial Abnormality

The terms *right* and *left atrial abnormality* are preferred to such labels as right and left atrial enlargement, hypertrophy, overload, and conduction delay, as the P-wave changes attributed to these states are not specific for just one, and substantial crossover exists (Table 7.1.1) [1]. Differentiation of these conditions based on the surface electrocardiogram is fraught with error and should generally be avoided.

Numerous studies have examined the sensitivity and specificity of various criteria for right and left atrial *enlargement* using a reference standard of either echocardiography or cardiac magnetic resonance imaging. These studies have uniformly shown poor sensitivity but good specificity for right atrial enlargement, whereas criteria for left atrial enlargement have reasonable sensitivity and specificity (Table 7.1.2) [2, 3, 4, 5].

Because the SA node resides in the right atrium, this chamber is activated first and is represented by the initial portion of the P wave. Subsequent left atrial activation comprises the terminal portion of the P wave. Consequently, right atrial abnormality affects the early P wave, while left atrial abnormality affects the latter portion. Of the two, only left atrial abnormality should prolong the *duration* of the P wave (Figure 7.1.1).

Right Atrial Abnormality

Right atrial abnormality produces a tall (greater than 0.25 mV), peaked P wave in lead II and may shift the P-wave axis rightward (greater than +75°) (Figure 7.1.2a). This results in a P wave that is larger in lead III than in lead I. In addition, the initial positive P-wave deflection in leads V1 and V2 is amplified (greater than 0.15 mV) (Figure 7.1.2b).

Left Atrial Abnormality

Left atrial abnormality manifests as P-wave prolongation (greater than or equal to 0.12 s) with notching of the P wave in leads with similarly directed right and left P wave forces (i.e. those without biphasic P waves). A delay of greater than 0.04 s between the peaks of the notched P wave increases the specificity of this finding to near 100% (Figure 7.1.3a) [4]. In lead V1, the increased left atrial forces pull the terminal (negative) portion of the P wave further downward, resulting in an amplitude deeper than 0.10 mV

Electrocardiogram in Clinical Medicine, First Edition. Edited by William J. Brady, Michael J. Lipinski, Andrew E. Darby, Michael C. Bond, Nathan P. Charlton, Korin Hudson, and Kelly Williamson.

Table 7.1.1 Atrial abnormality may result from atrial volume/pressure overload, hypertrophy, enlargement, or conduction delay.

Right atrial abnormality	Left atrial abnormality
• Acute pulmonary illness – Pulmonary embolism – Asthma exacerbation • Chronic pulmonary disease (e.g. COPD) • Chronic pulmonary hypertension • Structural heart disease – Atrial septal defect – Ebstein anomaly – Pulmonic stenosis – Tricuspid stenosis	• Cardiomyopathy – Dilated – Hypertrophic – Restrictive • Coronary artery disease • Systemic hypertension (chronic) • Valvular disease – Mitral stenosis or insufficiency – Aortic stenosis or insufficiency

COPD = chronic obstructive pulmonary disease.

Table 7.1.2 Diagnostic criteria for atrial abnormality.

Right Atrial Abnormality
- Tall (>0.25 mV), peaked P waves in frontal-plane leads (best seen in II, III, aVF)[a]
- P-wave amplitude >0.15 mV in lead V1 and/or V2
- P-wave duration <0.12 s (normal)
- May have P-wave axis +75° or further rightward

Left Atrial Abnormality
- Wide P waves (≥0.12 s)
- Notched P waves in frontal-plane leads (best seen in I, II, aVL, V5, V6; inter-peak distance >0.04 s)[a]
- Prominent terminal negative P-wave deflection in lead V1 (>0.10 mV, >0.04 s)
- May have P wave axis +15° or further leftward

Biatrial Abnormality
- Components of both right and left atrial abnormality
- Increased P-wave amplitude (>0.25 mV) and width (≥0.12 s) in frontal-plane leads
- Peaked P wave (positive amplitude >0.15 mV) with prominent terminal negative deflection in lead V1 (>0.10 mV and/or >0.04 s)
- Wide (≥0.12 s), notched P waves in frontal-plane or lateral transverse-plane (V5 or V6) leads with tall, peaked P wave (positive amplitude >0.15 mV) in V1 and/or V2

[a] Most specific criterion (sensitivity of criteria vary widely among studies).

and an increase in the duration of this negative deflection to greater than 0.04 s (Figure 7.1.3b) [6]. The P-wave axis is directed leftward (generally left of +15°), producing a P wave in lead I that is larger than that in lead III.

Biatrial Abnormality

Biatrial abnormality manifests as a combination of the findings seen with right atrial abnormality and left atrial abnormality. The limb leads may show a prolonged (greater than or equal to 0.12 s) P wave with increased amplitude

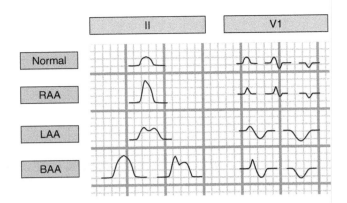

Figure 7.1.1 Atrial abnormality. Note the various P-wave morphologies seen with right, left, and bi-atrial abnormality in leads II and V1. Normal P-wave morphologies are also provided for comparison. RAA = right atrial abnormality, LAA = left atrial abnormality, BAA = biatrial abnormality.

(greater than 0.25 mV) (Figure 7.1.4). Another diagnostic criterion for biatrial abnormality requires a peaked P wave taller than 0.15 mV in lead V1 with a terminal portion deeper than 0.10 mV and/or wider than 0.04 s. Finally, a wide, notched P wave in the limb leads or lateral transverse-plane leads (V5 and V6), in combination with a tall (>0.15 mV), peaked P wave in the right precordial leads, also qualifies as biatrial abnormality.

Ectopic Atrial Foci

Atrial pacemakers distant from the SA node produce P waves of varying axis and morphology. These may be positive, biphasic, or negative in a given lead, depending on the particular location of the focus. If the pacemaker is low in the atria, the P wave will likely be negative in leads II, III, and aVF due to retrograde conduction away from the inferior leads (Figure 7.1.5).

Biphasic P Waves

Biphasic P waves are normal in leads V1 and V2 and may also be seen less commonly in leads III, aVL, and aVF; however, they should be completely positive or negative in the remaining leads (Figure 7.1.6). In the case of blocked conduction through Bachmann's bundle (which connects the right and left atria), an impulse generated in the superior right atrium in or around the SA node proceeds toward the AV node, then must cross to the left atrium and travel superiorly to activate the remainder of that chamber. This is known as interatrial block and often yields wide (at least 0.12 s) and biphasic (positive–negative) P waves in leads II, III, and aVF, as the left atrium is activated in a retrograde fashion away from those inferior leads [7]. Wide, notched P waves result from partial interatrial block in which conduction through Bachmann's bundle is slowed but not blocked entirely (Figure 7.1.7) [8, 9].

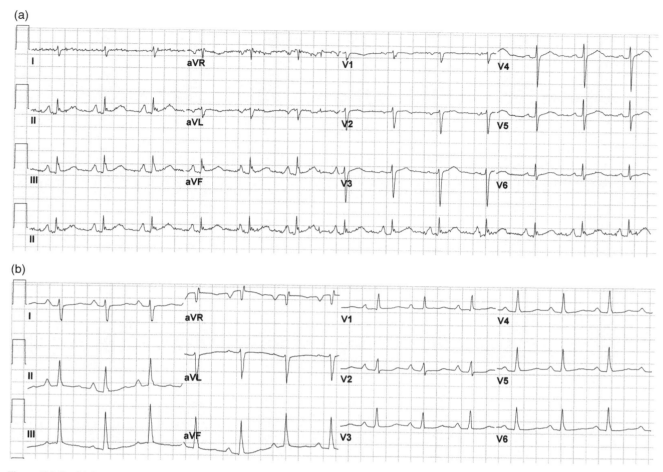

Figure 7.1.2 Right atrial abnormality. (a) Note the tall P waves ("P pulmonale" morphology) in lead II. Specifically, the amplitude of the upright P wave is >0.25 mV. In addition, the P-wave amplitude in lead III is greater than that in lead I, indicating a rightward shift of the P-wave axis. (b) Note the entirely positive P waves in leads V1 and V2 that are greater than 0.15 mV in amplitude.

Multifocal Atrial Tachycardia

Multifocal atrial tachycardia (MAT) is a chaotic atrial tachydysrhythmia that manifests with multiple (at least three) different P-wave morphologies that represent various atrial foci responsible for impulse generation. By definition, the ventricular rate must be greater than 100 bpm. Without a dominant focus in the SA node or atrial tissue, the rhythm may arise from anywhere in the atria, which leads to variability in the PP, PR, and RR intervals. This rhythm is most commonly seen transiently during periods of acute illness in patients with chronic lung disease (Figure 7.1.8). In order to differentiate this rhythm from atrial fibrillation, which is commonly seen in these same patients, an isoelectric baseline must be confirmed. If an isoelectric baseline is identified, and more than three P-wave morphologies exist, then the rhythm is a multifocal atrial rhythm. If no isoelectric baseline is present and it is difficult to identify distinct P waves, then the rhythm more likely represents atrial fibrillation.

The Normal PR Interval

The PR interval represents the time from the start of atrial activation to the onset of ventricular activation and can be shortened or lengthened by factors that affect the speed of conduction from the atria to the ventricles (Figure 7.1.9). It is measured from the start of the P wave through the start of the QRS complex and, therefore, includes both the P wave and the PR segment. The normal PR interval is 0.12–0.20 s (Figure 7.1.6). Infants and small children may have normal conduction with a PR interval shorter than this, though it is typically greater than 0.09 s.

The Abnormal PR Interval

Short PR Interval

An abnormally short PR interval results from conditions that allow faster conduction from the atria to the ventricles. This can occur with accessory conduction

(a)

(b)

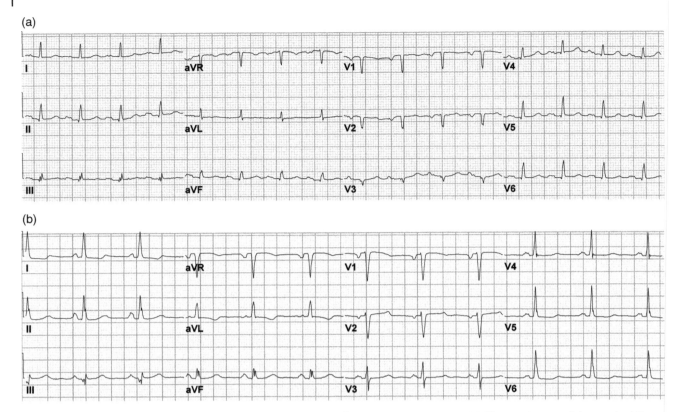

Figure 7.1.3 Left atrial abnormality. (a) Note the notched P wave ("P mitrale" pattern) in lead II. The two humps of the notched P wave are greater than 0.04 sec apart, which improves the specificity of this finding. (b) Note the deep and entirely negative P waves in lead V1. Some of the P waves in other leads are notched, but the distance between the humps is not greater than 0.04 sec, rendering this finding less reliable in confirming left atrial abnormality.

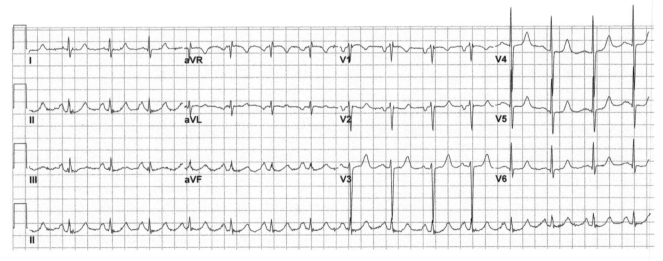

Figure 7.1.4 Biatrial abnormality. 70-year-old female with a history of diastolic heart failure presented with acute-on-chronic dyspnea. Biatrial enlargement was confirmed by echocardiography. Note the tall and wide P waves in lead II and the deep, almost entirely negative P waves in lead V1.

pathways that facilitate ventricular preexcitation by shortcircuiting normal conduction through the AV node or with exercise-induced sinus tachycardia. Other causes of a short PR interval likely to be seen on a resting ECG include junctional rhythms and ectopic atrial rhythms in which the site of atrial activation is in close proximity to the AV node (Table 7.1.3, Figure 7.1.10).

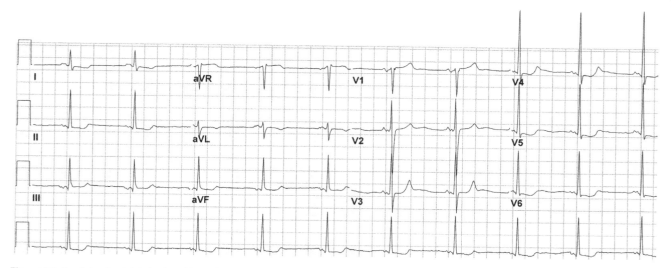

Figure 7.1.5 Ectopic atrial rhythm. Note the atypical P-wave morphology and axis. All of the P waves have the same morphology, suggesting that they all originate from the same ectopic focus.

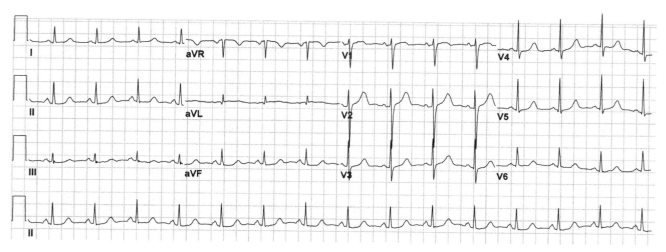

Figure 7.1.6 Normal P-wave morphology. Note the biphasic P waves in lead V1 and the negative P waves in lead aVR. Biphasic P waves would also be considered normal in leads V2, III, aVL, and aVF. The P wave duration is less than 0.12 sec, and the amplitude neither exceeds 0.25 mV in the frontal-plane leads nor 0.15 mV in the transverse-plane leads. Additionally, the PR interval is normal.

Figure 7.1.7 Interatrial block. Delayed conduction from the right atrium to the left atrium may manifest as changes in the P-wave morphology of the inferior leads. Partial interatrial block results in a prolonged (≥0.12 sec) P wave, often notched. Complete interatrial block causes retrograde atrial activation after the normal impulse reaches the tissue near the AV node. This retrograde activation is represented as a negative terminal deflection in the inferior leads. IAB = interatrial block.

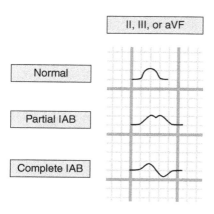

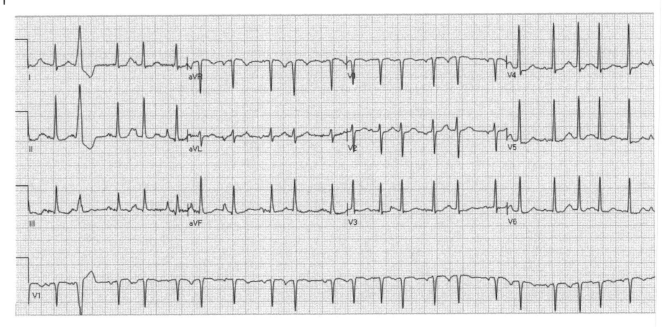

Figure 7.1.8 Multifocal atrial tachycardia (MAT). Note the irregular rhythm and multiple P-wave morphologies (at least 3 required for diagnosis).

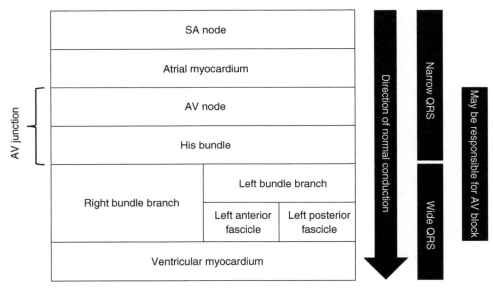

Figure 7.1.9 Normal atrioventricular conduction. Note that generation of an impulse from structures including and proximal to the His bundle can result in a narrow QRS complex (if no conduction delay is present distally), while those that originate distal to the His bundle produce a wide QRS complex. The "AV junction" refers to the AV node and His bundle. AV block can result from conduction delay or failure at any of the structures in the conduction system between the atrial and ventricular myocardia.

Preexcitation

Accessory pathways that allow for rapid conduction of atrial impulses to the ventricular myocardium result in a syndrome of ventricular preexcitation. One such example is the Wolff-Parkinson-White (WPW) pattern in which the so-called "bundle of Kent" allows for a portion of the ventricle to be activated sooner than the remainder of the ventricle that is dependent upon depolarization via the AV-His-Purkinje system. This yields a slurred QRS upstroke, known as a *delta wave,* which results in a shortened PR interval and (sometimes) a prolonged QRS interval (Figure 7.1.11). Individuals exhibiting these findings on a resting ECG are at risk for tachydysrhythmias.

Table 7.1.3 Causes of abnormal PR interval.

Short PR interval	Long PR interval[a]
• Exercise-induced sinus tachycardia	• Acute MI
• Junctional rhythms	– Anterior (usually permanent)
• Preexcitation	– Inferior (usually temporary)
• Thyrotoxicosis [10]	• Congenital heart disease
• Pheochromocytoma [11]	– Atrial septal defect
• Pompe disease [12]	– Ebstein anomaly
• Fabry disease [13]	• Connective tissue disease
	– Lupus (neonatal or adult) [14]
	– Marfan syndrome
	– Scleroderma
	• Hyperkalemia
	• Hypothermia
	• Hypothyroidism
	• Iatrogenic
	– Post ablation
	– Post valve surgery
	• Infection
	– Endocarditis
	– Lyme carditis [15]
	– Myocarditis
	– Toxoplasmosis
	• Infiltration
	– Amyloidosis
	– Sarcoidosis
	• Medications
	– Amiodarone
	– Beta-adrenergic receptor antagonists
	– Calcium channel antagonists[b]
	– Class IA and IC sodium channel antagonists
	– Digoxin
	• Neuromuscular disease (inherited)
	– Kearns-Sayre syndrome
	– Myotonic dystrophy [16]
	• Valve disease, calcific (aortic & mitral)

[a] The items listed can produce AV blocks of varying degrees.
[b] Non-dihydropyridine agents, such as diltiazem or verapamil
AV = atrioventricular; MI = myocardial infarction.

Similar preexcitation states are facilitated by Brechenmacher fibers, which extend from atrial tissue to the His bundle, and by James fibers, which serve as a bridge from the proximal AV node to the distal AV node. These both produce a short PR interval but no delta wave or widened QRS complex because the ventricular myocardium is ultimately activated through the His-Purkinje system; in such cases, at best, only the AV node is bypassed (Figure 7.1.12).

Ectopic Atrial Foci

Atrial impulses originating from ectopic sites distant from the SA node and near the AV node may also produce a short PR interval, simply due to the shorter distance for the impulse to travel prior to reaching the AV node. These are often labeled as having come from the AV junction (Figure 7.1.10).

Junctional Rhythms

If the electrical impulse is initiated within the AV junction (AV node or His bundle), conduction proceeds in both directions simultaneously – back up toward the atria and down toward the ventricles. If atrial activation occurs before ventricular activation, then a P wave may be seen, but it will appear immediately before the QRS complex and will likely be inverted, as the direction of conduction is away from the surface ECG leads. In many cases, the P wave is entirely obscured by the more dominant QRS complex, as ventricular activation often begins at the same time, or slightly before, atrial activation. In some cases, a P wave may even be seen in the terminal portion of the QRS complex, as the retrograde activation of the atria leads to depolarization, which occurs just after ventricular depolarization and in a direction away from the surface ECG leads (Figure 7.1.13). Certain types of junctional tachycardias produce similar findings, but clues other than the PR interval may be more helpful in guiding the clinician to these diagnoses.

Long PR Interval

First-Degree Atrioventricular Block

First-degree AV block is defined by a PR interval longer than 0.20 s with an otherwise normal appearing P wave of sinus origin. In addition, every P wave must be followed by a QRS complex, and every QRS complex is preceded by a P wave (Figure 7.1.14a and b). A variety of medical conditions and therapeutic agents are associated with PR prolongation (Table 7.1.3), and many of these conditions and medications may also lead to higher-degree AV blocks, which are discussed below. Asymptomatic and isolated first-degree AV block is of no immediate clinical significance.

Second-Degree Atrioventricular Block

Second-degree AV block differs from first-degree AV block in that not every P wave is followed by a QRS complex. There are two principal types of second-degree AV block – type I (Wenckebach or Mobitz type I) and type II (Mobitz type II).

In type I second-degree AV block, the PR interval progressively lengthens from beat to beat until a single QRS complex is dropped (Figure 7.1.15). That is, there is a P wave that is not followed immediately by a QRS complex.

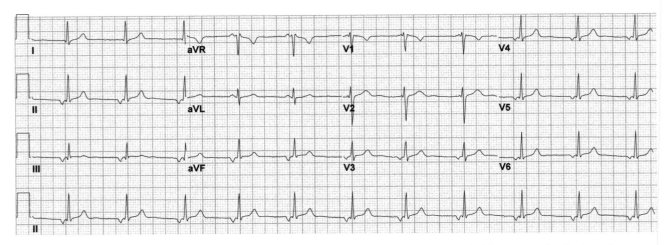

Figure 7.1.10 Ectopic atrial rhythm with short PR interval. This 16-year-old patient presented with a syncopal episode and was found to have an ectopic atrial rhythm with a short PR interval (0.10 sec). Repeat ECG several days later showed normal sinus rhythm with a normal PR interval.

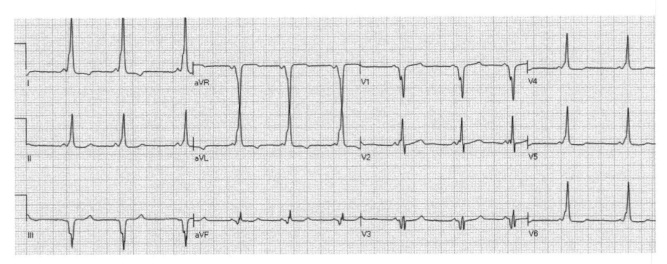

Figure 7.1.11 Wolff-Parkinson-White (WPW) pattern. Note the short PR interval, prolonged QRS interval, and prominent "delta wave." The latter is most easily seen in lead II and represents the ventricular preexcitation that defines this condition.

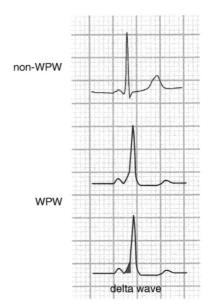

Figure 7.1.12 Ventricular preexcitation. The upper tracing is an example of a non-Wolff-Parkinson-White pattern of preexcitation in which the PR interval is shortened, but the QRS duration is normal and no delta wave is present. In this case, the accessory pathway delivers the impulse proximal to the ventricle after bypassing a portion of the normal conduction pathway. The middle and lower tracings show the classic pattern of WPW in which an atrioventricular accessory pathway results in a delta wave, a shortened PR interval, and a prolonged QRS duration.

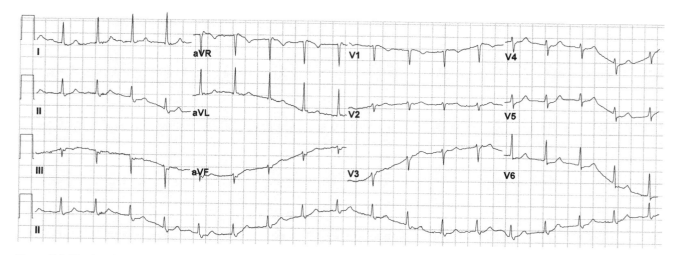

Figure 7.1.13 Accelerated junctional rhythm. Note the inverted P waves in the inferior leads that appear to merge with the end of the QRS complexes. Also, note the upright P waves (at the end of the QRS complexes) in lead aVR.

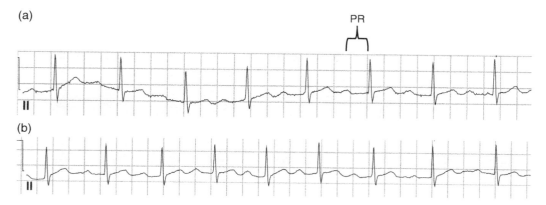

(a)

PR

(b)

Figure 7.1.14 (a) First-degree AV block. This 17-year-old male presented to the emergency department with complaint of palpitations. Note the prolonged PR interval, which measures 0.31 sec. (b) The PR interval shortens to 0.26 sec after the same patient engages in low-intensity exercise during the same visit. His PR interval was normal at a subsequent follow-up visit with cardiology. The cause for his first-degree AV block was not determined.

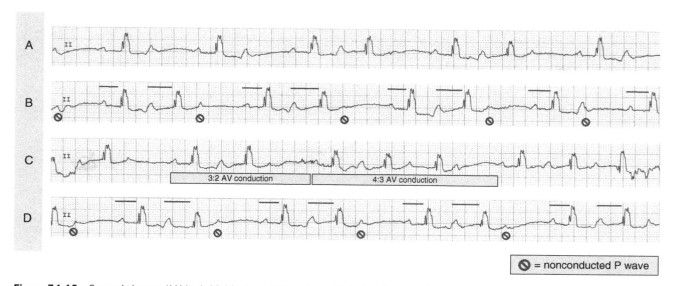

⊘ = nonconducted P wave

Figure 7.1.15 Second-degree AV block, Mobitz type I (Wenckebach). **Strip A** begins with second-degree AV block with 2:1 conduction, then displays Mobitz type I pattern. **Strip B** demonstrates 3:2 AV conduction with lengthening PR intervals until the third P wave in each series is dropped; it ends with reversion to 2:1 AV conduction. **Strip C** shows periods of both 3:2 and 4:3 AV conduction. **Strip D** shows consistent 3:2 AV conduction with the lengthening PR intervals and non-conducted P waves highlighted again.

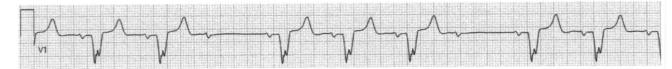

Figure 7.1.16   Second-degree AV block, Mobitz type II. This rhythm strip demonstrates a constant PR interval with failure to conduct every fourth beat. This would be described as 4:3 AV conduction, meaning that for every four atrial impulses, only three are conducted to the ventricles. Note that the QRS complexes are wide (left bundle branch block pattern), which is typical of Mobitz type II.

(a)

(b)

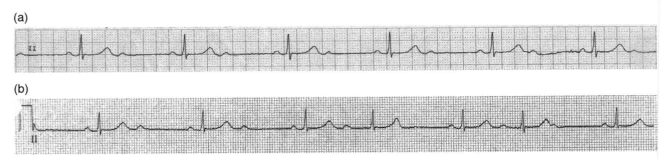

Figure 7.1.17   (a and b) Second-degree AV block with 2:1 AV conduction. Note that the first half of this strip does not allow differentiation between type I and type II second-degree AV block, but the latter half of the strip shows prolongation of the PR interval, followed by a non-conducted P wave, confirming a type I AV block.

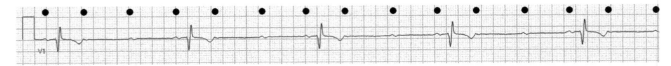

Figure 7.1.18   High-grade AV block with 3:1 conduction ratio. Note that there are three P waves for each QRS and that the PR interval of the conducted beats is constant. The fact that more than one consecutive P wave is not conducted renders this a "high-grade" or "advanced" AV block and differentiates it from a Mobitz II block. The black circles mark the P waves.

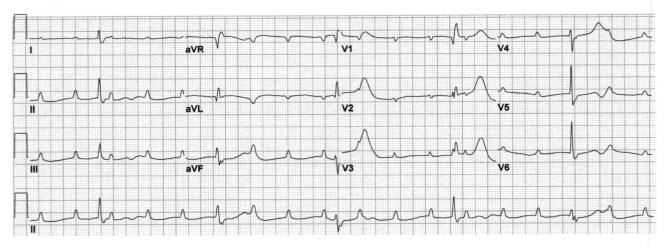

Figure 7.1.19   Third-degree AV block (complete heart block). This 67-year-old female presented to the emergency department after a syncopal episode and was experiencing periods of intermittent weakness and near syncope. This ECG was obtained during one of those periods and displays sinus tachycardia with complete heart block and a junctional escape rhythm with right bundle branch block. She was diagnosed with a non-ischemic cardiomyopathy of uncertain etiology and required permanent pacemaker placement.

The QRS duration is typically normal but may be wide, especially in conditions that also affect conduction via the His-Purkinje system or in the case of preexisting bundle branch block. The opposite is true of type II second-degree AV block in that the QRS complex is most often wide, but may be normal, as in the case of type II block at the His bundle (Figure 7.1.9).

In type II second-degree AV block, the PR interval is constant on every conducted beat, but not every P wave conducts to produce a QRS complex. The PR interval may be long or normal. The QRS complexes that do conduct are most often wide because the lesion is typically farther down the conduction system (usually in the bundle branches) than in type I block and, therefore, affects the QRS interval. In judging the severity of the block, it is useful to describe the conduction ratio in terms of the number of P waves generated to the number of QRS complexes that result. For example, if three of every four P waves are conducted, this would be described as an AV conduction ratio of 4 : 3 (Figure 7.1.16). Ratios of 4 : 3 or 3 : 2 are most common, but others may be seen. In addition, the ratio need not be constant over time, as a variety of dynamic factors influence AV conduction (e.g. sympathetic and parasympathetic tone, ischemia, circulating concentration of calcium channel or beta-adrenergic antagonists).

If the AV conduction ratio is seen to be 2 : 1, it is usually impossible to differentiate type I from type II second-degree AV block, as the progressive PR-interval lengthening that is characteristic of type I block cannot be seen (Figure 7.1.17a). Sometimes, a long rhythm strip reveals a variable conduction ratio over time. In this case, PR interval lengthening in consecutive cycles may be seen (Figure 7.1.17b). Because QRS complexes may be narrow or wide with either of these scenarios, QRS duration does not definitively identify the precise type of block, either. Autonomic influences that accelerate the atrial rate (e.g. anticholinergic medications, exercise) often improve AV conduction in the setting of type I block, while having no effect on, or potentially worsening, the conduction in type II block. On the contrary, vagal maneuvers may improve type II block by slowing the atrial rate and allowing more time for recovery of the infranodal conduction system between impulses. Demonstration of such changes in the severity of the block with these maneuvers may assist with the diagnosis, though expert consultation is advised.

So-called "high-grade" or "advanced" AV block can result from either type I or type II second-degree AV block and indicates significant risk for progression to complete heart block. Differentiation of the type of block that preceded the high-grade block (type I versus type II) is not immediately important. This condition is defined by an AV conduction ratio of 3 : 1 or greater. In other words, for every three sinus beats, only one QRS complex is seen (Figure 7.1.18). Similarly, a 4 : 1 AV conduction ratio would indicate that of four sinus beats, only one QRS complex results. Both the PR interval (of conducted beats) and the QRS duration in a high-grade block may be normal or prolonged.

Third-Degree Atrioventricular (Complete Heart) Block

In complete heart block, there is no meaningful communication between the atria and the ventricles (Figure 7.1.19). The atrial rate is independent of the ventricular rate, and the P waves and QRS complexes display no relationship to one another; this is referred to as AV dissociation. It is important to recognize, though, that third-degree AV block is but one type of AV dissociation; other types include junctional and ventricular tachycardias. The PP interval and the RR interval should be relatively constant, though the former may vary some as in the case of sinus arrhythmia. The PR interval, however, is variable. The QRS duration and ventricular rate are determined by the site of the escape focus. If this focus is within the His bundle, the QRS complex may be narrow, and the rate may be 40–60 bpm. Pacemakers distal to the His bundle typically generate a ventricular rate less than 40 beats per minute with wide QRS complexes.

Conclusion

While the P wave and PR interval are often overlooked as less important components of the electrocardiogram, when examined carefully, they can provide the clinician with critical information that directly impacts patient management. Indeed, close inspection of the P wave's morphology, amplitude, and duration, as well as its relation to the other components of the tracing (e.g. QRS complex and associated PR interval), reveals the anatomic focus of the rhythm in the majority of cases. This is certainly crucial for the electrocardiographic diagnosis and is often central to determining the origin of the patient's symptomatology.

References

1 Hancock, E.W., Deal, B.J., Mirvis, D.M. et al. (2009). AHA/ACCF/HRS recommendations for the standardization and interpretation of the electrocardiogram: part V: electrocardiogram changes associated with cardiac chamber hypertrophy: a scientific statement from the American Heart Association Electrocardiography and Arrhythmias Committee, Council on Clinical Cardiology; the American College of Cardiology Foundation; and the Heart Rhythm Society. *J. Am. Coll. Cardiol.* 53 (11): 992–1002.

2 Kaplan, J.D., Evans, G.T. Jr., Foster, E. et al. (1994). Evaluation of electrocardiographic criteria for right atrial enlargement by quantitative two-dimensional echocardiography. *J. Am. Coll. Cardiol.* 23 (3): 747–752.

3 Munuswamy, K., Alpert, M.A., Martin, R.H. et al. (1984). Sensitivity and specificity of commonly used electrocardiographic criteria for left atrial enlargement determined by M-mode echocardiography. *Am. J. Cardiol.* 53 (6): 829–832.

4 Tsao, C.W., Josephson, M.E., Hauser, R.H. et al. (2008). Accuracy of electrocardiographic criteria for atrial enlargement: validation with cardiovascular magnetic resonance. *J. Cardiovasc. Magn. Reson.* 10: 7.

5 Waggoner, A.D., Adyanthaya, A.V., Quinones, M.A., and Alexander, J.K. (1976). Left atrial enlargement. Echocardiographic assessment of electrocardiographic criteria. *Circulation* 54: 553–557.

6 Hopkins, C.B. and Barrett, O. Jr. (1989). Electrocardiographic diagnosis of left atrial enlargement. Role of the P terminal force in lead V1. *J. Electrocardiol.* 22 (4): 359–363.

7 Bayés de Luna, A., Platonov, P., Cosio, F.G. et al. (2012). Interatrial blocks. A separate entity from left atrial enlargement: a consensus report. *J. Electrocardiol.* 45: 445–451.

8 Ariyarajah, V., Asad, N., Tandar, A., and Spodick, D.H. (2005). Interatrial block: pandemic prevalence, significance, and diagnosis. *Chest* 128 (2): 970–975.

9 Bayés de Luna, A., Guindo, J., Viñolas, X. et al. (1999). Third-degree inter-atrial block and supraventricular tachyarrhythmias. *Europace* 1: 43–46.

10 Fadel, B.M., Ellahham, S., Ringel, M.D. et al. (2000). Hyperthyroid heart disease. *Clin. Cardiol.* 23: 402–408.

11 Huang, S.K., Rosenberg, M.J., and Denes, P. (1984). Short PR interval and narrow QRS complex associated with pheochromocytoma: electrophysiologic observations. *J. Am. Coll. Cardiol.* 3 (3): 872–875.

12 Jastrzebski, M. (2009). Short PR interval in Pompe disease. *J. Intern. Med.* 266: 571–572.

13 Aryana, A., Fifer, M.A., Ruskin, J.N., and Mela, T. (2008). Short PR interval in the absence of preexcitation: a characteristic finding in a patient with Fabry disease. *Pacing Clin. Electrophysiol.* 31 (6): 782–783.

14 Askanase, A.D., Friedman, D.M., Copel, J. et al. (2002). Spectrum and progression of conduction abnormalities in infants born to mothers with anti-SSA/Ro-SSB/La antibodies. *Lupus* 11 (3): 145–151.

15 van der Linde, M.R., Crijns, H.J., and Lie, K.I. (1989). Transient complete AV block in Lyme disease. *Chest* 96: 219–221.

16 Pelargonio, G., Dello Russo, A., Sanna, T. et al. (2002). Myotonic dystrophy and the heart. *Heart* 88: 665–670.

Additional Resources

Baltazar, R.F. (2009). *Basic and Bedside Electrocardiography*. Philadelphia: LWW.

Chan, T.C., Brady, W.J., Harrigan, R.A. et al. (eds.) (2005). *ECG in Emergency Medicine and Acute Care*. Philadelphia: Elsevier.

Goldberger, A.L., Goldberger, Z.D., and Schvilkin, A. (2013). *Clinical Electrocardiography: A Simplified Approach*, 8e. Philadelphia: Saunders.

Huszar, R.J. (2002). *Basic Dysrhythmias: Interpretation & Management*, 3e. St. Louis: Mosby.

Mirvis, D.M. and Goldberger, A.L. (2012). Electrocardiography. In: *Braunwald's Heart Disease: A Textbook of Cardiovascular Medicine*, 9e (ed. R.O. Bonow, D.L. Mann, D.P. Zipes and P. Libby), 126–167. Philadelphia: Saunders.

Surawicz, B. and Knilans, T.K. (eds.) (2008). *Chou's Electrocardiography in Clinical Practice*, 6e. Philadelphia: Saunders.

Wagner, G.S. (ed.) (2008). *Marriott's Practical Electrocardiography*, 11e. Philadelphia: LWW.

2

Differential Diagnosis of QRS Complex Abnormalities

Matthew Wilson, Michael Ybarra, and Munish Goyal

Department of Emergency Medicine, Georgetown University & MedStar Health, Washington, DC, USA

The QRS complex on the surface ECG represents ventricular depolarization of the myocardium as the electrical conduction moves infero-laterally through the heart. Ventricular depolarization normally lasts for 0.06–0.10 s and the QRS amplitude is typically less than 15 mm. In 725 healthy adult males, QRS duration ranged from 74 to 114 ms, with an average duration of 95 ms [1]. A prolonged QRS, more than 0.12 s in duration, signifies a conduction delay resulting from an anatomic, physiologic, iatrogenic, or toxicologic disruption of myocardial depolarization. Normal conduction varies somewhat with age. In children, who typically have a healthy conduction system, QRS prolongation of more than 100 ms may signify a conduction delay; whereas more than 34% of patients over 85 have a QRS prolongation in the form of a left bundle branch block (LBBB), reflecting underlying ventricular conduction delay [2]. Bundle branch blocks are described in detail later in this chapter.

Understanding the morphology of the normal QRS complex is essential to understanding the various pathologic alterations in its appearance. In a normal QRS complex the initial negative deflection, termed the "Q" wave, can be seen in I, aVL, and V4–V6 and is reflective of ventricular septal depolarization. This is followed by a positive deflection, termed the "R" wave, which reflects ventricular depolarization proceeding toward the infero-lateral leads and toward the precordial leads. The R wave is seen with progressing amplitude throughout the precordial leads V4–V6, which is termed R-wave progression. Finally, the second negative deflection to occur within the complex is termed the "S" wave and is reflective of depolarization of the high lateral wall of the left ventricle.

QRS Complex Abnormalities

The Large QRS Complex

An increased QRS amplitude (greater than 15 mm) is most commonly seen in ventricular hypertrophy, reflecting myocardial response of the right or left ventricle to longstanding increased afterload. Other causes of increased QRS amplitude to consider include hyperthyroidism [3], improper amplitude calibration of the ECG machine, or as a normal variant in young athletic individuals. The criteria for diagnosis of ventricular hypertrophy are discussed below.

Left Ventricular Hypertrophy

An increase in QRS amplitude has been correlated with ventricular hypertrophy by autopsy and imaging studies [4]. The ability to identify ventricular muscle hypertrophy is of significance in the maintenance of cardiovascular health and in the interpretation of acute ECG abnormalities. Various criteria have been developed to effectively identify ventricular hypertrophy and the sensitivity and specificity varies with different criteria as well as with patient age, gender, race, and body habitus [4]. A commonly used criterion involves calculation of the sum of the largest S-wave amplitude in V1 or V2 with the largest R-wave amplitude in V5 or V6. If this sum is greater than 35 mm, then the ECG is consistent with left ventricular hypertrophy (LVH) [4]. An additional criterion developed by Casale et al. identifies LVH when the sum of S in V3 and R in aVL is greater than 28 mm in men and greater than 20 mm in women [5] (Figure 7.2.1).

Electrocardiogram in Clinical Medicine, First Edition. Edited by William J. Brady, Michael J. Lipinski, Andrew E. Darby, Michael C. Bond, Nathan P. Charlton, Korin Hudson, and Kelly Williamson.

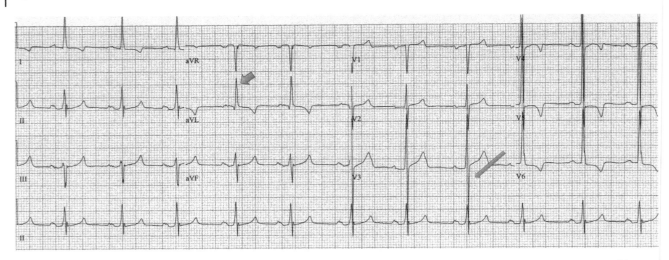

Figure 7.2.1   LVH by Casele Criteria with the sum of S wave in V3 (long arrow) and R wave in aVL (short arrow) greater than 28 mm.

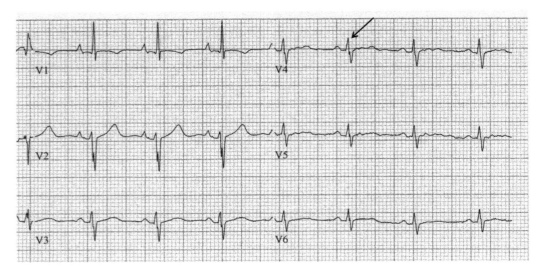

Figure 7.2.2   Right ventricular hypertrophy (RVH) demonstrated by an R wave greater than 6 mm in lead V1 (arrow).

Right Ventricular Hypertrophy

Identification of right ventricular hypertrophy (RVH) by ECG is more difficult than for LVH and the calculations have lower sensitivity. This is because of the larger mass of the left ventricle and its prominent position, which make it more "visible" to the standard-surface ECG leads. This means that significant RVH is necessary in order to be evident on the ECG as a rightward and anterior shift of the QRS vector. An inversion of the pattern seen in LVH can be reflective of RVH when the R wave is greater than 6 mm in V1 or S wave is greater than 10 mm in V5 or greater than 3 mm in V6 [4]. (Figure 7.2.2) Right-axis deviation should also be seen when considering the diagnosis of RVH. However, right-axis deviation alone is not a specific finding as it may also be seen as a normal variant or as a reflection of increased lung volume in chronic obstructive pulmonary disease (COPD) patients. In order to make the diagnosis of RVH the overall clinical picture is more important than in LVH given the lower sensitivity of electrocardiographic criteria [4].

The Small QRS Complex

A small QRS amplitude (less than 5 mm) is seen less often than the large amplitude QRS and its implications are somewhat less specific. It is most commonly seen in conditions that decrease conduction to the surface electrodes such as obesity, COPD (from an increased chest wall diameter) and in a few cardiac anatomical processes such as amyloidosis, pericardial effusion, and loss of myocardial muscle mass following infarction. It can also be seen in systemic disease states like hypothyroidism/myxedema [3]. For a large pericardial effusion, one may also see electrical alternans with rhythmical beat-to-beat variation in the

Figure 7.2.3 Electrical alternans- note both the generally low voltage QRS complexes as well as the alternating height of consecutive beats in the patient with a pericardial effusion. *Source:* Adapted with permission from LITFL ECG Library: http://lifeinthefastlane.com/ecg-library/electrical-alternans.

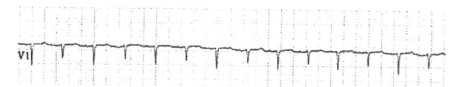

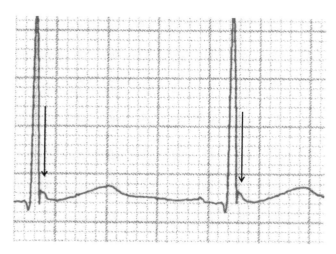

Figure 7.2.4 Osborn wave is a positive deflection occurring immediately following the QRS segment. It is usually a sign of profound hypothermia.

QRS amplitude reflective of the heart moving within the pericardial fluid (Figure 7.2.3).

The Wide QRS Complex

The widened QRS complex (greater than 120 ms) reflects a delay in ventricular conduction and has the broadest differential for clinicians. A widened QRS complex can occur in relatively benign conditions such as ectopic beats and ventricular paced rhythms, it can portend a risk for sudden cardiac death in the case of ventricular preexcitation, or it may be an ominous sign of a toxicologic emergency such as hyperkalemia or sodium channel blockade. It may also be seen in wide-complex tachydysrhythmias (discussed in a separate chapter), an incorrectly calibrated ECG machine, or in cases of severe hypothermia as the "J" wave or "Osborn wave" repolarization abnormality (Figure 7.2.4). Finally, QRS prolongation is seen in intraventricular conduction delays (bundle branch blocks), which are discussed in the next section of this chapter.

Ectopic Beats

Ectopic beats may arise from anywhere in the cardiac cycle. Premature atrial contractions (PACs) and premature junctional contractions (PJCs) are described elsewhere in this

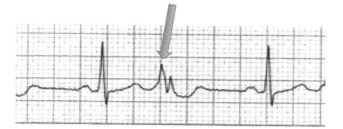

Figure 7.2.5 Ectopic beat: the arrow indicates a premature ventricular contraction or PVC. Note that there are normal sinus beats both preceding and following the wide, abnormal QRS complex.

text and arise from the atria and AV node, respectively. These ectopic beats tend to have narrow QRS morphologies. By contrast, a wide complex ectopic beat represents the premature depolarization of the ventricular myocardium. They can be identified by their irregular shape and widened QRS complex (greater than 120 ms). The widened QRS occurs because the electrical impulse does not originate from the SA node and does not follow the typical conduction system pathway. Because they are not responding to the underlying/intrinsic atrial rhythm, ectopic beats occur at irregular intervals. They are followed by a T wave that reflects ventricular repolarization, though these T waves also have an irregular appearance. Ectopic ventricular beats are then followed by a compensatory pause that represents the time required for the repolarization of the myocardium and is reflected on the ECG as a mild prolongation of the RR interval before resumption of sinus rhythm. Common causes of ectopic beats include electrolyte abnormalities, stimulants, medications, and underlying heart disease. They may also be seen as part of normal aging [6]. Ectopic beats have been described in 1% of normal patients on ECG and are seen during Holter monitoring in 40–75% of patients [7] (Figure 7.2.5).

Ventricular Paced Rhythm

Prolonged QRS complex duration may also be the result of ventricular pacing. With the initial (extrinsic) electrical impulse originating outside of the His-Purkinje system, delayed depolarization may occur across the ventricular myocardium, which will prolong the QRS complex to greater than 120 ms. Ventricular paced rhythms are

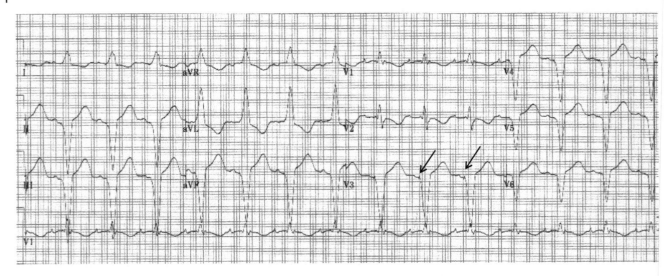

Figure 7.2.6 Ventricular paced rhythm- though the pacer spikes (arrows) may be difficult to identify in some cases, along with a broad QRS complex with discordant ST elevation (directed to the opposite side of the isoelectric baseline when compared to the QRS complex) in leads with a predominantly negative QRS, they can help identify the ventricular paced rhythm.

identifiable by vertical pacing spike at the beginning of the QRS complex [8] (Figure 7.2.6).

Preexcitation

According to the American Heart Association (AHA), ventricular preexcitation is defined by a PR interval less than 120 ms during sinus rhythm in adults, less than 90 ms in children, with slurring of initial portion of the QRS complex (also called the *delta wave*), which either interrupts the P wave or arises immediately after the P termination of the P wave [9]. This depolarization abnormality was initially described in 1930 when Wolff, Parkinson, and White described the "combination of bundle branch block, abnormally short PR interval, and paroxysms of tachycardia occurring in young, healthy patients with normal hearts" [10] (Figure 7.2.7).

The estimated prevalence of the Wolff–Parkinson–White (WPW) pattern is 0.1–0.3% [11], which is significant because these patients may develop episodes of symptomatic tachycardia. Tachydysrythmia occurs because conduction can travel both through the His-Purkinje pathway or the accessory pathway, represented on ECG by the delta wave. This bidirectional circuit allows rapid re-conduction of impulses from the atria to the ventricles and back, which can result in a symptomatic supraventricular tachycardia. In some cases, rapid conduction over the accessory pathway precipitates ventricular fibrillation and sudden death. The accessory pathway bypasses the protective AV node, which would otherwise act to limit the electrical activity that reaches the ventricle [11].

The WPW syndrome is often identified by the presence of a delta wave during normal conduction. It is more

difficult to identify during rapid reentry conduction. The delta wave may not even be seen in orthodromic AV reciprocating tachycardia where conduction proceeds along the normal conduction pathway but returns to the atria via the accessory pathway. In antidromic AV reciprocating tachycardia, atrial impulses are first conducted to the ventricle via the accessory pathway resulting in a prolonged depolarization and then return back to the atria along the bundle of His creating a wide complex tachycardia that appears similar to ventricular tachycardia [10].

The WPW syndrome and conduction abnormalities are discussed further elsewhere in this text.

Hyperkalemia

Hyperkalemia results in progressive conduction changes throughout the myocardium, which can create various abnormalities on ECG. With increasing intracellular potassium the concentration gradient for potassium is decreased, thus making the resting membrane potential of the myocardial cell more negative. This limits the number of available sodium channels for depolarization, which slows conduction through the myocardium, which is reflected on ECG by QRS prolongation [12] (Figure 7.2.8). The cardiovascular and ECG changes resulting from progressive hyperkalemia are described in Figure 7.2.9 but the development of these findings may occur at different serum concentrations depending on the rate of change in potassium [3].

Sodium Channel Blockade

There are a number of medications that cause sodium channel blockade in the cardiac myocytes. These drugs in overdose can be rapidly fatal. The effects of sodium channel

Figure 7.2.7 Wolf–Parkinson–White syndrome; preexcitation identified by the presence of a "delta" wave (see arrow), or slurred upstroke, during normal conduction.

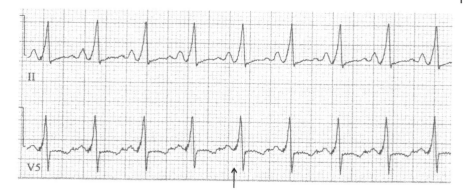

Figure 7.2.8 Hyperkalemia. Panel (a) demonstrates early hyperkalemia with tall, narrow, and peaked T waves (arrows). Panel (b) shows more severe changes with widened QRS complexes leading to the classic "sine wave" appearance.

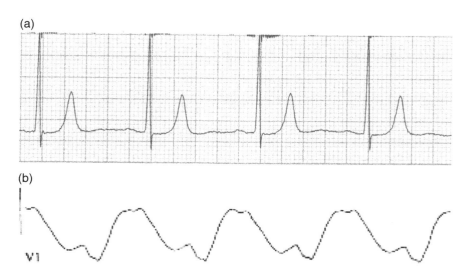

Figure 7.2.9 Expected ECG changes associated with elevated levels of serum potassium.

Potassium Level (mmol/l)	ECG Changes	Explanation
5.5–6.5	Tall, narrow, and peaked T waves	Only about one in five will have this classic appearance [4]
6.5–7.5	P wave widens and flattens and the PR segment lengthens	With rising potassium concentration the P wave may disappear
7.0–8.0	QRS Widening affecting all portions of the QRS complex	As the QRS continues to widen it may merge with the T Wave to creating a sine wave pattern (pre-terminal)
>8.0	Asystole, ventricular fibrillation, or a wide pulseless idioventicular rhythm	Death may result from these rhythms which reflect loss of sinoatrial conduction

blocking agents were initially described as "Quinidine-like" after Quinine, an early type 1A anti-arrhythmic derived from the bark of the cinchona tree. Now, the most well-known sodium channel blocking agents are the tricyclic antidepressants (Figure 7.2.10).

Pharmacologic blockade of the cardiac myocyte sodium channel current decreases the rate of depolarization, which is reflected as QRS prolongation on ECG. Severe blockade ultimately progresses to a sine wave pattern, asystole, or ventricular tachycardia, which is thought to result from the

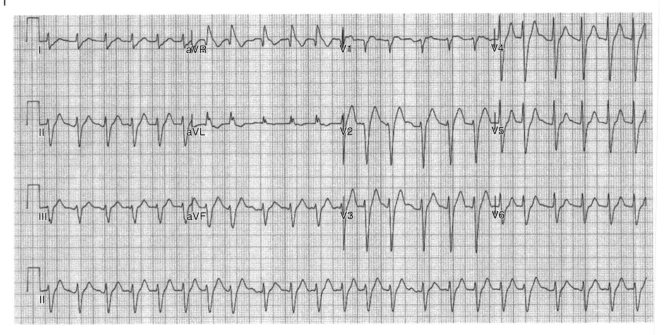

Figure 7.2.10 Sodium channel blockade- pharmacologic blockade of the cardiac myocyte sodium channel current decreases the rate of depolarization, which is reflected as QRS prolongation on ECG. *Source:* Reprinted with permission from LITFL ECG Library. http://lifeinthefastlane.com/resources/ecg-database.

slowing of intraventricular conduction to the point that reentrant tachycardia occurs. Sodium channel blockade also directly lowers cardiac inotropy resulting in profound, refractory hypotension [13].

Early recognition and treatment of a sodium channel blocking agent overdose is imperative for successful management. QRS prolongation from sodium channel blockade has been associated with arrhythmias and increased mortality [14]. ECG abnormalities precede symptomatology; seizures or ventricular arrhythmias are generally not seen if the QRS is less than 0.10 s whereas a QRS greater than 0.16 s is associated with ventricular arrhythmias [15]. An early sign of toxicity may be detected on ECG as rightward axis shift in the terminal 40 ms of the QRS complex in the frontal plane. This "may be reliably detected by a negative deflection of the final portion of the QRS complex in lead I (a deep S wave), and a positive deflection of the terminal portion of lead aVR (a large R wave)" [15]. This "R" in aVR, when 3 mm or more, has been associated with the development of seizures or arrhythmias after an acute tricyclic antidepressant overdose [16]. Patients with a tricyclic overdose have been shown to have a more rightward terminal 40 ms frontal plane QRS vector thought to be related to increased susceptibility of the right side of the heart to sodium channel blocking activity [17]. A list of medications with sodium channel blocking activity is found in Figure 7.2.11.

Sodium Channel Blockers
Antidysrhythmics:
Ajmaline, Aprindine, Cibenzoline, Disopyramide, Encainide, Flecainide, Lidocaine, Lorcainide, Mexiletine, Moricizine, Pilsicainide, Procainamide, Propafenone, Quinidine, Amiodarone
TCAs:
Amitriptyline, Desipramine, Imipramine, Nortriptyline, Maprotiline, Amoxapine
Sympathomimetics:
Cocaine
Antiepileptics:
Carbamazepine, Lamotrigine, Phenytoin
Antimalarials:
Chloroquine, Quinine
Antipsychotics/antidepressants:
Bupropion, Citalopram, Fluoxetine, Risperidone, Venlafaxine, Thioridazine
Anesthetics:
Bupivacaine, Procaine, Ropivacaine
Others:
Amodiaquine, Desethylamodiaquine, Diltiazem, Diphenhydramine, Dolasetron, Mesoridazine, Perhexiline

Figure 7.2.11 Medications with sodium channel blocking effects.

Intraventricular Blocks

One of the most common causes of a widened QRS is intraventricular block. In cases of intraventricular conduction delay or bundle branch block, QRS prolongation may reflect an underlying change in the intrinsic electrical conduction of the heart. Intraventricular conduction delay may occur acutely in the setting of myocardial infarction or may occur chronically with longstanding cardiovascular or systemic

Figure 7.2.12 Description of criteria for right and left bundle branch blocks.

Left Bundle Branch Block	Right Bundle Branch Block
Delay in conduction along the left bundle of His-Purkinje System	Delay in conduction along the right bundle of the His-Purkinje System
Prolonged QRS duration (> 120 ms)	Prolonged QRS duration (> 120 ms)
Broad, notched R wave in V5, V6, I, and aVL	RSR' is seen in leads V1 and V2 (R' represents the second positive repolarization of the QRS complex

Figure 7.2.13 Right bundle branch block as demonstrated by a prolonged QRS and RSR' pattern in leads V1 and V2.

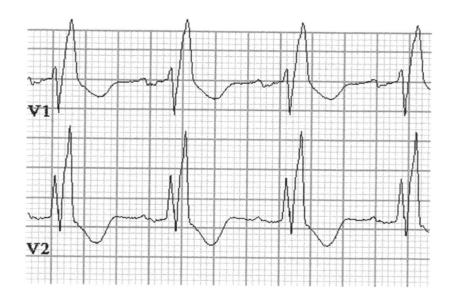

disease. Intraventricular blocks are categorized as right or LBBBs. Individual fascicles of the left bundle (anterior and posterior) may also be involved. A summary of characteristics for left and right bundle branch blocks is seen in Figure 7.2.12.

A right bundle branch block (RBBB) reflects a delay in conduction along the right bundle of the His-Purkinje system. A prolonged QRS (greater than 120 ms) is required for the diagnosis. Recall that when an R wave (the positive repolarization within the QRS complex) is seen twice it is termed an R' or "R prime" wave. The R' is wider than the initial R wave. In RBBB an rsr', rsR', or rSR' should be seen in leads V1 or V2 (Figure 7.2.13). The S wave is typically of greater duration than the R wave in leads I and V6. Finally, if the typical rsR' pattern is seen but there is no QRS prolongation then the pattern is described as an incomplete RBBB [9].

A LBBB (Figure 7.2.14) reflects a delay in conduction along the left bundle of the His-Purkinje system. In LBBB, the QRS is prolonged (greater than 120 ms) and a broad, notched or slurred R wave is seen in leads I, aVL, V5, and V6. Occasionally an RS pattern is seen in V5 and V6. A

LBBB is termed incomplete with the presence of the LBBB pattern in V4, V5, or V6 but a QRS of normal width [9].

The fascicular blocks reflect isolated conduction disturbances along the anterior or posterior fascicles of the left bundle. A left anterior fascicular block (LAFB, Figure 7.2.15) is diagnosed on ECG by the presence of left-axis deviation, a qR in aVL, and an R-peak time in lead aVL is 45 ms or more. A left posterior fascicular block (LPFB, Figure 7.2.16) is diagnosed on ECG by the presence of right-axis deviation, an rS pattern in leads I and aVL, and a qR pattern in leads III and aVF. A bifascicular block is the combination of two bundle branch blocks (RBBB and either LAFB or LPFB) and a trifascicular block (Figure 7.2.17) is a bifascicular block with the addition of first-degree AV block.

To conclude, there are many etiologies for QRS abnormalities, and many of them have serious etiologies, reflective of intrinsic heart disease, overdose, or lethal electrolyte abnormalities. The astute clinician must be able to differentiate the benign from the potentially deadly in a timely fashion by coupling ECG findings with the patient's clinical picture.

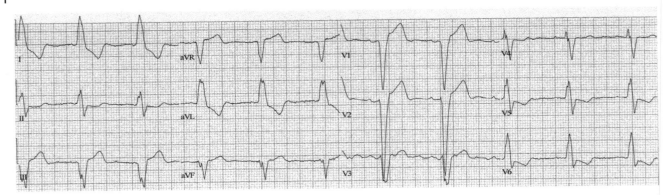

Figure 7.2.14 Left bundle branch block (LBBB with a wide QRS with a broad R wave in leads I, aVL, V5 and V6 and an RS pattern in leads V5 and V6.

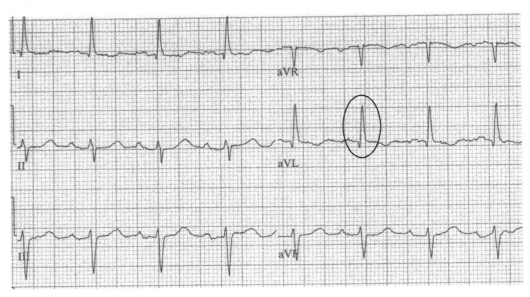

Figure 7.2.15 Left anterior fascicular block (LAFB) diagnosed by the presence of left axis deviation, a qR in lead aVL (circled), and a R peak time > 45 ms.

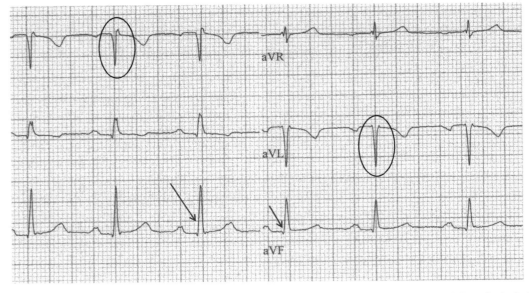

Figure 7.2.16 Left posterior fascicular block (LPFB) diagnosed on ECG by the presence of right-axis deviation, an rS pattern in leads I and aVL (circled), and a qR pattern in leads III and aVF (arrows).

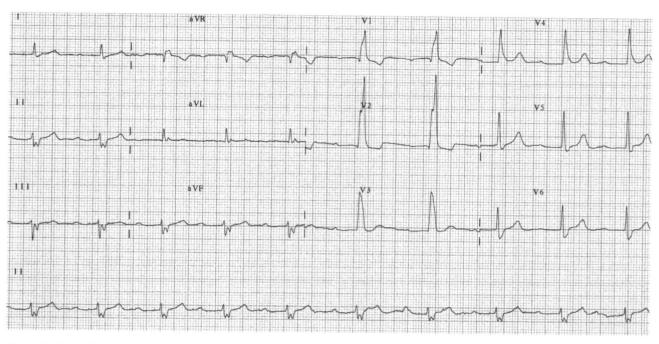

Figure 7.2.17 Trifascicular block is the presence of two intra-ventricular blocks (a RBBB and either a LAFB or LPFB) in the presence of a coexisting first-degree AV block. Here RBBB with LAFB and first-degree AVB. *Source:* Reprinted with permission from LITFL ECG Library. http://lifeinthefastlane.com/resources/ecg-database.

References

1 MacFarlane, P.W. and Lawrie, T.D.V. (1989). The normal electrocardiogram and vector cardiogram. In: *Comprehensive Electrocardiology: Theory and Practice in Health Disease* (eds. P.W. Macfarlane and T.D.V. Lawrie), 424–449. New York: Pergamon Press.

2 Samaras, N., Chevalley, T., Samaras, D., and Gold, G. (2010). Older patients in the emergency department: a review. *Ann. Emerg. Med.* 56 (3): 261–269.

3 Slovis, C. and Jenkins, R. (2002 June 1). ABC of clinical electrocardiography conditions not primarily affecting the heart. *BMJ* 324 (7349): 1320–1323.

4 Hancock, E.W., Deal, B.J. et al. (2009). AHA/ACCF/HRS recommendations for the standardization and interpretation of the electrocardiogram part V: electrocardiogram changes associated with cardiac chamber hypertrophy a scientific statement from the American Heart Association electrocardiography and arrhythmias committee, council on clinical cardiology; the American College of Cardiology Foundation; and the Heart Rhythm Society *Endorsed by the International Society for Computerized Electrocardiology. J. Am. Coll. Cardiol.* 53 (11).

5 Casale, P., Devereux, R., Kligfield, P. et al. (1985). Electrocardiographic detection of left ventricular hypertrophy: development and prospective validation of improved criteria. *J. Am. Coll. Cardiol.* 6: 572–580.

6 Hebbar, A.K. and Hueston, W.J. (2002 Jun 15). Management of common arrhythmias: part II. Ventricular arrhythmias and arrhythmias in special populations. *Am. Fam. Physician* 65 (12): 2491–2497.

7 Ng, A. (2006). Treating patients with ventricular ectopic beats. *Heart* 92: 1707–1712.

8 Barold, S. and Herweg, B. (2011). Usefulness of the 12-lead electrocardiogram in the follow-up of patients with cardiac resynchronization devices. Part I. *Cardiol. J.* 18 (5): 476–486.

9 Surawicz, B., Childers, R. et al. (2009). Recommendations for the standardization and interpretation of the electrocardiogram part III: intraventricular conduction disturbances a scientific statement from the American Heart Association Electrocardiography and Arrhythmias Committee, Council on Clinical Cardiology; the American College of Cardiology Foundation; and the Heart Rhythm Society *Endorsed by the International Society for Computerized Electrocardiology. Circulation* 119: e235–e240.

10 Rosner, M., Brady, W., Kefer, M., and Martin, M. (1999). Electrocardiography in the patient with the Wolff-Parkinson-White syndrome: diagnostic and initial therapeutic issues. *Am. J. Emerg. Med.* 17: 705–714.

11 Lerman, B. and Basson, C. (November 6, 2003). High-risk patients with ventricular preexcitation — a pendulum in motion. *NEJM* 349 (19).

12 Parham, W., Mehdirad, A., Biermann, K., and Fredman, C. (2006). Hyperkalemia revisited. *Tex. Heart Inst. J.* 33 (1): 40–47.

13 Koleck, P. and Curry, S. (Oct 1997). Medical toxicology: poisoning by sodium channel blocking agents. *Crit. Care Clin.* 13 (4).

14 Harmer, A.R., Valentin, J.P., and Pollard, C.E. (2011). On the relationship between block of the cardiac Na+ channel and drug-induced prolongation of the QRS complex. *Br. J. Pharmacol.* 164: 260–273.

15 Harrigan, R.A. and Brady, W.J. (1999 Jul). ECG abnormalities in tricyclic antidepressant ingestion. *Am. J. Emerg. Med.* 17 (4): 387–393.

16 Liebelt, E.L., Francis, P.D., and Woolf, A.D. (August 1995). ECG lead aVR versus QRS interval in predicting seizures and arrhythmias in acute tricyclic antidepressant toxicity. *Ann. Emerg. Med.* 26: 195–201.

17 Niemann, J.T., Bessen, H.A., Rothstein, R.J. et al. (1986). Electrocardiographic criteria for tricyclic antidepressant cardiotoxicity. *Am. J. Cardiol.* 57: 1154–1159.

3

Differential Diagnosis of ST Segment Changes

Korin Hudson[1] and Norine McGrath[2]

[1]*Department of Emergency Medicine, MedStar Georgetown University Hospital, Georgetown University School of Medicine, Washington, DC, USA*
[2]*Department of Emergency Medicine, Georgetown University & MedStar Health, Washington, DC, USA*

Introduction

On the standard 12-lead surface ECG, the ST segment represents the electrical activity that occurs between ventricular depolarization (QRS complex) and repolarization (T wave). The normal ST segment is isoelectric, that is, neither elevated nor depressed when compared to the baseline, defined by the preceding T–P segment (Figure 7.3.1). ST-segment elevation (STE) and depression may be caused by a number of conditions with a wide range of clinical significance and severity.

Describing ST-Segment Changes

The differential diagnosis of acute ST segment changes is broad (Table 7.3.1), and the astute clinician will use additional clues from the patient history, physical exam, and the ECG to help make the diagnosis. Closer analysis of the ST segment itself may be very helpful in ascertaining the etiology and diagnosis of the underlying syndrome. When evaluating both ST segment elevation and ST segment depression (STD) it is often helpful to describe the changes in terms of *distribution*, described by which anatomic leads reflect the abnormality, and *morphology*, including both the *contour* or shape as well as the *amplitude* of the ST segment.

The amplitude of the ST segment deviation is defined by the deviation in mm above or below the isoelectric baseline. When evaluating STE, it is important to remember that the total amount of ST segment elevation – that is, the total mm of elevation across all leads – will generally be greater in the patient who is suffering from an acute MI (AMI) than will be seen in the noninfarction patient. However, in some conditions the STE may be quite subtle (Figure 7.3.2).

The contour of the STD segment is generally described as upsloping or downsloping, referencing whether the wave is moving toward or away from the isoelectric baseline (moving left to right on the page). In general, when evaluating morphology of STD, upsloping STD is less often associated with an acute ischemic event while STD that is flat, horizontal, or parallel to the isoelectric baseline and down-sloping STD is more often associated with ACS (Figure 7.3.3). However, nonischemic etiologies may result in the flat or downsloping morphologies as well.

The morphology of STE is determined by considering the shape of the initial up-sloping portion of the ST segment beginning at the J-point (the junction point between the QRS complex and the ST segment) and ending at the apex of the T wave. The elevated ST segment can assume one of three distinct morphologies: concave, obliquely straight, or convex (Figure 7.3.4) While any of these morphologies may be associated with STEMI, the obliquely straight (Figure 7.3.4a) and/or convex STE (Figure 7.3.4b) are more frequently associated with STEMI, while the concave shape (Figure 7.3.4c) is less often associated with acute ischemic events. However, it is important to recall that concave STE may be seen in STEMI, particularly early in the course of an acute infarction [1–3].

The anatomic distribution of ST segment changes should be considered as well- though this criteria is less helpful in determining ACS from non-ACS syndromes. In general, more widespread STE is associated with nonischemic etiologies while localized changes, associated with anatomic or regional myocardial damage, occur more often in patients with ACS. Similarly, the anatomic distribution of STE/STD may provide clues to the diagnosis with specific patterns seen with certain conditions (i.e. bundle branch block, ventricular hypertrophy with strain pattern, and

Electrocardiogram in Clinical Medicine, First Edition. Edited by William J. Brady, Michael J. Lipinski, Andrew E. Darby, Michael C. Bond, Nathan P. Charlton, Korin Hudson, and Kelly Williamson.

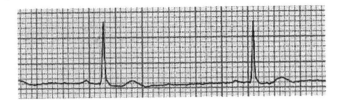

Figure 7.3.1 Normal sinus rhythm. Note the isoelectric ST segment that is neither elevated nor depressed when compared to the baseline.

Table 7.3.1 Clinical conditions that result in ST segment elevation or depression. Note that many conditions may result in both ST-segment elevation and ST-segment depression, occasionally in the same ECG. The affected leads may help guide diagnosis.

ST segment elevation	ST segment depression
Acute coronary syndrome (ACS)	Acute coronary syndrome (ACS)
ST segment myocardial infarction (STEMI)	Myocardial infarction • Non-ST elevation MI (NSTEMI) • Reciprocal changes • Posterior wall MI-depression in leads V1–V3 represents the ST elevation that would be seen if additional posterior oriented leads were placed.
Benign early repolarization (BER)	Myocardial ischemia
Prinzmetal's angina ("vasospastic angina")	Bundle branch block
Cardiomyopathy	Left ventricular hypertrophy
Bundle branch block (BBB)	Ventricular paced rhythm
Ventricular-paced rhythm	Nonischemic myocardial injury (e.g. cardiac contusion)
Left ventricular hypertrophy (LVH)	Post-electrical injury (including electrical cardioversion)
Left ventricular aneurysm	Digitalis
Acute pericarditis	Electrolyte abnormalities (e.g. hypokalemia)
Acute myocarditis	Tachycardia-related changes
Hyperkalemia	
Postelectrical injury (including electrical cardioversion)	
Nonischemic myocardial injury (e.g. cardiac contusion)	
Takasubo syndrome ("broken heart" syndrome)	
Preexcitation syndromes	
Central nervous syndrome (CNS) injury	
Brugada syndrome	
Hypothermia	

ventricular paced rhythms, as described below). However, the distribution of ST segment changes alone cannot rule out ACS and as with all ECG findings, the distribution of both STE and STD should be considered within the clinical context of the specific patient.

It is often helpful to consider the causes of STE and depression in two broad categories: ischemic and nonischemic. Ischemic causes of ST segment changes include all conditions related to acute coronary syndrome (ACS): unstable angina, non-ST elevation MI (NSTEMI), and ST elevation MI (STEMI). These are serious conditions requiring prompt recognition and appropriate intervention in order to avoid significant morbidity and mortality. Nonischemic etiologies of ST segment deviation are varied and range in significance and may represent normal variants or important clinical findings with potentially serious implications. The differential diagnosis of ischemic and nonischemic STE and depression will be discussed separately below.

Acute Coronary Syndrome and Related ST Segment Deviation

STE and STD that are associated with ACS deserve special attention here. In fact, in the evaluation of an ECG with ST segment changes, the astute clinician will often evaluate first for signs of ACS, the most serious of which is the acute STEMI, as this represents a "can't miss" diagnosis that requires prompt recognition and appropriate treatment. As noted above, at baseline the ST segment is flat, reflecting the isoelectric nature of the myocardium during the repolarization period. Ischemia reduces the membrane potential and shortens the action potential in the affected area causing a voltage gradient. Within minutes to hours following coronary vessel occlusion, alterations in the electrical potential of the myocytes may be reflected on the surface ECG as ST segment deviation.

An early finding of STEMI is the hyper-acute T wave, defined as a prominent, or large, T wave [4]. Acute T-wave changes are discussed at length elsewhere in this text; however, in short, it is thought that the decreased perfusion to the soon-to-infarct myocardium results in cellular injury and the release of potassium from damaged myocytes, which leads to a change in the electrical potential and ultimately to grossly enlarged T waves are seen in the impacted area. Hyper-acute T waves are often associated with elevation of the J point. These changes may be seen as soon as 1–2 minutes after onset of vessel occlusion. As the infarction progresses, the hyper-acute T wave is transient and quickly evolves into the elevation of the entire ST segment.

By definition, the diagnosis of STEMI requires the presence of STE of greater than or equal to 1 mm in the limb leads (leads I, II, and III) or augmented limb leads (AVL and AVF) and/or 2 mm in the precordial leads (V1–V6).

Figure 7.3.2 Panel (a) shows pronounced ST segment elevation and hyperacute T waves in the precordial leads while the ST segment changes in Panel (b) are more subtle.

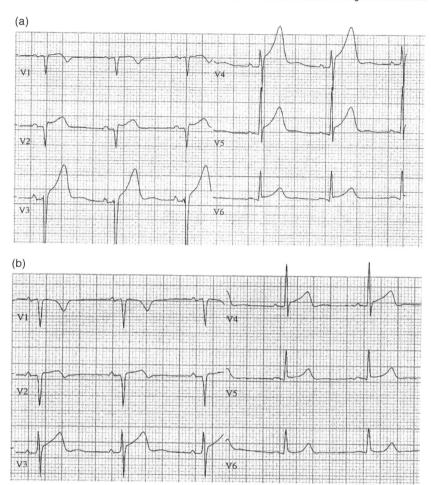

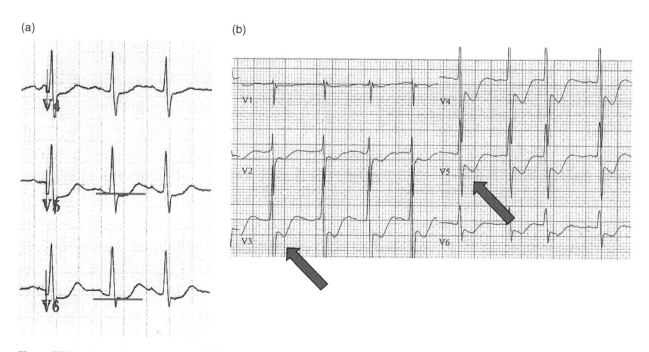

Figure 7.3.3 Panel (a) demonstrates ST depression that is flat (lines) while Panel (b) shows downsloping ST depression (arrows), both are typical of ACS.

(a)   (b)   (c)

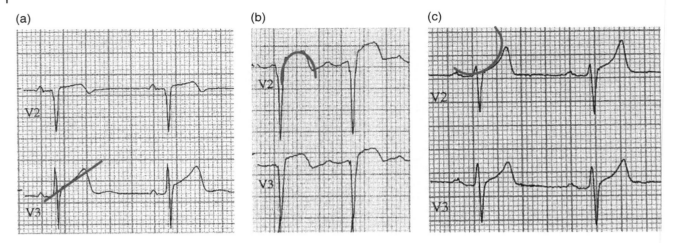

Figure 7.3.4 Note the different morphology, or shape of ST segment elevation (STE) in three patients all with acute ischemic disease. Panel (a) shows a pattern described as "obliquely straight" (see line). Panel (b) demonstrates a convex pattern of STE and Panel (c) depicts a concave pattern (see overlaying lines).

Table 7.3.2 Regional patterns of ST segment elevation; note that leads marked with * require either moving leads or applying leads that are not usually part of the standard surface 12-lead ECG. This use of additional ECG leads is described in depth elsewhere in this text.

Affected region of myocardium	Leads demonstrating STE
Anterior wall	V3–V4
Septal	V1–V2
Anterior/Septal	V1–V4
Lateral	V5–V6, I, AVL
Anterior/Lateral	V1–V6, I, AVL
Inferior	II, III, AVF
Posterior	V1, V2*, V7, V8, V9
Right ventricle	RV3-RV6*, occasionally V1

In addition, STE in at least two anatomically contiguous leads – that is, leads within the same anatomic region – is frequently seen in patients with STEMI and this finding is required to meet diagnostic criteria [5–7]. The anatomic distribution of STE in the setting of AMI may be helpful in assessing the affected area of myocardium and the presence of STE on the ECG, if related to STEMI, is indicative of ongoing ischemia. Regional patterns of STE are listed in Table 7.3.2.

Several ischemic conditions may lead to STD, such as ischemia without infarction, NSTEMI (aka, *subendocardial infarction*, or *non-Q wave MI*), posterior wall infarction, and so-called *reciprocal changes* associated with STEMI. When considering ECGs with confounding patterns in patients with chest pain, including the nonischemic patterns described below, STD is 69% sensitive and 93% specific for AMI [8]. Though STD is often present in the

anterior and/or inferior leads, STD does not necessarily localize to the affected anatomic area of myocardial damage and STD may be found in multiple leads on the ECG. In order to meet the diagnostic criteria for ACS, STD must be either horizontal or downsloping, and must be at least 1 mm at the J point.

In the case of a posterior wall AMI, because the standard surface 12-lead ECG only "views" the heart from the anterior aspect of the thorax, altered conduction in the myocardium in the posterior wall of the heart is represented as STD rather than elevation because the electrical impulses in the affected myocardium are directed away from the anterior surface leads. Characteristic ECG findings include the following, seen in leads V1–V3: (i) horizontal STD associated with tall, upright T waves, (ii) a tall, wide, R wave, and (iii) an R/S ratio greater than 1 in lead V2. The STD seen in these cases represents the infarction, which would be seen as STE if posterior leads were placed. An additional lead ECG may be useful in such cases, including the standard 12 leads, and adds posterior leads V7–V9 placed at the posterior axillary line, the mid-scapular line, and the medial scapular border respectively (Figure 7.3.5). STE greater than 1 mm in these posterior leads confirms the presence of posterior wall ischemia [9, 10].

The terms *reciprocal ST segment depression* or simply *reciprocal changes* are used to describe STD seen in the setting of STEMI. These reciprocal changes are defined by STD in leads that are separate and distant from the leads that demonstrate STE (Figure 7.3.6). These changes are sometimes described as *electrocardiographic mirroring* of transmural myocardial injury occurring on the opposite side of the heart. The morphology of this STD is either horizontal or downsloping and may be present in a single lead or may be more widely distributed in several leads. Reciprocal change is an important ECG concept to

(a)

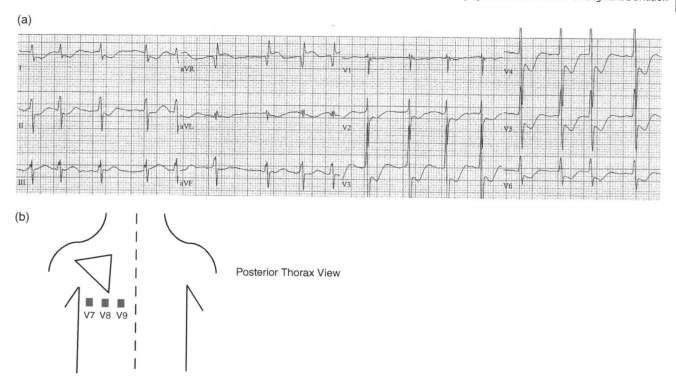

(b)

Posterior Thorax View

V7 V8 V9

Figure 7.3.5 Posterior wall MI. In Panel (a), note the downsloping STD across the precordial leads with a tall R wave and upright T waves. Panel (b) demonstrates the placement of posterior leads, V7, V8, and V9, which would demonstrate ST elevation in this scenario.

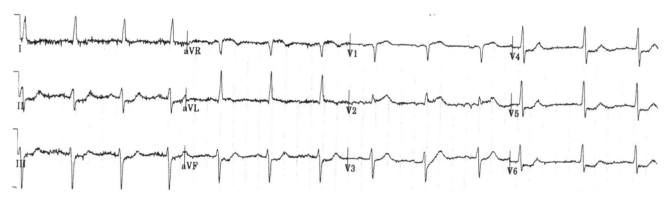

Figure 7.3.6 Reciprocal changes. In this patient with anterior ST elevation, note the ST segment depression inferior and lateral leads.

consider and recognize on the 12-lead ECG as it identifies patients with high-risk ACS and provides confirmation that a STEMI is in fact present. Reciprocal changes in the setting of STEMI identifies a patient with increased chance of cardiovascular complication, including heart block, malignant ventricular dysrhythmia, and cardiogenic shock, as well as increased risk for poor outcome – severe LV dysfunction or death. Furthermore, the presence of reciprocal changes on the ECG supports the diagnosis of ACS with very high sensitivity and positive predictive value.

In the patient with a clinical presentation consistent with ACS, special attention should be paid to the presence of ST segment changes in certain leads, particularly in lead AVL and AVR, which are often overlooked. STE of 1–1.5 mm in lead AVR suggests L main coronary artery obstruction. This finding may be present in the setting of any of the ACS syndromes and is associated with markedly higher mortality. The reperfusion of such lesions is best performed via percutaneous coronary intervention rather than through fibrinolysis. Furthermore, the ECG finding of STE in lead AVR is associated with significant risk of short-term adverse events, including malignant ventricular dysrhythmias, heart block, cardiogenic shock, and death [11] (Figure 7.3.7). In lead AVL, significant STD, especially that which is disproportionate to the size

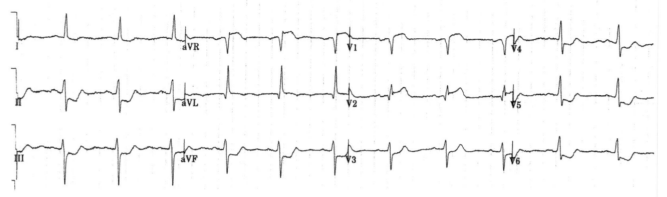

Figure 7.3.7 ST elevation in lead AVR, though subtle, as in this case of ACS, may be a marker of greater risk and higher mortality. Note also the widespread ST-segment depression. These reciprocal changes are a clue to an ischemic etiology.

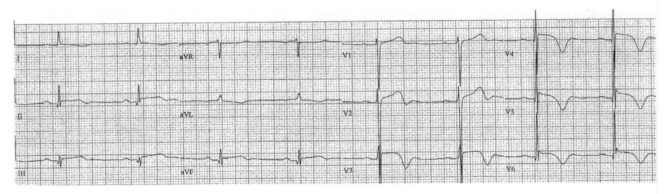

Figure 7.3.8 Takotsubo cardiomyopathy. Also known as *broken heart syndrome,* this condition is believed to occur due to overstimulation of the autonomic nervous system associated with abrupt emotional or psychological stressors. Though the coronary arteries are not direction affected, the left ventricle shape is altered with a narrowed neck and ballooned lower portion, which can affect LV function and can lead to heart failure.

of the QRS complex, may indicate an impending inferior wall ischemia [12].

It is important to recall that while ischemic disease is most frequently due to coronary artery disease (CAD) and acute vessel occlusion, in young patients without traditional CAD risk factors, several other conditions can lead to the similar chest pain syndromes. Takotsubo syndrome (Figure 7.3.8), Prinzmetal's angina, cocaine-induced vasospasm, and acute coronary artery dissection can all cause ST-segment changes and regional patterns due to regional hypoperfusion of the myocardium. These alternate etiologies should be considered in the appropriate clinical setting with an ECG concerning for ischemic injury.

Nonischemic Causes of ST-Segment Changes

Bundle Branch Block (BBB)

BBB are discussed at length elsewhere in this text. However, when evaluating ST-segment changes, it is important to recall that intraventricular conduction delay patterns,

including left and right bundle branch blocks (LBBB and RBBB), demonstrate ST-segment changes related with their altered electrical conduction. In the patient with BBB, the anticipated ST-segment and T-wave configurations follow the "Rule of Appropriate Discordance," which states that the ST segment and T wave should be directed opposite the major, terminal portion of the QRS complex. These ST segment changes are referred to as discordant STE and STD, respectively, and represent a "new normal" in the patient with BBB. Loss of this normal QRS-ST segment discordance in patients with a BBB may imply an acute process, such as an acute myocardial infarction, and should be considered in the patient who exhibits concerning symptoms.

Left BBB

In the patient with LBBB, the right precordial leads, V1–V3, have predominantly negative QRS complexes, with prominent S waves and STE with large, upright T waves. Simultaneously, the left-side leads, V5, V6, I, and AVL, will have prominent/monophasic R waves, STD, and T wave inversion. "Notching" of the R wave in lead V6 is also

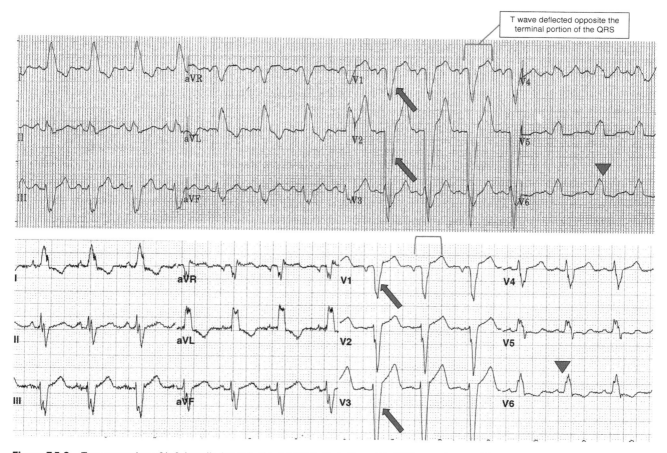

Figure 7.3.9 Two examples of left bundle branch block (LBBB). Note the wide QRS complexes with a prominent t S wave in V1 and V2 (arrows), the "appropriate discordance" (bracket) and the notched R wave in V6 (arrow head).

Table 7.3.3 Sgarbossa criteria ≥ 3 pts is 90% sensitive for STEMI (36% specific) [13].

Sgarbossa criteria for detecting AMI in the setting of LBBB	
ST elevation of ≥1 mm in a lead with a positive QRS (concordance)	5 points
ST depression ≥1 mm in lead V1, V2, or V3	3 points
ST elevation of ≥5 mm in a lead with a negative QRS (discordance)	2 points

common (Figure 7.3.9). LBBB is considered to be a *confounding pattern*; that is, one that reduces the diagnostic potential of the ECG to detect a STEMI. The Sgarbossa criteria (Table 7.3.3) are one set of guidelines that describe a method to evaluate for AMI in the presence of a LBBB. These criteria are specific, but not sensitive, in terms of their ability to diagnose STEMI in this setting.

Right BBB

In the patient with RBBB, the characteristic RSR', qR, or monophasic R wave in the right precordial leads (V1–V3) is

accompanied by discordant STD, which blends into an inverted T wave. Deep, wide, S waves in the left-sided leads may look like STD but are really slurred S waves due to the slower depolarization of the right side of the heart (Figure 7.3.10).

Ventricular-Paced Rhythms (VPRs)

Similar to BBB, VPR demonstrate wide QRS complexes associated with ST segment changes even in the nonischemic state. VPRs also follow the rule of appropriate discordance, exhibiting STD in leads with a predominantly positive QRS complex, and STE in leads with a predominantly negative QRS complex. The STE in VPR is usually concave. Pacer spikes may or may not be evident (Figure 7.3.11). As with BBB, as noted above, VPR may confound the diagnosis of STEMI. Serial ECGs and comparison to past ECGs may be useful to detect subtle changes in the patient with symptoms concerning for ACS. The Sgarbossa criteria, discussed above, may also be used in the setting of patients with implanted cardiac pacemakers and clinical scenarios suspicious for AMI. Discordant STE > 5 mm is the best predictor of STEMI in the patient with VPR.

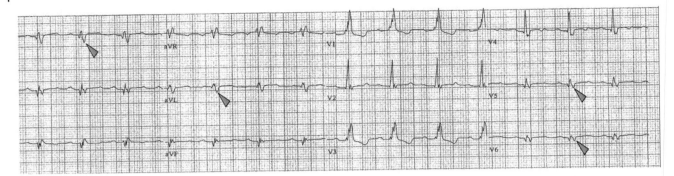

Figure 7.3.10 Right bundle branch block (RBBB). Note the RSR' ("M-shape") in V1 (arrow) as well as discordant ST segment depression and inverted T waves. Also the wide S waves in the lateral leads (I, AVL, V5, and V6; noted by arrow heads).

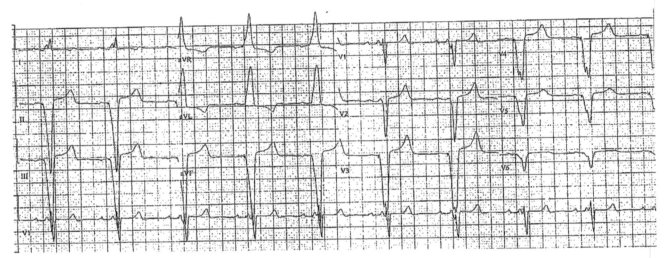

Figure 7.3.11 Ventricular paced rhythm (VPR). Note the wide QRS complexes associated with ST segment changes that follow the rule of appropriate discordance, with STD in leads with a predominantly positive QRS complex (i.e. AVR and AVL) and concave STE in leads with a predominantly negative QRS complex (i.e. V1–V4).

Ventricular Hypertrophy

Both right and left ventricular hypertrophy (RVH and LVH, respectively), most commonly resulting from longstanding hypertension, demonstrate ST segment changes as part of the classic "strain pattern" on the ECG. The ST-segment and T-wave changes associated with the classic strain pattern are seen in approximately 70% of patients with LVH [14] and are often misinterpreted as ACS. These changes include poor R-wave progression, concave STE (2–4 mm) with prominent T waves and large, negative QRS complexes in the right-mid precordial leads (V1–V3), and downsloping STD (>1 mm), J-point depression, and abnormal T waves in leads I, aVL, V5, and V6. In cases of RVH, STD may be seen in the right-sided leads, V1, and V2.

Of the many systems that have been proposed to diagnose LVH based on ECG findings, the Sokolow-Lyon criteria [15] is one of the most accurate and easy to use. Using this method, the largest S wave in either V1 or V2 is added to the size of the largest R wave in either V5 or V6, and LVH is considered to be likely when the sum is greater than 35 mm (Figure 7.3.12). Other ECG clues may help make the diagnosis, including: QRS widening, left atrial enlargement, and left axis deviation. However, none of these changes are required to make the diagnosis. As ventricular hypertrophy represents a chronic condition, all of the associate ECG changes are stable and consistent. Therefore, dynamic ECG changes should prompt the clinician to consider an acute condition.

Benign Early Repolarization

The syndrome of benign early repolarization (BER) is a common and nonpathologic finding that is considered a normal variant and not indicative of underlying cardiac disease, nor is it associated with a poor prognosis. This

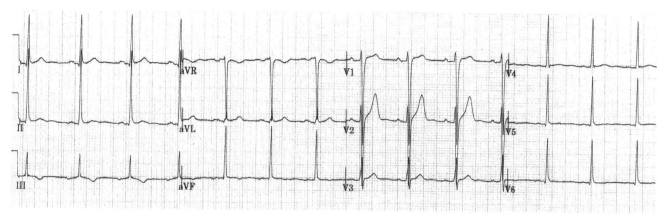

Figure 7.3.12 Left ventricular hypertrophy (LVH). Note the increased voltages throughout. In addition, the amplitude of S wave in V1 + R wave in V5 is >35 mm (Sokolow-Lyon criteria).

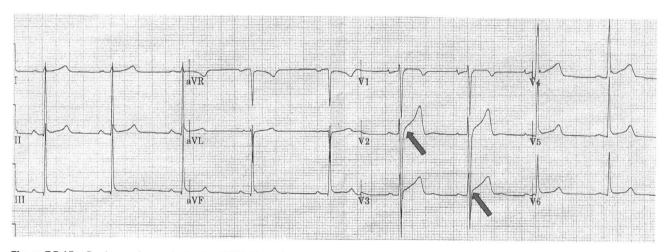

Figure 7.3.13 Benign early repolarization (BER). Note the characteristic ST elevation that begins at the J point (arrows).

pattern is usually found in younger individuals (<50 years old) and is more often seen in males and African Americans [16]. BER is a chronic pattern that lessens over time and is rarely seen after age 50. The ECG definition of BER includes (i) STE, (ii) upward concavity of the initial portion of the ST segment, (iii) notching or slurring of the J point, (iv) large, symmetric, concordant T waves, (v) diffuse or widespread STE, and (vi) relative temporal stability. The characteristic STE begins at the J point and is usually 0.5–3.5 mm in magnitude, though it can reach 5 mm in some cases. The precordial leads demonstrate greater magnitude of STE as compared to the limb leads. In general, the characteristic STE of BER appears as if the ST segment were lifted off the isoelectric baseline at the J point, while the normal concavity of the ST segment remains intact (Figure 7.3.13). While the findings decrease over years, they do not demonstrate changes over hours, days, or weeks. Therefore, dynamic ST segment changes associated with symptoms concerning ACS should prompt an evaluation for

an acute condition. Even younger patients, particularly those with chronic disease and/or multiple CAD risk factors, should be evaluated first for ischemic conditions in the appropriate clinical setting.

Acute Myocarditis/Pericarditis

Acute pericarditis, which is more correctly termed acute myopericarditis, is an acute, generally self-limited condition that results in diffuse inflammation of the pericardium and the superficial epicardium. This inflammation can produce a range of ECG abnormalities that may change throughout the course of the illness. These changes may include STE, T-wave inversion, and PR segment changes. The initial upsloping portion of the ST segment is most frequently concave, and STE is usually 1–3 mm in magnitude (rarely >5 mm) with a normal J point. These changes are generally diffuse and do not demonstrate a regional pattern,

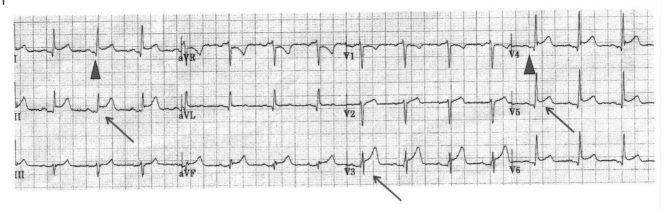

Figure 7.3.14 Acute myopericarditis. Note the PR depression (arrow heads) and the concave, upsloping ST elevation (arrows). These changes are diffuse and do not follow an anatomic/regional pattern.

nor are reciprocal changes seen. PR segment depression may also be identified, most commonly in leads II, III, AVF, and V6; PR segment elevation may be seen in lead AVR and is usually very apparent when present (Figure 7.3.14). PR depression is unlikely in AMI or BER and can help distinguish myopericarditis from these other conditions.

Ventricular Aneurysm

Though uncommon, ventricular aneurysms most often occur after large anterior wall infarctions, in patients who either do not come to medical attention or do not respond to appropriate therapies. Left ventricular aneurysm (LVA) is defined as the localized area of the infarcted myocardium which bulges outward during both systole and diastole. In most cases, the LVA is manifested on the ECG by varying degrees of STE of at least 1 mm, usually in the precordial leads, which persists more than four weeks after the AMI. The morphology of the elevated ST segment in LVA varies and may be concave, obliquely straight, or convex. STE is usually accompanied by Q waves, which indicate the completed MI. And though the STE may mimic an AMI, there are no reciprocal changes present. Furthermore, the T wave/QRS ratio may be used to help differentiate between LVA and STEMI. When the (Sum of the T-wave amplitude) ÷ (Sum of the QRS amplitude) in leads V1–V4 is >0.22 or if the ratio of T-wave amplitude to QRS amplitude in any single lead is >0.36, STEMI is favored. Alternately, a ratio less than 0.36 in all leads is indicative of LVA [17, 18].

Digitalis

The *digitalis effect* refers to ECG changes including STD that are more prominent in the inferior and anterior leads. The STD morphology in this condition is charac-

terized by a scooped appearance that results from a gradual downsloping of the initial limb, which is followed by an abrupt upsloping limb that returns to the baseline. The J point may be at the isoelectric baseline, or may be slightly depressed. In digitalis use, the STD is generally more globally distributed as compared to the more localized changes seen in ACS and other nonischemic conditions. Other ECG findings may be seen in the patient taking digitalis, including short QT, flattened, or inverted T waves, PR prolongation, and the presence of U waves. In addition, smooth, domed STE may be seen in leads I and AVR. It is important to note that while these ECG changes are seen in patients who are taking digitalis, they are not necessarily indicative of digitalis toxicity and are often seen in those with therapeutic levels. Also, as always, these findings must be used in conjunction with other clinical information as patients who take digitalis generally suffer from cardiac disease and even with a classic digitalis pattern, which in and of itself is not concerning, the patient is not excluded from having a AMI Figure 7.3.15.

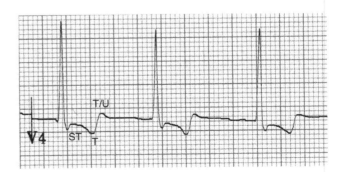

Figure 7.3.15 Digitalis effect. Note the depressed J point, downsloping ST segment, and biphasic T wave. *Source:* Image reproduced with permission from http://lifeinthefastlane.com/ecg-library/digoxin-effect.

Hypothermia

The ECG changes associated with hypothermia (defined as body temperature < 90 °F or 32.2 °C) typically involve the J point but may appear to be ST segment changes. In patients with severe hypothermia, the J point and the initial portion of the ST segment may be lifted off the isoelectric baseline. This may also be seen as positively directed notching at the terminal portion of the R wave that is best seen in leads with the most prominent R waves (V2–V4). This J wave, or Osborn wave, is very distinctive to the hypothermic patient and they are typically more prominent in patients with lower body temperatures. However, the presence of J waves in the hypothermic patient does not rule out the presence of acute ischemia, especially in the patient found down in the cold for unknown reasons. See Figure 7.5.8 in Section 7, Chapter 5 (Differential Diagnosis of Bradycardia) for a demonstration of ECG findings associated with hypothermia.

Hyperkalemia

The ECG findings associated with hyperkalemia are distinctive and may change rapidly as the patient's condition progresses and/or improves. These ECG changes are related to the rate of change of serum potassium rather than to the absolute value of the serum concentration and may be very different in patients with acute vs. chronic conditions. Initially, diffuse T wave changes are present that are seen as

prominent, narrow, symmetric T waves, which are typically described as *peaked*. As the condition worsens, J-point elevation with p*seudo-ST segment elevation*, may be seen. Upon further progression, the QRS complex may be widened, leading to an even greater appearance of STE. Ultimately, the entire QRS/ST/T wave complex may take on a characteristic sine wave pattern (Figure 7.3.16). In the early stages of hyperkalemia, though, it may be difficult to differentiate between hyperkalemia and AMI. It is important to remember that the hyperacute T waves of hyperkalemia tend to be narrower and more symmetric, and that in cases of hyperkalemia, the initial portion of the elevated ST segment is typically concave, rather than the obliquely straight or convex pattern that is often seen with AMI.

Brugada Syndrome

The Brugada syndrome, first described in 1992 [19] is encountered in patients with structurally normal hearts who often present with syncope or cardiac arrest without preceding symptoms. This syndrome presents electrocardiographically with an RBBB pattern and STE that is seen in the right precordial leads (V1, V2). The ECG changes associated with Brugada syndrome may have one of three characteristic appearances, seen in the right precordial leads (V1–V3): Type I includes pronounced J-point elevation (>2 mm) and STE, which is concave and downsloping followed by an inverted T wave (Figure 7.3.17); Type II demonstrates J-point

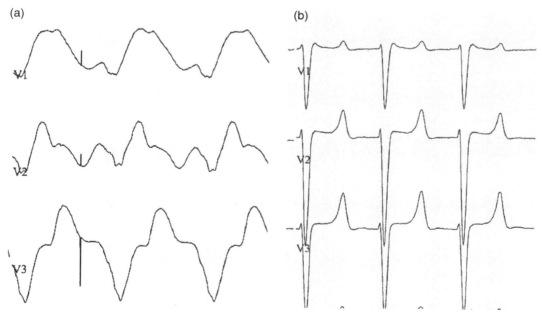

(a)   (b)

Figure 7.3.16 Hyperkalemia. Panel (a) shows the ECG of a dialysis patient who had missed several treatments, her potassium level on presentation was 8.5 mmol/l. Note the wide QRS complexes and sine wave appearance. Panel (b) is the ECG from the same patient after appropriate treatment. Note that the T waves are still prominent but the QRS duration and ST segments have returned to normal.

(a)　　　　　　　　　　　　　　　　　　(b)

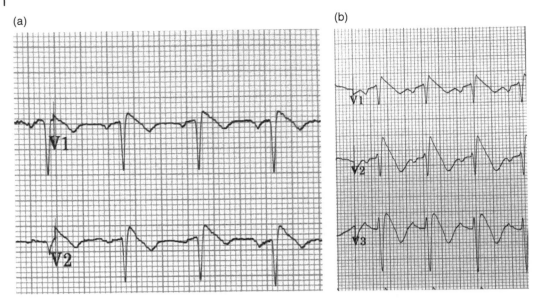

Figure 7.3.17 Brugada syndrome. Type I abnormality with coved STE and a negative T wave. *Source:* Panel (a) ECG courtesy of Dr. Muthuswamy and Dr. Greenman, Cooper University Hospital, Camden, NJ; Panel (b) ECG courtesy of Dr. Bowers, St. Louise Regional Hospital, Gilroy, CA.

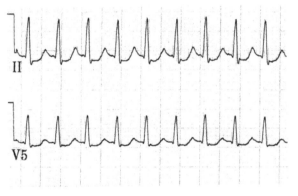

Figure 7.3.18 Tachycardia-related ST depression. Note the markedly elevated heart rate, depressed J point and upsloping ST segment.

elevation with STE >1 mm, which is convex (the "saddle type") and an upright or biphasic T wave; and Type III includes J-point elevation, "saddleback" STE >1 mm, and an upright T wave. Of these, only Type I is the only definitive diagnostic criteria based on ECG [20]. These patients are at significant risk of dysrhythmia-mediated sudden cardiac death even in the absence of myocardial ischemia and must be promptly identified and should be referred to a cardiologist immediately for defibrillator implantation.

Tachycardia-Related STD

Patients with supraventricular tachycardia, including sinus tachycardia, may demonstrate J-point depression with upsloping STD. This *rate-related* STD is not necessarily indicative of AMI (Figure 7.3.18). Nonischemic, tachycardia-related STD has been verified both in cases of new/spontaneous SVT, as well as in exercise treadmill tests. The STD associated with tachycardia is typically upsloping and has a depressed J point [21, 22].

CNS Injury

Certain severe intracranial injuries can lead to significant ST and T-wave changes on the ECG. This can include varying degrees of STE and/or diffuse T-wave inversion, so called *cerebral T waves*. In the moribund patient with ECG changes that include STE, one should consider whether a neurologic, rather than cardiac, etiology may be to blame (Figure 7.3.19).

Other Causes

Several other nonischemic conditions may cause ST segment changes, including cardiomyopathy, cardiac contusion, metabolic abnormalities, postcardiac arrest changes, and electrical injury (including electrical cardioversion). The patient and his/her ECG should be evaluated within the clinical context of their presenting symptoms to make the appropriate diagnosis.

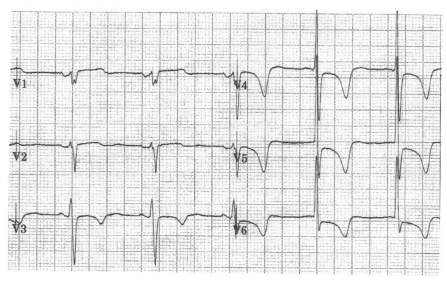

Figure 7.3.19 Cerebral T waves. Note the deep, inverted T waves in this patient with a severe subarachnoid hemorrhage.

References

1 Brady, W.J., Perron, A.D., and Ullman, E.A. (2002). ST segment elevation: a comparison of electrocardiographic features of AMI and non-AMI ECG syndromes. *Am. J. Emerg. Med.* 20: 609.

2 Brady, W.J., Syverud, S.A., Beagle, C. et al. (2001). Electrocardiographic ST segment elevation: the diagnosis of AMI by morphologic analysis of the ST segment. *Acad. Emerg. Med.* 8: 961–967.

3 Brady, W.J., Perron, A.D., Martin, M.L. et al. (2001). Electrocardiographic ST segment elevation in emergency department chest pain center patients: etiology responsible for the ST segment abnormality. *Am. J. Emerg. Med.* 19: 25–28.

4 Nable, J.V. and Brady, W.J. (2009). The evolution of electrocardiographic changes in ST-segment elevation myocardial infarction. *Am. J. Emerg. Med.* 27: 734–746.

5 Fesmire, F.M., Hahn, S., Jagoda, A.S. et al. (2006). American college of emergency physicians clinical policy: critical issues in the evaluation and management of adult patients with non–ST-segment elevation acute coronary syndromes. *Ann. Emerg. Med.* 48: 270–301.

6 Fesmire, F.M., Brady, W.J., Hahn, S. et al. (2006). American college of emergency physicians clinical policy: indications for reperfusion therapy in emergency department patients with suspected acute myocardial infarction. *Ann. Emerg. Med.* 48: 358–371.

7 O'Connor, R.E., Brady, W., Brooks, S.C. et al. (2010). Acute coronary syndromes: 2010 American Heart Association guidelines for cardiopulmonary resuscitation and emergency cardiovascular care. *Circulation* 122: s787–s817.

8 Brady, W.J., Perron, A.D., and Syverud, S.A. (2002). Reciprocal ST segment depression: impact of electrocardiographic diagnosis of ST segment elevation acute myocardial infarction. *Am. J. Emerg. Med.* 20: 35–38.

9 Zalinski, R.J., Cooke, D., Rydman, R. et al. (1993). Assessing the diagnostic value of an ECG containing leads V4R, V8 and V9: the 15-lead ECG. *Ann. Emerg. Med.* 22: 786–793.

10 Brady, W.J. (1998). Acute posterior wall myocardial infarction: electrocardiographic manifestations. *Am. J. Emerg. Med.* 16: 409–413.

11 Williamson, K., Mattu, A., Binder, A. et al. (2006). Electrocardiographic applications of lead AVR. *Am. J. Emerg. Med.* 24: 864–874.

12 Mariott, H.J.L. (1997). *Emergency Electrocardiography*, 28–40. Naples, FL: Trinity Press.

13 Sgarbossa, E.B., Pinski, S.L., Barbagelata, A. et al. (1996). Electrocardiographic diagnosis of evolving acute MI in the presence of left bundle-branch block. *NEJM* 334 (8): 481–487.

14 Chan, T.C., Brady, W.J. et al. (2005). *ECG in Emergency Medicine and Acute Care*. Elsevier Inc.

15 Sokolow, M. and Lyon, T.P. (1949). The ventricular complex in left ventricular hypertrophy as obtained by unipolar precordial and limb leads. *Am. Heart J.* 37: 161–186.

16 Eastaugh, J. (1989). The early repolarization syndrome. *J. Emerg. Med.* 7: 257–262.

17 Smith, S.W. (2005). T/QRS amplitude ratio best distinguishes the ST elevation of anterior left ventricular aneurysm from anterior acute myocardial infarction. *Am. J. Emerg. Med.* 23 (3): 279–287.

18 Smith, S. and Shroff, G. (2011 Oct). T/QRS Amplitude Ratio Is Significantly Higher in Acute Anterior ST-Elevation Myocardial Infarction Than in Previous Myocardial Infarction with Persistent ST Elevation (Left Ventricular Aneurysm Morphology): A Validation. *Annals of Emergency Medicine.* 1: 58(4).

19 Brugada, P. and Brugada, J. (1992). Right bundle branch block, ST elevation and sudden cardiac death: a distinct clinical and electrocardiographic syndrome; a multicenter report. *J. Am. Coll. Cardiol.* 20: 1391–1396.

20 Wilde, A.A., Antzelevitch, C., Borggrefe, M. et al. (2002 Nov 5). Study group on the molecular basis of arrhythmias of the European society of cardiology. Proposed diagnostic criteria for the Brugada syndrome: consensus report. *Circulation* 106 (19): 2514–2519.

21 Kastor, J.A. (2000). *Arrhythmias*, 2e. Philadelphia: WB Saunders.

22 Harrigan, R.A. and Chan, T.C. (2011). What is the ECG differential diagnosis of ST segment depression? In: *Critical Decisions in Emergency and Acute Care Electrocardiography* (eds. W.J. Brady and J.D. Truwit). Wiley Blackwell.

4

ECG Differential Diagnosis of T Wave and QT Interval Abnormalities

Sanjay Shewakramani[1] and Kari Gorder[2]

[1]*Department of Emergency Medicine, University of Cincinnati West Chester Hospital, University of Cincinnati School of Medicine, Cincinnati, OH, USA*
[2]*Department of Anesthesia, University of Cincinnati Hospital, University of Cincinnati School of Medicine, Cincinnati, OH, USA*

The T Wave

The T wave seen on the surface ECG represents the repolarization of the ventricular action potential. During depolarization, a wave of positive charge travels from the innermost layers of the myocardium to the periphery. The muscle then repolarizes in the opposite fashion, with a negative charge moving from the epicardium in toward the endocardium. As the charges are also opposite, the waveform is usually concordant with the QRS complex, resulting in an upright T wave in most leads [1].

Because the T wave is a direct reflection of ventricular response, it is a visible metric of the health and conductivity of the ventricular muscle [1]. This makes it an important tool for the clinician evaluating patients with potential cardiac complaints, as subtle changes in the T wave's amplitude or morphology can reflect significant cardiac compromise, as well as many other potentially life-threatening etiologies.

The T wave is classically broad, as ventricular repolarization is a slower process than the depolarization seen in the QRS complex. The T wave tends to have a gradual upstroke with a more rapid downstroke, causing a mild asymmetry [2], as is seen in Figure 7.4.1. Abnormalities of the T wave are described in terms of their morphology, and can be classified as prominent, biphasic, flat, or inverted [1].

Prominent T Waves

The amplitude of the T wave is usually most positive in the anterior leads, specifically V_2 or V_3 [1]. The upper limits of normal for positive T wave amplitude are 0.5 mV (5 mm on a standard ECG) in the limb leads and 1.0 mV (10 mm) in the precordial leads. Anything greater than 5 mm or 0.5 mV

is considered prominent [3]. Prominent T waves are most commonly caused by hyperkalemia or myocardial ischemia, although they can also be a normal variant seen with Benign Early Repolarization (BER) [3]. Table 7.4.1 demonstrates a list of the most common causes of prominent T waves.

Hyperkalemia

Peaked T waves are prominent T waves that are often the first ECG abnormality seen in patients with acute hyperkalemia. Classically, these T waves have a narrow base, a steep upstroke, and a symmetric downstroke. This rapid ascent and descent of the T wave result in a sharp, pointed apex, which is often described as looking like "it would hurt if you were to put your hand on it" (Figure 7.4.2). As demonstrated in these ECGs, with rising serum potassium levels, one can expect the amplitude of the T wave to increase, until further changes (including widening of the QRS complex and loss of the P wave) occur [4]. However, it is important to note that some patients, especially those on hemodialysis, may have no ECG changes despite critically high serum potassium levels due to their adaptation to chronic hyperkalemia [5].

Myocardial Infarction

The first ECG abnormality noted during an ST segment-elevated myocardial infarction (STEMI) may actually be something other than the classic ST segment changes. Isolated prominent or peaked T waves – which in this setting are referred to as hyperacute T waves [6] – generally arise within a few minutes of coronary artery occlusion. They may persist for 5–30 minutes, after which they are usually replaced by ST elevation [7]. Typically, these

Electrocardiogram in Clinical Medicine, First Edition. Edited by William J. Brady, Michael J. Lipinski, Andrew E. Darby, Michael C. Bond, Nathan P. Charlton, Korin Hudson, and Kelly Williamson.

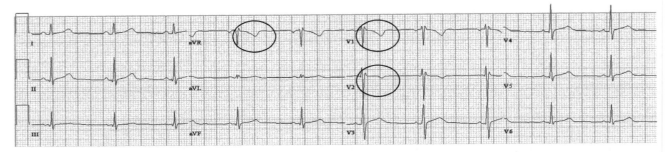

Figure 7.4.1   Normal ECG. Note the asymmetric T waves as well as the expected T-wave inversions (circled) in aVR, V1, and V2.

Table 7.4.1   Etiologies of prominent T waves.

Common	Less Common
Hyperkalemia (peaked)	Valvular heart disease
Acute myocardial infarction (hyperacute)	Mitral stenosis
Prinzmetal's angina	
Benign early repolarization (BER)	Paced rhythms
Myocardial ischemia	Idiopathic hypertrophic subaortic stenosis
Left ventricular hypertrophy (LVH)	Mitral valve prolapse
Bundle branch block (BBB)	Cor pulmonale
Pericarditis	Central nervous system (CNS) disease
	Hyperthyroidism
	Exercise
	Anemia
	Acidosis

Source: adapted from [3].

hyperacute T waves occur in the anteroseptal leads (V_1–V_4), have a broader base than those seen with hyperkalemia, and are often slightly asymmetric, typically with a more gradual upstroke and more rapid downstroke (Figure 7.4.3) [3]. When these peaked T waves are accompanied by ST segment depression in the precordial leads, they are referred to as de Winter T waves and are associated with acute LAD occlusion. This pattern may persist or develop into a "classic" STEMI [7].

Benign Early Repolarization

BER, an idiopathic variant seen most often in young, healthy patients, is a benign and common condition occurring in about 1% of the population. However, distinguishing the morphology of BER from the other causes of prominent T waves is very important [8, 9]. First, BER is almost exclusively seen in patients under the age of 50, which makes it an unlikely diagnosis in older adults. While the ECG of a

patient with BER may look very similar to that of a patient suffering from an acute myocardial infarction (AMI), the T waves seen in BER have a broad base and are asymmetric, with a slow upstroke and a more rapid downstroke. This gives their summit a more "rounded" appearance [3].

As seen in Figure 7.4.4, these T waves are usually most pronounced in the precordial leads [8]. The concave nature of the ST segment in BER is another key distinguishing feature that differentiates it from an acute myocardial infarction, which typically produces a convex or straight ST segment. Another subtle diagnostic difference seen in BER include a notching or "slurring" of the J-point, seen in leads III, aVF and V6. Finally, patients suffering from AMI often demonstrate reciprocal changes (ST depression) elsewhere in the ECG [3], while patients with BER exhibit no such reciprocal changes. Table 7.4.2 provides a summary of classic findings associated with the three most common causes of prominent T waves.

T-Wave Inversions

As mentioned earlier, the T wave is normally upright in most leads. However, inverted T waves are expected in lead aVR, and can often also be seen in leads III and V_1 in healthy adults [10]. In fact, an upright T wave in V1 is generally considered abnormal, and is a strong predictor of coronary artery disease [11]. Inverted T waves are common yet nonspecific signs of myocardial ischemia. They are defined as any T wave with negative amplitude, as seen in Figure 7.4.5. They can be further classified as "deep negative" (−0.5 to −1.0 mV or 5–10 mm on a standard ECG) and "giant negative" (more negative than −1.0 mV or greater than 10 mm). T-wave inversions can be either dynamic or fixed, which illustrates the importance of reviewing old ECGs [1]. New or transient T-wave inversion is generally a sign of acute, ongoing ischemia. If these T waves return to their normal morphology after the event resolves, they may be referred to as "dynamic" T-wave changes. By contrast, chronic T-wave inversion is typically seen in patients who have suffered ischemia in the past, and can accompany Q waves. Particular attention should be paid when upright T

(a)

(b)

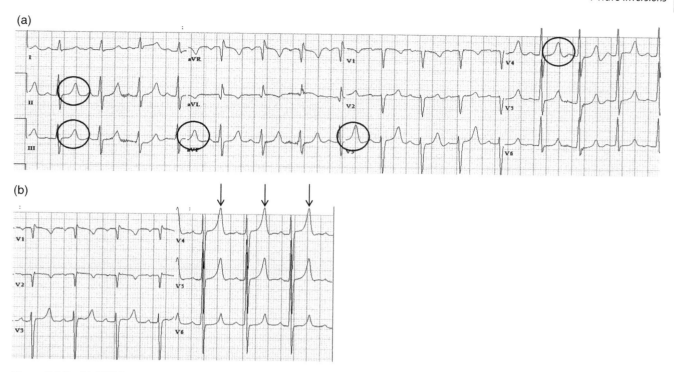

Figure 7.4.2 (a) ECG from a patient with a serum potassium of 6.5 mEq/L. Note the prominent T waves (circled) in the limb leads as well as V3 and V4. (b) ECG for the same patient, now with a serum potassium of 7.4 mEq/L. Note the peaking (arrows) of the T waves in V4 and V5, with the associated "sharp" apex.

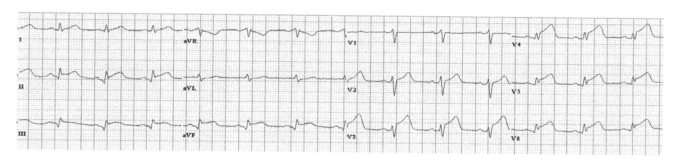

Figure 7.4.3 A patient with an ST-elevation myocardial infarction. Note the prominent slightly asymmetric T waves with the broad base in almost all of the precordial leads. Also note the convexity of the ST segment.

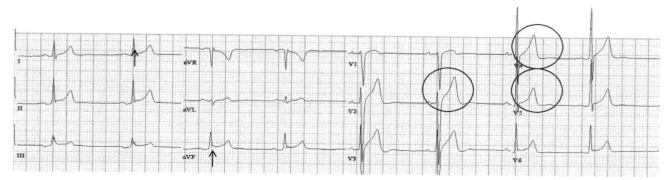

Figure 7.4.4 A patient with benign early repolarization (BER). Note the concave appearance of the upstroke (circles) as well as J-point elevation (arrows), and lack of reciprocal changes.

Table 7.4.2 Classic characteristics of commonly encountered prominent T waves.

	Symmetry	Base	Other
Acute myocardial infarction	Usually asymmetric	Broad	• Reciprocal changes present • Convex ST segment • Evolving (dynamic Changes
Hyperkalemia	Symmetric	Narrow	• Sharp apex; "peaked" appearance
Benign early repolarization (BER)	Asymmetric	Broad	• Concave ST segment elevation, less than 25% of the T wave height in lead V6 • No reciprocal or dynamic changes

(a)

(b)

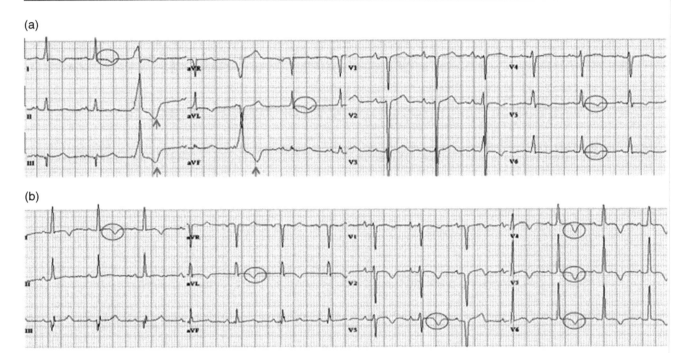

Figure 7.4.5 (a) A patient with anterolateral T wave inversions (circled), which are non-specific, but nonetheless concerning. (b) T-wave inversions laterally (circled), as well as deeper T-wave inversions with ectopic beats (arrows).

waves are seen in a patient with a history of fixed T-wave inversions. This "pseudonormalization" of the T wave may indicate active myocardial ischemia, but could easily be interpreted as normal if comparison to old ECGs is not made [12].

Any cardiopulmonary pathology that causes strain or ischemia to the heart can cause inverted T waves [1]. Table 7.4.3 lists the various causes of T-wave inversions, many of which can be life-threatening. In fact, the presence of abnormal T waves (inverted or flattened) has been correlated with increased morbidity and mortality [14]. However, it is also important to note that 15% of healthy patients have ECGs with T-wave abnormalities [15], and as mentioned earlier, inverted T waves can be expected in leads aVR, V1, and III. Moreover, as mentioned previously, an upright T wave in V1 should be considered abnormal, and is associated with coronary artery disease.

Deep and Giant T-Wave Inversions

Deep and giant T-wave inversions are rare, caused by only a handful of etiologies (Table 7.4.4), but can be evidence of significant underlying pathology. For example, patients with hypertrophic cardiomyopathy may display deep T-wave inversions (Figure 7.4.6) although findings of left ventricular hypertrophy and repolarization abnormalities are more common [1]. Non-ST segment elevation myocardial infarctions (NSTEMIs) and large pulmonary emboli can also cause deepened T waves (Figure 7.4.7) [16]. Post-tachycardia syndrome is an ECG abnormality characterized by diffuse deep T-wave inversions and can be seen after an episode of paroxysmal tachycardia. The ECG changes often resolve over time, and can be seen in patients with normal coronary arteries [17]. Finally, deep and giant T-wave inversions can be seen in patients suffering

Table 7.4.3 Causes of T-wave inversion.

Primary T-wave inversion (due to repolarization abnormalities)	Secondary T-wave inversion (due to QRS changes)
Normal variants • Juvenile T-wave pattern • Early repolarization	Bundle branch block (BBB)
Myocardial ischemia or infarction • Ongoing or past	Wolf-Parkinson-White (WPW) syndrome
CNS events	Ventricular paced rhythms
Ventricular overload • Classic strain patterns (e.g. LVH) • Apical hypertrophic cardiomyopathy	Ventricular ectopic beats
Post-tachycardia T-wave pattern	Idiopathic global T-wave inversions
Digitalis effect	Acute myocarditis
	Acute pulmonary embolism

Source: adapted from [13].

Table 7.4.4 Causes of deep T-wave inversions.

• CNS disorders
  – Cerebral T waves
• Hypertrophic cardiomyopathy
• Anterior myocardial ischemia or infarction
• Pulmonary embolism
• Post-tachycardia syndrome

from intracranial hemorrhage, and are often referred to as "cerebral T waves." These changes are thought to be secondary to sympathetic stimulation, and can also occur in patients without any evidence of preexisting coronary artery disease [18]. They tend to be wider and deeper than giant T-wave inversions due to alternate causes. Figure 7.4.8 shows an example of deep T-wave inversion seen in a patient suffering brainstem herniation after a subarachnoid hemorrhage before and after surgical decompression was performed.

Biphasic T Waves

Biphasic T waves, or T waves with an initial deflection opposite to their terminal deflection, are most commonly seen in the anterior leads. When present with a terminal downward deflection, they are highly suggestive of myocardial ischemia. In this setting, repeat ECG analysis often shows evolution of biphasic T waves to T-wave inversions [19]. Hypokalemia can also cause biphasic T waves, classically with a terminal upward deflection. It is thought the terminal upward deflection may actually represent a U wave, which may often be seen as a distinct entity following the T wave in patients with severe hypokalemia [20].

Wellens Syndome

Wellens syndrome describes a specific ECG pattern of inverted of biphasic T waves that is highly suggestive of a critical stenosis of the proximal left anterior descending (LAD) coronary artery. Specifically, deep or giant (seen in the more common Wellens Type A) or biphasic (Wellens Type B) T-wave inversions are noted in leads V2 and V3. (Figure 7.4.9) [21]. The downslope of the biphasic T wave is

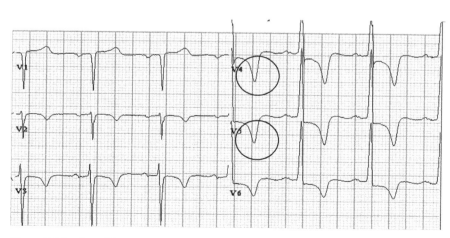

Figure 7.4.6 Deep T-wave inversions (circled) due to hypertrophic obstructive cardiomyopathy.

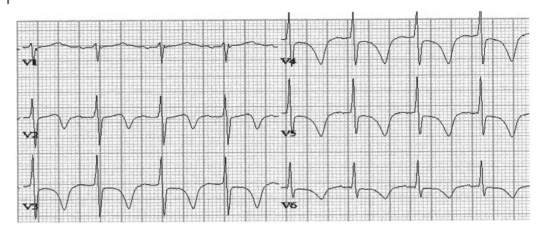

Figure 7.4.7 Deep T-wave inversions (throughout precordial leads) due to NSTEMI.

(a)

(b)

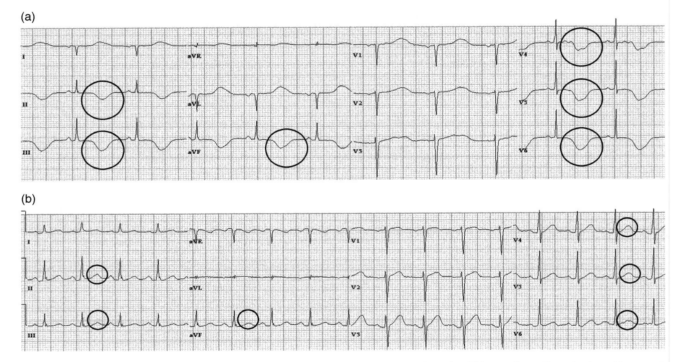

Figure 7.4.8 (a) Cerebral T waves (circled), seen in a patient herniating due to a subarachnoid hemorrhage. Note the broad base and the depth of the T waves. (b) Resolution of the cerebral T waves after surgical decompression. Note that the previously wide and inverted T waves are now smaller, narrower, and upright.

typically steep and symmetric. It is important to note that these changes are often seen when the patient is not having active chest pain or an anginal equivalent; Wellens syndrome indicates inadequate perfusion which may be waxing and waning. Any of these abnormalities should alert the treating physician of the possibility of impending myocardial infarction, and aggressive treatment, including anticoagulation and catheterization, should be considered [22].

T-Wave Flattening

T-wave flattening is a relatively nonspecific finding on ECG. It is often idiopathic in nature, but can be secondary to electrolyte abnormalities and myocardial ischemia. Even though it is relatively common, T-wave flattening has been positively correlated with a higher rate of morbidity and mortality [14]. A list of causes of T-wave flattening can be found in Table 7.4.5.

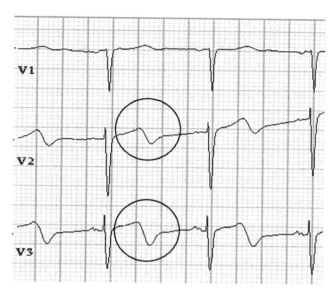

Figure 7.4.9 Biphasic T waves anteriorly (circled) are concerning for Wellens syndrome, Type B.

Table 7.4.5 Causes of T-wave flattening.

- Myocardial ischemia
- Thick chest wall
- Emphysema or chronic obstructive pulmonary disease (COPD)
- Pericardial effusion
- Constrictive pericarditis
- Hypothyroidism
- Hypoadrenalism
- Hypocalcemia
- Hypokalemia

The QT Interval

The QT interval represents the time from the first moment of ventricular depolarization (the beginning of the QRS complex) to the last moment of ventricular repolarization (the end of the T wave) [23]. Accurately calculating the QT interval can be a difficult task. The interval will vary depending on a multitude of factors unique to the individual being monitored. Most notably, the QT interval is inversely proportional to the heart rate: it shortens during times of tachycardia and lengthens when the patient is bradycardic [24]. Therefore, the QTc (corrected QT) interval is often used to standardize the measurement, and is most often calculated by the Bazett formula: $QT_c = QT/\sqrt{(R\text{-}R\ interval)}$, which standardizes the QT interval for a heart rate of 60 bpm. Even when this correction is used, it can still be inaccurate during tachycardia (>100 bpm) and extreme bradycardia (<50 bpm)

Table 7.4.6 Methods for calculating QTc.

Bazett:	$QT_c = \dfrac{QT}{\sqrt{RR}}$
Friderica:	$QT_c = \dfrac{QT}{\sqrt[3]{RR}}$
Sagie:	$QT_c = QT + 0.154(1 - RR)$

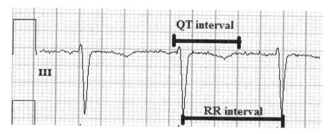

Figure 7.4.10 A patient with a prolonged QT. Note the width of the R–R interval. The QT segment is longer than half of the R–R interval, suggesting QT prolongation.

[25]. Other formulas to calculate the QTc have been developed (see Table 7.4.6), but the Bazett formula continues to be most often used in practice, as it is the simplest [26]. Along with changes in heart rate, an individual's QT interval can fluctuate due to changes in sympathetic tone. For this reason, QT prolongation is more pronounced early in the morning, with stress or during exercise [27].

On gross examination of an ECG, QT prolongation is suggested when its length is more than half of the R–R interval (Figure 7.4.10). However, this *gestalt method* is not entirely reliable, especially when the pulse is less than 70 beats per minute [28]. Additionally, even though most ECG machines automatically calculate the QT and QTc intervals, they have been found to be somewhat unreliable. Therefore, when QT prolongation is being entertained as a diagnosis, the QTc interval should be manually calculated by the physician, using the average of three to five QTc values on consecutive beats, as some beat-to-beat variation is expected [24]. There is debate regarding which lead to use when measuring the QT interval, as measurement can vary by as much as 20 ms between leads. Some sources advise measuring QT interval where it is longest (usually V2 or V3), whereas other groups have suggested measuring it in a limb lead (II), where the end of the T wave can clearly be seen [23]. The authors' preference is to use a limb lead to calculate the QT interval, assuming that the end of the T wave can be easily identified.

A normal QT interval is between 330 and 440 ms, and when corrected for heart rate, the QTc is considered prolonged if greater than 440 ms in men or 460 ms in women [29]. While QT prolongation is frequently discussed, a short QT interval can also be problematic, and is defined as a QT < 350 ms in males and < 360 ms in females [30].

QT Prolongation

QT Prolongation – defined as a QTc of greater than 440 ms in men or 460 ms in women – can be acquired or hereditary, and represents a repolarization phase that is abnormally long. The importance of QT prolongation, no matter the etiology, is the increased risk of torsades de pointes (TdP) with resultant syncope (if nonsustained) or sudden death. A longer QT interval provides a larger window for a random abnormal depolarization of myocytes (known as an early afterdepolarization) to occur during repolarization, which is the most common trigger for TdP. A QTc greater than 0.50 seconds puts the patient at significant risk for TdP. Therefore, the analysis of the QT interval is extremely important when evaluating any patient, but especially one presenting with palpitations, presyncope, syncope, or cardiac arrest [24].

A number of conditions and medications can prolong the QT interval (Figure 7.4.10), and a combination of multiple etiologies is often responsible for the prolonged QT interval. Common culprits seen in the hospital or emergency setting include antipsychotics, antibiotics, and electrolyte abnormalities. The definitive treatment for any patient with an acquired prolonged QT interval is to correct the underlying problem; the treating physician should remove or reverse any medications or metabolic conditions which may be responsible for the abnormality. In the case of a medication-induced prolonged QT interval, it is important to note that there is usually a dose dependent effect, so patients with supratherapeutic levels of any of these medications are at even further risk of morbidity and mortality [31]. Please see Table 7.4.7 for a list of common medications and individual factors which can prolong the QT interval.

Table 7.4.7 Causes of QT prolongation.

Medications	Individual Factors
Antiarrhythmics • Type III: amiodarone, sotalol, ibutilide • Type IA: quinidine, procainamide, flecanide	Female gender
Calcium channel blockers • Diltiazem, verapamil	Electrolyte abnormalities • Hypokalemia • Hypomagnesemia
Psychiatric medications • TCAs • Antipsychotics: haloperidol, droperidol, ziprasidone • SSRIs: fluoxetine, paroxetine, sertraline • Lithium	Structural heart disease • Cardiomyopathy • Congestive heart failure • Ischemia
Antihistamines • Diphenhydramine, hydroxyzine	Bradycardia • HR < 50 bpm
Antibiotics/Anti-viral • Amantadine • Fluoroquinolones • Fluconazole • Azithromycin	Renal dysfunction
Anti-retrovirals	Hepatic dysfunction
Miscellaneous • Methadone • Vasopressin • Ondansetron	Genetic mutations

Source: From: De Ponti [32].

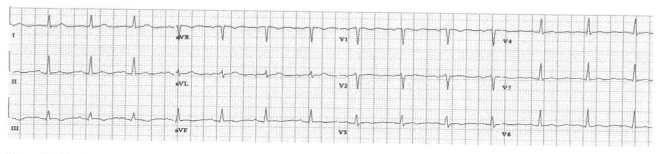

Figure 7.4.11 The QT_c in this patient was 0.35 seconds, serum calcium was markedly elevated.

Congenital Long QT Syndrome

Congenital long QT syndrome (LQTS) is due to a genetic mutation that results in a channelopathy [33]. It has a prevalence of approximately 1 in 5000 [34] and is more commonly diagnosed in women [35]. However, 2.5% of healthy individuals may have a mildly prolonged QT interval [36]. Therefore, QTc alone cannot be used to make a diagnosis of LQTS, and other ECG characteristics are used to make the diagnosis.

The T waves in patients with LQTS tend to be abnormal, and often have a biphasic or notched appearance [37]. Additionally, patients with LQTS often display "T wave alternans," or an alternation in T wave amplitude or polarity from beat to beat [38]. Finally, QT dispersion, or significant variation of QTc from lead to lead, is often noted on the ECG of patients with LQTS. This phenomenon is highly correlated with the development of ventricular arrhythmias [39]. Thus, one must include LQTS in the differential diagnosis when treating the otherwise healthy child or adult who presents with syncope or cardiac arrest, especially when they occur in the setting of exercise, when sympathetic surge can further prolong the QT interval further.

Short QT Interval

A short QT interval (Figure 7.4.11) is defined as a QT_c < 350 ms in males and < 360 ms in females. As opposed to a prolonged QT interval, there are a limited number of causes for a shortened QT interval (see Table 7.4.8), but it can be seen as a normal variant in up to 2% of the population [40].

Table 7.4.8 Causes of short QT interval.

- Electrolyte abnormalities
  - Hypercalcemia
  - Hyperkalemia
- Hyperthermia
- Acidosis
- Digitalis
- Myocardial ischmia
- Increased vagal tone

The most common acquired cause of QT shortening is hypercalcemia, often due to hyperparathyroidism, renal failure, or certain metastatic cancers. QT shortening is rarely life-threatening if it is due to an acquired cause, and treatment should be targeted toward the underlying metabolic abnormality. However, when the QTc is less than 330 ms, severe and potentially life-threatening arrhythmias – specifically atrial and ventricular fibrillation – can and do occur [41].

Congenital Short QT Syndrome

Although a congenital short QT syndrome (SQTS) was only recently discovered in 2000, it is just as dangerous as LQTS, as it can also cause life-threatening dysrhythmias [42]. Like LQTS, SQTS is due to a genetic abnormality of cardiac ion channels, and the diagnosis is made only after acquired causes are ruled out. The QTc intervals in these patients commonly range between 0.22 and 0.36 seconds, and the T wave often appears immediately after the QRS complex [43].

References

1 Rautaharju, P.M., Surawicz, B., and Gettes, L.S. (2009). AHA/ACCF/HRS recommendations for the standardization and interpretation of the electrocardiogram. *J. Am. Coll. Cardiol.* 53 (11): 982–991.

2 Baynes de Luna, A. (1993). *Clinical Electrocardiography; A Textbook.* New York: Futura Publishing Company.

3 Somers, M.P., Brady, W.J., Perron, A.D. et al. (2002). The prominent T wave: electrocardiographic differential diagnosis. *Am. J. Emerg. Med.* 20 (3): 243–251.

4 Mattu, A., Brady, W.J., and Robinson, D.A. (2000). Electrocardiographic manifestations of hyperkalemia. *Am. J. Emerg. Med.* 18 (6): 721–729.

5 Aslam, S., Friedman, E.A., and Ifudu, O. (2002). Electrocardiography is unreliable in detecting potentially lethal hyperkalemia in hemodialysis patients. *Nephrol. Dial. Trasplant.* 17 (9): 1639–1642.

6 Marx, J.A., Hockberger, R.S., Walls, R.M. et al. (eds.) (2002). *Rosen's Emergency Medicine: Concepts and Clinical Practice*, 1019. Philadelphia, PA: Mosby.

7 De Winter, R.J., Verouden, N.J.W., Wellens, H.J.J., and Wilde, A.A.M. (2008). A new sign of proximal LAD occlusion. *N. Engl. J. Med.* 359: 2071–2073.

8 Brady, W.J. (2006). ST segment and T wave abnormalities not caused by acute coronary syndromes. *Emerg. Med. Clin. North Am.* 24: 91–111.

9 Mehta, M.C. and Jain, A.C. (1995). Early repolarization on scalar electrocardiogram. *Am J Med Sci* 309: 305–311.

10 Hayden, G.E., Brady, W.J., Perron, A.D. et al. (2002). Electrocardiographic T-wave inversion: differential diagnosis in the chest pain patient. *Am. J. Emerg. Med.* 20 (3): 252–262.

11 Schimpf, R., Wolpert, C., Gaita, F. et al. (2005). Short QT syndrome. *Cardiovasc. Res.* 67: 357–366.

12 Simon, A., Robins, L.J.H., Hooghoudt, T.H.E. et al. (2007). Pseudonormalisation of the T wave: old wine? *Neth. Hear. J.* 15: 257–259.

13 Hayden, G.E., Brady, W.J., Perron, A.D. et al. (2002 May 1). Electrocardiographic T-wave inversion: differential diagnosis in the chest pain patient. *The American journal of emergency medicine.* 20 (3): 252–262.

14 Kannel, W.B., Anderson, K., McGee, D.L. et al. (1987). Nonspecific electrocardiographic abnormality as a predictor of coronary heart disease: the Framingham Study. *Am. Heart J.* 113: 370–376.

15 Yamazaki, T., Myers, J., and Froelicher, V.F. (2005). Prognostic importance of isolated T-wave abnormalities. *Am. J. Cardiol.* 95: 300–304.

16 Pillarisetti, J. and Gupta, K. (2020). Giant inverted T waves in the emergency department: case report and review of differential diagnoses. *J. Electrocardiol.* 43: 40–42.

17 Katz, A.M. (1995). Post-tachycardia T-wave syndrome. *N. Engl. J. Med.* 332: 161.

18 Goldstein, D.S. (1979). The electrocardiogram in stroke: relationship to pathophysiological type and comparison with prior tracings. *Stroke* 10: 253–258.

19 Channer, K. and Morris, F. (2002). Myocardial ischaemia. *Br. Med. J.* 321: 1023–1026.

20 Manno, B.V., Hakki, A.H., Iskandrian, A.S. et al. (1983). Significance of the upright T wave in precordial lead V1 in adults with coronary artery disease. *J. Am. Coll. Cardiol.* 1 (5): 1213–1215.

21 De Zwann, C., Bar, F.W., and Wellens, H.J.J. (1982). Characteristic electrocardiographic pattern indicating a critical stenosis high in left anterior descending coronary artery in patients admitted because of impending myocardial infarction. *Am. Heart J.* 103 (4): 730–736.

22 Tandy, T.K., Bottomy, D.P., and Lewis, J.G. (1999). Wellens' Syndrome. *Ann. Emerg. Med.* 33 (3): 347–351.

23 Davey, P.P. (2000). Which lead for Q-T interval measurements? *Cardiology* 94 (3): 159–164.

24 Al-Khatib, S.M., Allen LaPointe, N.M., Kramer, J.M. et al. (2003). What clinicians should know about the QT interval. *JAMA* 289 (16): 2120–2127.

25 Funck-Brentano, C. and Jaillon, P. (1993). Rate-corrected QT interval: techniques and limitations. *Am. J. Cardiol.* 72: 17B.

26 Sagie, A., Larson, M.G., Goldberg, R.J. et al. (1992). An improved method for adjusting the QT interval for heart rate (the Framingham heart study). *Am. J. Cardiol.* 70: 797–801.

27 Brenyo, A.J., Huang, D.T., and Aktas, M.K. (2012). Congenital long and short QT syndromes. *Cardiology* 122: 237–247.

28 Baltazar, R.F. (2009). *Basic and Bedside Electrocardiography*, vol. 13. Baltimore, MD: Lippincott Williams & Wilkins.

29 Moss, A.J. (1993). Measurement of the QT interval and the risk associated with QTc interval prolongation: a review. *Am. J. Cardiol.* 72: 23B.

30 Patel, C., Yan, G., and Antzelevitch, C. (2010). Short QT syndrome: from bench to bedside. *Circ.: Arrhythm. Electrophysiol.* 3: 401–408.

31 Kao, L.W. and Furbee, R.B. (2005). Drug induced QT prolongation. *Med. Clin. N. Am.* 89: 1125–1144.

32 De Ponti, F. (2002). Safety of non-antiarrhythmic drugs that prolong the QT interval or induce torsade de pointes: an overview. *Drug Saf.* 25 (4): 263–286.

33 Hedley, P.J., Jorgensen, P., Schlamowitz, S. et al. (2009). The genetic basis of long QT and short QT syndromes: a mutation update. *Hum. Mutat.* 30: 1486–1511.

34 Goldenberg, I., Zareba, W., and Moss, A.J. (2008). Long QT syndrome. *Curr. Probl. Cardiol.* 33: 629–694.

35 Imboden, M., Swan, H., Denjoy, I. et al. (2006). Female predominance and transmission distortion in the long-QT syndrome. *N. Engl. J. Med.* 355: 2744–2751.

36 Goldenberg, I., Horr, S., Moss, A.J. et al. (2011). Risk for life-threatening cardiac events in patients with genotype-confirmed long-QT syndrome and normal-range corrected QT intervals. *J. Am. Coll. Cardiol.* 57: 51–59.

37 Zhang, L., Timothy, K.W., Vincent, G.M. et al. (2000). Spectrum of ST-T wave patterns and repolarization parameters in congenital long-QT syndrome: ECG findings identify genotypes. *Circulation* 102: 2849.

38 Burattini, L., Zareba, W., Rashba, E.J. et al. (1998). ECG features of microvolt T-wave alternans in coronary artery disease and long QT syndrome patients. *J. Electrocardiol.* (31 Suppl): 114.

39 Shah, M.J., Wieand, T.S., Rhodes, L.A. et al. (1997). QT and JT dispersion in children with long QT syndrome. *J. Cardiovasc. Electrophysiol.* 8: 642.

40 Mason, J.W., Ramseth, D.J., Chanter, D.O. et al. (2007). Electrocardiographic reference ranges derived from 79,743 ambulatory subjects. *J. Electrocardiol.* 40: 228.

41 Cross, B., Hamoud, M., and Link, M. (2011). The short QT syndrome. *J. Interv. Card. Electrophysiol.* 31: 25–31.

42 Giustetto, C., Di Monte, F., Wolpert, C. et al. (2006). Short QT syndrome: clinical findings and diagnostic-therapeutic implications. *Eur. Heart J.* 27: 2440.

43 Hanna, E.B. and Glancy, D.L. (2011). ST-segment depression and T-wave inversion: classification, differential diagnosis, and caveats. *Cleve. Clin. J. Med.* 78 (6): 404–414.

5

Bradycardia

B. Elizabeth Delasobera[1] and Tress Goodwin[2]

[1] *Department of Emergency Medicine, Georgetown University & MedStar Health, Washington, DC, USA*
[2] *Department of Emergency Medicine & Pediatrics, Children's National Hospital, George Washington School of Medicine, Washington, DC, USA*

Bradycardia Basics

Definition of Bradycardia

Bradycardia is defined as any heart rate that is less than 60 bpm. When the rhythm originates from the SA node but is slower than 60 bpm it is called sinus bradycardia. However, many other bradycardic rhythms exist in which the rhythm does not originate from the SA node. A strategy for defining these bradycardic rhythms is described here.

Differential Diagnosis of Bradycardia

Bradycardia can be caused by many different etiologies, ranging from benign to life threatening. Many young, athletic patients have a normal sinus bradycardia that develops solely based on their age and/or their fitness level. Other causes of sinus bradycardia include medications (e.g. beta blockers, or other anti-sympathomemetics), ischemia, hypothermia, thyroid disease, or electrolyte abnormalities. Nonsinus bradycardias may also be due to medications, ischemia, hypothermia, or electrolyte abnormalities, but they can also be caused by intrinsic changes with the conduction system that occurs with age. Figure 7.5.1 lists a differential diagnosis of several of the most common causes of bradycardia.

Bradycardia Rhythms

Sinus Bradycardia

Sinus bradycardia (Figure 7.5.2) is defined by a rate less than 60 bpm originating from the SA node; made evident by the presence of a normal appearing P wave before each QRS, and a QRS after every P wave. The QRS is normal appearing and narrow. Sinus bradycardia is usually a normal variant seen in the healthy, young, athletic population. This occurs because athletes have a higher stroke volume due to heart muscle conditioning, and therefore require fewer beats to generate the same cardiac output. Sinus bradycardia also occurs in many healthy individuals during sleep. However, sinus bradycardia is not always a normal variant and can be seen with ischemia, hypothermia, hypoglycemia, hypothyroidism, conduction abnormalities, or as a side effect of medications such as beta blockers, calcium channel blockers, digoxin, opioids, or organophosphates (Figure 7.5.3).

Junctional Bradycardia

Junctional bradycardia (Figure 7.5.4) occurs with the rhythm is generated from a focus in the AV junction and typically leads to a rate between 40 and 60 beats/minute. This can occur when the usual pacemaker site (such as the SA node and/or atrial foci) are no longer present or active. Most often with junctional bradycardia there are no P waves at all; however, retrograde P waves may be present, representing atrial depolarization moving superiorly from the AV node and away from the surface ECG leads. These often appear as inverted P waves and may have a short PR interval. Alternately, these P waves may be buried in the QRS complex, or they may appear as a notch in the terminal portion of the QRS. This is described further elsewhere in this text.

Idioventricular

When all pacemaking centers above the ventricles have failed or when there is a complete block below the AV node such that the ventricular myocardium does not receive a signal from the SA or the AV node, a site within the

Electrocardiogram in Clinical Medicine, First Edition. Edited by William J. Brady, Michael J. Lipinski, Andrew E. Darby, Michael C. Bond, Nathan P. Charlton, Korin Hudson, and Kelly Williamson.
© 2021 John Wiley & Sons Ltd. Published 2021 by John Wiley & Sons Ltd.

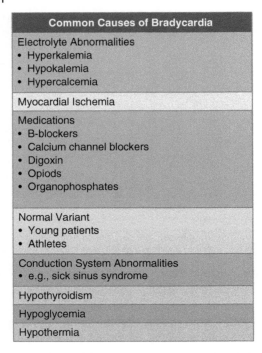

Common Causes of Bradycardia
Electrolyte Abnormalities • Hyperkalemia • Hypokalemia • Hypercalcemia
Myocardial Ischemia
Medications • B-blockers • Calcium channel blockers • Digoxin • Opiods • Organophosphates
Normal Variant • Young patients • Athletes
Conduction System Abnormalities • e.g., sick sinus syndrome
Hypothyroidism
Hypoglycemia
Hypothermia

Figure 7.5.1 Differential diagnosis of bradycardia.

ventricles assumes the pacemaker role. The resulting rhythm is referred to as an idioventricular rhythm (Figure 7.5.5). The intrinsic ventricular rate is generally 20–40 bpm. The QRS complex is wide, and often bizarre in appearance, representing a cell-to-cell transmission of the electrical signal.

Sinoventricular Rhythm with Hyperkalemia

Markedly high serum potassium levels may lead to characteristic rhythm disturbance described as a sinoventricular rhythm. As potassium levels rise, progressive changes in the ECG occur, which can lead to sinoventricular rhythm and ultimately to ventricular fibrillation and death. The

first of these changes is the development of tall, symmetric, peaked T waves across the entire ECG. These differ from the hyperacute T waves seen in the setting of acute ischemia where peaked T waves are usually more broad-based and are seen in an anatomical distribution only. As the potassium level continues to elevate, the PR interval becomes longer and the P waves become flat. Eventually, if left untreated, the QRS complex widens and then peaked T waves and wide QRS complexes become almost indistinguishable. If the hyperkalemia persists, the QRS then merges, with the T wave forming a sine wave pattern (sinoventricular rhythm, Figure 7.5.6), which is usually a slow rhythm. This can ultimately lead to ventricular fibrillation and death if untreated.

Hypokalemia

Low potassium also can cause ECG changes, including bradycardia. The main changes that can be seen are ST depression, flat T waves, U waves, and bradycardia (Figure 7.5.7).

Hypothermia

ECG changes are often seen when body temperatures drop below 30 °C. In general, everything on the ECG slows down. The segments and intervals all become prolonged (PR, QRS, QT, etc.), leading to a sinus bradycardia. Slow atrial fibrillation is also commonly seen. J waves or Osborn waves following the QRS are also pathognomonic for hypothermia (Figure 7.5.8).

Rhythms That Can Be Slow

The following rhythms are reviewed in depth in other chapters, but it is important to review these again in the context of bradycardia, as they can all present with rates

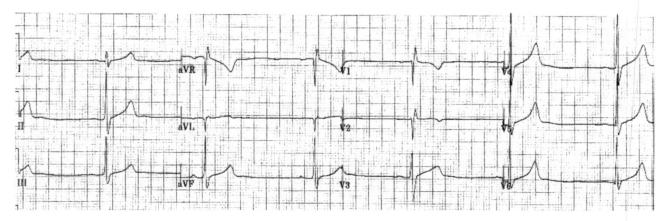

Figure 7.5.2 Sinus bradycardia in a healthy elite athlete; heart rate 38 bpm.

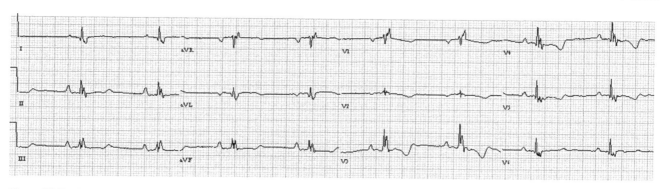

Figure 7.5.3 Sinus bradycardia with an underlying right bundle branch block (RBBB) in an elderly patient on a beta-blocker medication.

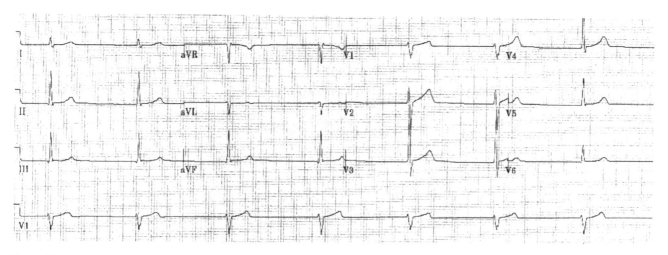

Figure 7.5.4 Junctional bradycardia: note the absence of P waves in this slow, narrow complex rhythm.

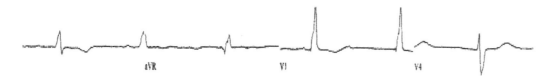

Figure 7.5.5 Idioventricular; note the absence of P waves and the bizarre-looking QRS complexes in this extremely slow rhythm, also referred to as a *ventricular escape rhythm*.

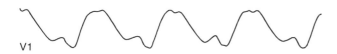

Figure 7.5.6 Sinoventricular rhythm with hyperkalemia; see the classic sine wave pattern in this V5 rhythm strip from a patient with critically high potassium levels after several missed dialysis sessions.

less than 60 bpm. Treatment for these rhythms should be focused on the clinical status of the patient, and any underlying etiology, ensuring adequate perfusion to end organs, regardless of the heart rate. The oft-heard phrase

"treat the patient, not the rhythm" certainly applies in many of these cases.

Slow Atrial Fibrillation

While atrial fibrillation is typically associated with a ventricular rate of 110–160, patients with underlying atrial fibrillation can develop a bradycardia, "Slow atrial fibrillation" is an irregularly irregular rhythm with a ventricular rate <60. The most common causes of slow atrial fibrillation (Figure 7.5.9) include hypothermia, sinus node dysfunction, and side effects of medications such as antiarrhythmics (e.g. digoxin) or AV nodal blockers (beta blockers or

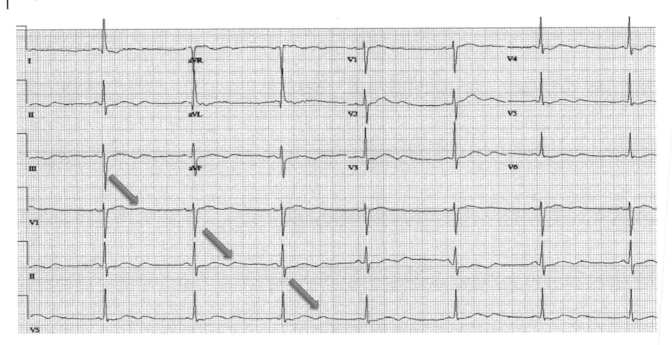

Figure 7.5.7 Sinus bradycardia with U waves (arrows shown in single lead rhythm strips) due to hypokalemia.

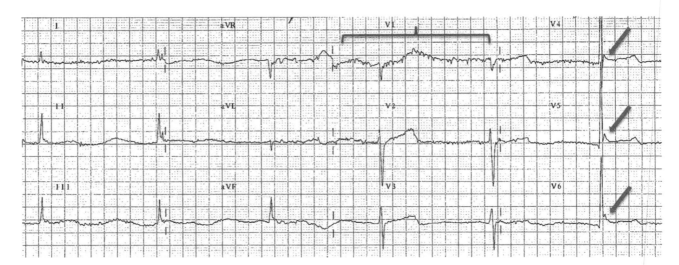

Figure 7.5.8 Sinus bradycardia due to hypothermia; demonstrating bradycardia, J waves/ Osborn waves (arrows), and shivering artifact (braces). *Source:* Adapted with permission from http://lifeinthefastlane.com/ecg-library/basics/hypothermia.

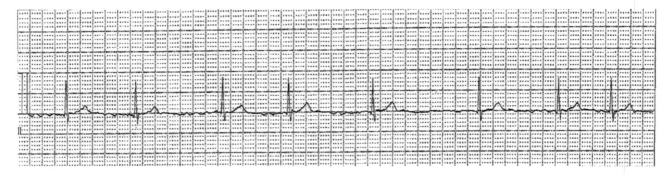

Figure 7.5.9 Slow atrial fibrillation with a heart rate less than 60 bpm. Note the absence of discrete P waves.

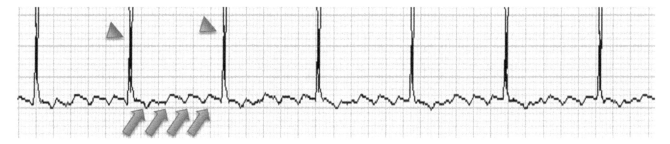

Figure 7.5.10 Slow atrial flutter, 5:1 block. Note that there are four flutter waves (arrows) for each QRS complex (arrow head).

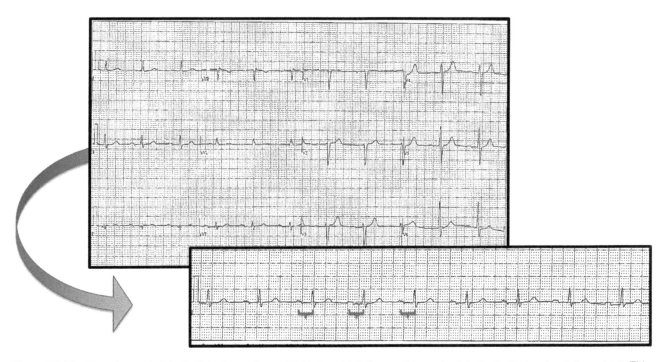

Figure 7.5.11 First-degree AV block. Note the prolonged PR interval (>0.2 sec or 1 large box), indicated in the inset figure here. This PR interval is consistent from beat to beat.

calcium channel blockers). Given that many patients with atrial fibrillation are one or a combination of these drugs, the clinician should maintain high suspicion for medication side effects as the cause of bradycardia in patients with known atrial fibrillation.

Slow Atrial Flutter

Though atrial flutter is often associated with a rate of 150 in a 2:1 block, defined by the number of flutter waves occurring for each QRS complex (by convention, the number of flutter waves seen between QRS complexes, plus 1). However, if the block occurs with a ratio of 4:1 or 5:1, the

rate would be 75 and 60, respectively. Figure 7.5.10 shows atrial flutter with a 5:1 block. Atrial flutter with variable block could also produce bradycardic rates. As with atrial fibrillation, medications are the likely cause of bradycardia in a patient with atrial flutter.

AV Blocks

Atrioventricular (AV) blocks, also called simply *heart blocks*, are defined by a delay or interruption in conduction between the atria and the ventricles. While the heart rates can be variable, heart blocks are often a cause of bradycardia with rates of less than 60 bpm.

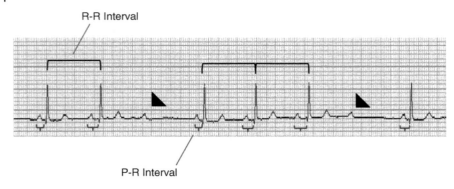

Figure 7.5.12 Second-degree AV block, Type I (Weneckebach). Note that the PR interval lengthens for each consecutive conducted beat while the R-R interval remains consistent, but that there are characteristic "dropped beats" where P waves are not followed by a QRS complex (arrow heads).

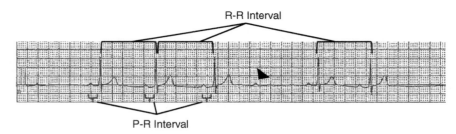

Figure 7.5.13 Second-degree AV block, type 2. The PR interval and RR interval are consistent for each conducted beat, but note the presence of P waves without a subsequent QRS complex, which represent nonconducted or "dropped" beats (arrow heads).

First-Degree AV Block

First-degree AV block occurs when conduction through the AV node is slowed, defined by a PR interval longer than 200 msec (Figure 7.5.11). Though conduction is slow through the AV node, each atrial depolarization is followed by a ventricular depolarization and therefore every P wave is followed by a QRS complex and every QRS complex is preceded by a P wave. Because the pacemaker site is constant, typically the SA node, the PR interval is regular from beat to beat. Possible causes of first-degree AV block include: AV nodal blocking agents or antiarrhythmics, increased vagal tone, inferior MI, mitral valve surgery, myocarditis (e.g. Lyme disease) hypokalemia. First-degree AV block may also have no recognized cause and therefore is also considered a normal variant. This rhythm is stable and does not require specific treatment. As in sinus bradycardia, treatment for a first-degree AV block should be directed toward the clinical status of the patient (e.g. symptomatic hypotension) and not for the heart rate specifically.

Second-Degree AV Block: Mobitz Type 1 (Wenckebach)

Second-degree AV block Type I, also known as Wenckebach rhythm, or Mobitz type I is defined by a progressive PR interval prolongation from beat to beat, ultimately leading

to a nonconducted P wave (Figure 7.5.12). That is, a P wave that is not followed by a QRS complex. Because heart rate is defined by the number of ventricular contractions, this can lead to an overall bradycardic rate. The possible etiologies of Mobitz Type 1 are very similar to first degree AV block and include AV nodal blocking agents or antiarrhythmics, increased vagal tone, inferior MI, myocarditis, and cardiac surgery. This is also a stable rhythm, and treatment should be based on clinical status.

Second-Degree AV Block: Mobitz Type 2

Second-degree AV Block type 2 is a rhythm in which the PR interval remains unchanged from beat to beat for a time, until there is a nonconducted P wave and a *dropped beat* (Figure 7.5.13). As in second-degree type 1 block, this occurs when an atrial depolarization fails to conduct via the AV node and hence there is no QRS complex and no ventricular depolarization to follow it. Immediately following the nonconducted P wave, the cycle resets and there is another P wave, followed by a QRS complex. The ratio of conducted P waves to nonconducted P waves may be variable. Again this can present as a form of bradycardia. This is considered an unstable rhythm due to the fact that it can progress to complete heart block and has increased mortality compared to a Mobitz Type 1 block. Possible etiologies include AV nodal blocking agents or antiarrhythmics,

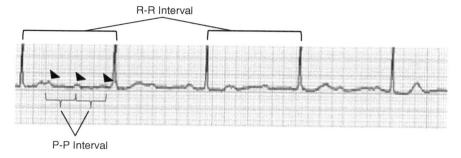

R-R Interval

P-P Interval

Figure 7.5.14 Third-degree (or complete) heart block. Note that though the P—P interval is consistent and the R-R interval is consistent, they are not equal and the P waves (arrow heads) and QRS complexes bear no direct relationship to each other (though one may obscure the appearance of the other); they are "dissociated."

hyperkalemia, anterior MI, cardiac surgery (especially surgery near the septum such as mitral valve repair), autoimmune, or inflammatory conditions such as lupus or rheumatic fever, or infiltrative disease such as sarcoidosis or amyloidosis.

Third-Degree or Complete Heart Block

In third-degree or complete heart block, there is no meaningful communication between the atria and the ventricles. Also known as AV dissociation, both the atria and the ventricles are depolarizing in a regular fashion. However, they do so without relation to each other (Figure 7.5.14). That is, there is a regular P—P interval and a regular R-R interval, but the atrial rate and ventricular rate may vary widely. This represents significant disease in the cardiac conduction system and of all of the heart blocks, complete heart block is the most likely to present with profound bradycardia. Depending on the site of escape focus, the rate and QRS complex width will vary. A rhythm that arises from a site near the bundle of His will have a narrow complex rhythm with a rate of 40–60 bpm, while rhythms arising from sites distal to the His bundle are more likely to

have a wide complex with a rate of 40 bpm or less. Causes of complete heart block include AV nodal blocking agents, inferior MI. However there are cases that are considered to be idiopathic as well. Third-degree heart block is unstable and patients are at high risk of sudden cardiac death. The risk of death is mostly due to the fact that patients can develop polymorphic ventricular tachycardia when significant bradycardia is present. In addition they are often significantly bradycardic and hypotensive due to the significant bradycardia.

Conclusion

In conclusion, it is important for the astute clinician to consider the differential diagnosis for bradycardia, and to know the management options, depending on the underlying cause of the bradycardia. Hyper- or hypokalemia, hypercalcemia, hypothermia, hypoglycemia, hypothyroid, medication toxicity, ischemia, and sick sinus syndrome are all important things to consider. In addition, it is important to be able to recognize sinus bradycardia from heart block and to be able to identify the various types and degrees of heart block, as some of these rhythms are more inherently unstable than others.

Additional Resources

Baltazar, R.F. (2009). Basic and bedside electrocardiography, vol. 13. Baltimore, MD: Lippincott Williams & Wilkins.

Da Costa, D., Brady, W.J., and Edhouse, J. (2008). Bradycardias and atrioventricular conduction block. In: *ABC of Clinical Electrocardiography*, (ed. Morris, F., Brady, W., and Camm, A.J.), 9–13. Malden: John Wiley & Sons, Incorporated.

Link, M.S., Homoud, M.K., Wang, P.J., and Estes, N.A. (2002). Cardiac arrhythmias in the athlete: the evolving role of electrophysiology. *Curr Sports Med Rep.* 1 (2):75–85.

Mattu, A., and Brady, W.J. (2008). ECGs for the emergency physician 2. Blackwell Publishing.

Mirvis, D., and Goldberger, A. (2011). Electrocardiography. In: *Braunwald's Heart Disease – A Textbook of Cardiovascular Medicine*, 9e (ed. R. Bonow, D.L. Mann, D.P. Zipes, and P. Libby), 126–165. Philadelphia: Elsevier.

Parham, W., Mehdirad, A., Biermann, K., and Fredman, C. (2006). Hyperkalemia revisited. *Tex. Heart Inst. J.* 33 (1): 40–47.

Semelka, M., Gera, J., and Usman, S. (2013). Sick sinus syndrome: a review. *Am Fam Physician.* 87 (10):691–696.

Sepehrdad, R., Paulsen, J., and Amsterdam, E.A. (2012). The ECG that came in from the cold. *Am J Med.* 125 (3): 246–248.

Surawicz, B., Knilans, T.K., and Chou, T.-C. (2008). *Chou's electrocardiography in clinical practice : adult and pediatric* (6th ed.). Philadelphia, PA: Saunders/Elsevier.

Tintinalli, J.E., Cline, D., and American College of Emergency Physicians (c2012). Arrhythmia Management. In: *Tintinalli's Emergency Medicine Manual.* New York: McGraw-Hill Education.

6

Rhythms Presenting with Normal Rate

Robert Katzer[1] and Janet Smereck[2]

[1]*Department of Emergency Medicine, University of California, Irvine, CA, USA*
[2]*Department of Emergency Medicine, Georgetown University & MedStar Health, Washington, DC, USA*

Definitions and Clinical Considerations

A normal heart rate, reassuring to the clinician, may be present in a multitude of electrocardiographic scenarios, both physiologic and pathologic. A heart rate greater than 100 beats per minute (bpm) defines tachycardia and less than 60 bpm defines bradycardia; therefore normal rate falls between 60 and 100 bpm [1]. The definition of "normal" assumes a resting state, as heart rate is expected to increase under circumstances such as exercise, fever and hypovolemia, and decrease during sleep [2]. Moreover, the "athletic heart" beats more efficiently, and the resting heart rate of well-conditioned individuals may be less than 60 bpm as a normal physiologic adaptation to the increased stroke volume produced by an athletically strengthened myometrium [3].

Normal heart rate is not a static phenomenon; it represents a balance between sympathetic and parasympathetic reflexes [4]. Variability of the heart rate indicates a healthy cardiovascular system; a decrease in heart rate variability is found with aging, autonomic neuropathies including diabetes, intrinsic heart disease such as congestive heart failure, and pharmacologic agents, particularly digoxin [5, 6].

Age-based definitions of what constitutes a normal rate should be taken into account when managing pediatric patients. Although this chapter does not discuss the nuances of the pediatric electrocardiogram, a study of healthy newborns in the first 10 days of life found wide variability in resting heart rates, 82−175 bpm [7]. Age-based normal rates for pediatric patients are presented in Figure 7.6.1 [8].

The following rhythms, both regular and irregular, may present with a normal rate. Regular rhythms include normal sinus rhythm, AV nodal and junctional rhythms, first-degree AV block, accelerated idioventricular rhythm, and atrial flutter, which may be regular or irregular.

Irregular rhythms include sinus arrhythmia, sinus rhythm with atrial, junctional, or ventricular ectopic beats, atrial fibrillation and atrial flutter. The second-degree AV blocks may occasionally present with rates sufficient to be considered normal. Additionally, paced rhythms are typically set to normal rate and may be regular or irregular depending on whether the pacing is complete or intermittent.

Regular Rhythms

Normal Sinus Rhythm

The normal resting rate of depolarization of the sinus node in adults is 72 bpm. Normal sinus rhythm (Figure 7.6.2) originates from the sinoatrial node, the natural "pacemaker" of the heart. This is represented by the P wave, which precedes atrial activation. This is followed by AV nodal conduction, electrically represented by the P-R interval. The QRS complex represents electrical conduction through the His-Purkinje tracts to activate ventricular depolarization. The presence of conduction delays or blocks may be seen as a widening of the QRS complex. Repolarization is represented by the T wave.

First-Degree AV Block

In a normally conducted beat, an electrical impulse passes from the atria to the ventricles through the A-V bundle, the bundle of His, and the Purkinje fibers to the ventricles. The normal conduction time through the atria, represented on the surface ECG as the period between the beginning of the P wave and the beginning of the QRS complex, is about 0.16 seconds. Prolonged conduction greater than 0.2 seconds is defined as delayed conduction, also known as first-degree

Electrocardiogram in Clinical Medicine, First Edition. Edited by William J. Brady, Michael J. Lipinski, Andrew E. Darby, Michael C. Bond, Nathan P. Charlton, Korin Hudson, and Kelly Williamson.

Age	Normal Heart Rate (beat per min)
0–1 month	100–205
1–6 months	105–175
6–12 months	90–160
1–3 years	80–150
3–6 years	70–120
6–12 years	60–110
12–15 years	60–100
>16 years	60–100
Highly Trained Athlete	40–60

Figure 7.6.1   Age-based normal rates for pediatric patients.

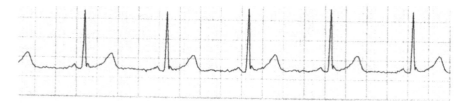

Figure 7.6.2   Normal sinus rhythm. Note the normal and consistent intervals and waveforms.

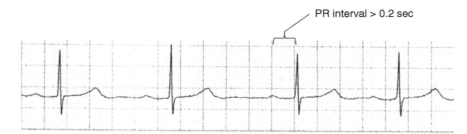

PR interval > 0.2 sec

Figure 7.6.3   Normal sinus rhythm with first degree A-V block, rate 60 bpm; note the prolonged PR interval.

AV block (Figure 7.6.3). Although not requiring treatment, this finding may represent disease of the AV bundle due to scarring, ischemia, or rheumatic heart disease.

Accelerated Junctional Rhythm

Junctional rhythms typically fall within the intrinsic rate of the AV nodal pacer, 40–60 bpm, but may be accelerated due to altered vagal tone due to myocardial ischemia, sick sinus syndrome or digoxin toxicity. P waves may or may not be evident on the surface ECG and are often inverted as they result from retrograde impulses (which conduct away from the surface ECG leads) from the AV junction back toward the atria. They may exist just prior to, buried within, or following the QRS complex. In the absence of aberrant conduction, the QRS will be narrow (Figure 7.6.4).

Irregular Rhythms

Sinus Arrhythmia

Sinus arrhythmia (Figure 7.6.5) is the most frequently seen cardiac arrhythmia and represents an exaggeration of the normal rate variation that occurs with the respiratory cycle. Heart rate increases with inspiration and decreases with expiration due to sympathetic and parasympathetic signals to the sinus node produced by changes in intrathoracic pressure which affect the volume of venous return to the atria [9]. This may be accentuated in clinical scenarios that cause hypovolemia and is commonly seen in healthy individuals with mild-to-moderate dehydration, who may experience symptoms of palpitations or lightheadedness.

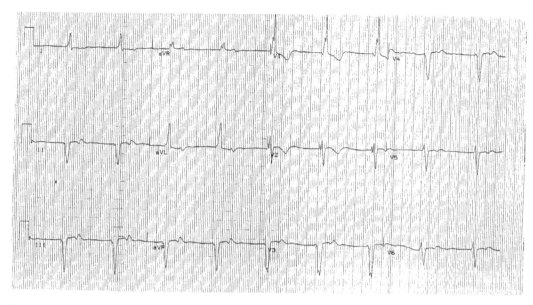

Figure 7.6.4   Accelerated junctional rhythm. Note the absence of P waves in this rhythm with a normal rate and narrow QRS complex.

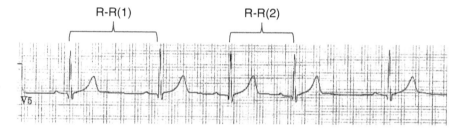

Figure 7.6.5   Sinus arrhythmia. Note that the R-R interval is slightly different from beat to beat and R-R(1) is longer than R-R(2) in this rhythm with an underlying rate of 62 bpm.

Sinus arrhythmia is defined as greater than 10% variation in R-R interval between the longest and shortest cycle lengths, or when the variation between the longest and shortest cycle length exceeds 120 ms.

Atrio-Ventricular Blocks

Delays in conduction through the atrioventricular (AV) node may manifest with varying degrees of conduction failure. Disease in the nodal conducting pathways, increased vagal tone, and numerous pharmacologic agents, including digoxin, beta blockers and some calcium channel blockers, may slow or block nodal conduction. While these rhythms frequently present with slow rates, any of the AV blocks (particularly first- and second-degree) may present with normal rates, and the rhythms are generally irregular. First-degree AV block has already been discussed; the higher-grade AV blocks are discussed in detail in Section 3, Chapter 2.

Premature Atrial Contractions (PAC)

PACs are defined as narrow complex beats that sporadically occur earlier than anticipated within an otherwise normal cardiac cycle. The P-wave morphology in the ectopic beats is distinct from that of the underlying sinus rhythm because the ectopic P waves originate from a site in the atria outside of the SA node. In the absence of underlying aberrant conduction through the AV node or ventricular conduction system, the P waves are usually followed by a narrow QRS complex that matches the underlying rhythm.

The PR interval may be lengthened or shortened depending on the location of the atrial ectopic focus. An ectopic focus that leads to extremely premature P wave may result in a blocked PAC, that is, an extremely premature P wave with no subsequent QRS complex, due to the refractory period of the His-Purkinje system, AV node, or myocardium. Similarly, the P wave may also occur so prematurely

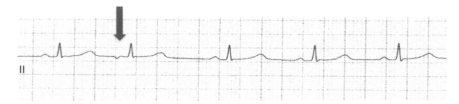

Figure 7.6.6 Normal sinus rhythm with premature atrial contraction (PAC) occurring in the second beat. Note the inverted P wave (arrow), which precedes the premature beat, indicating an ectopic atrial focus.

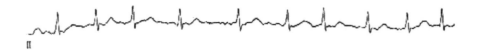

Figure 7.6.7 Atrial fibrillation, average rate 87 bpm. Note the absence of organized and consistent P waves and no consistent R-R interval.

that it is buried in the preceding T wave. The pause demonstrated after a PAC is not fully compensatory because the atrial impulse resets the SA node during the PAC. This can be observed by noting that the duration of a sinus beat and the following PAC is shorter than that of two consecutive sinus beats (Figure 7.6.6).

Most PACs are idiopathic and are not clinical significance. Electrolyte abnormalities such as hypokalemia may cause increased myocardial irritability producing atrial ectopic beats. Conditions such as congestive heart failure or pulmonary hyptertension, which increase atrial pressure, are also associated with increased frequency of PACs. Finally, pharmacologic agents such as digoxin, nicotine, caffeine, thyroid hormones, and anti-arrhythmic agents may also stimulate the formation of atrial ectopic beats.

Atrial Fibrillation with Normal Rate

Atrial fibrillation, present in 5% of adults older than 65, is classically described as an "irregularly irregular" rhythm. This arrhythmia stems from uncoordinated or chaotic atrial depolarization, leading to an absence of organized P waves on the ECG. These waves, which are best visualized in lead V1, do not exhibit consistent morphology [10]. The typical fibrillatory rate is in the 400s, and when these fibrillatory waves demonstrate amplitudes of at least 0.5 mm, the rhythm is described as coarse atrial fibrillation. Otherwise, the rhythm is referred to as fine atrial fibrillation. In the absence of aberrant ventricular conduction, the QRS duration will be normal. However, the lack of a regular atrial pacemaker leads to irregular ventricular response, seen as R-R intervals which vary from beat to beat. The ventricular rate may vary from quite slow to very rapid; yet

many patients will present with atrial fibrillation with a normal rate (Figure 7.6.7).

Atrial fibrillation is further categorized into paroxysmal (self-terminating), persistent (which may still respond to cardioversion, reverting to a sinus rhythm with appropriate treatment), and permanent. Atrial fibrillation may be seen in association with hypertension, myocardial infarction, coronary artery bypass surgery, and alcohol abuse [11]. The ventricular rate may be influenced by current medications including digitalis, beta blockers, and calcium channel blockers.

While a full discussion of the management of atrial fibrillation is beyond the scope of this chapter, options include both rate control and rhythm control. Rhythm control is accomplished via chemical or electrical cardioversion, and rate control may be achieved by a number of pharmacologic means, particularly short-acting calcium channel blockers and beta blockers [12].

Atrial Flutter

Atrial flutter results from the irritability of a single focus in the atria, usually at the root of the SVC and IVC. This irritability may be due to any one of a number of etiologies, including: MI, surgery, SA node disease, digitalis toxicity, or pulmonary disease. Atrial flutter is characterized by "sawtooth" P waves ("flutter waves"), which are noted most readily on the inferior precordial leads as downward deflecting, with a steeper upstroke than downstroke. Though the atrial rate is typically 250–350 BPM, this rate may be slower under circumstances that slow atrial conduction. Because of the refractory period of the AV node, only a limited number of impulses are transmitted through to the ventricles. Atrial flutter is often defined by the ratio

(a)

(b)

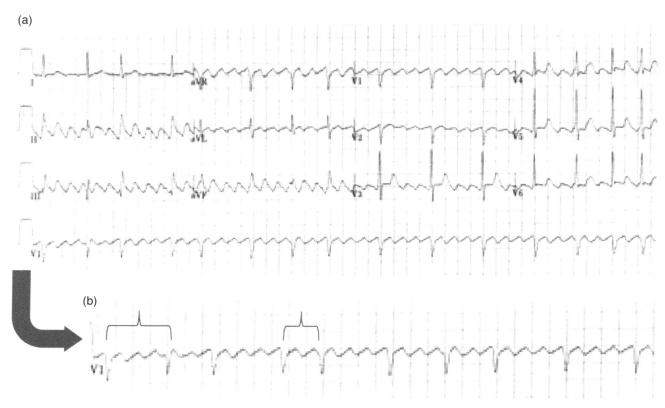

Figure 7.6.8   Atrial flutter with variable block. Note the characteristic "sawtooth" waves more visible in certain leads (panel a). Note that the ratio of flutter waves to QRS complexes varies from beat to beat (as demonstrated in panel b).

of flutter waves to QRS complexes. By convention, this is described as the number of flutter waves seen between QRS complexes plus 1 (as it is assumed that due to the regular nature of the flutter waves, one is obscured by the QRS complex). Atrial flutter often presents with a consistent ratio, the most common being 2 : 1; however, it may also present with variable conduction, in which the number of flutter waves between QRS complexes varies from beat-to-beat (Figure 7.6.8). The arrhythmia is typically paroxysmal and may start and stop abruptly without pharmacologic intervention.

Wandering Atrial Pacemaker or Multifocal Atrial Rhythm

Wandering atrial pacemaker and multifocal atrial rhythm are terms used to describe a rhythm that demonstrates at least three distinct P-wave morphologies and a rate of 60–100 bpm. Unlike atrial fibrillation, the baseline with this rhythm is isoelectric and distinct P waves are present. The P waves originate in various locations within the atria and/or SA node and often demonstrate varying PR intervals. This rhythm may result from varying vagal tone or irritability of the myocardium. Multifocal atrial

rhythms may also present with rates greater than 100 bpm, then referred to as multifocal atrial tachycardia. This is usually secondary to chronic pulmonary disease and strain on the atria.

Ventricular Extrasystoles

Premature ventricular contractions (PVCs) are caused by electrical foci in the ventricles, which produce depolarization and contraction ahead of the sinus node pacemaker. PVCs are demonstrated by large abnormal QRS complexes of different morphology and often different polarity from the intrinsic sinus rhythm. PVCs are both wide and of high voltage because the two ventricles are depolarized sequentially rather than simultaneously. In most cases, the T wave following the PVC has an electric polarity opposite the QRS complex because the relatively slow conduction of the impulse through the cardiac muscle causes the area, which depolarizes first also to be the first to repolarize.

Because the premature beat may result in decreased time for ventricular filling, the stroke volume will be less and the pulse wave may not be palpable, leading to a pulse deficit or perception of a "skipped beat." A compensatory

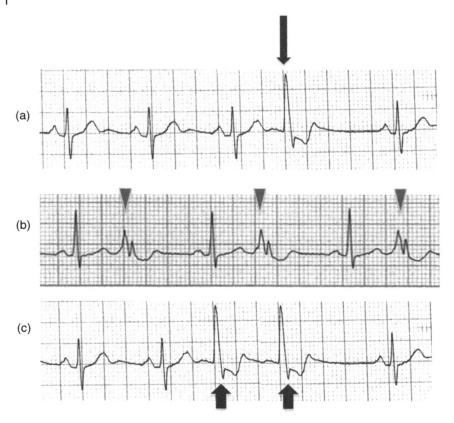

Figure 7.6.9 Ectopy. Panel a shows normal sinus rhythm with a single PVC seen in the fourth beat (arrows). Note the compensatory pause, which follows the premature beat. Panel b shows Bigeminy: PVCs on every other beat (arrow heads). Panel c shows a couplet, two consecutive PVCs (short arrows).

pause usually follows a PVC, due to retrograde conduction through the AV node, which makes it refractory to the next sinus impulse; the normally generated P wave may be buried within the PVC. Retrograde conduction through the atria may produce abnormal or inverted P waves, which may follow the QRS, blocking the next normal sinus node impulse [13] (Figure 7.6.9).

When a ventricular premature beat follows each sinus beat, ventricular bigeminy is produced and may be self-perpetuating because the compensatory pause precipitates the next PVC after the next sinus beat. When two sinus beats are repetitively followed by a PVC, trigeminy is present, and when three sinus beats are repetitively followed by a PVC, quadrigeminy is present.

Ventricular extrasystoles are produced under similar circumstances to atrial premature beats, including ischemia, electrolyte disturbances, nicotine, caffeine, and other stimulant drugs. They are present in 1–4% of the general population and in the absence of ischemic or structural heart disease have a benign prognosis; however, in the presence of acute myocardial infarction they are associated with an increased risk of sudden death [14, 15].

Paced Rhythms

The type of paced rhythm, and, as a result, its interpretation, depends on two major considerations: the type of pacemaker and its current setting. The three major types of pacemaker are atrial, ventricular, and dual chamber. Although biventricular pacers are at times used for patients with bundle branch block, ejection fraction less than 35%, and severe congestive heart failure, the term *dual chamber pacemaker* usually refers to a device that paces both the right atrium and ventricle.

The most basic pacemaker coding system consists of three letters. The first identifies the chamber that the unit will pace: A for atrium, V for ventricle, or D for dual. The second identifies the chamber that the unit will sense using the same letter representations. The third letter indicates the action that the unit will take when it senses an impulse in the indicated chamber. Potential responses include triggering a paced impulse, inhibiting one, or generating synchronous impulses to both the atria and ventricle. Demand pacemakers typically have a built-in refractory period of about 0.4 seconds from the most recent sensed impulse or the most recent pacer delivered impulse.

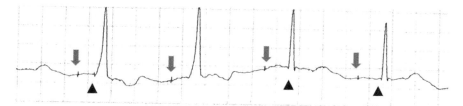

Figure 7.6.10 AV sequential pacemaker. Note the pacer spikes just before the P waves (arrows) and just before the QRS complexes (arrow heads).

The presence of a 0 in any of the letter locations indicates that current function is turned off. These settings are made to the pacemaker device via a communicating device that is placed above the chest.

When approaching the ECG of a patient with a pacemaker, the provider should first determine whether the patient is currently utilizing their native rhythm or if the pacemaker is generating impulses. To do this, they should search for the vertical pacer spikes. Unipolar leads are typically 20 mm in amplitude and bipolar leads are 5 mm. If there are no spikes then it is likely that the sensing portion of the function is responding to impulses by inhibiting. It may also be possible that this is a result of the pacemaker not functioning correctly. Common paced rhythms are as follows. Atrial paced rhythm displays a pacer spike just before the P wave, followed by a native-appearing QRS. Ventricular-paced rhythms display a pacer spike just before the QRS followed by a QRS in a left bundle branch block (LBBB) pattern. Dual chamber paced rhythms will display a spike prior to both the P and QRS waves (Figure 7.6.10).

References

1 Hall, J. (2011). Cardiac arrhythmias and their electrocardiographic interpretation, Chapter 13. In: *Guyton and Hall Textbook of Medical Physiology*, 12e, 143–153.

2 Boriata Perez, A. and Serratosa Fernandez, L. (1998). The athlete's heart: most common electrocardiographic findings. *Revista Española de Cardiología* 51: 356–368.

3 Acharya, U., Kannathal, N., Sing, O. et al. (2004). Heart rate analysis in normal subjects of various age groups. *Biomedical Engineering Online* 3: 24.

4 Wagner, G., Lim, T., Strauss, D., and Simlud, J. (2014). Interpretation of the normal electrocardiogram. In: *Marriott's Practical Electrocardiography*, 12e (eds. G. Wagner and D. Strauss), 47–68.

5 Mirvis, D. and Goldberger, A. (2011). Electrocardiography, Chapter 13. In: *Braunwald's Heart Disease – A Textbook of Cardiovascular Medicine*, 9e (eds. Bonow, R, D.L. Mann, D.P. Zipes and P. Libby), 126–165. Philadelphia: Elsevier Saunders.

6 Singh, J., Larson, M., O'Donnell, C. et al. (1999). Heritability of heart rate variability: the Framingham heart study. *Circulation* 99: 2251–2254.

7 Southall, D., Richards, J., Mitchell, P. et al. (1980). Study of cardiac rhythm in healthy newborn infants. *British Heart Journal* 43: 14–20.

8 Custer, J.W. and Rau, R.E. (eds.) (2008). *Johns Hopkins: Harriet Lane Handbook*, 18e. Philadelphia, PA: Mosby Elsevier Inc.

9 Goldberger, A (2012). *Clinical Electrocardiography: A Simplified Approach*, 8e. Philadelphia: Elsevier Saunders.

10 Chan, T.C., Brady, W.J., Harrigan, R.A. et al. (2004). *ECG in Emergency Medicine and Acute Care*, 1e. Philadelphia, PA: Mosby.

11 Allessie, M.A., Boyden, P.A., Camm, A.J. et al. (2001). Pathophysiology and prevention of atrial fibrillation. *Circulation* 103: 769.

12 Gutierrez, C. and Blanchard, D. (2011). Atrial fibrillation: diagnosis and treatment. *American Family Physician* 83: 61–68.

13 Kennedy, H., Whitlock, J., Sprqgue, M. et al. (1985). Long term follow up of asymptomatic healthy subjects with frequent and complex ventricular ectopy. *The New England Journal of Medicine* 312: 193–197.

14 Bigger, J., Dresdale, R., Heissenbuttel, R. et al. (1977). Ventricular arrhythmias in ischemic heart disease: mechanism, prevalence, significance and management. *Progress in Cardiovascular Diseases* 19: 255–300.

15 Moss, A., Davis, H., Camilla, J. et al. (1979). Ventricular ectopic beats and their relation to sudden and non sudden cardiac death after myocardial infarction. *Circulation* 60: 998–1003.

7

Narrow Complex Tachycardia

David J. Carlberg and Rahul Bhat

Department of Emergency Medicine, Georgetown University & MedStar Health, Washington, DC, USA

Introduction

Narrow complex tachycardias (NCTs) are cardiac rhythms that are defined by their rates of greater than 100 beats per minute (bpm) and QRS complexes on electrocardiogram (ECG) of less than 120 ms. This chapter summarizes the NCTs and their ECG diagnosis. With rare exception, NCTs arise proximal to the ventricles and are classified as supraventricular tachycardias (SVTs); however, not all SVTs have narrow QRS complexes. It is important to note that most of the rhythms in this chapter can become wide complex in the setting of an accessory pathway or aberrant conduction through the AV node and/or the His-Purkinje system as in the case of a bundle branch block. These wide complex SVTs, such as SVT with a bundle branch block, are discussed elsewhere in this text.

The impact of NCT is extremely variable, so early and accurate diagnosis is important to guide appropriate evaluation, management, and disposition [1]. In their most benign forms, NCTs are asymptomatic or cause minimal discomfort, but in their most dangerous forms, they can cause syncope, hypotension, angina, tachycardia-related cardiomyopathy, congestive heart failure, and, much less commonly, death [2, 3]. Clinical differentiation among various NCT is frequently simple, especially at heart rates closer to 100 bpm. However, rhythm differentiation can be more challenging, particularly as heart rates increase [4, 5]. Incorrect diagnosis and treatment of NCT may also result in complications [5]. Based on the rhythm and its etiology, as well as the clinical scenario, management may range from reassurance to pharmacologic therapy, electrical cardioversion, and/or acute inpatient admission. Therefore, it is important that a wide variety of medical personnel understand the ECG diagnosis of NCT.

Mechanisms for NCTs

NCTs are caused by three different mechanisms, 1) reentry, 2) enhanced/abnormal automaticity, and 3) triggered activity. Understanding these mechanisms may help the provider determine the type of rhythm, the underlying etiology, and potential treatments.

Reentry

Reentry is the most common cause of narrow complex tachydysrhythmias [6]. For reentry to occur, there must be at least two separate functional or anatomic pathways that can conduct an electrochemical signal. During normal cardiac function the electrochemical signal travels through both pathways from the atria toward the ventricles. This is called anterograde conduction. The two pathways frequently have different refractory periods after transmitting the signal, thus an early beat, such as a premature atrial contraction (PAC) or premature ventricular contraction (PVC), can encounter one pathway blocked with the other available for impulse conduction. As the impulse is being conducted via the available pathway, the refractory period for the previously blocked pathway ends and it becomes available for conduction. When the impulse reaches the point where the two pathways merge, it is picked up by the previously refractory pathway and travels toward the initial source, in a retrograde fashion. This establishes a circuit through the two pathways. The impulse continues to travel anterograde through one branch and retrograde through the other [3, 6].

Reentrant circuits causing NCTs can occur in one of three ways: (i) entirely within the atria, (ii) entirely within the atrioventricular (AV) node, or (iii) via the AV node and

Electrocardiogram in Clinical Medicine, First Edition. Edited by William J. Brady, Michael J. Lipinski, Andrew E. Darby, Michael C. Bond, Nathan P. Charlton, Korin Hudson, and Kelly Williamson.

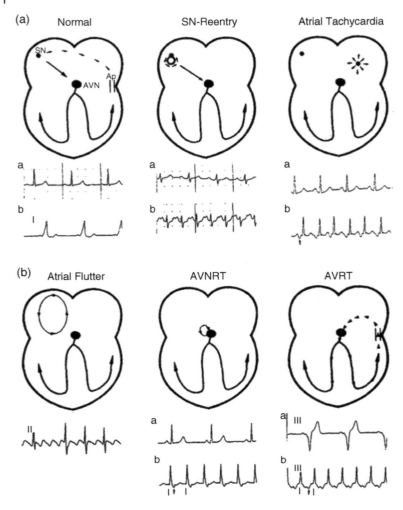

(a)　Normal　　SN-Reentry　　Atrial Tachycardia

(b)　Atrial Flutter　　AVNRT　　AVRT

Figure 7.7.1 Classification of narrow complex tachycardia based on ECG characteristics. *Source:* Reproduced with permission from Ref. [3].

an accessory conduction pathway between the atria and the ventricles (Figure 7.7.1). Microreentry occurs when the reentrant circuit is anatomically small, and macroreentry occurs when the reentrant circuit is anatomically large [3].

Atrial flutter, atrial fibrillation, sinus node reentrant tachycardia, AV nodal reentrant tachycardia (AVNRT), and AV reciprocating tachycardia (AVRT) occur through reentry.

Enhanced and Abnormal Automaticity

Enhanced automaticity is defined as an increased rate of activation by cardiac fibers that have intrinsic pacemaker activity. *Abnormal automaticity* is defined as the acquisition of pacemaker activity by cardiac tissue that usually does not have it. Abnormal automaticity usually occurs in the setting of diseased myocardium [6]. Sinus tachycardia as well as certain atrial and junctional tachycardias can be caused by enhanced and abnormal automaticity.

Triggered Activity

Triggered activity is caused by after-depolarizations during the repolarization phase of the cardiac cycle. Early after depolarizations lead to the wide complex unstable tachycardia known as torsades de pointes, while late after depolarizations, which are rarer, lead to the narrow complex atrial tachycardia seen in digoxin toxicity [6].

Approach to NCT

In any patient with NCT, rhythm determination is vital (Figure 7.7.2). A patient's cardiac rhythm may provide an important diagnostic clue to determining the underlying medical condition. Furthermore, correct diagnosis of rhythm is crucial for correct treatment as certain NCTs require pharmacologic AV nodal blockade or cardioversion,

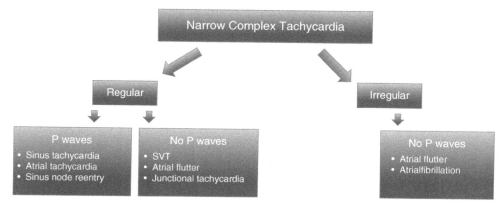

Figure 7.7.2 Classification of narrow complex tachycardia based on ECG characteristics.

some require long-term anticoagulation, while other rhythms require no treatment other than treating the underlying cause. In the best-case scenario, without accurate rhythm determination the provider risks missing an opportunity for treatment. In the worst-case scenario, he or she risks doing harm by providing inappropriate treatment.

Determining Regularity

The first step in rhythm differentiation is determining whether the heart rate is regular or irregular. Regular R-R intervals are seen in sinus tachycardia, sinus node reentrant tachycardia, atrial tachycardia, AVRNT, AVRT, and atrial flutter with a fixed block. Irregular R-R intervals are seen in atrial fibrillation, multifocal atrial tachycardia (MAT), atrial flutter with variable block, and sinus rhythms with frequent premature atrial or ventricular contractions, as well as physiologic sinus arrhythmia.

At slower rates, determining R-R interval regularity is frequently simple and can easily be done with the naked eye or with calipers. However, as the rate increases, and especially at rates above 150 bpm, this determination becomes more difficult. One potential way to improve accuracy in differentiating between regular and irregular rhythms on ECG is to print the ECG at double speed. The standard ECG prints at 25 mm/s, meaning that each small box represents 0.04 s. Printing the ECGs of rapid NCTs at 50 mm/s has been shown to improve the diagnosis of many rhythms, including atrial fibrillation. This faster printing means that fewer QRS complexes are printed on each sheet, theoretically enhancing irregularity if it is present. This faster printing may also help improve visualization of P waves and flutter waves [5].

Determining Sinus Rhythm

The next step in differentiating NCT is determining whether a rhythm is sinus in origin. Sinus tachycardias

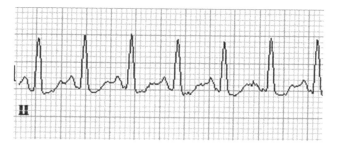

Figure 7.7.3 Sinus tachycardia. Note the regular narrow complex rhythm with a rate of 160 bpm with consistent, regular P waves and no beat-to-beat variability.

have a P wave prior to each QRS and a QRS after each P wave (see Figure 7.7.3). P waves in sinus tachycardia are upright in leads II, III, and aVF. Occasionally atrial tachycardias will also have upright P waves in leads II, III, and aVF, and these can be difficult to differentiate from sinus tachycardias, and may need an invasive electrophysiology study to distinguish the source of tachycardia [1].

Evaluating P-Wave Presence and Morphology

Examination for P-wave presence and morphology is the next step in rhythm determination. P waves are present in sinus tachycardia, atrial tachycardia, sinus node reentry tachycardia, and MAT. P waves in sinus tachycardia, sinus node reentry tachycardia, and sometimes atrial tachycardia are upright in the inferior leads (II, III, and aVF). The axis of the P wave in atrial tachycardia is dependent on the location of origin of the beat within the atria (Figure 7.7.4) [7]. MAT features at least three different P-wave morphologies, as the beats arise from various locations within the atria.

P waves are absent in atrial fibrillation, atrial flutter, and junctional tachycardia, however in atrial flutter, the flutter waves are frequently mistaken for P waves when there is 2:1 conduction (Figure 7.7.5) [1].

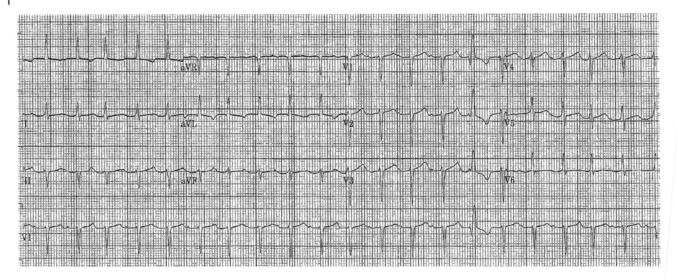

Figure 7.7.4 Atrial tachycardia. Note the similar appearance to sinus tachycardia. On a surface ECG, these two entities are difficult to distinguish, and the differentiation is largely based on axis of the P wave that in sinus tachycardia will be upright in the inferior leads, but may be upright or inverted in the inferior leads in atrial tachycardia depending on the origin of the atrial activity.

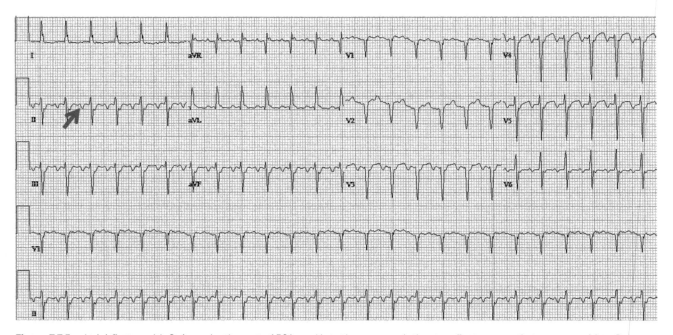

Figure 7.7.5 Atrial flutter with 2:1 conduction, rate 150 bpm. Note the arrow pointing to a flutter wave that can resemble a P wave.

Onset and Variability

Two other clues that can be helpful in differentiating among the NCTs are the rhythm onset and variability. The onset of a tachycardia may be captured by a portable rhythm monitor in the outpatient setting, or it may be captured by telemetry in the ED or inpatient setting. It would be rare to capture the onset via a standard ECG. Both sinus tachycardias and atrial tachycardias generally have a warm-up and a warm-down phase, characterized by gradual onset and gradual cessation, whereas many reentrant tachycardias, such as AVRT and AVNRT, have both an abrupt onset and termination.

Evaluating the heart rate variability is also a useful tool in differentiating among the regular NCTs. The heart rate in sinus tachycardia is variable, even when the heart rate is very fast. The heart rate may be 130 at one time point, 136 a few seconds later, and 124 a few seconds after that. Conversely, the heart rate in atrial flutter with fixed block,

AVRT, and AVNRT remain stable. If the heart rate is 145, it will generally remain within a few beats of that for extended periods of time.

Sinus Node Tachycardias

Sinus Tachycardia

Sinus tachycardia is a sinus rhythm with conduction proceeding in the regular fashion from the SA node through the ventricles, the AV node and the His-Purkinje system. There are upright P waves in leads II, III, and aVF and the ventricular rate is over 100 bpm. It is the most common NCT seen in clinical practice [1], and it generally occurs in response to a physiologic stress, such as exercise, fever, pain, or hypovolemia. It may also be caused by endocrinopathies, sympathomimetic drugs, and anticholinergic drugs [4, 7], as well as pulmonary embolism. Sinus tachycardia rarely exceeds 200 bpm; thus, if the rate is higher, other etiologies should be considered [2, 4]. The heart rate in sinus tachycardia increases and decreases gradually [4, 6], and the heart rate should decrease in response to treatment of the underlying process [6]. P-wave morphology in sinus tachycardia should be the same as it is when the patient is in normal sinus rhythm, however the height of the P wave may increase slightly as the heart rate increases [4]. As the heart rate increases, the PR interval will also shorten, and with very fast rhythms, the P wave may merge with the preceding T wave [4]. Both atrial flutter with 2:1 block and atrial tachycardia are misinterpreted as sinus tachycardia. However, atrial flutter usually has a very fixed rate at about 150 bpm, and atrial tachycardia often has a different P-wave axis [6] (see Figure 7.7.3).

Inappropriate Sinus Tachycardia

Inappropriate sinus tachycardia is sinus tachycardia without an obvious physiologic cause [2, 3]. It is not caused by an underlying structural heart disease [3], and it occurs most frequently in women [2, 3]. Patients with inappropriate sinus tachycardia will frequently have rapid increases in their heart rates with mild physiologic stresses [3]. Inappropriate sinus tachycardia is a diagnosis of exclusion [3], and portable outpatient rhythm monitoring will frequently show persistent daytime tachycardia with heart rate normalization at night [2].

Sinus Node Reentrant Tachycardia

Occasionally a reentrant phenomenon occurs within the sinus node. The sinus node reentrant tachycardia gener-
ated by this has the same appearance as sinus tachycardia. P waves have the same morphology and axis, and P waves occur before each QRS complex. Unlike sinus tachycardia, sinus node reentrant tachycardia has a sudden onset and termination, has a consistently regular rate, and is not caused by an acute physiologic stress [4]. At fast rates, the P wave may be buried in the preceding QRST complex [7], but locating the P wave is usually not difficult, as the rate is usually between 130 and 140 bpm [4].

Atrial Tachycardias

Atrial Tachycardia

Atrial tachycardia is a relatively infrequent NCT [3] that arises from an ectopic focus within an atrium but outside of the SA node. This typically occurs as a result of enhanced automaticity, reentry, or triggered activity. The rate ranges from 120 to 300 bpm. Potential causes include cardiomyopathy, pulmonary disease, ischemic heart disease, rheumatic heart disease, sick sinus syndrome, and digoxin toxicity [4]. Reentrant mechanisms for atrial tachycardias are frequently associated with atrial scarring from prior surgery [7]. Atrial tachycardia, even when reentrant, should not respond to a trial dose of adenosine because the rhythm does not involve the AV node [3]. Untreated incessant atrial tachycardia may lead to tachycardia-induced dilated cardiomyopathy [4].

Atrial tachycardias arise from the left atrium and the right atrium with approximately equal frequency [8]. Atrial tachycardia arising near the SA node may be difficult to differentiate from a sinus rhythm because both may share the same axis (Figure 7.7.6) [1].

Multifocal Atrial Tachycardia

MAT is defined as a rhythm with an atrial rate of over 100 bpm in the setting of organized, discrete, nonsinus P waves having at least three different morphologies in the same ECG lead (Figure 7.7.7) [8]. As the rate does not generally exceed the refractory period of the AV node, all atrial beats are conducted and both the atrial and ventricular rhythms are irregular. In fact, the PP, PR, and RR intervals are all irregular [8]. Enhanced automaticity is the mechanism behind MAT [4]. Diagnosis of MAT can be difficult for even experienced providers. One retrospective study showed that only 22% of patients hospitalized with MAT had their ECG interpreted correctly upon admission [9]. MAT is sometimes mistaken for atrial fibrillation [3], but the two can be differentiated by the presence of an isoelectric baseline

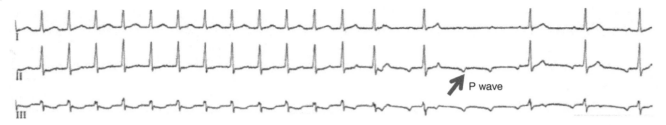

Figure 7.7.6 Atrial tachycardia with carotid massage. At times P waves can be difficult to visualize, but with vagal maneuvers or AV nodal blocking agents, they may appear (arrow).

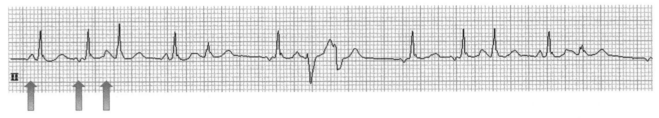

Figure 7.7.7 Multifocal atrial tachycardia. Note the different P wave morphologies (arrows). At least three distinct P wave morphologies are required to make the diagnosis.

between P waves in MAT [4, 8]. Also in MAT, despite the variable P wave axis and morphology, there is a P wave before every QRS complex, which can help the clinician differentiate MAT from atrial fibrillaton. Some authors debate whether the requirement for heart rate over 100 bpm is too restrictive for the diagnosis of MAT, as some patients with decompensated pulmonary or cardiac disease have multifocal atrial rhythms with heart rates of less than 100 bpm. These rhythms are sometimes called slow MATs or multifocal atrial rhythms. These slower rhythms are important to differentiate from those caused by wandering atrial pacemakers, as their clinical significance is different. A patient with wandering atrial pacemaker is usually asymptomatic and not medically decompensated [8].

MAT is a relatively uncommon rhythm, occurring in 0.36% of patients admitted to the hospital [8]. It occurs most frequently in elderly patients with active co-morbid medical conditions, including lung disease, heart disease, and metabolic disorders [3, 8, 9]; 60 % of MAT cases occur in patients with clinically important pulmonary disease [8]. Despite the low frequency of MAT, the morbidity of patients with this rhythm is high. The overall in-hospital mortality rate for patients with MAT is 45%, and the mortality rate for patients with concomitant chronic obstructive pulmonary disease and MAT has been reported as high as 80% [9].

Atrial Flutter

Atrial flutter is an NCT caused by a macroreentrant circuit, generally within the right atrium. Atrial flutter is actually divided into two categories: typical and atypical flutter

[10]. Atypical flutter is a heterogeneous category of atrial macroreentry and may occur anywhere within the atria. Atypical flutter may be due to surgical scarring, or a variety of abnormal conduction pathways [10]. The atrial rate of atypical flutter is generally 340–430 bpm [7]. Its diagnosis, evaluation, and treatment are much less understood than typical flutter [10]. This chapter focuses primarily on typical flutter.

Typical flutter is caused by a specific combination of conduction blocks and slowed conduction within the right atrium that predispose to reentry phenomena [11]. The conduction blocks that set up the reentry circuit are [1] the tissue between the superior vena cava and the inferior vena cava, known as the crista terminalis, and [2] the tissue between the inferior vena cava and the coronary sinus, known as the Eustachian ridge [8, 10–12]. These two areas of block plus slow conduction through the atrial tissue between the tricuspid valve and the inferior vena cava provide suitable conditions for the development and continuation of a reentrant loop in the right atrium [7]. The left atrium is not needed for completion of the circuit; it is secondarily activated by the signal cycling through the right atrium [7]. Classically, current moves counterclockwise through this circuit, causing the typical pattern of negative flutter waves in the inferior leads and in V6, with upright flutter waves in lead V1 [7, 11]. When current moves clockwise through the circuit, it is called reverse typical flutter, and demonstrates either sine-wave or upright flutter waves in the inferior leads [11].

In typical flutter, the atrial rate usually ranges from 250 to 350 bpm [6]. Because the AV node cannot conduct at the

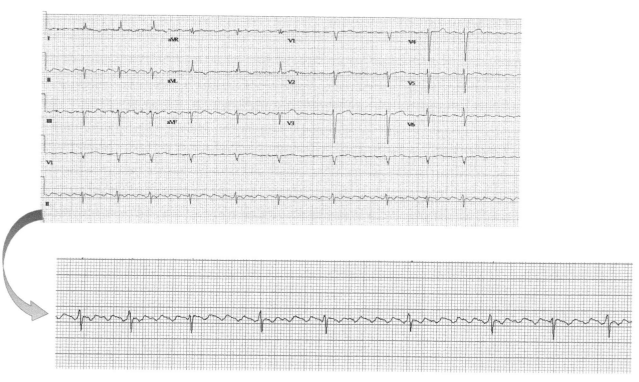

Figure 7.7.8 Atrial flutter with variable block. Note how the ratio of flutter waves to QRS complexes changes from beat to beat.

rate attained by the atria, atrial flutter most often presents with a 2:1, 3:1, or 4:1 block [6, 7]. When a variable block is present (Figure 7.7.8), the ventricular rate is irregular [8]. In the presence of a fixed block, however, the overall heart rate should have minimal variation [6]. In a patient with an invariable heart rate of approximately 150 bpm (such as the example shown in Figure 7.7.6), atrial flutter should be strongly considered as an etiology [6].

At faster rates, it can be difficult to differentiate sinus tachycardia from paroxysmal SVT or atrial flutter with 2:1 conduction. One clue suggesting atrial flutter is that its surface ECG has no isoelectric point in lead II. This is because the circuit courses parallel to the base of the atrium, so the flutter current is always moving toward or away from lead II [6]. Other methods to help differentiate between atrial flutter and other rhythms include looking at the patient's underlying pathophysiology. If a patient has a fever or is volume depleted or is undergoing some other type of physiologic stress, this could suggest that the rhythm is a reactive sinus tachycardia. It is important to note, however, that a patient undergoing an acute physiologic stress could still be in atrial flutter. When the ventricular rate is near 150 bpm, flutter waves often blend with the T wave of the preceding QRS complex, making atrial flutter difficult to differentiate from other rhythms. Slowing AV node conduction and thus

ventricular response with vagal maneuvers may reveal flutter waves [6]. Adenosine may also be used as a diagnostic tool. While adenosine treats paroxysmal SVTs by breaking the reentrant loop at the AV node, in atrial flutter the effect of temporarily halting conduction through the AV node is to cause QRS complexes to transiently disappear, often unmasking the underlying atrial flutter waves (Figure 7.7.9).

Atrial Fibrillation

Atrial fibrillation, first described by Maimonides in 1187, is the most common sustained cardiac arrhythmia seen in clinical practice [13, 14]. Its clinical importance cannot be understated as it has a prevalence of approximately 2.3 million cases in the United States and it leads to 15–20% of ischemic strokes [13]. Atrial fibrillation is frequently idiopathic, but it may also be caused by hypertension, ischemic heart disease, valvular disease, cardiomyopathy, lung disease, thyroid disease, sepsis, surgery, alcohol abuse, and adrenergic drugs [2].

Both reentry and enhanced automaticity have been proposed as mechanisms for atrial fibrillation [8, 14, 15]. The most commonly accepted and best understood mechanism is a specific type of reentry called the *multiple wavelet hypothesis*, in which wavelets of current travel through

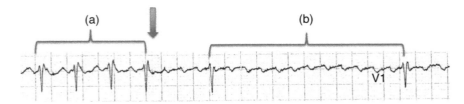

Figure 7.7.9 Atrial flutter with 2:1 conduction (a), which may have been misidentified as supraventricular SVT and was treated with adenosine (arrow). Note the nodal blockade unmasks the underlying flutter waves (b).

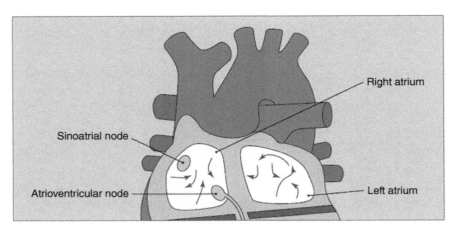

Figure 7.7.10 Atrial fibrillation multiple wavelets form of reentry. Arrows indicate chaotic electrical activity within the atria. Reproduced with permission from [4].

the atrial myocardium in various reentrant loops (Figure 7.7.10) [4, 7]. When more wavelets are present, there is a higher likelihood that they will self-propagate and the rhythm will continue [7]. When the atria have a larger tissue mass for the wavelets to travel in, there is a higher likelihood for wavelet induction and sustainability. Thus, patients with atrial enlargement are at higher risk for atrial fibrillation [7].

On the surface ECG, wavelets that cause atrial fibrillation are seen as uncoordinated atrial activation that is manifested as random, low amplitude, variable deflections from the expected isoelectric point [8, 15]. These deflections are either fine or coarse, with coarse deflections potentially suggesting atrial enlargement [6]. When the ventricular rate is over 100 bpm, the rhythm is classified as atrial fibrillation with rapid ventricular response.

During atrial fibrillation the atrial activation rate is 350–700 bpm [6, 7]. Because the AV node cannot transmit at such a high frequency due to its refractory period, the ventricles do not attain these high rates (Figure 7.7.11). In the setting of a healthy conducting system without pharmacologic AV nodal blockade, the ventricular response rate is variable and should be 100–200 bpm resulting in an irregularly irregular rhythm [6]. A lower response rate should prompt consideration of a diseased AV node [6].

The QRS complex should remain narrow unless there is an underlying conduction abnormality such as a bundle branch block or accessory pathway. When the heart rate is either very fast or very slow, atrial fibrillation may appear regular [2]. Calipers may help highlight irregularity in these cases. Also, when the heart rate is very fast, the clinician can double the ECG printing speed from 25–50 mm/s, which may accentuate irregularity [5].

Atrial fibrillation is further categorized by the duration of time a patient is in the rhythm. Paroxysmal atrial fibrillation occurs when the rhythm self-terminates within seven days of onset. It usually arises from atrial tissue surrounding the pulmonary veins. Atrial fibrillation is considered *persistent* when it lasts for longer than seven days and recurrent if there are two or more episodes of atrial fibrillation regardless of the duration. Atrial fibrillation becomes *permanent* when it is proven refractory to rhythm control or when clinicians decide on a long-term rate control strategy [13, 16]. As atrial fibrillation evolves from paroxysmal to persistent to permanent, the atria undergo a remodeling

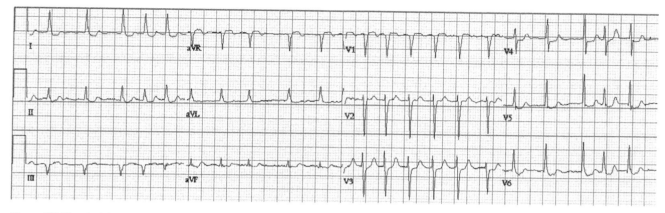

Figure 7.7.11 Atrial fibrillation with rapid ventricular response (137 bpm). Note the lack of consistent P waves as well as the irregular nature of the R-R interval.

process that predisposes the tissue to continued atrial fibrillation [13, 14].

Reentrant Tachycardia Involving the AV Node

AV Nodal Reentry Tachycardia

AVNRT is the most common of the reentrant tachycardias involving the AV node, accounting for over 70% of such cases [7]. This rhythm is more common in young people and occurs more frequently in women [2, 3, 17]. For an AVNRT to develop, two separate pathways are required within the AV node or in the perinodal tissue [3, 7]. One pathway, generally anterior, is characterized by fast conduction and a relatively long refractory period, while the other pathway, generally posterior, is characterized by slow conduction and a relatively short refractory period. When a PAC occurs while the fast pathway is refractory but the slow pathway is not, the atrial signal travels anterograde through the slow pathway. If the fast pathway is no longer refractory when the signal reaches the point where the two pathways have merged, the signal will travel retrograde through the fast pathway, creating a micro reentrant loop [17]. The signal also continues traveling anterograde through the conducting system and activates the ventricles. Similarly, if a PVC occurs, it may travel retrograde through the AV node and set up a similar conduction loop. If the onset of AVNRT is captured on ECG, there will frequently be a prolonged PR interval immediately after the PAC that triggers the rhythm because this signal travels down the slow pathway instead of the fast [18]. Since the ventricle is activated through the normal conduction pathway, the QRS complex is narrow unless there is a preexisting intra-ventricular conduction delay, such as a bundle branch block. The ventricular rate in AVNRT can range from 100 to 280 bpm, and averages 170 bpm [6, 7]. The reentrant loop causes retrograde activation of the atria, but since the atria are generally activated by the fast pathway, the atria and ventricles depolarize nearly simultaneously so the retrograde P wave is usually lost in the QRS complex, but may be visible (Figure 7.7.12). Occasionally the retrograde P wave can be seen at the end of the QRS complex [6, 7, 18]. When this occurs, it is seen best as a pseudo R′ wave in lead V1 and as pseudo S waves in leads II, III, and AVF [7, 18].

Ten percent of the time in AVNRT, the conduction is reversed [3] such that the signal travels anterograde through the fast pathway and retrograde through the slow pathway. For this to occur, the fast pathway also must be the one with the short refractory period [7]. In this case, retrograde atrial activation occurs via the slow pathway and a retrograde P wave is more likely to be visible after the QRS complex [6, 7].

AV Reentry Tachycardia

AVRT is similar to AVNRT, except only one limb of the reentrant loop goes through the AV node. The other limb is an anatomically distinct accessory pathway between the atria and the ventricles. This accessory pathway, when visible on ECG during sinus rhythm as a short PR interval and a delta wave, is indicative of Wolff-Parkinson-White syndrome (Figure 7.7.13). The delta wave represents early activation of the ventricular muscle fibers by the accessory pathway. Some accessory pathways, however, can only transmit in a retrograde fashion, and therefore are not demonstrated on a surface ECG during sinus rhythm. These are called concealed accessory pathways [3, 7, 18].

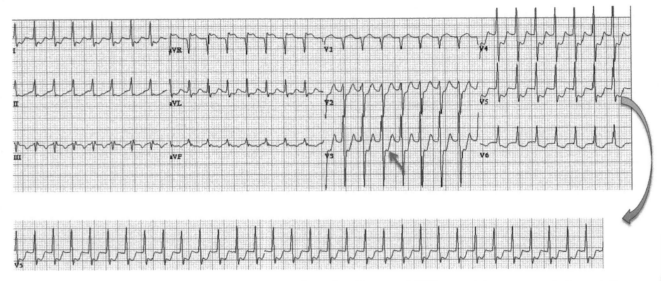

Figure 7.7.12 AVNRT: Note the regular narrow complex tachycardia with a rate of 195 bpm and the presence of retrograde P waves (arrow).

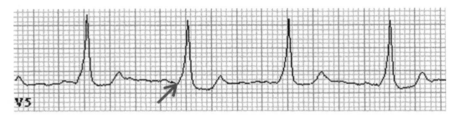

Figure 7.7.13 Wolf-Parkinson-White syndrome: Seen here at a normal rate. Note the presence of delta wave during sinus rhythm (arrow), which represents preexcitation of ventricular fibers via fast accessory pathway. The delta wave may be more difficult to see at rapid rates.

Orthodromic AVRT is triggered by a PAC that occurs when the accessory pathway is refractory but the AV node is not. The signal from the PAC travels down the AV node, through the conducting system, and into the ventricular tissue. If the accessory pathway has completed its refractory period, the signal travels from the ventricle to the atrium via the accessory pathway and establishes the macro reentrant circuit [17]. In the absence of a bundle branch block, the QRS complex is narrow because the ventricle is activated through conducting system. The rate of orthodromic AVRT may range from 140 to 280 bpm, and the rate of AVRT is generally faster than that of AVNRT [6]. Antidromic AVRT can also occur, but creates a wide complex tachycardia because the ventricle is activated through the accessory pathway and not through the conducting system (Figure 7.7.14). Antidromic AVRT is beyond the scope of this chapter.

As in AVNRT, there is retrograde activation of the atria in AVRT; however, in orthodromic AVRT this occurs via the accessory pathway. Because the accessory pathway generally features slow conduction, retrograde P waves are generally seen on ECG [3, 6, 7, 18]. These P waves generally follow the QRS complex by 70 ms or more, and may present as a notch in the T wave (Figure 7.7.15) [18]. P waves are generally inverted in the inferior leads because the signal travels from the peri-ventricular atrial tissue to the rest of the atria [6, 7, 18].

Differentiating AVRT and AVNRT can be difficult, and sometimes is only possible in the electrophysiology lab. The presence of QRS alternans, defined as a variation in the QRS amplitude by over 1 mm in the presence of a relatively fixed heart rate, suggests AVRT. This is especially true when the ventricular rate is under 180 BPM. At higher

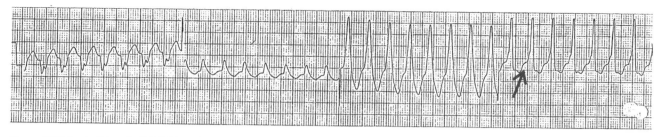

Figure 7.7.14 Antidromic AVRT: Note the delta waves (arrow) that can help differentiate this tachycardia from ventricular tachycardia.

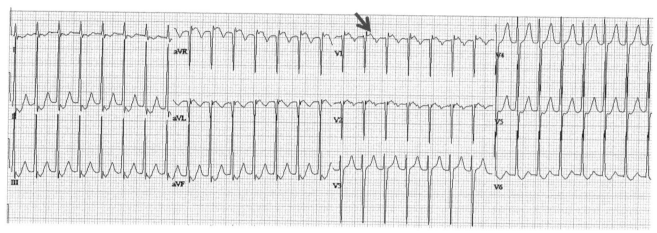

Figure 7.7.15 Orhtodromic AVRT: Note the notching of the T wave (arrow), which represents a retrograde P wave via the slow accessory pathway.

rates, AVNRT may also show QRS alternans [3, 7]. The presence of ST elevation in lead AVR also suggests the possibility of AVRT over AVNRT, but only with a sensitivity of 71% and a specificity of 70% [19].

Compared to AVNRT, AVRT patients are generally younger and have a male predominance [2].

Junctional Tachycardia

Junctional tachycardia is a relatively rare tachycardia that arises from within the AV node or the bundle of His [6]. It features a narrow QRS complex and causes retrograde atrial activation, so it may be associated with retrograde P waves either before or after the QRS complex (Figure 7.7.16) [3, 6]. However, these P waves are frequently buried in the QRS complex [6].

Junctional tachycardia has a gradual onset, as it can be caused by enhanced automaticity or triggered activity [6]. Its rate is generally 70–130 BPM [6]. In adults, junctional tachycardia is caused by acute myocardial infarction, valvular surgery, and digoxin toxicity [3, 6]. In children it is caused by underlying heart disease and surgical correction of congenital heart defects [3, 6].

Conclusions

While NCTs are frequently simple to diagnose, the differential diagnosis may be challenging and the rhythms may arise from a number of underlying conditions. A good understanding of the pathophysiology and ECG diagnosis of these rhythms can help the clinician make the most appropriate diagnostic and therapeutic interventions.

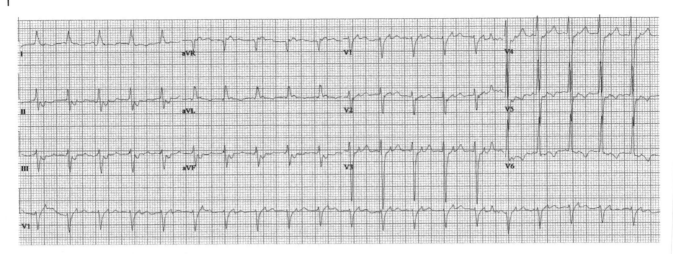

Figure 7.7.16 Junctional tachycardia: Note the regular narrow complex tachycardia with the absence of P waves preceding the QRS complexes or flutter waves.

References

1 Kireyev, D., Fernandez, S.F., Gupta, V. et al. (2012). Targeting tachycardia: diagnostic tips and tools. *J. Fam. Pract.* 61 (5): 258–263.

2 Linton, N.W.F. and Dubrey, S.W. (2009). Narrow complex (supraventricular) tachycardias. *Postgrad. Med. J.* 85: 546–551.

3 Xie, B., Thakur, R.K., Shan, C.P., and Hoon, V.K. (1998). Clinical differentiation of narrow QRS complex tachycardias. *Emerg. Med. Clin. North Am.* 16 (2): 295–330.

4 Goodacre, S. and Irons, R. (2002). ABC of clinical electrocardiography: atrial arrhythmias. *BMJ* 324 (7337): 594–597.

5 Accardi, A.J., Miller, R., and Holmes, J.F. (2002). Enhanced diagnosis of narrow complex tachycardias with increased electrocardiograph speed. *J. Emerg. Med.* 22 (2): 123–126.

6 Stahmer, S.A. and Cowan, R. (2006). Tachydysrhythmias. *Emerg. Med. Clin. North Am.* 24 (1): 11–40.

7 Obel, O.A. and Camm, A.J. (1997). Supraventricular tachycardia: ECG diagnosis and anatomy. *Eur. Heart J.* 18 (Supplement C): C2–C11.

8 Kastor, J.A. (1990). Multifocal atrial tachycardia. *N. Engl. J. Med.* 322 (24): 1713–1717.

9 McCord, J. and Borzak, S. (1998). Multifocal atrial tachycardia. *Chest* 113 (1): 203–209.

10 Cosio, F.G., Martin-Penato, A., Pastor, A. et al. (2003). Atypical flutter: a review. *Pacing Clin. Electrophysiol.* 26 (11): 2157–2169.

11 Sawhney, N.S., Anousheh, R., Chen, W.C., and Feld, G.K. (2009). Diagnosis and management of typical atrial flutter. *Cardiol. Clin.* 27 (1): 55–67.

12 Waldo, A.L. (2002). Mechanisms of atrial flutter and atrial fibrillation: distinct entities or two sides of a coin? *Cardiovasc. Res.* 54 (2): 217–229.

13 Beck, H. and See, V.Y. (2012). Acute management of atrial fibrillation: from the emergency department to cardiac care unit. *Cardiol. Clin.* 30 (4): 567–589.

14 Iwasaki, Y.K., Nishida, K., Kato, T., and Nattel, S. (2011). Atrial fibrillation pathophysiology: implications for management. *Circulation* 124 (20): 2264–2274.

15 Gutierrez, C. and Blanchard, D.G. (2011). Atrial fibrillation: diagnosis and treatment. *Am. Fam. Physician* 83 (1): 61–68.

16 Stiell, I.G. and Macle, L. (2011). CCS atrial fibrillation guidelines committee. Canadian cardiovascular society atrial fibrillation guidelines 2010: management of recent-onset atrial fibrillation and flutter in the emergency department. *Can. J. Cardiol.* 27 (1): 38–46.

17 Fox, D.J., Tischenko, A., Krahn, A.D. et al. (2008). Supraventricular tachycardia:diagnosis and management. *Mayo Clin. Proc.* 83 (12): 1400–1411.

18 Lowenstein, S.R., Halperin, B.D., and Reiter, M.J. (1996). Paroxysmal supraventricular tachycardias. *J. Emerg. Med.* 14 (1): 39–51.

19 Williamson, K., Mattu, A., Plautz, C.U. et al. (2006). Electrocardiographic applications of lead aVR. *Am. J. Emerg. Med.* 24 (7): 864–874.

8

Wide Complex Tachycardia

Scott Young[1] and Rachel Villacorta Lyew[2]

[1] Department of Emergency Medicine, Madigan Army Medical Center, Tacoma, WA, USA
[2] Department of Emergency Medicine, Tripler Army Medical Center, Honolulu, HI, USA

Introduction to Wide Complex Tachycardia

Evaluating an ECG showing a wide complex tachycardia (WCT) can be a disconcerting event for any provider, regardless of experience level. The differential diagnosis is broad, and patients often have unstable vital signs associated with their arrhythmia and/or their underlying medical condition. The ability to make a timely interpretation of these ECGs can facilitate rapid and appropriate treatment, which may truly mean the difference between life and death. If approached in a systematic manner, any provider can accurately determine the rhythm, narrow the differential diagnosis, and make decisions that can ultimately improve outcomes in this challenging patient population.

This chapter will discuss the differential diagnosis of WCT, including a systematic way to distinguish between ventricular tachycardia (VT) and supraventricular tachycardia (SVT) with aberrant conduction.

Before considering specific rhythms and a differential diagnosis for WCT, it is important to understand some key terminology and features that are used in defining and differentiating WCTs (Table 7.8.1). A QRS complex is considered wide when it is greater than 120 ms in duration, or wider than 3 "small boxes" on a standard ECG. This increase in the width of the QRS occurs because either (i) the arrhythmogenic focus is outside the normal conduction system, or (ii) there are conduction abnormalities present within the His-Purkinje fibers. The rate associated with a WCT is greater than 100 beats per minute (bpm). A ventricular rhythm with a rate of 50–120 bpm can be referred to as an accelerated idioventricular rhythm, overlapping with the definition of WCT [1] but will not be discussed at length here.

The QRS axis, or the direction of depolarization when all cardiac electrical signals are averaged together, is measured in degrees. The degrees of the QRS axis are like a clock face, where 0° corresponds to 3 o'clock (the patient's left), +90° to 6 o'clock (the patient's feet), +180° to 9 o'clock (the patient's right), and −90° to 12 o'clock (the patient's head). A normal QRS axis ranges from −30 to +90°. In a WCT, the axis can deviate either left or right, depending on the origin of the arrhythmia. The morphology of a WCT refers to the shape of the QRS complex. The term *monomorphic* implies that all of the QRS complexes have a similar shape implying a single focus for electrical activity. When a WCT demonstrates constantly changing QRS morphology and/or axis, it is termed *polymorphic*. Identifying the morphology of the QRS complex represents the first step in differentiating WCTs.

Figure 7.8.1 offers a flow chart to consider the classification of WCT based on electrocardiographic features. This chapter will discuss these features and the differential diagnosis of WCT.

Monomorphic WCT

Ventricular Tachycardia

VT is the most common cause of WCT and the most deadly (Figure 7.8.2). VT is generally defined by three or more continuous beats from a ventricular focus. While nonsustained VT is a common problem and often asymptomatic, sustained VT – that is, lasting longer than 30 seconds, may require immediate intervention due to hemodynamic instability. The clinical significance of nonsustained VT is dependent on its association with structural heart disease such as myocardial scarring, hypertrophy, or valvular

Electrocardiogram in Clinical Medicine, First Edition. Edited by William J. Brady, Michael J. Lipinski, Andrew E. Darby, Michael C. Bond, Nathan P. Charlton, Korin Hudson, and Kelly Williamson.

disease. VT represents a "can't miss" diagnosis and should be the assumed rhythm when evaluating WCT until proven otherwise.

Several electrical phenomena can be found on the ECG that are unique to VT(Figure 7.8.3). A *fusion beat* occurs when a supraventricular beat and a beat beginning within the ventricles coincide to produce a hybrid complex. They indicate that two foci are firing nearly simultaneously, and will typically produce a beat with intermediate width (90–120 ms) and a different morphology than complexes

Table 7.8.1 Features that define wide complex tachycardia (WCT).

Defining Features of Wide Complex Tachycardia

Ventricular rate > 100 bpm.

QRS duration >120 ms.

More than three small boxes on standard ECG paper.

QRS deviation to the left or to the right.

Deviation will depend on the origin or focus of ectopic rhythm.

Monomorphic rhythm indicates single focus.

Polymorphic rhythm indicates multiple ectopic foci.

stemming from a single focus. A *capture beat* is formed when a depolarization impulse of supraventricular origin is able to capture the ventricles during a ventricular dominated arrhythmia. It is typically seen as a normal QRS complex following a P wave that occurs in the middle of a wide complex dysrhythmia, such as VT. *Atrioventricular (AV) dissociation* may arise from a number of different conditions, including VT. When AV dissociation is present in the setting of VT, the atria and ventricles are being controlled by independent pacemakers, but the conduction system between the two may still be functional. When VT is the source of the WCT, the ventricular rate is typically the same or faster than the atria [2]. Rarely in AV dissociation a properly timed atrial beat, known as a *capture beat*, can pass through the normal conduction system, and an impulse from the ectopic ventricular focus can travel in retrograde fashion to the atria [3]. This is distinct from the AV dissociation seen in complete heart block where an impulse originating in the atria cannot pass through the AV node into the His-Purkinje fibers. *Concordance* is present when the QRS complexes in all six precordial leads are entirely positive (monophasic R waves) or entirely negative (monophasic qS waves). If a

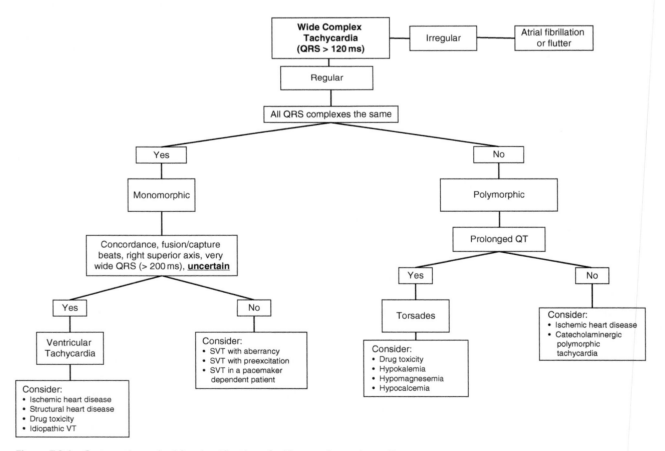

Figure 7.8.1 Systematic method for classification of wide complex tachycardia.

(a)

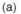

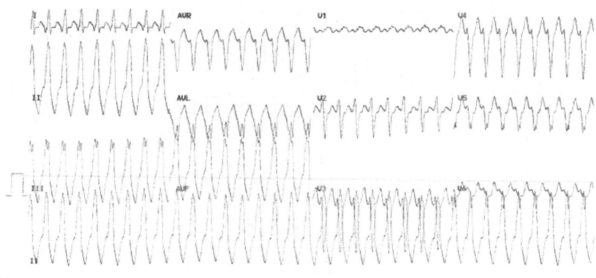

(b)

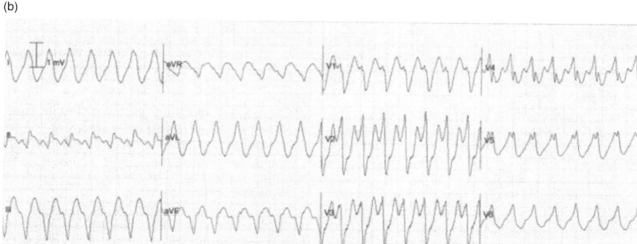

Figure7.8.2 (a and b) Both panels show ventricular tachycardia. Note the fast rate, the wide QRS complexes and the QRS complexes that all have the same morphology indicating a single focus.

single precordial lead has a biphasic QRS complex, concordance is not present. The presence of positive or negative concordance is greater than 90% specific for VT, but only 20% sensitive. Therefore the absence of concordance does not rule out VT [4].

The QRS axis, duration, and morphology can also help to establish VT as the cause of a WCT. If the focus of the arrhythmia is in the left ventricle, it will cause a delay in conduction to the right ventricle producing a right bundle branch block (RBBB) morphology. A WCT with a RBBB appearance and an axis left of −30° (superior axis) suggests VT. If the VT origin is in the right ventricle, a left bundle branch block (LBBB) like rhythm will result with an

axis to the right of +90° (inferior axis) [3]. Generally speaking, the wider a QRS complex is, the more likely it is to be VT in origin. An RBBB-like and LBBB-like WCT with QRS durations greater than 140 and 160 ms, respectively, suggests VT [3, 5].

Supraventricular WCT

Understanding the pathophysiology of WCT with supraventricular origin versus a VT is essential for appropriate management. For a wide QRS complex to be generated from above the AV node, there is usually one of three broad categories of abnormal conduction: a fixed or

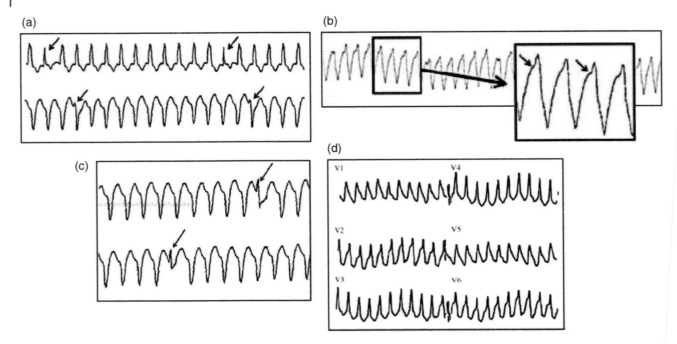

Figure 7.8.3 ECG findings in ventricular tachycardia. Panel a shows a *fusion beat* (arrows). Panel b shows a *capture beat* (arrows). Panel c shows *AV dissociation* with dissociated P waves (arrows) buried in the QRS complexes. Panel d shows *positive concordance* with positively oriented QRS complexes in all precordial leads. *Source:* Reprinted with permission from Ref. [24].

functional bundle branch block, aberrant conduction, or conduction via an accessory pathway. The diagnosis of "SVT with aberrancy" is often referenced in the literature and includes all three etiologies [6].

In the case of a fixed bundle branch block, the wide QRS complexes are the result of abnormalities in the His-Purkinje conduction system. Necrosis, fibrosis, calcification, infiltrative lesions and impaired vascular supply can all lead to conduction abnormalities in the His-Purkinje fibers [7]. Because of the abnormality in the conduction system, there is a delay in the depolarization of the myocardium supplied by the dysfunctional left or right bundle branch, resulting in a widened QRS complex as the electrical complex propagates in a cell-to-cell fashion through the respective ventricle. Bundle branch blocks are described in depth elsewhere in this text.

A true aberrant intraventricular conduction abnormality is the functional result an arriving supraventricular impulse during the relative refractory period, or may be rate related malfunction when the heart rate exceeds a characteristic maximum for a particular patient [7]. At this point, the conducting fibers have not fully recovered from the previous electrical stimulus and are unable to conduct the impulse. These patients will often have an underlying normal sinus rhythm, with a normal QRS duration, prior to the onset of the SVT. Aberrancy may be due to concealed retrograde penetration from a premature ventricular complex (PVC)

originating in the ventricle, rendering the bundle branch refractory to subsequent beats [8]. Several other conditions may predispose the conduction system to this situation by prolonging the refractory period including hyperkalemia, underlying His-Purkinje fiber abnormalities and certain anti-arrhythmic medications.

When an accessory conduction pathway is present, premature activation of the ventricles occurs due to a tract of anomalous conducting tissue. This tract allows impulses to bypass the AV node, producing a shorter PR interval (less than 0.12 seconds). This accessory pathway also bypasses the normal His-Purkinje conduction system and causes eccentric activation of the ventricles and a WCT [3].

There are many different types of accessory pathways including nodoventricular, atriofascicular, and intranodal bypass tracts. The Bundle of Kent is the most common AV bypass tract. It is an embryologic defect during AV septation, which produces a band of myocytes that bridge the AV junction. Two directional loops are possible over these accessory conduction pathways. (Figure 7.8.4) An *orthodromic conduction loop* generates a narrow complex arrhythmia in which the antegrade impulse is conducted through the AV node with the usual slowing through the normal conduction tissues. The retrograde reentrant portion of the circuit is conducted through the accessory pathway. An *antidromic conduction loop* results in a wide complex arrhythmia as the antegrade impulse is conducted

(a)

(b)

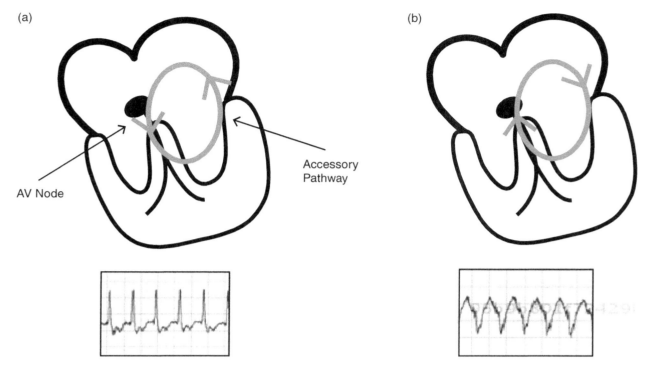

AV Node

Accessory
Pathway

Figure 7.8.4 Orthodromic (Panel a) and Antidromic (Panel b) reentry loops; because ventricular activation occurs via the accessory pathway in the antidromic loop the resulting rhythm is a wide QRS complex tachycardia. *Source:* Reprinted with permission from Ref. [24].

through the accessory pathway directly to the ventricles, bypassing the intraventricular conduction system. The retrograde loop is then conducted through the AV node.

These two processes are collectively termed atrioventricular reentrant tachycardia (AVRT). In AVRT, the accessory pathway is required for activation and maintenance of the tachycardia. Ventricular activation across the Kent bundle (thus an antidromic loop) produces the classic form of preexcitation WCT known as the Wolff-Parkinson-White (WPW) syndrome, definitively described in 1930 [9]. In WPW, the early excitation of the ventricles results in a shortened PR interval and slurred upstroke of the QRS wave, known as the delta wave. WPW is described in depth elsewhere in this text.

In some cases, the accessory pathway is not responsible for initiation or maintenance of the WCT. Instead, it acts as a route for atrial and ventricular activation. This situation can occur in several atrial and ventricular dominated arrhythmias, which may lead to a WCT.

Atrial fibrillation may occur in as many as one-third of patients with the WPW syndrome [10]. The focus of the arrhythmia is in the atria, and classically the ECG will show an irregularly irregular rhythm. However, once the rate surpasses 180 BPM it may appear to be regular on a standard speed ECG. Atrial fibrillation in the presence of the WPW syndrome can lead to ventricular rates

approaching or exceeding 300 beats/min, which may degrade rapidly to ventricular fibrillation [6]. This phenomenon is quite uncommon though, and the incidence of sudden cardiac death in patients with WPW is thought to be a rare event [11].

Similar to atrial fibrillation, atrial flutter is produced and sustained in the atria, but an accessory pathway can conduct impulses to the ventricles. A unique aspect of atrial flutter is the potential for a one to one conduction of impulses, where each atrial beat produces a wide complex ventricular beat. When this occurs, the resulting WCT can be difficult to differentiate from VT. Atrial flutter conducted over an accessory pathway is also at risk for degeneration to ventricular fibrillation.

AV nodal reentrant tachycardia (AVNRT) occurs when the reentry pathway is near or within the AV nodal tissue. When AVNRT takes place in the presence of the WPW syndrome, a WCT can result from impulses traveling directly down the accessory pathway to the ventricles.

Other Etiologies

In addition to structural myocardial pathology, WCT may result from more global etiologies affecting action potentials such as medications, toxins, electrolyte disturbances, or as a result of aggressive resuscitation after cardiac arrest. Cardiac conduction is exquisitely sensitive to substances that affect the cardiac sodium channels, resting membrane potentials, and ventricular repolarization. When there is a disturbance that affects any one of these variables, a WCT may result.

Cardiac voltage-gated sodium channels reside in the cell membrane and open in response to depolarization of the cell. There are a wide range of medications and electrolyte abnormalities that can create a blockade of these transmembrane sodium channels, either as a therapeutic end state or as an unintended side effect. Sodium channel blockade creates a delay of sodium entry into the cardiac myocyte during phase 0 of depolarization, resulting in a slowed upslope of depolarization and the QRS complex widening [6]. Additional effects of this blockade include slowed intraventricular conduction, unidirectional block, development of a reentrant circuit and VT.

Tricyclic antidepressants (TCAs) achieve their therapeutic effects through the reuptake inhibition of norepinephrine, serotonin, and dopamine at pre-synaptic terminals of the central nervous system. However, there are major pharmacologic effects that result in toxicity of the cardiovascular system. Potassium efflux blockage prolongs phase 3 of the myocardial action potential resulting in QT interval prolongation. TCA's also prolong the phase 0 myocardial depolarization by inhibiting the fast sodium channels resulting in a widened QRS complex [6]. The pathognomonic ECG finding in a TCA poisoned patient demonstrates a WCT with a prominent S wave in lead I and R' wave in lead aVR (Figure 7.8.5).

(a)

(b)

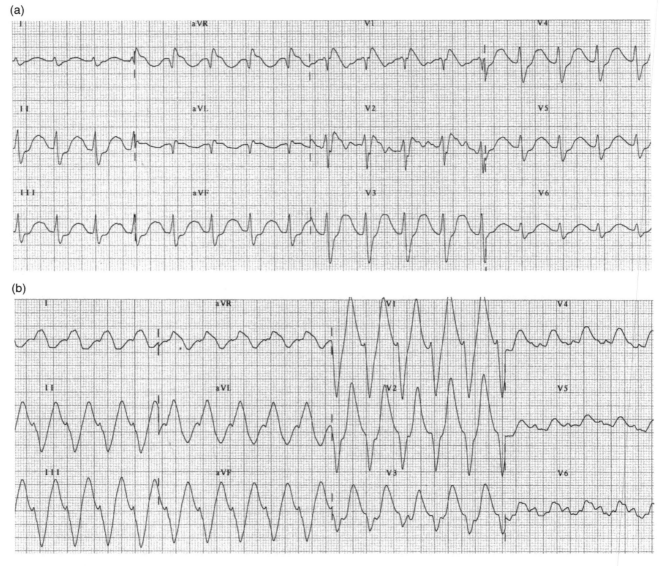

Figure 7.8.5 Tricyclic antidepressant toxicity. Panel a shows early TCA toxicity with a prominent R' wave in aVR Panel b shows worsening TCA cardiotoxicity with marked QRS widening. *Source:* Reprinted with permission from: http://lifeinthefastlane.com.

Antihistamines such as diphenhydramine are another example of common medications with significant cardiac toxicity. ECG changes resulting from diphenhydramine poisoning are a result of its ability to block fast sodium channels. This produces tachycardia, wide QRS complexes, terminal alterations of the QRS complex, and right axis deviation with R′ wave in aVR and S wave in leads I and aVL.

Hyperkalemia greatly disrupts cardiac resting membrane potential. With progressive hyperkalemia, an increased proportion of sodium channels are inactivated by the resting membrane depolarization created by the potassium ions. This causes the atrial myocytes to become unexcitable, leading to a decrease in P wave amplitude and depressing the intraventricular conduction velocity. These changes are manifested on the ECG as a widened QRS (Figure 7.8.6).

After a cardiac arrest a patient may demonstrate various arrhythmias, ranging from bradycardias, narrow complex tachycardias, and WCTs. The WCT may be a result of an acute bundle branch dysfunction from the arrest itself, the administration of defibrillating electrical shocks, from the ischemic event that precipitated the arrest, or from the ischemia induced by the administration of epinephrine or other vasopressors [12]. The arrhythmia created by the resuscitation itself usually resolves within 15–30 minutes after the return of spontaneous circulation as opposed to those arrhythmias created by ongoing ischemia and electrolyte abnormalities. Additionally, an accelerated idioventricular rhythm may be seen in the setting of reperfusion, typically after an acute myocardial infarction. This is thought to be due, in part, to ischemia induced mitochondrial dysfunction [13]. As previously mentioned, the rhythm resembles a monomorphic VT but has a rate <100–120 bpm. This "reperfusion arrhythmia" is generally transient, lasting minutes, and does not require any specific treatment.

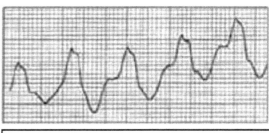
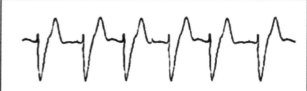

Figure 7.8.6 Hyperkalemia. Both panels show wide QRS complexes in patients with elevated serum potassium levels. *Source:* Reprinted with permission from Ref. [24].

Differentiating VT from Supraventricular WCT

One of the many challenges in evaluating a WCT is differentiating true VT from SVT with aberrancy (SVTAB). Old ECGs can be helpful when available but as previously mentioned, some patient's with a true aberrancy will often have an underlying normal sinus rhythm with a narrow QRS. While no method for differentiating the two rhythms is perfect, there are several clues that can lead the astute provider toward the correct ECG interpretation.

- Heart rate alone is not enough to differentiate the two; both VT and SVT with aberrant conduction may have moderate or profound tachycardia [5].
- VT will typically result in a left- or right-axis deviation. A "northwest" (or right superior) axis between −90° and 180°, seen as a net negative QRS voltage in leads I and AVF, strongly favors VT [14]. A normal axis, between −30° and +90°, is more likely to be associated with a SVT.
- The QRS in VT will typically be very wide, with a duration of >160 ms. With the exception of hyperkalemia and the presence of some drugs, the QRS will likely be less than 140–160 ms in SVTAB [3, 5].
- Concordance is strongly suggestive of VT. Rarely SVT with LBBB aberrancy will appear to have negative concordance, but the QRS complexes will likely show R waves in the lateral leads. The presence of concordance is greater than 90% specific for VT, but the lack of concordance is not a sensitive finding [4].
- Certain QRS morphology patterns can indicate the origin of the arrhythmia. An rSR′ noted in V1, resembling a RBBB pattern, suggests SVTAB. A single R wave ≥0.04 ms in V1 or a qR in V6, similar to a LBBB, indicates VT [5].
- The presence of capture beats, fusion beats, or evidence of AV dissociation, as noted above, is strongly suggestive of VT.

Several criteria and algorithms have been developed to help differentiate VT and SVTAB with varying levels of sensitivity and specificity. The Brugada criteria, one of the more commonly used methods, demonstrates a sensitivity of 89% and a specificity of 59%. The Vereckie criteria has shown a sensitivity of 87% and a specificity of 48% [15]. In 2010 Dr. Brugada et al. published a single finding, R-wave peak time in lead II (RWPT), with a positive likelihood ratio of 34.8 for determining the presence of VT [16]. RWPT is determined by measuring the time from the beginning of the QRS in lead II to the first change in electrical polarity, either the nadir of the Q wave or the peak of the R wave (in the absence of a Q wave). Unfortunately, the application of these criteria in a clinical setting has been demonstrated to miss 7–21% of cases of VT [17].

Due to the potentially lethal consequences of missing VT, a WCT should always be treated as VT until proven otherwise. Medications for the treatment of VT are generally not harmful if the WCT is supraventricular in origin, but the reverse is not true. Pharmacologic management of a WCT presumed to be SVT with aberrancy but actually originates in the ventricles could have disastrous consequences.

Polymorphic WCTs

Polymorphic ventricular tachycardia (PVT) is defined as a VT with an unstable, varying QRS complex in any single ECG lead (Figure 7.8.7). Variation in both the R-R interval

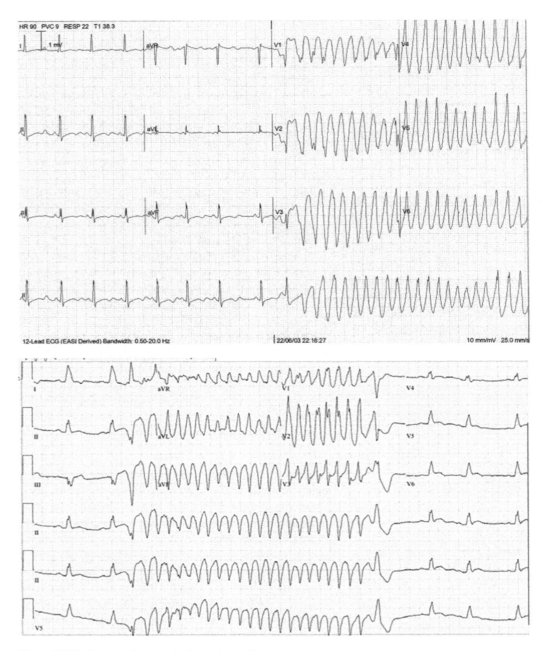

Figure 7.8.7   Polymorphic ventricular tachycardia.

and electrical axis are also noted features of this ventricular dysrhythmia. PVT demonstrates the following ECG characteristics [14]:

- Wide QRS complex (>120 ms)
- Changing R-R intervals (ranging 200–400 ms) with a rate of 150–300 bpm
- QRS complexes that have different morphology and an axis that changes frequently, if not from beat to beat.

PVT syndromes, unlike monomorphic VT, are often associated with sudden death. Spontaneous PVT is most commonly due to coronary vascular disease or nonischemic cardiomyopathy, and is found in 20–25% of prehospital cardiac arrest patients as the initial rhythm that then degenerates to VF. However, nonstructural abnormalities may be present at the molecular level that predispose those affected to this arrhythmia. Polymorphic VT not associated with coronary artery disease or cardiomyopathy is rare and can be classified based on the association with a normal or prolonged QT interval.

Prolonged QT Interval

Torsades de pointes (TdP, Figure 7.8.8) is the manifestation of PVT associated with prolongation of the QT interval. Nearly one in five prehospital cardiac arrest patients with PVT will demonstrate TdP [14]. TdP has many descriptive synonyms include cardiac ballet, atypical VT, transient recurrent ventricular fibrillation, swinging VT, and pleomorphic VT. These all refer to the characteristic ECG appearance of the "twisting of points," which may require longer rhythm strips to visualize the true pattern. The QRS complex varies in amplitude, appearing to oscillate around an isoelectric baseline.

A prolonged QT is defined by the corrected QT interval (QTc) of greater than 440 ms in men and 460 ms in women. An increased risk of TdP has been shown with a QTc

interval of greater than 500 ms, but no true threshold has been established for the development of an arrhythmia [18]. Prolonged repolarization of the cardiac action potential, caused by an increase in inward sodium currents or a decrease in outward potassium currents, leads to the characteristic ECG changes. Abnormalities of the QT interval are discussed at length elsewhere in this text.

Normal QT Interval

Catecholaminergic polymorphic ventricular tachycardia (CPVT) is a PVT associated with a normal QT interval and occurs in the absence of structural cardiac abnormalities [20]. It is a genetic disorder, often referred to as familial CPVT, and has been linked to two different gene mutations [19, 21]. These alterations are manifested by intracellular calcium overload and delayed afterdepolarizations, which occur during phase 4 of the action potential [22]. Afterdepolarizations are abnormal cardiac myocyte depolarizations that interruption the normal action potential and can lead to aberrant ventricular activation [23]. CPVT is associated with stress and physical exertion, and patients will typically present with exercise induced syncope or sudden death [20]. These patients will usually have an underlying sinus rhythm on ECG, making the diagnosis challenging under resting conditions.

Conclusion

A WCT can result from a number of etiologies including structural heart disease, accessory conduction pathways and exposure to certain medications. Differentiating between ventricular and supraventricular etiologies of WCT can be challenging, and no method is 100% accurate. Due to the potential lethality of VT and other ventricular dysrhythmias, clinically a WCT should always be considered VT until proven otherwise.

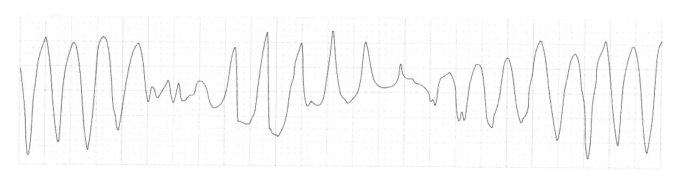

Figure 7.8.8 Torsades de pointes. Note the polymorphic appearance of the QRS complexes and the "twisting of the points," the changing axis. *Source:* Reprinted with permission from: http://cdn.lifeinthefastlane.com/wp-content/uploads/2011/11/TDP1.jpg (accessed 23 September 2014).

References

1 Riera, A., Barros, R.B., de Sousa, F. et al. (2010). Accelerated Idioventricular rhythm: history and chronology of the main discoveries. *Indian Pacing and Electrophysiology Journal* 10 (1): 40–48.

2 Braunwald, E (2001). Atrioventricular dissociation. In: *Heart Diseases: A Textbook of Cardiovascular Medicine* (eds. Zipes, DP, E. Braunwald and P. Libby). Philadelphia, PA: WB Saunders Co.

3 Wellens, H. (2001). Ventricular tachycardia: diagnosis of broad QRS complex tachycardia. *Heart* 86 (5): 579–585.

4 Miller, J.M., Hsia, H.H., Rothman, S.A., and Buxton, A.E. (2000). Ventricular tachycardia versus supraventricular tachycardia with aberration: electrocardiographic distinctions. In: *Cardiac Electrophysiology from Cell to Bedside* (eds. J. Jalife and D.P. Zipes), 696. Philadelphia: W.B. Saunders.

5 Gupta, A.K. and Thakur, R.K. (2001). Wide QRS complex tachycardias. *The Medical Clinics of North America* 85 (2): 245–266, ix-x.

6 Hollowell, H., Mattu, A., Perron, A.D. et al. (2005). Wide-complex tachycardia: beyond the traditional differential diagnosis of ventricular tachycardia vs supraventricular tachycardia with aberrant conduction. *The American Journal of Emergency Medicine* 23 (7): 876–889.

7 Surawicz, B., Macfarlane, P., Wellens, H. et al. (2009). AHA/ACCF/HRS recommendations for the standardization and interpretation of the electrocardiogram: part III: intraventricular conduction disturbances: a scientific statement from the American Heart Association electrocardiography and arrhythmias committee, council on clinical cardiology; the American College of Cardiology Foundation; and the Heart Rhythm Society: endorsed by the International Society for Computerized Electrocardiology. *Circulation* 119 (10): e235–e240.

8 Neiger, J.S. and Trohman, R.G. (2011). Differential diagnosis of tachycardia with a typical left bundle branch block morphology. *World Journal of Cardiology* 3 (5): 127–134.

9 Wolff, L., Parkinson, J., and White, P.D. (2006). Bundle-branch block with short P-R interval in healthy young people prone to paroxysmal tachycardia. *Annals of Noninvasive Electrocardiology* 11 (4): 340–353.

10 Campbell, R.W., Smith, R.A., Gallagher, J.J., et al. (1977). Atrial fibrillation in the preexcitation syndrome. *The American Journal of Cardiology* 40 (4): 514–520.

11 Obeyesekere, M.N., Leong-Sit, P., Massel, D., et al. (2012). Risk of arrhythmia and sudden death in patients with asymptomatic preexcitation: a meta-analysis. *Circulation* 125 (19): 2308–2315.

12 Barlotta, K.S., Holstege, C., Brady, W.J., and Mattu, A. (2006). Apparent wide complex tachycardia after ventricular fibrillation cardiac arrest in patients with ST-segment elevation myocardial infarction. *The American Journal of Emergency Medicine* 24 (3): 362–367.

13 Akar, F.G. Aon, M. A., Tomaselli, G.F., and O'Rourke, B. (2005). The mitochondrial origin of postischemic arrhythmias. *The Journal of Clinical Investigation* 115 (12): 3527–3535.

14 Hudson, K.B. Brady, W.J., Chan, T.C., et al. (2003). Electrocardiographic manifestations: ventricular tachycardia. *Journal of Emergency Medicine* 25 (3): 303–314.

15 Vereckei, A., Duray, G., Szénási, G., et al. (2007). Application of a new algorithm in the differential diagnosis of wide QRS complex tachycardia. *European Heart Journal* 28 (5): 589–600.

16 Pava, L.F., Perafán, P., Badiel, M., et al. (2010). R-wave peak time at DII: a new criterion for differentiating between wide complex QRS tachycardias. *Heart Rhythm* 7 (7): 922–926.

17 Szelenyi, Z., Duray, G.Z., Katona, G., et al. (2013). Comparison of the "real-life" diagnostic value of two recently published electrocardiogram methods for the differential diagnosis of wide QRS complex tachycardias. *Academic Emergency Medicine* 20 (11): 1121–1130.

18 Bednar, M.M., Harrigan, E.P., Anziano, R.J., et al. (2001). The QT interval. *Progress in Cardiovascular Diseases* 43 (5 Suppl 1): 1–45.

19 Priori, S.G., Napolitano, C., Tiso, N., et al. (2001). Mutations in the cardiac ryanodine receptor gene (hRyR2) underlie catecholaminergic polymorphic ventricular tachycardia. *Circulation* 103 (2): 196–200.

20 Priori, S.G., Napolitano, C., Memmi, M., et al. (2002). Clinical and molecular characterization of patients with catecholaminergic polymorphic ventricular tachycardia. *Circulation* 106 (1): 69–74.

21 Lahat, H., Eldar, M., Levy-Nissenbaum, E., et al. (2001). Autosomal recessive catecholamineor exercise-induced polymorphic ventricular tachycardia: clinical features and assignment of the disease gene to chromosome 1p13-21. *Circulation* 103 (23): 2822–2827.

22 Nakajima, T., Kaneko, Y., Taniguchi, Y., et al. (1997). The mechanism of catecholaminergic polymorphic ventricular tachycardia may be triggered activity due to delayed after depolarization. *European Heart Journal* 18 (3): 530–531.

23 Wehrens, X.H., Lehnart, S.E., Huang, F., et al. (2003). FKBP12.6 deficiency and defective calcium release

channel (ryanodine receptor) function linked to exercise-induced sudden cardiac death. *Cell* 113 (7): 829–840.

24 Brady, W.J. (2011). *Cardiovascular Problems in Emergency Medicine: A Discussion-Based Review*, CTEM – Current Topics in Emergency Medicine, 2e (ed. S. Grossman). Wiley-Blackwell.

Additional Resources

Anttonen, O., Junttila, M.J., Rissanen, H., et al. (2007). Prevalence and prognostic significance of short QT interval in a middle-aged Finnish population. *Circulation* 116 (7): 714–720.

Chiang, C.E. and Roden, D.M. (2000). The long QT syndromes: genetic basis and clinical implications. *Journal of the American College of Cardiology* 36 (1): 1–12.

Funck-Brentano, C. and Jaillon, P. (1993). Rate-corrected QT interval: techniques and limitations. *The American Journal of Cardiology* 72 (6): 17B–22B.

Gilmour, R.F. Jr. (2004). Early afterdepolarization-induced triggered activity: initiation and reinitiation of reentrant Arrhythmias. *Heart Rhythm* 1 (4): 449–450.

Kobza, R., Roos, M., Niggli, B., et al. (2009). Prevalence of long and short QT in a young population of 41,767 predominantly male Swiss conscripts. *Heart Rhythm* 6 (5): 652–657.

Maisel, W.H., Kuntz, K.M., Reimold, S.C., et al. (1997). Risk of initiating antiarrhythmic drug therapy for atrial fibrillation in patients admitted to a university hospital. *Annals of Internal Medicine* 127 (4): 281–284.

Mason, J.W., Ramseth, D.J., Chanter, D.O., et al. (2007). Electrocardiographic reference ranges derived from 79,743

ambulatory subjects. *Journal of Electrocardiology* 40 (3): 228–234.

Roden, D.M. (2004). Drug-induced prolongation of the QT interval. *The New England Journal of Medicine* 350 (10): 1013–1022.

Segal, O.R., Chow, A.W., Wong, T. et al. (2007). A novel algorithm for determining endocardial VT exit site from 12-lead surface ECG characteristics in human, infarctrelated ventricular tachycardia. *Journal of Cardiovascular Electrophysiology* 18 (2): 161–168.

Vincent, G.M. et al. (1992). The Spectrum of symptoms and QT intervals in carriers of the gene for the long-QT syndrome. *New England Journal of Medicine* 327 (12): 846–852.

Viskin, S. Zeltser, D., Ish-Shalom, M., et al. (2004). Is idiopathic ventricular fibrillation a short QT syndrome? Comparison of QT intervals of patients with idiopathic ventricular fibrillation and healthy controls. *Heart Rhythm* 1 (5): 587–591.

Yang, T. and Roden, D.M. (1996). Extracellular potassium modulation of drug block of IKr. Implications for torsade de pointes and reverse use-dependence. *Circulation* 93 (3): 407–411.

Index

Note: Page numbers in *italic* refer to figures, those in **bold** refer to tables.

Electrocardiogram in Clinical Medicine, First Edition. Edited by William J. Brady, Michael J. Lipinski, Andrew E. Darby, Michael C. Bond, Nathan P. Charlton, Korin Hudson, and Kelly Williamson.
© 2021 John Wiley & Sons Ltd. Published 2021 by John Wiley & Sons Ltd.